C. Stephen Foster
Maite Sainz de la Maza

The Sclera

Foreword by Frederick A. Jakobiec

With 134 Illustrations and 33 Color Plates

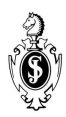

Springer-Verlag
New York   Berlin   Heidelberg   London   Paris
Tokyo   Hong Kong   Barcelona   Budapest

C. Stephen Foster, MD
Associate Professor of Ophthalmology
Harvard Medical School
Director, Immunology and Uveitis Service
Massachusetts Eye and Ear Infirmary
Boston, MA 02114
USA

Maite Sainz de la Maza, MD, PhD
Assistant Professor of Ophthalmology
Central University of Barcelona
08036 Barcelona
Spain

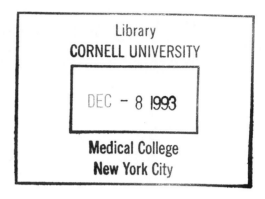
Cover illustration: The eye of a patient with rheumatoid arthritis who has developed pro-gressively destructive necrotizing scleritis.

Library of Congress Cataloging-in-Publication Data
Foster, C. Stephen (Charles Stephen), 1942–
    The sclera/C. Stephen Foster and Maite Sainz de la Maza.
       p. cm.
    Includes bibliographical references and index.
    ISBN 0-387-94058-8.—ISBN 3-540-94058-8
    1. Sclera—Diseases. I. Maza, Maite Sainz de la. II. Title.
    [DNLM: 1. Scleritis. 2. Sclera.   WW 230 F754s 1993]
    RE328.F67   1993
    617.7′ 19—dc20
    DNLM/DLC
    for Library of Congress   93-10235

Printed on acid-free paper.

Production coordinated by TechEdit Production Services and managed by Ellen Seham; manufacturing supervised by Vincent Scelta.
Typeset by Best-set Typesetter Ltd., Chai Wan, Hong Kong.
Color separations by Best-set Typesetter Ltd., and color printing by New England Book Components.
Printed and bound by Braun-Brumfield, Inc., Ann Arbor, MI.
Printed in the United States of America.

9 8 7 6 5 4 3 2 1

ISBN 0-387-94058-8 Springer-Verlag New York Berlin Heidelberg
ISBN 3-540-94058-8 Springer-Verlag Berlin Heidelberg New York

To our parents:
  Carson and Martha Foster
  Julio and Teresa Sainz de la Maza

Foreword

Over the past five years, in sharing patients with him, following his research, and benefitting from his teaching, I have come to marvel at Dr. Stephen Foster's mind, dedication, and productivity. No one has a richer or more challenging clinical practice, has approached his clinical care with more critical questioning, or has produced as much useful clinical and basic research in his field.

Steve has kept meticulous clinical records with elegant photographic documentation, which serve as the basis for the creation of this treatise. He has been fortunate in his co-author, Dr. Sainz de la Maza, who initially inveigled Steve to participate in this project and then set herself the enormous task of repairing the lacuna occasioned by the nonavailability of the classic text by Watson and Hazelman, *The Sclera and Systemic Disorders*. Steve has taken great pride in the trainees who have passed through his fellowship program, and has methodically tried to select them from around the world in order to extend the influence of his clinical and research traditions. Dr. Sainz de la Maza, who practices academic ophthalmology in Barcelona, Spain, is a superb exemplar of the fruits of this strategy; the ophthalmic communities, both American and international, are in their debt for producing this textbook.

I have read many of the chapters in this textbook, and they augment one's impressions of Steve's high standards of scholarship and originality. Steve has also generously noted that the Massachusetts Eye and Ear Infirmary's unique resources are very much embedded in the content of this book. I have had several in-depth discussions with Steve and Dr. Sainz de la Maza regarding pathogenetic concepts of scleritis, auto-immune diseases, and vasculitis, and have personally profited from those dialogues. Now trainees, general ophthalmologists, specialists, and particularly patients far and wide will benefit from the dissemination of this unique database and codification of the principles of clinical management. My admiration for Steve's work, which was great from a distance when I was in New York, has simply mushroomed in proximity to him in Boston.

I am pleased to contemplate that this textbook will bring him and his accomplishments closer to the entire ophthalmic community.

Frederick A. Jakobiec, M.D.
Henry Willard Williams Professor of Ophthalmology
Professor of Pathology, and
Chairman of Ophthalmology
Harvard Medical School

Chief of Ophthalmology
Massachusetts Eye and Ear Infirmary

Preface

The sclera composes 80% of the geographic extent of the exterior confines or wall of the eyeball, yet it receives relatively little attention in the ophthalmic literature. This is understandable, given the fact that disorders of the sclera are not common and the fact that, when relatively minor problems of the sclera do develop, healing without consequence is the usual outcome. After all, a scar in the sclera is of little importance, because the sclera is an opaque structure. Such a scar in the cornea, or an opacity in the lens or vitreous, or a scar in the macula, of course, carries infinitely more visual significance. But it is exactly this rarity of significant scleral problems, coupled with the profound systemic implications that some inflammatory disorders of the sclera carry, that makes studies of the sclera and its disorders important. Indeed, a substantial proportion of individuals who develop serious scleral inflammation are discovered to have an occult systemic disease; in *The Sclera and Systemic Disorders* Watson and Hazleman* emphasized that 27% of patients who develop necrotizing scleritis are dead within 5 yr from a systemic, vasculitic lesion. Watson and Hazleman also emphasized that because of the comparative rarity of scleral disease, the diagnosis is often missed, and 40% of eyes reported in one series of enucleated eyes had had a primary diagnosis of scleritis.

We have written this book because the finest book ever written on this subject, *The Sclera and Systemic Disorders*, by Watson and Hazleman (published in 1976 by W.B. Saunders, Philadelphia, as Volume 2 in their series, *Major Problems in Ophthalmology*), has been out of print, unavailable through any source whatsoever, since 1985. Dr. Sainz de la Maza was frustrated by this; she could find no copies of this magnificent book in the medical library in Barcelona. Watson gave me his last copy of the book, which he obtained from the attic of his home, and inscribed to me "with all best wishes." It is this rare treasure that our efforts try to emulate. The two books are different in style, organization, patient populations that form the basis of the material, and, to a small degree, point of view. But in many respects the books are quite similar: our

---

*Watson PG, Hazleman BL: *The Sclera and Systemic Disorders*, WB Saunders, Philadelphia, 1976.

experiences corroborate theirs, and the philosophies born of those separate experiences are identical.

We began with all that we had learned from Watson and Hazleman and built on that excellent foundation. The basis of our experience springs from the Immunology Service at the Massachusetts Eye and Ear Infirmary, which was begun in 1977, and which has been devoted to the study and care of patients with any inflammatory problem related to the eye, from the lids to the optic nerve. The first Research Fellow joined the service in 1980, and the first Clinical Fellow arrived in 1984. Between 1977 and 1992 approximately 45,000 patient visits have occurred, approximately 6000 new patients have been evaluated, and 40 Ocular Immunology Fellows have been trained in the Service. Dr. Sainz de la Maza was one of those Fellows, and in the course of training she developed a special interest in and affinity for patients with scleritis. It was her initiative that was at the heart of the genesis of this project, and it is entirely through her efforts that this project has been successfully completed.

Our hope is that this book will serve as a resource for residents in ophthalmology, for cornea and immunology fellows in training, and for those ophthalmologists in practice and on faculties who have an interest in patients with diseases of the sclera. The majority of the book is devoted to scleral inflammation, because scleritis represents, by far, the most common scleral disorder encountered in ophthalmic practice, and because of the profound systemic implications of scleritis. The references at the end of each chapter, although not exhaustive, are generous in number and should provide the reader with more than enough original source material for further reading. Finally, for those who have access to a copy of the book by Watson and Hazleman, we would enthusiastically encourage you to read their book as well as this one.

Acknowledgments

We acknowledge the help, patience, and understanding provided by our patients in the course of treatment. This book, which is based on their personal experiences, would not exist without them. So, too, we gratefully acknowledge the generosity of referring physicians throughout New England: not only have they referred patients, with all their varieties of ocular inflammatory disorders, to the Immunology Service, but they have allowed us to care for them longitudinally as well.

The physicians who have chosen to spend additional years training in ocular immunology deserve special thanks. In the course of their training, they assumed increasing amounts of responsibility in the care of our patients, and without their help much of the work that has been done would not have been finished. These individuals are listed separately on the following page. The research associates and laboratory technicians of the Hilles Immunology Laboratory and of the Rhoads Molecular Immunology Laboratory are also gratefully acknowledged. These individuals include Drs. Robin Campbell, Peter Wells, and Soon Jin Lee, and Carolyn DiSiena, Lou Ann Caron, Beverly Rice, Tom Ihley, James Dutt, Tong Zhen Zhao, Victor Correa, and Jane Lui.

Anterior segment and posterior segment photographers Kit Johnson and Phil Ruderman, and retinal photographers Jeff Napoli, Martha Cunningham, Ann Elias-Dreiker (CRA), and Alice George are responsible for most of the clinical illustrations that are included in this book, and we are grateful to them for the fine quality of their work. Similarly, we acknowledge Lauri Cook for her superb medical illustrations and Richard Fleischer for his help in making publication prints. The personnel of the Immunology Service, technicians, nurses, and secretaries, are also acknowledged for their help in running an efficient operation, which allows us to accomplish the day's work.

Fellows of the Ocular Immunology Service, Massachusetts Eye and Ear Infirmary

Former Fellows

LESLIE FUJIKAWA, M.D., Associate, University of the Pacific
RICHARD WETZIG, M.D., Private Practice, Colorado Springs, CO
JAMES KALPAXIS, M.D., Private Practice, San Antonio, TX
ROBIN CAMPBELL, Ph.D., Industry (Burroughs-Wellcome)
INGER SANDSTROM, M.D., Assoc. Professor, Karolinska Institute, Sweden
PAUL THOMPSON, M.D., Assoc. Professor, University of Montreal, Canada
RICHARD BAZIN, M.D., Assoc. Professor, Lasoli University, Quebec, Canada
PETER WELLS, Ph.D., Industry (Upjohn Pharmaceuticals)
LYE PHENG FONG, M.D., Assoc. Professor, University of Melbourne, Australia
MICHAEL RAIZMAN, M.D., Assoc. Professor, Tufts University, Boston, MA
E. MITCHEL OPREMCAK, M.D., Assoc. Professor, Ohio State University
GURINDER SINGH, M.D., Private Practice, Anaheim, CA
BARRY GOLUB, M.D., Assoc. Professor, SUNY Stonybrook
JOSEPH TAUBER, M.D., Assist. Professor, University of Missouri, Kansas City
HUM CHUNG, M.D., Assoc. Professor, Seoul University, Seoul, Korea
MAITE SAINZ DE LA MAZA, M.D., Assist. Professor, University of Barcelona, Spain
THANH HOANG-XUAN, M.D., Assoc. Professor, University of Paris, France
MANDI ZALTAS, M.D., Fellow in Glaucoma, Boston, MA
NEIL TOLCHIN, M.D., Resident in Ophthalmology
EUGENE LIU, M.D., Resident in Ophthalmology
MARGARITA CALONGE, M.D., Assist. Professor, University of Valladolid, Spain
JOHN BAER, M.D., Assoc. Professor, University of Maryland
ALEJANDRO GARCIA RODRIGUEZ, M.D., University of Monterey, Mexico
TUYET MAI PHAN, M.D., Private Practice, Los Angeles, CA
RAMZI HEMADY, M.D., Assist. Professor, University of Maryland
RICHARD TAMESIS, M.D., University of Nebraska
SARKIS SOUKASIAN, M.D., Private Practice, Lahey Clinic, Burlington, MA
MANFRED ZIERHUT, M.D., Assist. Professor, Tubingen University, Germany
NADA JABBUR, M.D., Resident in Ophthalmology, George Washington University
XIN XIN CAI, M.D., Ph.D. Program, Tufts University, Boston, MA
MARTIN FILIPEC, M.D., Assoc. Professor, University of Prague, Czechoslovakia
SOON JIN LEE, Ph.D., Assist. Professor, University of Missouri
RON NEUMANN, M.D., Director of Immunology Research, Pharmos Corp., Israel
NEAL BARNEY, M.D., Assist. Professor, University of Wisconsin

HELEN WU, M.D., Assist. Professor, Tufts University, Boston, MA
ARND HEILIGENHAUS, M.D., Assist. Professor, University of Essen, Germany
ADAM KAUFMAN, M.D., Assist. Professor, University of Cinncinnatti
AMYNA MERCHANT, M.D., Resident in Ophthalmology
VICTOR CORREA, Ph.D., Fellow, Harvard Medical School
ALEJANDRO BERRA, Ph.D., Chairman, Dept. of Immunology, University of
   Moron, Buenos Aires, Argentina
ELISABETH MESSMER, M.D., Resident in Ophthalmology, University of Munich,
   Germany
ZHENGZHI LI, M.D., Research Assoc., St. Louis University
YONCA AKOVA, M.D., Assist. Professor, University of Ankara, Turkey

Current Fellows

ALEJANDRO GARCIA RODRIGUEZ, M.D., Mexico
MIGUEL PEDROZA-SERES, M.D., Mexico
ALBERT VITALE, M.D., USA
LEON LANE, M.D., USA
JESUS MERAYO-LLOVES, M.D., Spain
WILLIAM POWER, M.D., Ireland
RENATO NEVES, M.D., Brazil
WILLIAM AYLIFFE, M.D., England

Contents

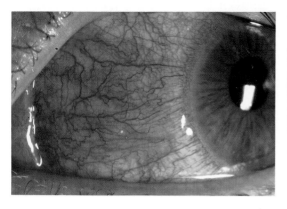

FIGURE 3.1. Episcleritis. Note the vascular dilatation of conjunctival vessels, and superficial episcleral and deep episcleral vascular plexuses. There is no underlying scleral edema or loss of sclera, and the eye appears bright red.

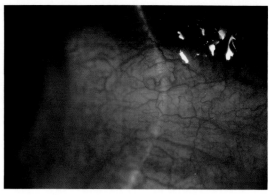

FIGURE 3.19. Slit-lamp photomicrograph, patient with scleritis. Note the displacement, anteriorly, of the slit beam as it sweeps across an area of scleral edema underlying the dilated vessels of the conjunctiva and the superficial and deep episcleral vascular plexuses.

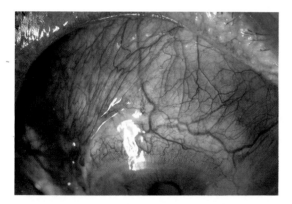

FIGURE 3.2. Scleritis. Note the bluish-red appearance of the inflamed eye, owing to the loss of some of the scleral fibers under the conjunctiva and episcleral tissue.

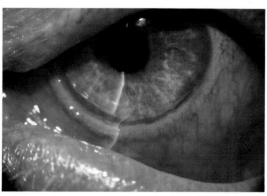

FIGURE 3.22. Peripheral corneal ulcer in a patient with diffuse anterior scleritis (slit-lamp photomicrograph). Note the presence of a peripheral corneal ulcer extending from approximately 3:30 clockwise to 8:30.

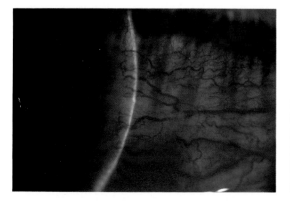

FIGURE 3.18. Slit-lamp photomicrograph, patient with episcleritis. Note that there is no displacement of the slit beam from underlying scleral edema.

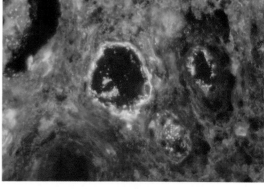

FIGURE 3.32. Immunofluorescence photomicrograph: conjunctival biopsy, patient with scleritis. Anti-IgG antibody has been used. Note the presence of IgG in the vessel wall, indicating the presence of inflammatory microangiitis. (Magnification, ×28.)

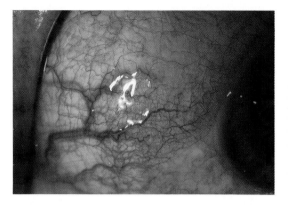

FIGURE 4.1. Episcleritis prior to instillation of 10% phenylephrine drops.

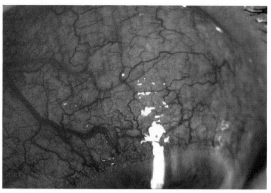

FIGURE 4.4. Scleritis. Note the slightly violaceous character of the inflammation. The patient complains of pain, and the globe is tender to palpation through the upper lid.

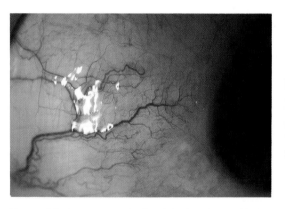

FIGURE 4.2. Same eye as in Fig. 4.1 after the instillation of 10% phenylephrine drops. Note the dramatic reduction in the inflamed appearance of the globe, because of the vasoconstrictor effect on the episcleral vascular plexuses, indicating that this patient probably has episcleritis rather than true scleritis.

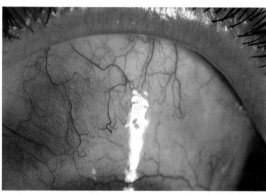

FIGURE 4.5. Same eye as in Fig. 4.4, 2 years after the photograph in Fig. 4.4 was taken. The scleritis has been successfully treated and has been held in remission for 1 year. Note, however, the areas of scleral loss with uveal "show" through the remaining scleral fibers.

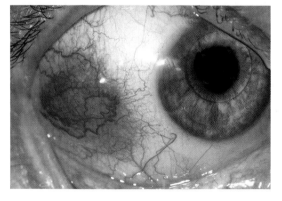

FIGURE 4.3. Nodular episcleritis. The nodule is mobile, that is, not incorporated into sclera or part of sclera.

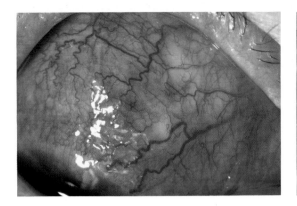

FIGURE 4.6. Patient with necrotizing scleritis prior to instillation of 10% phenylephrine.

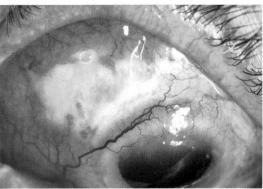

FIGURE 4.14. Necrotizing scleritis. Note not only the loss of sclera, but also the pronounced vascularity in the area.

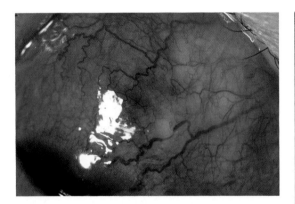

FIGURE 4.7. Same eye as in Fig. 4.6, 10 min after instillation of 10% phenylephrine drops. Note that the degree of clinical inflammatory signs is virtually unchanged, indicating that this patient's inflammation, even in areas outside the focus of frank necrotizing scleritis, represents true scleritis.

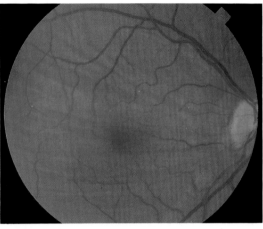

FIGURE 4.22. Fundus photomicrograph of patient with posterior scleritis. Note the choroidal folds, as shown by the alternating light and dark lines.

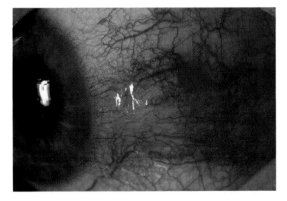

FIGURE 4.12. Nodular scleritis. This nodule is incorporated into sclera, indeed, is part of the sclera and, therefore, is immobile as one tries to palpate and move it.

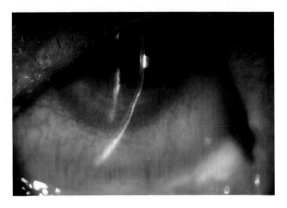

FIGURE 4.34. Slit-lamp photomicrograph. Note the area in the inferior cornea of peripheral corneal thinning in this patient, who has had multiple bouts of diffuse anterior scleritis.

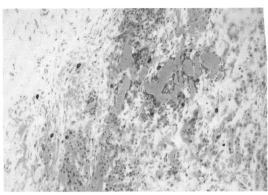

FIGURE 5.5. Scleral biopsy of a specimen from a patient with scleritis. Note the large number of purple-stained cells in the specimen, the mast cells. (Magnification, ✕40; alkaline Giemsa stain.)

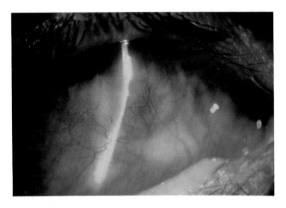

FIGURE 4.36. Slit-lamp photomicrograph: peripheral sclerosing keratitis. Note the peripheral keratitis with associated neovascularization and opacification of the peripheral cornea in this patient, who has had chronic anterior scleritis.

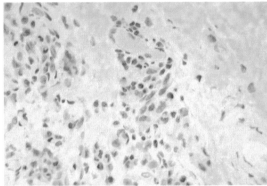

FIGURE 5.6. Scleral biopsy, Note the striking presence of eosinophils in this specimen. (Magnification, ✕60; hematoxylin–eosin stain.)

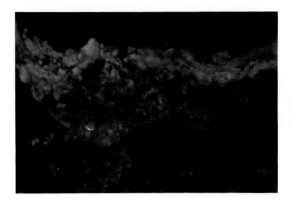

FIGURE 5.8. Immunofluorescence microscopy: specimen is from a patient with scleritis. The antibody is anti-dermatan sulfate antibody. Note (in comparison to Fig. 5.9) the dramatic reduction in the presence of dermatan sulfate in the scleritis specimen.

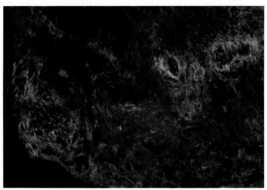

FIGURE 5.10. Immunofluorescence microscopy: scleral biopsy from a patient with scleritis. Note (particularly in relationship to Fig. 5.11) the relative lack of bright staining, except around the vessels, indicating a relative paucity of chondroitin sulfate in this scleral specimen. (Magnification, x40.)

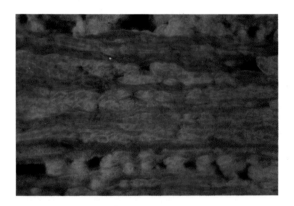

FIGURE 5.9. Immunofluorescence microscopy: biopsy of normal sclera. Antibody is anti-dermatan sulfate antibody. Note the large amount of bright apple-green fluorescence, indicating rather large amounts of dermatan sulfate in normal sclera. (Magnification, x100.)

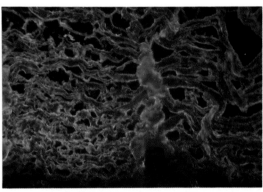

FIGURE 5.11. Immunofluroescence microscopy: normal sclera. Antibody is anti-chondroitin sulfate antibody. Note the relative abundance of bright apple-green fibrils, indicating a relatively large amount of chondroitin sulfate in normal sclera. (Magnification, x40.)

FIGURE 5.15, Scleral biopsy of patient with scleritis. Note the inflammatory microangiopathy, with clustering of inflammatory cells around the vessel. Because the vessel lacks a true vascular wall, however, the criteria typically used by general pathologists to declare the presence of a true vasculitis cannot be used in analyzing these specimens. (Magnification, x60; hemaloxylin–eosin stain.)

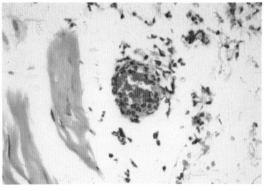

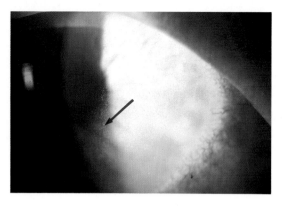

Figure 5.28. Forty-nine-year-old man with scleritis and associated keratitis. Note the feathery central advancing edge of the keratitis (arrow).

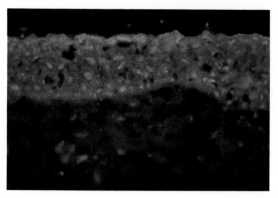

Figure 5.30. Immunofluorescence microscopy: conjunctival biopsy from the same patient illustrated in Figs. 5.28 and 5.29. Antibody is anti-herpes simplex virus antibody. Note the striking positivity of the nuclei in the epithelial cells and in some of the keratocytes, indicating the presence of herpes simplex virus in the tissue.

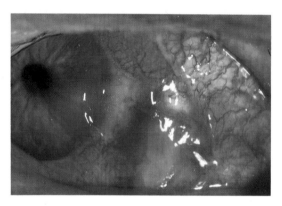

Figure 5.29. Same patient as in Fig. 5.28: different area and view. Note the intense scleritis.

Figure 5.31. Negative control for the anti-herpes antibody immunohistochemical staining, eliminating the first (anti-herpes) antibody in a two-step, indirect immunofluorescence technique. This negative control is important: it makes it clear that the findings shown in Fig. 5.30 are indeed true positives.

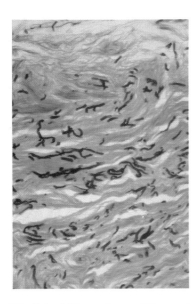

FIGURE 5.33. Scleral biopsy from a 67-year-old patient with necrotizing scleritis, which developed following trauma to the right eye, inflicted by a cow's tail. Scleral biopsy has been stained with Gomori methenamine silver stain. Note the large number of filamentous fungi (black) in this scleral biopsy specimen.

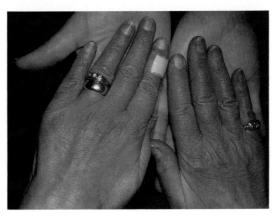

FIGURE 6.8. Hands of a patient with systemic lupus erythematosus and Raynaud's phenomenon. The patient's hands had been exposed to the cold just prior to her arriving in the clinic, and they were markedly blanched during the exposure to the cold. They were painful then and were still painful at the time that this photograph was taken, with venous dilatation producing the dramatic, bluish color of the fingers, particularly those of the right hand.

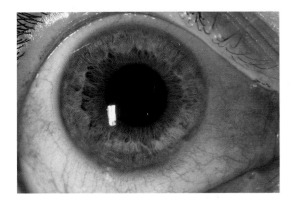

FIGURE 6.5. Keratoconjunctivitis sicca. Rose bengal dye (1%) has been instilled into the cul-de-sac. Note the punctate staining of the conjunctival epithelium in the interpalpebral fissure.

1
Structural Considerations of the Sclera

1.1. Introduction

The sclera, the dense connective tissue that encloses about five-sixths of the eye, is remarkable for its strength and for the firmness with which it maintains the shape of the globe. It aids in the maintenance of intraocular pressure, provides attachment sites for the extraocular muscles, and protects the intraocular structures from trauma and mechanical displacement.

To appreciate these normal functions and to understand the pathogenesis of inflammatory and noninflammatory diseases of the sclera, one must acquire some knowledge of the development, anatomy, and physiology of the sclera. A brief description of these areas follows.

1.2. Development of the Sclera

1.2.1. Prenatal Development: Ultrastructural Studies

1.2.1.1. First Week

In placental mammals, the fertilized zygote is transformed by cleavage cell division into a solid mass of cells with the appearance of a mulberry called morula. The cells then rearrange, becoming organized as a group of centrally placed cells, the inner cell mass, completely surrounded by a layer of cells, the outer cell mass. The cells of the inner cell mass are attached at one pole of the morula; they eventually develop into the tissues of the embryo. The cells of the outer cell mass become flattened; they eventually develop into the trophoblast. The space between inner and outer cell mass forms a central cavity, the blastocystic cavity, after which the embryo is called a blastocyst.

1.2.1.2. Second Week

During the second week of development, some of the cells of the inner cell mass become detached from the inner surface and give rise to a cavity, the primitive yolk sac. The remaining cells give rise to another cavity, the amniotic cavity, and to a bilaminar embryonic disk, consisting of a single upper layer of columnar cells, the epiblast, and a single lower layer of flattened cells, the hypoblast. The cells of the outer cell mass form the trophoblast, which divides into two layers, the inner cytotrophoblast and the outer syncytiotrophoblast.

1.2.1.3. Third Week

Early in the third week, a thick linear band of epiblast, called the primitive streak, appears caudally in the midline of the dorsal aspect of the embryonic disk. The cranial end of the primitive streak is swollen and is known as the primitive knot. The primitive streak gives rise to the mesoblast, which spreads to form a layer between the epiblast and hypoblast. This new layer is called the embryonic mesoderm and the process by which the bilaminar embryonic disk becomes trilaminar is called gastrulation. At the end of gastrulation, the cells that remain in the epiblast form the outer layer or embryonic ectoderm. Some mesoblastic cells displace the hypoblastic cells laterally, forming the layer known as the embryonic endoderm. Hence, the epiblast is the source of embryonic ectoderm, embryonic mesoderm, and most, if not all, of embryonic endoderm.

A solid cord of cells grows cranially from the primitive knot to the prochordal plate between ectoderm and endoderm, forming a midline cord known as the notochord. The notochord induces the thickening of the overlying ectoderm between the procordal plate and the primitive knot, forming the neural plate. Shortly after its appearance, the neural plate invaginates along the long axis of the embryo to form the neural groove. The lateral walls of the groove are called the neural folds and the edges of the folds form the neural crest. By the end of the third week, the inner neural folds begin to fuse, forming the neural tube, which will give rise to the central nervous system. The process of fusion starts in the future embryonic neck and extends toward the cranial and caudal ends of the embryo. The cranial end of the neural tube will form the forebrain, midbrain, and hindbrain; the remainder of the tube will form the spinal cord.

The mesoderm down the center of the embryo differentiates into the paraxial mesoderm, the intermediate mesoderm, and the lateral mesoderm; the paraxial mesoderm divides into dense condensations or somites, each of which differentiates into sclerotome, dermatome, and myotome. The mesoderm in the head and neck areas (cranial mesoderm) also undergoes differentiation but the segmentation results in contiguous loose condensations or somitomeres.[1,2] These mesodermal condensations are located close to the neural crest cell population, forming a neural crest–mesoderm interface.[1,2] The neural crest and the mesoderm form the mesenchyme, which is a population of loosely arrayed stellate or fibroblast-shaped cells.

1.2.1.4. Fourth Week

The eye develops early in the fourth week as an evagination from the ventrolateral aspect of the neural tube or neuroectoderm, at the level of the forebrain in the diencephalon (Fig. 1.1). The end of the evagination become slightly dilated to form the optic vesicle. Neural crest cells cover the convex surface of the vesicles or neuroectoderm and partially isolate them from the dorsal, cranial, lateral, and ventral surface ectoderm, and from the caudomedial paraxial mesoderm. At the same time, a small area of surface ectoderm overlying each optic vesicle thickens, forming the lens placode (Fig. 1.2), which invaginates to become the lens vesicle.

1.2.1.5. Fifth Week

Each optic vesicle then invaginates to form the double-layered optic cup of neuroectoderm, which is surrounded by neural crest, mesecto-

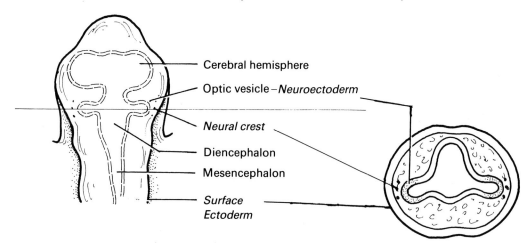

- Cerebral hemisphere
- Optic vesicle – *Neuroectoderm*
- *Neural crest*
- Diencephalon
- Mesencephalon
- *Surface Ectoderm*

FIGURE 1.1. Diagrams of longitudinal and transverse sections of the fourth-week embryo, showing the neuroectodermal evagination from the ventrolateral aspect of the neural tube at the level of the forebrain in the diencephalon to form the optic vesicle.

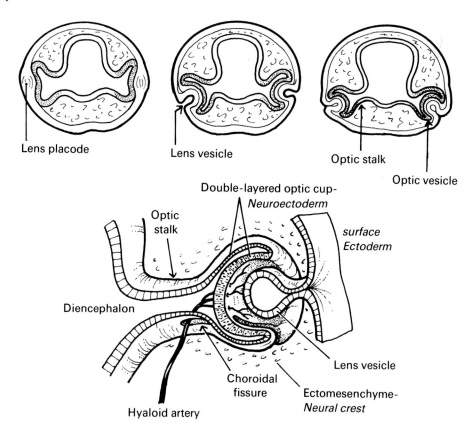

FIGURE 1.2. Diagrammatic representation of the formation of the lens placode (left transverse section) during the fourth week of embryo development (development of the optic vesicle during week 4 is shown in Fig. 1.1). Rapid, subsequent, se-quential development of the lens vesicle, the optic stalk, and (as shown in greater detail in Fig. 1.3) the double-layered optic cup of neuroectoderm is shown.

derm, or ectomesenchyme. The neuroectoderm gives rise to the pigment layer and the neural layer of the retina, the fibers and glia of the optic nerve, and the smooth muscle of the iris (Fig. 1.3) (Table 1.1). The surface ectoderm forms the corneal and conjunctival epithelium, the lens, the lacrimal gland, the tarsal glands, and the epidermis of the eyelids. The neural crest (or mesectoderm, or ectomesenchyme, also of ectodermal origin), forms the choroid, the iris, the ciliary musculature, part of the vitreous, the corneal stroma, the corneal endo-thelium, the trabecular meshwork, the optic nerve meninges, and almost all of the sclera. The mesoderm contributes only to the striated extraocular muscles, the vascular endothelia, and a small, temporal portion of the sclera.[3,4]

The sclera, therefore, is of dual origin, reflecting the location of the neural crest–mesodermal interface. Like the sclera, other connective tissues are of neural crest–mesodermal origin; they include cartilage, bones, ligaments, tendons, dermis, leptomeninges, and perivascular smooth muscle[1]; this may explain, at least in part, the frequent association of sclera and joints in many systemic diseases.

The differentiation of neural crest cells into sclera and choroid is induced by the retinal pigment epithelium.[5-7] In developmental colo-bomas, the defective pigment epithelium fails to induce development of the sclera and the choroid; the sclera remains thin and may develop internal staphylomas. The sclera, as well as the pigment epithelium and the choroid, also re-quires the presence of the developing lens for normal growth and change in shape, structure, and function.[2]

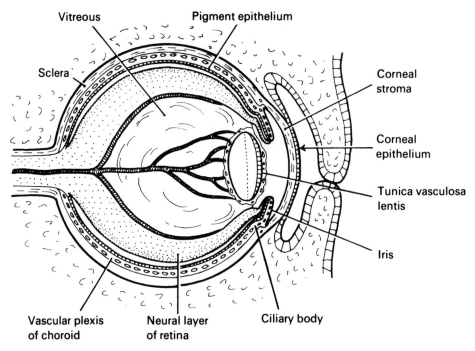

FIGURE 1.3. Further development of the eye (week 5). The neuroectoderm has now given rise to the pigment layer and to the neural layer of the retina, the fibers and glia of the optic nerve, and the smooth muscle of the iris. The lens vesicle has completely separated and is now a distinct, unattached entity within the developing globe, and the hyaloid artery has developed further throughout the vitreous and to the posterior aspect of the lens vesicle. The vascular plexus of the choroid has now developed, as has the primative sclera. The surface ectoderm has formed corneal and conjunctival epithelium, lens, lacrimal gland, and tarsal glands, as well as the epidermis of the skin. The neural crest mesectoderm has formed the choroid, the iris, the ciliary musculature, part of the vitreous, the corneal stroma and corneal endothelium, the trabecular meshwork, the optic nerve meninges, and the sclera. The mesoderm contributes only to the striated extraocular muscles and vascular endothelium and to a small temporal portion of the sclera.

TABLE 1.1. Embryology of ocular structures.

Neuroectoderm	Surface ectoderm	Neural crest	Mesoderm
Retina	Corneal epithelium	Choroid	Striated extraocular muscles
Fibers of optic nerve	Conjunctival epithelium	Iris	Vascular endothelia
Glia of optic nerve	Lens	Ciliary musculature	Small portion of the sclera
Smooth muscle of iris	Lacrimal gland	Part of vitreous	
	Tarsal glands	Corneal stroma	
	Epidermis or eyelids	Corneal endothelium	
		Optic nerve meninges	
		Most of sclera	

The sclera differentiates from anterior to posterior and from inside to outside.[8-10] Electron microscopy studies on human embryos and fetuses show that the developmental process has already started in the region destined to become the limbus by the sixth week, and progresses backward to the equator by the eighth week, and to the posterior pole by the twelfth week[2,10]; by the fourth month, the scleral spur appears as circularly oriented fibers,[2] and by the fifth month, scleral fibers crisscross around the axons of the optic nerve, thus forming the lamina cribrosa.[10] *Cytodevelopmental events* are characterized by a loss of free ribosomes and polysomes, an increase in the amount of rough-surfaced endoplasmic reticulum and Golgi complex components, and a decrease in glycogen granules and lipid deposits; *intercellular substance–developmental events* are characterized by an increase in the number and average diameter of collagen fibrils and in the amount of elastic deposits with electron-translucent central cores. By the beginning of week 10.9 there are no more differences between the inner and outer portions of the sclera. By week 13 there are no more differences between the anterior and posterior portions of the sclera. By week 24, the fetal sclera has the same ultrastructural characteristics as the adult sclera.

1.2.1.6. Sixth Week

The differentiation of periocular mesenchymal cells into fibroblasts has already started by week 6.4.[10] At this stage, the late mesenchymal cells or very early fibroblasts do not show pronounced differences between the anterior and posterior portions of the globe, except for the nuclei, the number of glycogen granules, and the number of lipid vacuoles; the cells in the anterior portion possess elongated nuclei and many glycogen granules and lipid vacuoles, whereas the cells of the posterior portion possess round-to-oval nuclei and few glycogen granules and lipid vacuoles. The late mesenchymal cells or very early fibroblasts contain many free ribosomes and polyribosomes, as well as immature rough-surfaced endoplasmic reticulum and Golgi complex. The intercellular space is filled with patches of immature collagen with an average diameter of 27 to 29 nm (range, 22 to 35 nm) without banding. There are no elastin deposits.

1.2.1.7. Seventh Week

By week 7.2, the cells of the anterior portion have more developed, rough-surfaced endoplasmic reticulum and Golgi complex and have fewer ribosomes and polyribosomes. The intercellular space in the outer portion is wider than in the inner portion; the number and average diameter (30 to 40 nm; range, 24 to 46 nm) of

collagen fibrils have increased in both locations in comparison with week 6.4. Immature elastin deposits consisting of microfibrillar components can be recognized for the first time. The cells of the posterior portion have more ribosomes and polyribosomes and less mature rough-surfaced endoplasmic reticulum and Golgi complex than do the cells of the anterior portion. The intercellular space in the posterior portion reveals fewer collagen fibrils than does the intercellular space in the anterior portion. There are no elastin deposits.

1.2.1.8. Ninth Week

By week 9.7, the cells of the inner anterior portion exhibit more glycogen granules and more elastin deposits than do the cells of the outer anterior portion. The number and average diameter (50 to 58 nm; range, 42 to 68 nm) of collagen fibrils have increased in both locations in comparison with week 7.2. The cells of the posterior portion have more cytoplasmic processes and rough-surfaced endoplasmic reticulum, and the intercellular spaces have more collagen fibrils and elastin deposits, in comparison with week 7.2.

1.2.1.9. Tenth Week

By week 10.9, the cells of the anterior portion have more developed rough-surfaced endoplasmic reticulum and Golgi complex, and fewer glycogen granules, than they had in week 9.7. The intercellular space has more collagen fibrils and elastin deposits in comparison with week 9.7. By this stage, the only difference between anterior and posterior portions is that the posterior area has fewer collagen fibrils than the anterior area.

1.2.1.10. Thirteenth Week

By week 13, the cells again exhibit more developed rough-surfaced endoplasmic reticulum and Golgi complex, and fewer glycogen granules, than do cells in week 10.9. Because collagen and elastin have increased in comparison with week 10.9, the volume ratio between cells and intercellular material is about 1 : 1. The average diameter of collagen fibrils in this stage is 62 to 74 nm (range, 50 to 84 nm).

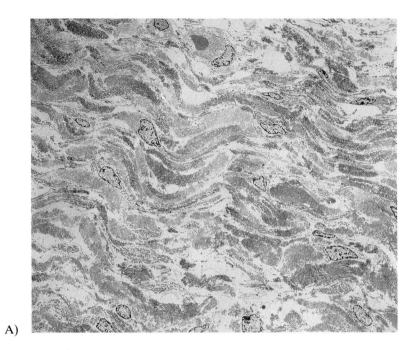

A)

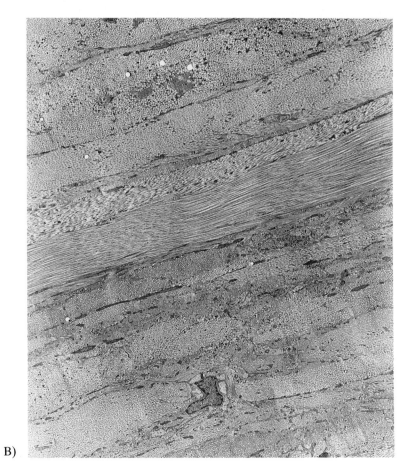

B)

1.2.1.11. Sixteenth Week

By week 16, the diameter of the collagen fibrils has increased in comparison with week 13. Our own transmission electron microscopy studies on human fetal and adult sclera showed that there are still differences between week 16 (Fig. 1.4A) and adult sclera (Fig. 1.4B); fetal sclera did not show the packed and dense, intermingled arrangements of collagen bundles with few fibroblasts of the adult sclera. Other characteristics of this stage are further enlargement of the rough-surfaced endoplasmic reticulum, complete loss of glycogen granules, and more elastin deposits.

1.2.1.12. Twenty-Fourth Week

By week 24, the sclera has the same ultrastructural characteristics as the adult sclera. The average diameter of the collagen fibrils is 94 to 102 nm (range, 84 to 102 nm), which is the average diameter of adult sclera. Mature elastin deposits exhibiting electron-translucent central cores also can be found.

Defects in synthesis of extracellular matrix components during scleral development at any of these stages may account for scleral abnormalities, including Marfan syndrome, osteogenesis imperfecta, pseudoxanthoma elasticum, Ehlers-Danlos syndrome, congenital myopia, and nanophthalmos.

1.2.2. Prenatal Development: Immunohistochemical Studies

Our own studies on immunolocalization of extracellular matrix components in human fetal and adult scleral specimens contribute to the understanding of scleral developmental events. The indirect immunofluorescence technique was performed on anterior and posterior portions of human fetal (13 to 22 weeks of gestation) and adult (52 to 73 years of age) sclera, using monoclonal antibodies against the collagens (types I to VII), the proteoglycans (heparan sulfate, dermatan sulfate, chondroitin sulfate, and hyaluronic acid), and the basement membrane glycoproteins (fibronectin, vitronectin, laminin). No marked differences in extracellular matrix component staining were found between the anterior and posterior portions of the sclera by week 16 and onward.

1.2.2.1. Collagens

Immunofluorescence studies localized collagen types I, III, IV, V, and VI in human fetal and adult scleral specimens; collagen types II and VII were not present. Collagen type I staining increased steadily from fetus to adult; the diffuse pattern seen in week 13 sclera became more fibrillar by week 16, the individual fibrils were larger by week 19, an extensive network of positive fibrils was evident by week 22, culminating in a diffuse presence in adult sclera. Collagen type III was moderately abundant, diffuse, and showed little change from 13 weeks to 73 years. Collagen type IV showed a pattern of granular positivity following individual fibrils at 13 weeks, decreasing steadily through 16, 19, and 22 weeks (Fig. 1.5). Adult sclera revealed only subtle type IV positivity, except for its dramatic presence in the blood vessels. Collagen type V staining was present in diffuse, moderate amounts in fetal scleral tissue; adult sclera showed a fine granular pattern along the edges of the collagen bundles. The amount of collagen type VI increased from fetal to adult scleral tissue, and the pattern became more striated in appearance.

Studies on tissue distribution of collagen type VIII in anterior and posterior human fetal (16 to 27 weeks) sclera showed an abundance in posterior fetal sclera; it gradually decreased and eventually disappeared in equatorial fetal sclera. Collagen type VIII showed a linear or fibrous pattern in anterior and posterior human adult sclera.[11]

FIGURE 1.4. (A and B) Transmission electron microscopy photomicrographs (×4000) of human fetal sclera, week 16 of development. Note the highly cellular nature of the fetal sclera (A) compared to the adult sclera (B) and the densely packed, intermingled arrangement of collagen bundles in the adult sclera (B) compared to the 16-week fetal sclera (A).

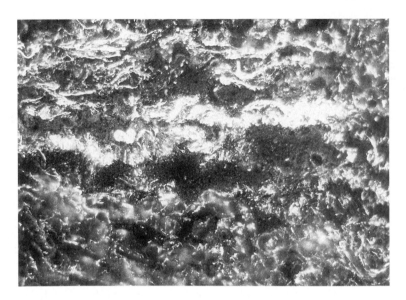

FIGURE 1.5. Immunofluorescence microscopy (using anti-collagen type IV antibody) of week 13 fetal sclera. The relatively abundant amount of collagen type IV seen in this 13-week fetal specimen steadily decreased throughout fetal development and was nearly absent in adult sclera, with the exception of its presence in the vascular walls.

Studies on tissue distribution of collagen type XII at the corneoscleral angle of the embryonic avian eye showed positive staining around the scleral ossicles and the scleral cartilages.[12]

1.2.2.2. Proteoglycans

Proteoglycans are macromolecular core proteins covalently attached to at least one sulfated glycosaminoglycan side chain. The glycosaminoglycan (GAG) chain consists of a hexosamine (D-galactosamine or D-glucosamine) and galactose units (keratan sulfate) or a hexuronic acid (L-iduronic acid or D-glucuronic acid). Chondroitin sulfate and dermatan sulfate are galactosaminoglycans and heparan sulfate is a glucosaminoglycan. Glycosaminoglycans are not homogeneous even within a given GAG because of the variability in sulfate substitutions and chain lengths.

Attempts to organize GAG terminology more clearly have resulted in the coinage of new terms for some of the GAGs, including lumican, decorin, versican, aggrecan, syndecan, and so on. In truth, however, a truly coherent new classification system for the GAGs must await additional studies and consensus.

The biological roles of GAGs are varied and multiple in nature. The most obvious roles in cornea and in sclera include support and organization, but it is clear that maintenance of corneal clarity is also a prime GAG function, as is directed cellular interactions and protein binding. The small, large, and even very large GAGs are soluble, and they interact in highly specific ways with specific sites on collagen fibrils. They maintain the "correct" spacing (and hence hydration) between fibrils. It should come as no surprise, then, that cornea and sclera present different GAG profiles.

We analyzed the glycosaminoglycans dermatan sulfate, chondroitin sulfate, hyaluronic acid, and heparan sulfate in human fetal and adult scleral specimens. Dermatan sulfate was present in moderate amounts through the different gestational periods, and chondroitin sulfate always stained intensely, without much difference between 13-week and adult sclera. In contrast, staining of hyaluronic acid changed from moderate at 13 weeks to mild at 22 weeks; this then subsided, and adult sclera showed only a subtle positivity. Heparan sulfate was identified in human fetal and adult sclera in small amounts.

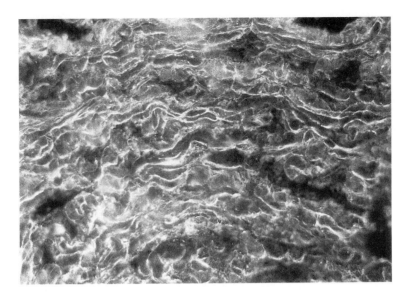

FIGURE 1.6. Immunofluorescence microscopy (using anti-fibronectin antibodies) of 13-week fetal sclera. Note the reticular pattern of the large amount of fibronectin present in the sclera. Fibronectin is nearly absent in adult sclera.

1.2.2.3. Glycoproteins

Fibronectin, vitronectin, and laminin were identified in human fetal and adult scleral specimens. Fibronectin staining changed from an intense reticular pattern at 13 weeks to a dramatic fibrillar pattern at 16 weeks; staining then decreased at 22 weeks and was subtle in adult sclera (Fig. 1.6). These findings indicate that, as in other organs during embryogenesis, fibronectin changes may play a major role in directing developmental events. Like fibronectin, vitronectin staining also decreased from fetal to adult scleral tissue. Laminin staining was subtle at 13 weeks and disappeared at 16 weeks and onward, except for its dramatic presence in the blood vessels.

1.2.3. Postnatal Development and Age-Related Changes

The postnatal sclera is relatively thin and somewhat translucent, allowing the blue color of the underlying uvea to show through. During the first 3 years of life, the sclera is also relatively distensible; thus increased intraocular pressure in cases of infantile glaucoma can cause buphthalmos. The sclera thickens gradually, becoming opaque and more rigid.[13] It also gradually enlarges as the eye grows during childhood and puberty.

In elderly individuals, scleral distensibility decreases, making stretching secondary to glaucoma unlikely. However, ectasias (localized protrusions of thin sclera) or staphylomas (localized protrusions lined by uveal tissue) may appear in areas where injury or inflammation has caused scleral thinning. Other age-related changes are a decrease in water content, a decrease in the amount of proteoglycans, and the subconjunctival deposition of lipids. The lipids, composed of cholesterol esters, free fatty acids, triglycerides, and sphingomyelin, give the sclera a yellowish color. Cholesterol esters and sphingomyelin show the greatest increase in volume with age.[14,15] Calcium phosphate is deposited in small rectangular areas just anterior to the insertions of medial and lateral rectus muscles. These areas, about 1 mm wide, may become translucent, revealing the bluish or brownish color due to the underlying uvea; they are called senile scleral plaques and usually occur in individuals over 70 years of age.[16]

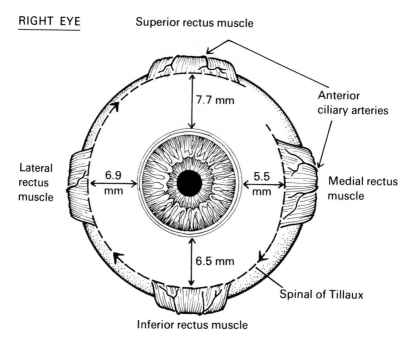

FIGURE 1.7. Diagrammatic representation of the relative positions of the insertions of the horizontal and vertical rectus muscles, illustrating the spiral of Tillaux.

1.3. Anatomy

1.3.1. Gross and Microscopic Anatomy

The scleral shell forms part of a circle averaging 22 mm in diameter.[13] Scleral thickness varies from 0.3 mm immediately behind the insertion of the rectus muscles to 1.0 mm near the optic nerve. It measures 0.4 to 0.5 mm at the equator, 0.6 mm where the tendons of the rectus muscles attach, and 0.8 mm adjacent to the limbus.[17] Traumatic scleral rupture usually occurs at the insertion of rectus muscles, at the equator, or in an area parallel to the limbus opposite from the site of the impact.

The outer surface of the sclera is smooth except where the tendons of the extraocular muscles insert. The insertions of the rectus muscles are progressively more posterior, following a pattern described by Tillaux and hence called the spiral of Tillaux (Fig. 1.7). The medial rectus inserts 5.5 mm posterior to the limbus, the inferior rectus 6.5 mm, the lateral rectus 6.9 mm, and the superior rectus 7.7 mm. The insertions of the superior oblique and inferior oblique muscles are posterior to the equator (Fig. 1.8). The long tendon for the superior oblique muscle inserts superiorly and slightly laterally; the line of insertion is convex posteriorly and laterally. The inferior oblique muscle inserts posterolaterally. Because this muscle has no tendon, the muscular fibers attach directly; the line of insertion is convex superiorly and laterally. The most posterior point lies 5 mm temporal to the optic nerve, external to the macula.

Tenon's capsule, the fascial sheath of the eyeball, is closely connected to the outer portion of the sclera or episclera by delicate lamellae, particularly where it fuses with the muscle tendon insertions anteriorly and with the optic nerve dural sheath posteriorly. Tenon's capsule lies anteriorly between two vascular layers: the conjunctival plexus and the episcleral plexus, both of which nourish it.

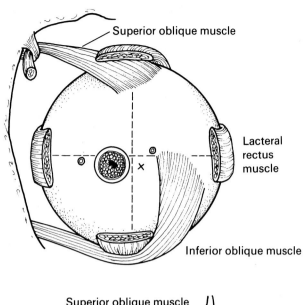

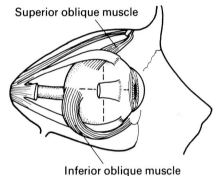

FIGURE 1.8. Diagrammatic representation of the insertions of the superior oblique and inferior oblique muscles.

1.3.1.1. Scleral Foramina

The sclera is an incomplete sphere that terminates anteriorly at the anterior scleral foramen surrounding the cornea, and posteriorly at the posterior scleral foramen surrounding the optic nerve canal.

1.3.1.1.1. Anterior Scleral Foramen

The anterior scleral foramen has an elliptical appearance externally (horizontal diameter of 11.6 mm and vertical diameter of 10.6 mm) and a circular appearance internally (diameter of 11.6 mm); it is not a discontinuity in the outer coat of the eye but is an anatomical concept of the sclera without the cornea. The sclera meets and merges with the cornea at the anterior scleral foramen, forming the corneoscleral junction, where the irregular scleral fibers tend to bend with the regular corneal lamellae. The corneoscleral junction is an area measuring about 1.5 to 2 mm wide; the concave scleral side is formed by the external scleral sulcus in its outer surface and by the internal scleral sulcus in its inner surface (Fig. 1.9). The external layers of the internal scleral sulcus merge with the stroma of the cornea. The internal layers of the internal scleral sulcus contain the trabecular meshwork and Schlemm's canal

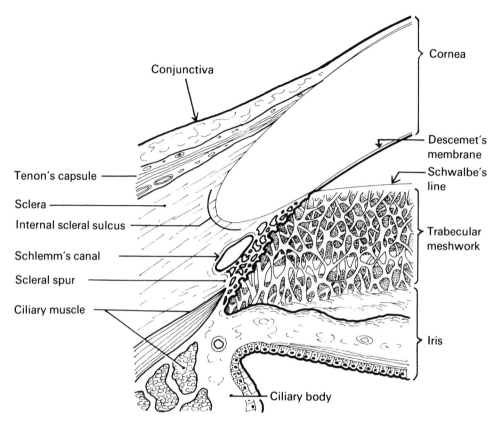

FIGURE 1.9. Diagrammatic representation of the corneoscleral junction in longitudinal section, illustrating the watch glass-like insertion of cornea into sclera, and the relationships between sclera, peripheral cornea, conjunctiva, and Tenon's capsule, the canal of Schlemm, and the trabecular meshwork and iris.

anteriorly, and the scleral spur posteriorly; the trabecular meshwork merges with Descemet's membrane. Because the scleral spur attaches to the meridional ciliary muscle, tension on the scleral spur by the muscle opens the trabecular meshwork.[3,18]

The corneoscleral junction can be best distinguished in a gross specimen of an enucleated eye after refrigeration, because the cornea thickens and opacifies whereas scleral thickness is not modified; however, it is indistinguishable in microscopic sections because of the similar structure of cornea and sclera.

1.3.1.1.2. Posterior Scleral Foramen

The sclera allows the passage of the optic nerve through the posterior scleral foramen. The site of this perforation is located 3 mm medial to the midline and 1 mm below the horizontal meridian. The outer two-thirds of the scleral fibers continue backward, fusing with the dural and arachnoid sheaths of the optic nerve (Fig. 1.10). The inner third of the scleral fibers cross the posterior scleral foramen in a sieve-like manner, forming the lamina cribrosa.[19] The lamina is slightly concave facing inward. The openings, lined by bundles of scleral fibers covered by glial tissue, are short canals that provide a passage for the axons of the optic nerve. Myelination of the axons stops at the lamina cribrosa before entering the inner retina. One of the openings in the lamina is larger than the rest and permits the passage of the central retinal artery and vein. Because the lamina cribrosa is a relatively weak area, it is bowed

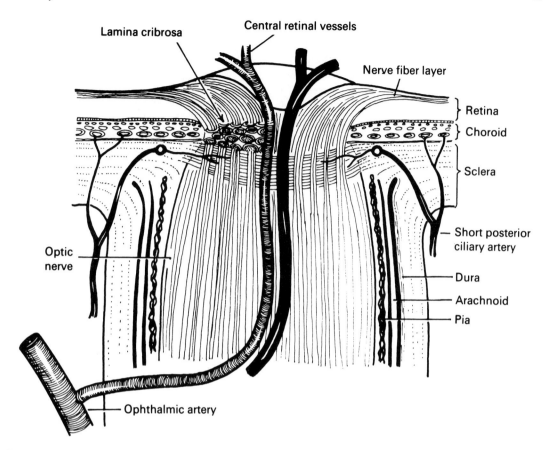

FIGURE 1.10. Diagrammatic representation of the optic nerve as it passes through the posterior scleral foramen, and the relationship of the ophthalmic artery and vein, as well as the short posterior ciliary arteries.

posteriorly in glaucomatous eyes, forming a cupped disk.

1.3.1.2. Layers of the Sclera

The sclera may be divided into three layers: the episclera, the scleral stroma, and the lamina fusca.

1.3.1.2.1. Episclera

The episclera forms the superficial aspect of the sclera and merges with the underlying scleral stroma. The episclera consists of loosely arranged bundles of collagen, intermingled with fibroblasts, occasional melanocytes, proteoglycans, and glycoproteins. Collagen bundles are thinner, fibroblasts are plumper, and ground substance is more plentiful than in the sclera. The episclera has a rich blood supply anteriorly, where it lies closely connected with the subconjunctival tissue, the rectus muscle insertions, and Tenon's capsule. These vessels are mainly derived from the anterior ciliary arteries and, although usually inconspicuous, may be prominent when the tissue is inflamed. The posterior ciliary arteries serve as the source of the equatorial and posterior episcleral vessels. The episclera becomes progressively thinner toward the back of the eye.

1.3.1.2.2. Scleral Stroma

The scleral stroma consists of collagen bundles associated with a few elastic fibers. Between the bundles are a few fibroblasts with occasional melanocytes. Collagen bundles, larger in diameter than those in the episclera, vary in thickness and form whorls and loops. Although they usually run parallel with the surface, many crisscross freely with each other, forming a feltlike structure. Because of the interlacing of the collagen bundles, the sclera presents a dull white color. Near the cornea and the optic nerve canal, the bundles tend to run in concentric circles. In other portions, they form patterns of loops running mainly in a meridional direction. This arrangement permits adjustment to the changes in intraocular pressure and to the stress produced by the extraocular muscles.

1.3.1.2.3. Lamina Fusca

The lamina fusca is the portion of the sclera that is adjacent to the uvea; collagen bundles become smaller and the number of elastic fibers is increased. A large number of melanocytes is present, giving to this portion a faintly brown color. The lamina has grooves that provide a passage for the ciliary vessels and nerves. It is separated from the outer aspect of the choroid by a potential space, the perichoroidal space, filled by fine collagen fibers that provide a weak attachment between both layers.

1.3.1.3. Blood Supply and Emissary Canals

The elegant dissections performed by Leber in 1903 form the foundation of our current understanding of the ocular anterior segment circulation.[20] Anatomical techniques involving India ink injections[21] and vascular casting, using neoprene and methyl methacrylate,[22–24] combined with scanning electron microscopy,[25–27] confirmed Leber's findings and provided a unique static method for three-dimensional analysis of the ocular microvasculature. Anterior segment fluorescein angiography,[28–32] low-dose fluorescein anterior segment angiography,[33] low-dose fluorescein anterior segment videoangiography,[34] and fluorescein anterior segment videoangiography with a scanning angiographic microscope[35] helped in the study of circulatory dynamics of the anterior segment

circulation, such as flow direction and flow velocity.

1.3.1.3.1. Vascular Distribution

Results of studies using static anatomical techniques show that the blood supply of the anterior segment of the eye has distinctive characteristics. Except for the perforating vessels, the sclera is a relatively avascular structure. It has a low metabolic requirement because of the slow turnover rate of its collagen. The episcleral blood supply is derived mainly from the anterior ciliary arteries anterior to the insertions of the rectus muscles and from the long and short posterior ciliary arteries posterior to these insertions. Scleral stroma contains capillary beds but is supplied by the episcleral and, to a lesser degree, choroidal vascular networks.

The arteries, veins, and nerves traverse the sclera through emissary canals.[36] These canals or passageways are separated from the sclera by a thin layer of loose connective tissue. There are more emissary canals superiorly at 12 o'clock and inferiorly at 6 o'clock than nasally and temporally. The fewest occur in the temporal quadrant. Emissary canals provide a passageway for extraocular extensions of intraocular tumors.[37]

On the surface of the eye, the muscular arteries, which arise from the ophthalmic artery, run forward as the anterior ciliary arteries. The anterior ciliary arteries pass through the sclera just in front of the insertions of the rectus muscles in a slightly oblique direction from posterior to anterior. Each rectus muscle has two anterior ciliary arteries, except the lateral rectus muscle, which has only one (Fig. 1.7). The seven anterior ciliary arteries meet via their lateral branches 1 to 5 mm behind the limbus and form the anterior episcleral arterial circle, which feeds the limbal, anterior conjunctival, and anterior episcleral tissues (Fig. 1.11). The anterior episcleral arterial circle broadly resolves into limbal arcades, an anterior conjunctival plexus, a superficial episcleral plexus, and a deep episcleral plexus (Fig. 1.12). Limbal arcades and anterior conjunctival plexus usually share their origins and form the most

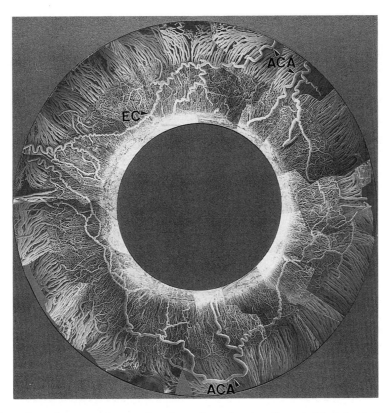

FIGURE 1.11. Scanning electron micrograph of a vascular cast, showing the formation of the major vascular plexuses of the anterior segment. The anterior ciliary arteries (ACA) meet via their lateral branches 1 to 5 mm behind the limbus and form the anterior episcleral arterial circle (EC), which feeds the limbal, anterior conjunctival, and anterior episcleral tissues.

superficial layer of vessels. The superficial episcleral plexus lies within the parietal layer of the episclera and anastomoses at the limbus with the conjunctival plexus, branches of the same plexus, and with the deep episcleral plexus (Fig. 1.13). The deep episcleral plexus lies within the visceral layer of the episclera and anastomoses with branches of the same plexus. In addition, extensions of the remaining anterior ciliary arterial branches perforate the limbal sclera through emissary canals and meet the long posterior ciliary arteries in the ciliary muscle to form the major arterial circle of the iris (Fig. 1.14). The anterior episcleral arterial circle and the major arterial circle of the iris communicate by scleral perforating anterior ciliary arterial branches, which do not form a capillary bed in the sclera but rather provide nutrients to the uveal tract (Fig. 1.15).

The limbal venous circle collects blood from the anterior conjunctival veins and limbal arcades, and drains into radial episcleral collecting veins. The episcleral collecting veins also receive blood from anterior episcleral veins and perforating scleral veins. Perforating scleral veins emerge from Schlemm's canal, from which they receive aqueous humor. They penetrate the sclera through different emissary canals than do the arteries. These canals, over the ciliary body, often also carry the ciliary nerves. As the episcleral collecting veins run posteriorly across the sclera, they form the anterior ciliary veins, which leave the anterior surface of the globe over the rectus muscles.

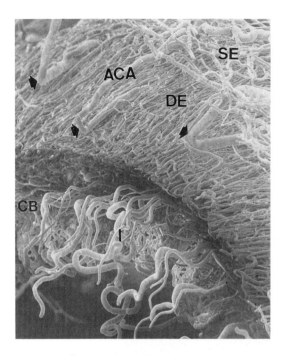

FIGURE 1.12. Scanning electron micrograph (×40) of a vascular cast of the anterior vascular plexuses of the eye. Note that the anterior ciliary arteries (ACA) bend toward the major iris arterial circle (arrows) anterior to the ciliary body (CB) and the iris (I). The superficial episcleral plexus (SE) and the deep episcleral plexus (DE) communicate via connecting vessels.

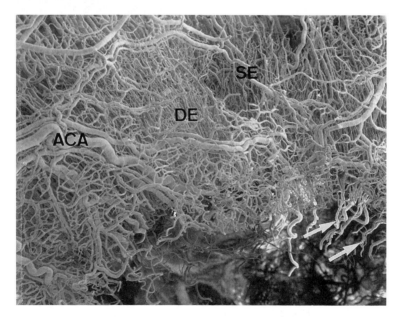

FIGURE 1.13. Scanning electron micrograph (×24) of a vascular cast. Iris vessels (white arrows) are seen posterior to the anterior ciliary artery (ACA) and its branches, as well as the superficial episcleral (SE) and deep episcleral (DE) plexuses and their interconnectors.

The two long posterior ciliary arteries (medial and lateral), which also arise from the ophthalmic artery, enter the sclera 3.6 mm nasal to the optic nerve and 3.9 mm temporal to the optic nerve (Figs. 1.14 and 1.16). The arteries, together with the nerves, traverse the sclera

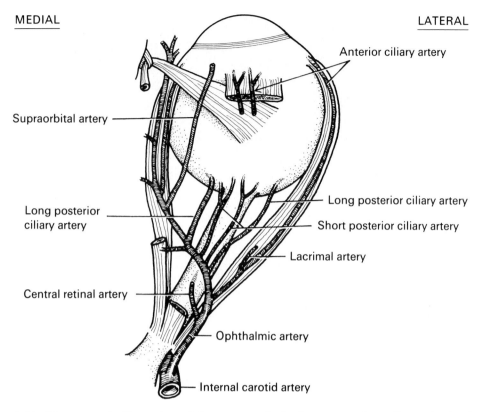

FIGURE 1.14. Diagrammatic illustration of the vascular supply to the globe, showing the relationships between the internal carotid, ophthalmic, central retinal, long posterior ciliary, lacrimal, short posterior ciliary, and anterior ciliary arteries.

through emissary canals in an oblique manner, from posterior to anterior, and enter the suprachoroidal space at the equator. They run forward to give arterial supply to the ciliary body and the iris. In addition, they meet the anterior ciliary arteries to form the major arterial circle of the iris. The major arterial circle of the iris is located in the stroma of the ciliary body and gives arterial supply to the iris. Surgery on the vertical, but not the horizontal, rectus muscles may give rise to ischemic defects in the iris.[26,28,29] This finding seems to indicate that the anterior ciliary arteries contribute to the iris supply and that this contribution is critical in sectors of the globe that receive inadequate long posterior ciliary artery perfusion (vertical meridian). The superior and inferior anterior uvea are, therefore, at greater risk of ischemia after superior and inferior anterior ciliary occlusion following ligation of the respective muscles. The greater prevalence of emissary canals containing perforating anterior ciliary arteries in the vertical meridia[36] may compensate for this deficit.

Posterior to the equator the sclera is perforated obliquely by the emissary canals for the vortex veins (Fig. 1.17). Each eye usually contains from four to seven veins. Vortex veins drain the venous system of the choroid, ciliary body, and iris. One or more veins are in each quadrant. The superior vortex veins exit 8 mm posterior to the equator, close to the most posterior edge of the insertion of the superior oblique muscle. The inferior vortex veins exit 6 mm posterior to the equator.

The short posterior ciliary arteries arise from the ophthalmic artery as it crosses the optic nerve. After dividing into 10 to 20 branches, they perforate the sclera around the entrance of the optic nerve (Fig. 1.18) and supply the

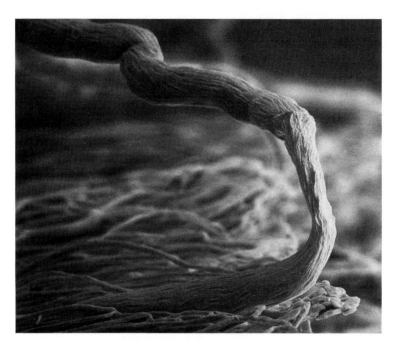

FIGURE 1.15. Scanning electron micrograph (×100) of a vascular cast of a scleral perforating anterior ciliary arterial branch connecting the anterior episcleral arterial circle and the major arterial circle of the iris.

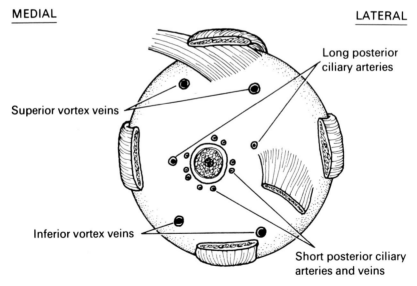

FIGURE 1.16. Diagrammatic representation of the sites of perforation of the sclera by the long and short posterior ciliary arteries, the short posterior ciliary veins, and the inferior and superior vortex veins.

MEDIAL   LATERAL

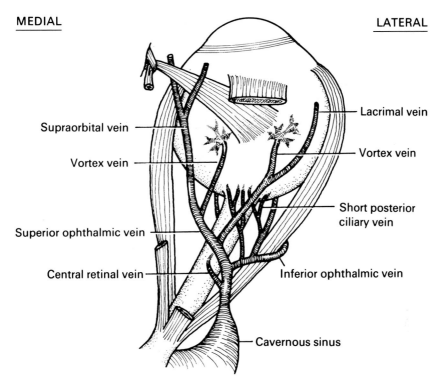

FIGURE 1.17. Diagrammatic representation of the relationships between the lacrimal, vortex, short posterior ciliary, inferior ophthalmic, central retinal, supraorbital, and superior ophthalmic veins.

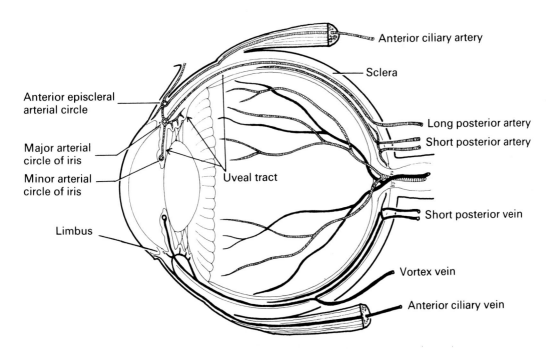

FIGURE 1.18. Diagrammatic representation of a transverse section of the globe, illustrating another view of the relationships between the short posterior ciliary, long posterior ciliary, and anterior ciliary arteries and the short posterior ciliary, anterior ciliary, and vortex veins.

choroid as far as the equator of the eye. The vessels pass directly to the choroid without forming a capillary bed in the sclera. Some of the branches in the sclera run toward the equator and anastomose with the branches of the long posterior ciliary arteries to supply the posterior episclera. However, this posterior episcleral plexus is so thin that it gives a poor supply to the underlying sclera in the equator. Most of the nutrient requirements of the sclera in this area are supplied by the choroidal circulation. Some of the branches of the short posterior ciliary arteries around the optic disk form the incomplete vascular circle of Zinn-Haller near the inner scleral rim. The emissary canals for the short ciliary vessels, arteries and veins, may be perpendicular, oblique, or spiral.

1.3.1.3.2. Circulatory Dynamics

The classic, static anatomical techniques have provided the foundation for our knowledge of the blood supply of the anterior segment of the eye (described in the preceding section). However, the direction of flow in these vessels, studied by circulatory dynamic techniques such as anterior segment fluorescein angiography, has excited controversy. Some studies support the traditional view[20] that the anterior ciliary artery flow is from the region of the rectus muscles toward the inside of the eye, providing major perforating contributions to the intraocular circulation.[35,38–40] This centripetal distribution is supported by corrosion plastic castings of the ocular vasculature, in which perforating anterior ciliary arteries divide extensively within the anterior uvea,[24,26,41] and by the fact that anterior segment ischemia may arise from surgery on the vertical but not horizontal rectus muscles (the vertical meridian of the anterior uvea is insufficiently perfused by the long posterior ciliary artery).[28,29] Other studies suggest that the anterior episcleral circulation is supplied by retrograde or centrifugal flow in the perforating ciliary arteries derived from the long posterior ciliary arteries.[31,32,34,42,43] Some investigators have argued that this retrograde flow represents emissary veins that drain the deep circulations of the anterior uvea into the superficial episcleral venous system.[21,30,44]

Others believe that it results from deficiencies in photographic and conventional videocamera techniques.[35] The resolution of this controversy will require further studies.

1.3.1.4. Nerve Supply

The posterior ciliary nerves perforate the sclera around the optic nerve. The many short posterior ciliary nerves supply the posterior region of the sclera, whereas the two long posterior ciliary nerves supply the anterior portion. Because the sclera receives a profuse sensory innervation, scleral inflammation may cause severe pain. In addition, because the extraocular muscles have their insertions in the sclera, the pain may increase with the ocular movement.

A branch of the long posterior ciliary nerve (intrascleral nerve loop of Axenfeld) may loop out through the sclera in the region of the ciliary body, forming a clinically visible nodular elevation 4 to 7 mm posterior to the limbus. These nerve loops are found in 12% of the eyes as a normal anatomical variation and are usually associated with blood vessels. It is sometimes of clinical significance because the nerves are occasionally accompanied by pigmented chromatophores, which may produce a pigmented spot on the sclera. They can be slightly painful if they lie in the episclera. Because such a nerve loop may be mistaken for a melanotic tumor or for a foreign body, it must be included in the differential diagnosis of primary or metastatic malignant melanoma occurring in this region.[45] They obviously should not be removed.

1.3.2. Ultramicroscopic Anatomy

1.3.2.1. Sclera

The sclera is composed of dense bundles of collagen, few elastic fibers, few fibroblasts, and a moderate amount of amorphous ground substance (proteoglycans and glycoproteins) (Fig. 1.19).

Collagen bundles consist of long, branched fibrils with a macroperiodicity of about 64 nm (range, 35 to 75 nm) and a microperiodicity of 11 nm. Unlike the uniform corneal collagen, the collagen fibrils in sclera vary in diameter,

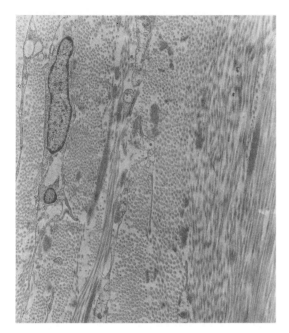

FIGURE 1.19. Transmission electron micrograph of adult human sclera (×11,000). Note the fibroblast, the collagen bundles, both longitudinal and transverse, with variable-diameter fibrils forming bundles more irregularly arranged than is seen in the cornea.

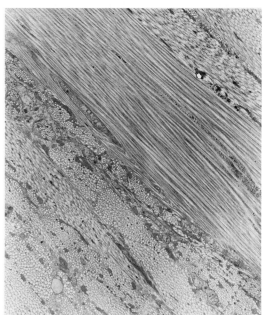

FIGURE 1.21. Transmission electron micrograph of adult sclera (×26,000). Note the periodicity in the longitudinal fibers and the variable fibril diameter in the transverse bundles.

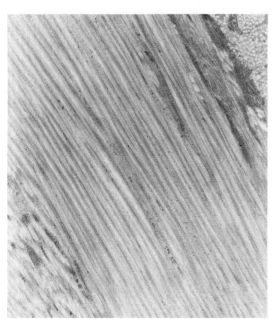

FIGURE 1.20. Transmission electron micrograph of human sclera (×26,000). Transverse section of collagen bundles in the sclera. The macroperiodicity is approximately 64 nm.

ranging from 28 to 300 nm, and their arrangement in the individual bundles is more random than in the cornea.[46–49] Collagen bundles in sclera vary in diameter, ranging from 0.5 to 6.0 μm, and form complex and irregular branching patterns, curving around the muscular insertions and the optic nerve (Figs. 1.20 and 1.21). Collagen bundles in the outer region are thinner (0.5 to 2 μm) than those in the inner region; they usually run in a lamellar fashion, whereas those in the inner region are interwoven randomly, forming irregular and intermingled arrangements.[49,50] These arrangements may account for the rigidity and flexibility against changes in intraocular pressure and for the opacity of the sclera.

The fibrils at the emissary canals run parallel to the direction of the canal. Few of these fibrils attach to the wall of the vessel or nerve in the canal. A small number of fine elastic fibers (10 to 12 nm in diameter) lie parallel to the collagen fibrils.[49,51]

Flat stellate or spindle-shaped cells, the fibroblasts, are few in number along the bundles

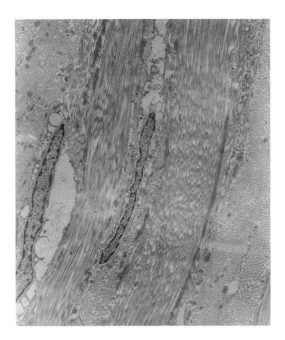

FIGURE 1.22. Transmission electron micrograph of human adult sclera (×17,750). Note the flat, spindle-shaped cells with long nuclei containing marginated chromatin. These fibroblasts are in a state of relative metabolic quiescence.

of collagen (Fig. 1.22). The long axis of the cell (and the large elliptical nucleus) is parallel to the surface.[37] The nucleus has one or two nucleoli and the chromatin is sparse. Quiescent fibroblasts contain a relative scanty cytoplasm with long mitochondria, a small Golgi complex, a few cisternal profiles of granular endoplasmic reticulum, and occasional small fat droplets. During growth or repair, however, the Golgi complex and the granular endoplasmic reticulum become prominent. The fibroblast elaborates the precursors of the amorphous ground substance components as well as the fibrillar proteins such as collagen and elastin. Following secretion the fibrils lie on the cell surface while full maturation into fibers occurs.

The amorphous ground substance, composed of proteoglycans and glycoproteins, fills intercellular and interfibrillar spaces. Proteoglycans, demonstrated by cuprolinic blue stain, are fine filaments approximately 54 nm in length and

5 nm in diameter, they are localized around, along, and radiating from the collagen fibrils.[52]

1.3.2.2. Vessels

Our own transmission electron microscopy studies on human adult sclera showed that episcleral vessels, as capillaries and postcapillary venules, are continuous and had simple walls consisting of endothelial cells attached to an underlying basement membrane secreted by them, and a discontinuous layer of pericytes (Figs. 1.23–1.25). The endothelial cells, irregular in shape, had a cytoplasm with mitochondria, rough-surfaced endoplasmic reticulum, smooth-surfaced endoplasmic reticulum, Golgi apparatus, and pinocytotic vesicles. Endothelial cells interconnect through thin areas of more or less tortuous interendothelial clefts composed of adjacent cell membranes. The basement membrane, almost parallel to the outer contour of the endothelial cells, consists of one to several dense layers with a less dense zone filling the

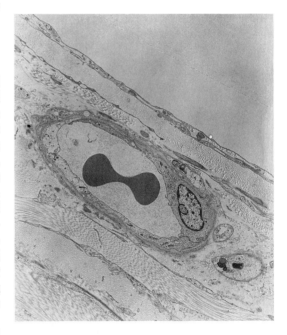

FIGURE 1.23. Transmission electron micrograph of human adult episcleral tissue (×7500). Episcleral vessel (transverse section) with discontinuous pericyte support, and typical microvascular endothelium, are visible. A red blood cell is seen in the lumen.

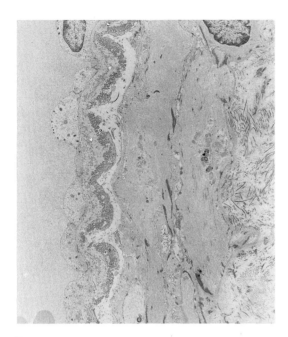

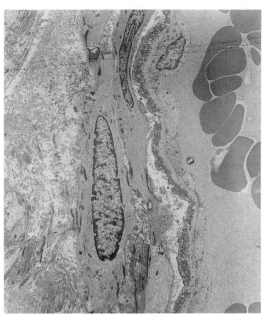

FIGURE 1.24. Transmission electron micrograph of human adult sclera ($\times$17,750), episcleral vessel. Note the continuous, thin vascular basement membrane and the lack of a vascular wall other than that formed by the endothelial cell, basement membrane, and the pericyte.

FIGURE 1.25. Transmission electron micrograph of human adult sclera ($\times$7500). Superficial scleral vessel, with red blood cells in the lumen, endothelial cells lining the vessel, and supporting pericyte cytoplasm are visible. Note the scleral fibroblasts and collagen underlying the vessel.

space between them. Pericytes are attached to the basement membrane, often with one or more dense zones between them and the endothelial cell; their cytoplasm contains endoplasmic reticulum, mitochondria, Golgi apparatus, pinocytotic vesicles, and fine filaments. No smooth muscle cells are present. Bundles of collagen fibrils adjacent to the vessel walls merge into the surrounding connective tissue.

Episcleral and conjunctival vessels in monkeys have an identical morphology.[53] Episcleral and conjunctival vessels are permeable to tracer molecules such as fluorescein-labeled dextrans of different molecular weight or horseradish peroxidase injected into the blood stream or into the anterior chamber[53,54]; tracers escape from the vessel lumen by crossing the thin interendothelial clefts. It can equally be expected that the aqueous humor that reaches the episcleral and conjunctival vessels through Schlemm's canal and collector channels can

diffuse freely into the episcleral loose connective tissues and the subconjunctival spaces across the walls of these permeable vessels.

1.4. Biochemistry

Collagen forms 75% of the dry weight of the sclera, as determined by quantitation of 4-hydroxyproline in acid hydrolysates of the total tissue.[55] Collagen type I is the predominant type, whereas type III is found in smaller amounts.[56–58] There is no difference in the collagen content or collagen type in sclera between anterior and posterior segments of the eye.[56]

Elastin content, estimated by desmosine and isodesmosine analysis, forms less than 2% of the dry weight of the sclera.[59]

Proteoglycans, determined by uronic acid analysis, constitute 0.7 to 0.9% of the dry weight of the sclera.[55] Proteoglycans are composed of glycosaminoglycan chains linked to a protein core. The most abundant glycosaminoglycan in sclera is dermatan sulfate, followed by chondroitin sulfate and hyaluronic acid.[60,61] Little heparan sulfate and no keratan sulfate is present. Regional analysis shows that the sclera around the optic nerve is the area richest in dermatan sulfate, the sclera around the equator is the richest in hyaluronic acid, and the sclera around the fovea is the richest in chondroitin sulfate.[61]

Glycoproteins such as fibronectin and vitronectin also can be detected in sclera. Laminin has not been found,[58] except in vessels.

The water content of sclera ranges from 65 to 75%. The sclera appears opaque if the water content is maintained between 40 and 80% but becomes transparent if it falls below 40% or rises above 80%.[55]

1.5. Immunohistochemistry

We studied the immunolocalization of extracellular matrix components in human adult sclera, using monoclonal antibodies against the collagens, proteoglycans, and glycoproteins.

Collagen types I, III, V, and VI stained intensely in extravascular sclera, whereas collagen types II and VII were not identified. Collagen type IV was almost absent except for its dramatic presence in blood vessels (see Chapter 5). Studies on tissue distribution of collagen type VIII in human sclera showed a linear or fibrous pattern of intense staining in anterior and posterior human adult sclera.[11]

The most abundant glycosaminoglycans in sclera were dermatan sulfate and chondroitin sulfate; hyaluronic acid and heparan sulfate also were present, although in small amounts.

The glycoproteins fibronectin and vitronectin were identified in scleral specimens. Laminin was absent in extravascular sclera but was dramatically represented in vessel walls.

Scleral blood vessels showed the presence of collagen types IV, V, and VI, the glycosaminoglycans heparan sulfate and chondroitin sulfate, and the glycoproteins fibronectin and laminin in endothelial cell basement membranes.

1.6. Biomechanics

By virtue of its rigidity or poor distensibility, the sclera provides a stable viscoelastic system for the globe. This property appears to be dependent, at least in part, on the glycosaminoglycan water-binding properties: the higher the water-holding capacity of the glycosaminoglycan, the more distensible the sclera. The adult sclera exhibits a biphasic response to a sudden force: a rapid lengthening is followed by a slow stretching.[62-64] However, like most viscoelastic systems, the sclera will stretch proportionately more with small pressure changes. The sclera will stretch with initial elevations of intraocular pressure, therefore small increases in intraocular volume at low pressure result in small increases in intraocular pressure. As the pressure increases, the resistance to further stretching also increases, and therefore small increases in intraocular volume at high pressures result in large increases in intraocular pressure. Following severe transient stretching of the sclera, as in acute glaucoma, scleral distensibility returns to the baseline levels prior to the increase in intraocular pressure.

Scleral distensibility is an important consideration when methods of intraocular pressure measurement are studied. The indentation method results in a significant increase in intraocular volume; the applanation method does not. In some eyes with increased scleral distensibility (e.g., as produced by inflammatory diseases, high myopia, or retinal detachment surgery), the indentation measurement method will result in a false low reading because the sclera will stretch to accommodate the pressure of the tonometer.

Scleral distensibility decreases with age.[65] This property appears to depend, at least in part, on the degree of hydration of connective tissue; highly hydrated tissues such as embryonic skin or fetal cornea are highly distensible, whereas adult tissues become more rigid as their water-holding capacity decreases.[66-69] Posterior sclera is more distensible than anterior sclera, and the choroid is more distensible than the sclera; the latter helps explain why the choroid forms redundant folds in orbital or choroidal tumors, ocular hypotony, and sub-retinal neovascularization.

1.7. Molecular Structure

Scleral connective tissue consists of cells and extracellular matrix. The cells, or fibroblasts, play a critical role in the synthesis and organization of the matrix elements. The extracellular matrix is composed of fibrillar proteins such as collagen and elastin, and of amorphous ground substance such as proteoglycans and glycoproteins. The specific turnover rate of the scleral matrix by fibroblasts and the degradative enzymes they secrete (collagenases, elastases, proteoglycanases, and glycoproteinases) is unknown, but collagen fibrils have a slower turnover rate than proteoglycans.[70] Healing of scleral wounds, based on a delicate balance of fibroblast matrix synthesis and enzyme matrix degradation, is a slow process, taking months or years, and the area of the wound can always be identified histologically by the abrupt change in scleral collagen fiber orientation and disorganization that persists throughout the life of the individual.[71]

1.7.1. Collagen

Collagen types I, III, IV, V, VI, and VIII have been identified in scleral tissue. Each collagen molecule is composed of three polypeptide α chains containing triple-helical and globular domains.[72,73] The triple-helical regions have a repeating triplet amino acid sequence, summarized as $(Gly-X-Y)_n$, where X and Y are often proline and hydroxyproline, respectively. The presence of glycine at every third residue, with the exception of short sequences at the ends of the chain, contributes to the triple-helical conformation. Interchain hydrogen bonds, especially with the hydroxyl groups of hydroxyproline, stabilize the triple-helical structure.

Collagen biosynthesis by scleral fibroblasts is a complex process consisting of several specific intracellular steps. Each polypeptide pro-α chain is a distinct gene product.[74–76] The pro-α chains, assembled in the lumen of the rough endoplasmic reticulum, undergo hydroxylation of specific proline and lysine residues by the action of prolyl-3-hydroxylase, prolyl-4-hydroxylase, and lysyl hydroxylase. Subsequent to hydroxylation, some of the hydroxylysine residues become glycosylated by the action of glycosyltransferases. After completion of the synthesis, the pro-α chain has two globular domains, the NH_2 terminal and the COOH terminal. Following alignment of three polypeptide pro-α chains, interchain and intrachain disulfide bonds form at the COOH-terminal propeptides, stabilizing and facilitating helix formation. Procollagen type I contains interchain disulfide bonds within the COOH-terminal propeptides. Procollagen type III contains interchain disulfide bonds within the NH_2-terminal propeptides as well. Disulfide bonds within the NH_2-terminal propeptides form after helix formation.[77] The assembled triple-helical procollagen types I and III molecules are secreted into the extracellular space, where the terminal propeptides are proteolytically removed. The resulting molecules have a remarkable tendency for spontaneous formation of fibrils.[78]

1.7.2. Elastin

Small but important amounts of the fibrillar protein elastin are synthesized by scleral fibroblasts as part of the extracellular matrix. Elastin is composed primarily of nonpolar hydrophobic amino acids such as alanine, valine, isoleucine, and leucine, and contains little hydroxyproline and no hydroxylysine. It also contains two unique amino acids, desmosine and isodesmosine, which serve to cross-link the polypeptide chains. Studies on genomic elastin clones from chick embryo aortas indicate that the rate of elastin synthesis is controlled at the level of transcription.[73]

1.7.3. Proteoglycans

Proteoglycans are complex molecules, synthesized by scleral fibroblasts and consisting of a core protein of varying length to which glycosaminoglycan chains are covalently linked. Glycosaminoglycans are long-chain, unbranched, linear polymers of repeating disaccharide units. One constituent of the unit is an Nacetylated amino sugar, which may or may not be sulfated, and the other is a uronic acid. The high molecular weight proteoglycan molecule is composed of 1 or 2 to more than 100 glycos-aminoglycan chains with a potential of giving more than 10,000 negatively charged groups per proteoglycan molecule.[79,80] During syn-thesis, assembly of the protein core and initiation of the glycosaminoglycan chain occur together in the rough endoplasmic reticulum. One or two different types of glycosaminoglycan chains attach to the core protein at one end and radiate from it in a bottle-brush configuration.[79]

At least four types of glycosaminoglycans have been detected in scleral tissue.[61] Dermatan sulfate, chondroitin sulfate, heparan sulfate, and hyaluronic acid largely compose the amorphous ground substance present in the intercellular and interfibrillar spaces of the sclera. Dermatan sulfate consists of sulfated N-acetylgalactosamine and two different types of uronic acid, glucuronic acid and iduronic acid; chondroitin sulfate consists of sulfated N-acetylgalactosamine and glucuronic acid; heparan sulfate consists of sulfated N-acetylglucosamine and two different types of uronic acid, glucuronic acid and iduronic acid; hyaluronic acid consists of N-acetylglucosamine and glucuronic acid (it is not linked to a core protein and lacks a sulfate group).

Proteoglycans interact with collagen deter-mining the organization and size of collagen fibrils.[81-84] They also interact with glycoproteins such as fibronectin. Most of these interactions are mediated by the glycosaminoglycan com-ponent although some are mediated by the core protein of proteoglycan.[85,86] The decrease in collagen fibril arrangement and increase in collagen fibril size in the area of transition from cornea to sclera coincide with the disappearance of keratan sulfate and the appearance of highly sulfated galactosaminoglycans, such as der-matan sulfate and chondroitin sulfate.[60] Pro-teoglycans maintain the proper anatomical structure of the collagen fibrils and protect them from attack.[70] Proteoglycans also func-tion as modulators of growth factors such as fibroblast growth factor or transforming growth factor.[81]

1.7.4. Glycoproteins

Although collagen, elastin, and proteoglycans are technically glycosylated proteins, the term *glycoprotein* is primarily used for molecules composed of oligosaccharide with a mannose core N-glycosidically linked to asparagine. The glycoprotein fibronectin has been detected in sclera as part of the amorphous ground substance.[58]

Fibronectin is a high molecular weight mole-cule synthesized by scleral fibroblasts. It con-sists of two similar subunits joined near their COOH termini by disulfide bonds.[87] Each subunit can be divided into a number of globular domains that have specific binding charac-teristics. There are binding sites for fibrin, heparin, bacteria, collagen, DNA, cell mem-branes, and a variety of other macromolecules. Fibronectin is thought to be important in the organization of the pericellular and intercellular matrix by its ability to bind to collagen, fibro-blasts, and glycosaminoglycans.[88,89] Antibodies directed against the collagen-binding domain of fibronectin have been shown to inhibit collagen fibril deposition.[90] Fibronectin has also been found to play a role in host defense, presumably by its ability to interact with C1q component of complement, fibrin, bacteria, and DNA.[91-93] Characterization of fibronectin cDNA clones indicates that only a single fibro-nectin gene exists; but multiple forms of cellular fibronectin are generated by alternative splicing of mRNA.[94-96] These alternatively spliced forms appear to have differential functions in embryogenesis, defense, wound healing, and homeostatic cell maintenance.

Laminin, a glycoprotein found in basement membranes, consists of three polypeptide chains—A (440 kDa) and B$_1$ and B$_2$ (each 220 kDa)—linked via disulfide bonds to form an asymmetric cross-structure.[97] Laminin pos-sesses multiple functional sites that mediate its interactions with cells, such as endothelial cells, and with other extracellular matrix components, such as glycosaminoglycans, nonintegrin pro-teins, and integrins.[98] Cells and extracellular matrix proteins interact with laminin via specific surface receptors. Laminin participates in promotion of cell adhesion, growth, migration, and differentiation, as well as assembly of basement membranes.[99]

The fact that laminin is the first extracellular matrix protein to appear in development emphasizes its importance in the intricate process of tissue organization.[97]

1.7.5. Matrix-Degrading Enzymes

Collagenase, elastase, proteoglycanase, and glycoproteinase are enzymes capable of degrading the matrix components. Some of these enzymes are synthesized by the scleral fibroblasts themselves, whereas others are secreted by inflammatory cells such as neutrophils and macrophages.

Collagenase degrades cross-linked type I and type II collagen fibrils by attacking the collagen molecule at one specific locus one-quarter of the distance from the COOH terminal. Two fragments, TC_A and TC_B, three-quarters and one-quarter of the collagen molecule, respectively, are generated. These fragments denature spontaneously at temperatures greater than 33°C, are phagocytosed, and become susceptible of further attack in the lysosomes by proteinases such as cathepsins B and N. Collagen degradation in normal and inflamed tissues depends on the balance between the collagenase and its inhibitors.[100] The protein core of the proteoglycans must be broken by proteoglycanases for the collagenase to come into contact with the underlying collagen.[70]

Elastase is a powerful proteinase that, unlike collagenase, lacks specificity. It degrades not only elastin but also other components of the extracellular matrix, such as collagen and proteoglycans. The neutrophil and macrophage elastases may be important in degrading elastin in inflammatory reactions.[101]

The core protein and link proteins of proteoglycans are degraded by proteoglycanases. The fragments are further degraded in the pericellular area by other proteinases such as cathepsin B. Glycosaminoglycan peptides are phagocytosed and further degraded in the lysosomes by proteinases such as cathepsin D. Subsequent attacks by different exoenzymes

result in monosaccharide residues and free sulfate.[102] Fibronectin can be degraded by a wide variety of glycoproteinases, including trypsin, chymotrypsin, pepsin, elastases, and cathepsin G and D.[103]

1.7.6. Fibroblast Growth Regulation

Human fibroblasts require growth factors for DNA synthesis. Fibroblast growth factors can be classified either as "competence" factors or "progression" factors.[104] The competence factors, including platelet-derived growth factor (PDGF) and fibroblast growth factor, render cells in G_0 or G_1 phase ready for DNA synthesis stimulation.[104,105] The progression factors, including somatomedins A and C and insulin growth factor, stimulate DNA synthesis in competent cells.[104–106] Other known fibroblast growth factors, including interleukin 1 (IL-1) and T cell-derived fibroblast growth factor, cannot be considered as either competence or progression factors and remain unclassified.[107–110] Specific receptors on fibroblasts for PDGF and IL-1 have been identified.[104,105,107,108] Recombinant interferon γ may stimulate or suppress fibroblast growth, depending on culture conditions.[111,112]

Summary

Almost all of the sclera is of neural crest origin, except a small temporal portion formed from mesoderm. The developmental process of the sclera is directed from anterior to posterior and from inside to outside. Scleral differentiation has already started in the region destined to become the limbus by the sixth week, and progresses backward to the equator by the eight week, and to the posterior pole by the twelfth week. There are no more differences between the inner and outer portions of the sclera by the beginning of week 10.9, and between the anterior and posterior portions of the sclera by week 13. The fetal sclera has the same ultrastructural characteristics as the adult sclera by week 24.

Human fetal and adult sclera is formed by collagen types I, III, IV, V, VI, and VIII, by the glycosaminoglycans dermatan sulfate, chondroitin sulfate, hyaluronic acid, and heparan sulfate, and by the glycoproteins fibronectin, vitronectin, and laminin. Collagen types I and VI increase steadily from fetus to adult, collagen type III shows little change through the gestational periods, and collagen type IV decreases steadily through 16, 19, and 22 weeks, revealing only subtle positivity in adult sclera except for its dramatic presence in the vessels; the staining pattern of collagen type V is diffuse in fetal sclera but is granular along the edges of the collagen bundles in adult sclera; collagen type VIII staining is intense in posterior fetal and adult sclera and anterior adult sclera but is negative in anterior fetal sclera. Dermatan sulfate and chondroitin sulfate are present in moderate and large amounts, respectively, through the different gestational periods; in contrast, hyaluronic acid changes from a moderate staining at 13 weeks to a subtle positivity in adult sclera; heparan sulfate is present in human fetal and adult sclera in small amounts. Fibronectin, vitronectin, and laminin are present at 13 weeks but steadily disappear onward, except for their presence in the vessels. Fibronectin and laminin may play a major role in directing developmental events.

The postnatal sclera is relatively distensible, thin, and somewhat translucent, allowing the blue color of the underlying uvea to show through. The sclera thickens gradually, becoming opaque and more rigid. In elderly individuals, the sclera shows a decrease in scleral distensibility, water content, and amount of proteoglycans, and an increase in amount of lipids and calcium phosphate.

Gross anatomical studies show that the scleral shell is an incomplete sphere, averaging 22 mm in diameter, that terminates anteriorly at the anterior scleral foramen surrounding the cornea, and posteriorly at the posterior scleral foramen surrounding the optic nerve canal. Its thickness varies from 0.3 mm immediately behind the insertion of the rectus muscles to 1.0 mm near the optic nerve. The sclera may be divided into three layers: the episclera, the scleral stroma, and the lamina fusca. It is a relatively avascular structure but is supplied by the episcleral and, to a lesser degree, choroidal vascular networks. The episcleral blood supply is derived mainly from the anterior ciliary arteries anterior to the insertions of the rectus muscles and from the long and short posterior ciliary arteries posterior to these insertions. The sclera receives a profuse sensory innervation; the short posterior ciliary nerves supply the posterior region of the sclera whereas the two long posterior ciliary nerves supply the anterior portion.

Microscopic and ultramicroscopic anatomical studies show that the sclera is composed of dense bundles of collagen, few elastic fibers, few fibroblasts, and a moderate amount of amorphous ground substance (proteoglycans and glycoproteins). Episcleral vessels, as capillaries and postcapillary venules, are continuous and have simple walls consisting of endothelial cells attached to an underlying basement membrane secreted by them, and a discontinuous layer of pericytes.

The cells, the fibroblasts, and the degradative enzymes they secrete (collagenases, elastases, proteoglycanases, and glycoproteinases) play a critical role in the synthesis and organization of the matrix elements.

References

1. Noden DM: Periocular mesenchyme: neural crest and mesodermal interactions. In Tasman W, Jaeger EA (Eds): *Duanes Foundations of Clinical Opthamology*, Lippincott, Philadelphia, 1991, pp 1–23.
2. Snell RS, Lemp MA: *Clinical Anatomy of the Eye*, 1st ed. Blackwell Scientific Publications, Boston, 1989.
3. Ozanics V, Jakobiec FA: Prenatal development of the eye and its anexa. In Tasman W, Jaeger EA (Eds): *Duane's Foundations of Clinical Opthamology*, Lippincott, Philadelphia, 1982, pp 1–93.
4. Johnston MC, Noden DM, Hazelton RD, Conlombre JL, Conlombre AJ: Origins of avian ocular and periocular tissues. Exp Eye Res 29:27, 1979.
5. Ozanics F, Rayborn M, Sagun D: Some aspects of corneal and scleral differentiation of the primate. Exp Eye Res 22:305, 1976.

6. Newsome DA: Cartilage induction by retinal pigmented epithelium of the chick embryo. Dev Biol 27:575, 1972.
7. Stewart PA, McCallion DJ: Establishment of the scleral cartilage in the chick. Dev Biol 46:383, 1975.
8. Duke-Elder S, Cook CH: Normal and abnormal development. In Duke-Elder S (Ed): *System of Ophthalmology*, Vol 3, Part 1. C.V. Mosby, St. Louis, 1963, pp 1–77.
9. Weale RA: *A Biography of the Eye*. Lewis, London, 1982.
10. Sellheyer K, Spitznas M: Development of the human sclera. A morphological study. Graefe's Arch Clin Exp Ophthalmol 226:89, 1988.
11. Tamura Y, Konomi H, Sawada H, *et al.*: Tissue distribution of type VIII collagen in human adult and fetal eyes. Invest Ophthalmol Vis Sci 32:2636, 1991.
12. Sugrue SP: Immunolocalization of type XII collagen at the corneoscleral angle of the embryonic avian eye. Invest Ophthalmol Vis Sci 32:1876, 1991.
13. Spencer WH: Sclera. In Spencer WH (Ed): *Ophthalmic Pathology*, 3rd ed. W.B. Saunders, Philadelphia, 1985, pp 389–422.
14. Broekhuyse RM, Kuhlmann ED: Lipids in tissues of the eye. VI. Sphingomyelins and cholesterol esters in human sclera. Exp Eye Res 14:111, 1972.
15. Broekhyse RM: The lipid composition of aging sclera and cornea. Ophthalmologica 171:82, 1975.
16. Cogan DG, Kuwabara T: Focal senile translucency of the sclera. Arch Ophthalmol 62:604, 1959.
17. Vannas S, Teir H: Observations on structure and age changes in the human sclera. Acta Ophthalmol 38:268, 1960.
18. Moses RA, Grodzki WJ Jr: The scleral spur and scleral roll. Invest Ophthalmol Vis Sci 16:925, 1977.
19. Anderson DR: Ultrastructure of human and monkey lamina cribrosa and optic nerve head. Arch Ophthalmol 82:800, 1969.
20. Leber T: Die cirkulations-und Ernährungsverhältnisse des Auges. In Saemisch T (Ed): *Graefe-Saemisch Handbuch der Gesamten Augenheilkunde*, 2nd ed. Wilhelm Engelmann, Leipzig, 1903, pp 1–101.
21. Kiss F: Der Blutkreislauf der Auges. Ophthalmologica 106:225, 1943.
22. Ashton N: Anatomical study of Schlemm's canal and aqueous veins by means of neoprene casts. Br J Ophthalmol 35:291, 1951.
23. Ashton N: Anatomical study of Schlemm's canal and aqueous veins by means of neoprene casts. II. Aqueous veins. Br J Ophthalmol 36:265, 1952.
24. Ashton N, Smith R: Anatomical study of Schlemm's canal and aqueous veins by means of neoprene casts. III. Arterial relations of Schlemm's canal. Br J Ophthalmol 37:577, 1953.
25. Van Buskirk EM: The canine eye: the vessels of aqueous drainage. Invest Ophthalmol Vis Sci 18:223, 1979.
26. Morrison JC, Van Buskirk EM: Anterior collateral circulation in the primate eye. Ophthalmology 90:707, 1983.
27. Fryczkowski AW, Sherman MD, Walker J: Observations on the lobular organization of the human choriocapillaris. Intern Ophthalmol 15:109, 1991.
28. Hayreh SS, Scott WE: Fluorescein iris angiography. II. Disturbances in iris circulation following strabismus operation on the various recti. Arch Ophthalmol 96:1390, 1978.
29. Virdi PS, Hayreh SS: Anterior segment ischemia after recession of various recti: an experimental study. Ophthalmology 94:1258, 1987.
30. Bron AJ, Easty DL: Fluorescein angiography of the globe and anterior segment. Trans Ophthalmol Soc UK 90:339, 1970.
31. Ikegami M: Fluorescein angiography of the anterior ocular segment. I. Hemodynamics in the anterior ciliary arteries. Acta Soc Ophthalmol Jpn 78:39, 1974.
32. Talusan ED, Swartz B: Fluorescein angiography: demonstration of flow pattern of anterior ciliary arteries. Arch Ophthalmol 99:1074, 1981.
33. Meyer PA, Watson PG: Low dose fluorescein angiography of the conjunctiva and episclera. Br J Ophthalmol 71:2, 1987.
34. Meyer PA: Patterns of blood flow in episcleral vessels studied by low-dose fluorescein videoangiography. Eye 2:533, 1988.
35. Ormerod LD, Fariza E, Hughes GW, Doane MG, Webb RH: Anterior segment fluorein videoangiography with a scanning angiographic microscope. Ophthalmology 97:745, 1990.
36. Norn MS: Topography of scleral emissaries and sclera-perforating blood vessels. Acta Ophthalmol (Copenhagen) 63:320, 1985.
37. Torczynski E: Sclera. In Jakobiec FA (Ed): *Ocular Anatomy, Embryology, and Teratology*. Harper & Row, Philadelphia, 1982, pp 587–599.

38. Brancato R, Frosini R, Boshi M: L'Angiografia superficiale a fluorescein del bulbo oculare. Ann Ottal Clin Ocul 95:433, 1969.

39. Laatikainen L: Perilimbal vasculature in glaucomatous eyes. Acta Ophthalmol 111(suppl): 54, 1971.

40. Raitta C, Vannas S: Fluorescein angiographic features of the limbus and perilimbal vessels. Ear Nose Throat J 50:58, 1971.

41. Shimizu K, Ujie K: [Structure of Ocular Vessels.] Igaku-Shoin, Tokyo, 1978.

42. Watson PG, Bovey E: Anterior segment fluorescein angiography in the diagnosis of scleral inflammation. Ophthalmology 92:1, 1985.

43. Meyer PA: The circulation of the human limbus. Eye 3:121, 1989.

44. Amalric P, Rebière P, Jourdes JC: Nouvelles indications de l'angiographie fluoresceinique du segment anterieur de l'oeil. Ann Ocul 204:455, 1971.

45. Crandall AS, Yanoff M, Schaffer DB: Intrascleral nerve loop mistakenly identified as a foreign body. Arch Ophthalmol 95:497, 1977.

46. Fine BS, Yanoff M: 76 cornea and sclera. In Hagerstown MD (Ed): Ocular Histology, 2nd ed. Harper & Row, Philadelphia, 1979, pp 161–193.

47. Hogan MJ, Alvarado JA, Weddell JE: Histology of the Human Eye. W.B. Saunders, Philadelphia, 1971.

48. Jakus MA: Ocular Fine Structure: Selected Electron Micrographs. Little, Brown, Boston, 1964.

49. Komai Y, Ushiki T: The three-dimensional organization of collagen fibrils in the human cornea and sclera. Invest Ophthalmol Vis Sci 32:2244, 1991.

50. Curtin BJ, Iwamoto T, Renaldo DP: Normal and staphylomatous sclera of high myopia. Arch Ophthalmol 97:912, 1979.

51. Kanai A, Kaufman HE: Electron microscopic studies of the elastic fiber in human sclera. Invest Ophthalmol Vis Sci 11:816, 1972.

52. Young RD: The ultrastructural organization of proteoglycans and collagen in human and rabbit scleral matrix. J Cell Sci 74:95, 1985.

53. Raviola G: Conjunctival and episcleral blood vessels are permeable to blood-borne horseradish peroxidase. Invest Ophthalmol Vis Sci 24:725, 1983.

54. Cole DF, Monro PAG: The use of fluorescein-labelled dextrans in investigation of aqueous humor outflow in the rabbit. Exp Eye Res 23:571, 1976.

55. Dische J: Biochemistry of connective tissues of the vertebrate eye. Int Rev Connect Tissue Res 5:209, 1970.

56. Keeley FW, Morin JD, Vesely S: Characterization of collagen from normal human sclera. Exp Eye Res 39:533, 1984.

57. Lee RE, Davidson PF: Collagen composition and turnover in ocular tissues of the rabbit: Exp Eye Res 32:737, 1981.

58. Tengroth B, Rehnberg M, Amitzboll T: A comparative analysis of the collagen type and distribution in the trabecular meshwork, sclera, lamina cribrosa and the optic nerve in the human eye. Acta Ophthalmol (Copenhagen) 63(suppl 173):91, 1985.

59. Moses RA, Grodzki WJ, Starcherd BC, Galione MJ: Elastic content of the scleral spur, trabecular meshwork, and sclera. Invest Ophthalmol Vis Sci 17:817, 1978.

60. Borcherding MS, Blacik LJ, Sittig RA, Bizzell JW, Breen M, Weinstein HG: Proteoglycans and collagen fiber organization in human corneoscleral tissue. Exp Eye Res 21:59, 1975.

61. Trier K, Olsen EB, Ammitzbøll T: Regional glycosaminoglycan composition of the human sclera. Acta Ophthalmol (Copenhagen) 68:304, 1990.

62. St Helen R, McEwen WK: Rheology of the human sclera. I. Anelastic behavior. Am J Ophthalmol 52:539, 1961.

63. Richards RD, Tittel PG: Corneal and scleral distensibility ratio on enucleated human eyes. Invest Ophthalmol Vis Sci 12:145, 1973.

64. Curtin BJ: Physiopathologic aspects of scleral stress-strain. Trans Am Ophthalmol Soc 67:417, 1969.

65. Friberg TR, Lace JW: A comparison of the elastic properties of human choroid and sclera. Exp Eye Res 47:429, 1988.

66. Bettelhein FA, Ehrlich SH: Water vapor sorption of mucopolysaccharides. J Physiol Chem 67:1948, 1963.

67. Loewi G, Meyer K: The acid mucopolysaccharides of embryonic skin. Biochim Biophys Acta 27:456, 1958.

68. Gregory JD, Damle SP, Covington HI, Citron C: Developmental changes in proteoglycans of rabbit corneal stroma. Invest Ophthalmol Vis Sci 29:1413, 1988.

69. Caparas VL, Cintrom C, Hernandez-Neufeld MR: Immunohistochemistry of proteoglycans in human lamina cribrosa. Am J Ophthalmol 112:489, 1991.

70. Watson PG, Hazelman BL: *The Sclera and Systemic Disorders*. W.B. Saunders, London, 1976.

71. Edelhauser HF, Van Horn DL, Records RE: Cornea and sclera. In Duane TD, Jaeger EA (Eds): *Biomedical Foundations of Ophthalmology*, Vol 2. Harper & Row, Philadelphia, 1982, Ch 4, pp 1–26.

72. Kivirikko KI, Myllyla R: Biosynthesis of collagens. In Piez KA, Reddi AH (Eds): *Extracellular Matrix Biochemistry*. Elsevier, New York, 1984, Ch 3, pp 83–112.

73. Postlethwaite AE, Kang AH: Fibroblasts. In Gallin JI, Goldstein IM, Snyderman R (Eds): *Inflammation: Basic Principles and Clinical Correlates*. Raven, New York, 1988, pp 747–774.

74. Chu ML, De Wet W, Bernard M, Ding JF, Morabito M, Myers J, Williams C, Ramirez F: Human pro-α_1(I) collagen gene structure reveals evolutionary conservation of a pattern of introns and exons. Nature (London) 310:337, 1984.

75. Chu ML, De Wet W, Bernard M, Ramirez F: Isolation of cDNA and genomic clones encoding human pro-α_1(III) collagen. J Biol Chem 260:2315, 1985.

76. Chu ML, Weil D, De Wet W, Bernard M, Sippola M, Ramirez F: Isolation of cDNA and genomic clones encoding human pro-α_1(III) collagen. Partial characterization of the 3' end region of the gene. J Biol Chem 260:4357, 1985.

77. Seyer JM, Kang AH: Structural proteins: collagen, elastin and fibronectin. In Kelley WN, Harris E Jr, Ruddy S, Sledge CB (Eds): *Textbook of Rheumatology*. W.B. Saunders, Philadelphia, 1985, pp 211–230.

78. Tresltad RL, Birk DE, Silver FH: Collagen fibrillogenesis in tissues, in solution, and from modeling: a synthesis. J Invest Dermatol 79:109, 1982.

79. Brandt KD: Glycosaminoglycans. In Kelley WN, Harris E Jr, Ruddy S, Sledge CB (Eds): *Textbook of Rheumatology*. W.B. Saunders, Philadelphia, 1985, pp 237–250.

80. Heinegard D, Paulson M: Structure and metabolism of proteoglycans. In Piez KA, Reddi AH (Eds): *Extracellular Matrix Biochemistry*. Elsevier, New York, 1984, pp 277–322.

81. Mathews MB, Deckers L: The effect of acid mucopolysaccharide proteins on fibril formation from collagen solutions. Biochem J 109:517, 1969.

82. Toole BP, Lowther D: Dermatan sulphate protein: isolation from and interaction with collagen. Arch Biochem 128:567, 1968.

83. Trelstad RL, Hayashi K, Toole BP: Epithelial collagens and glycosaminoglycans in the embryonic cornea: macromolecular order and morphogenesis in the basement membrane. J Cell Biol 62:815, 1974.

84. Gelman RA, Blackwell J: Collagen–mucopolysaccharide interactions at acid pH. Biochim Biophys Acta 342:254, 1974.

85. Ruoslahti E, Yamaguchi Y: Proteoglycans as modulators of growth factor activities. Cell 64:867, 1991.

86. Ruoslahti E: Proteoglycans in cell regulation. J Biol Chem 264:13369, 1989.

87. Hynes R: Molecular biology of fibronectin. Annu Rev Cell Biol 1:67, 1985.

88. Kleinman HK, Klebe RJ, Martin GR: Role of collagenous matrices in adhesion and growth of cells. J Cell Biol 88:473, 1981.

89. Yamada KM, Kennedy DW, Kimata K, Pratt PM: Characteristics of fibronectin interactions with glycosaminoglycans and identification of active proteolytic fragments. J Biol Chem 255:6055, 1980.

90. McDonald JA, Kelley DG, Broekelmann TJ: Role of fibronectin in collagen deposition: Fab' to the gelatin-binding domain of fibronectin inhibits both fibronectin and collagen organization in fibroblast extracellular matrix. J Cell Biol 92:485, 1982.

91. Kuusela P: Fibronectin binds to *Staphylococcus aureus*. Nature (London) 276:719, 1978.

92. Menzel EJ, Smolen JS, Liotta L, Reid KBM: Interaction of fibronectin with C1q and its collagen-like fragment. FEBS Lett 129:188, 1981.

93. Zardi L, Siri A, Carnemolla B, Santi L, Bardner WD, Hoch SO: Fibronectin: a chromatin-associated protein? Cell 18:649, 1979.

94. Kornblihtt AR, Vibe-Pedersen K, Baralle FE: Isolation and characterization of cDNA clones for human and bovine fibronectins. Proc Natl Acad Sci USA 80:3218, 1983.

95. Tamkun JW, Schwarzbauer JE, Hynes RO: A single rat fibronectin gene generates three different mRNAs by alternative splicing of a complex exon. Proc Natl Acad Sci USA 81:5140, 1984.

96. Vibe-Pedersen K, Kornblihtt AR, Petersen TE: Expression of a human α-globulin/fibronectin gene hybrid generates two mRNA by alternative splicing. EMBO J 3:2511, 1984.

97. Mecham RP: Receptor for laminin on mammalian cells. FASEB J 5:2538, 1991.
98. Albelda SM, Buck CA: Integrins and other cell adhesion molecules. FASEB J 4:2868, 1990.
99. Kleinman HK, Cannon FB, Laurie GW: Biological activities of laminin. J Cell Biochem 27:317, 1987.
100. Wooley DE: Mammalian collagenases. In Piez KA, Reddi AH (Eds): *Extracellular Matrix Biochemistry*. Elsevier, New York, 1984, pp 119–151.
101. Gosline JM, Rosenbloom J: Elastin. In Piez KA, Reddi AH (Eds): *Extracellular Matrix Biochemistry*. Elsevier, New York, 1984, pp 191–226.
102. Sandy JD, Brown HLG, Lowther DA: Degradation of proteoglycan in articular cartilage. Biochim Biophys Acta 543:536, 1978.
103. Hakomori S, Fukuda M, Sekiguchi K, Carter WB: Fibronectin, laminin, and other extracellular glycoproteins. In Piez KA, Reddi AH (Eds): *Extracellular Matrix Biochemistry*. Elsevier, New York, 1984, pp 229–264.
104. Scher CD, Shepard RC, Antoniades HN, Stiles CD: Platelet-derived growth factor and the regulation of the mammalian fibroblast cell cycle. Biochim Biophys Acta 560:212, 1979.
105. Stiles CD, Capone GT, Scher CD, Antoniades HN, Van Wyk JJ, Pledger WJ: Dual control of cell growth by somatomedins and platelet-derived growth factor. Proc Natl Acad Sci USA 76:L279, 1979.

106. Moses AC, Nissley SP, Rechler MM, Short A, Podskalny JM: The purification and characterization of multiplication stimulating activity (MSA) from media conditioned by a rat liver cell line. In Geordano G, Van Wyk JJ, Minuto F (Eds): *Somatomedins and Growth*. Academic Press, New York, 1979, pp 45–59.
107. Postlethwaite AE, Lachman LB, Kang AH: Induction of fibroblast proliferation by interleukin-1 derived from human monocytic leukemia cells. Arthritis Rheum 27:995, 1984.
108. Schmidt JA, Mizel SB, Cohen D, Green I: Interleukin 1, a potential regulator of fibroblast proliferation. J Immunol 128:2177, 1982.
109. Postlethwaite AE, Kang AH: Induction of fibroblast proliferation by human mononuclear derived proteins. Arthritis Rheum 26:22, 1983.
110. Wahl SM, Wahl LM, McCarthy JB: Lymphocyte-mediated activation of fibroblast proliferation and collagen production. J Immunol 121:942, 1978.
111. Brinkerhoff CE, Guyre PM: Increased proliferation of human synovial fibroblasts treated with recombinant immune interferon. J Immunol 134:3142, 1985.
112. Duncan MR, Berman D: Gamma interferon is the lymphokine and beta interferon the monokine responsible for inhibition of fibroblast collagen production and late but not early fibroblast proliferation. J Exp Med 162:516, 1985.

2
Immunological Considerations of the Sclera

Scleritis remains an enigmatic disease. Attempts to demonstrate a specific antigen associated with scleral vessel and tissue damage, or to reproduce suggested underlying pathogenic mechanisms in experimental animal models, have not yielded consistent abnormalities. The prevailing consensual view, however, based on the available evidence, is that disordered immune responses leading to vessel and tissue damage are central to the pathogenesis of scleritis. The histopathological and immunofluorescence detection of immune complex inflammatory microangiopathy in affected scleral biopsy specimens,[1] the frequent association of scleritis with systemic autoimmune diseases associated with circulating immune complexes (rheumatoid arthritis, systemic lupus erythematosus, or polyarteritis nodosa),[1-3] the favorable response of scleritis to immunosuppressive agents,[2,3] and the absence of vascular perfusion in severe types of scleritis, as determined by anterior segment fluorescein angiography,[4] all suggest that scleritis represents an autoimmune process mediated by a localized immune complex inflammatory microangiopathy or type III hypersensitivity reaction. The histopathological finding of a chronic granulomatous inflammation characterized predominantly by macrophages and T lymphocytes in scleritis biopsy specimens suggests that a cellular immunity dysfunction or type IV hypersensitivity reaction also may play a role.[1]

The prevailing hypothesis, based on the aforementioned data and on autoimmunity investigations, is that development of scleritis entails the interaction of genetically controlled mechanisms with environmental factors, such as infectious agents (e.g., virus) or trauma. Genetic predisposition coupled with the triggering event gives rise to an immune process that damages the vessels through immune complex deposition in vessel "walls" and subsequent complement activation (type III hypersensitivity). Persistent immunological injury leads to granuloma formation (type IV hypersensitivity). In certain systemic vasculitic diseases, circulating immune complexes may deposit in episcleral and scleral perforating vessels, particularly if they have suffered a previous insult (mild infection, trauma), as well as in other vessels or tissues of the body.

This chapter reviews the immunological considerations of the sclera, emphasizing the issues of relevance regarding the pathogenic mechanisms of scleritis.

2.1. General Immune Response Considerations

To appreciate the pathophysiology of scleritis, it is necessary to understand how components of the immune response act and are controlled. An immune response is the result of a complex network of cellular interactions against a foreign agent or antigen that involves innate and adaptive components of the immune system.[5]

The innate immune system consists mainly of cells such as neutrophils, macrophages, and natural killer cells, and of soluble factors such as complement and lysozyme. The innate immune system acts as a first line of defense against foreign invaders. This natural or innate or primitive immune response is not specific for a given antigen (does not need specific recognition), does not require central processing, and does not improve with repeated encounter (does not have cellular memory).

The adaptive immune system, consisting of cells such as T and B lymphocytes, and of soluble factors such as antibodies and cytokines, acts if the first defenses against antigen have not been sufficient to eliminate the foreign substance rapidly. The adaptive immune response is characterized by the relatively unique characteristics of specific recognition, central processing, cellular memory, and discrimination between self and nonself. Through evolution, humans have developed the ability to recognize myriads of foreign antigens through antigen-specific cells.

The adaptive immune response has three components: (1) the afferent arc, in which immunocompetent cells are exposed to an antigen, recognize the specific antigen, and become sensitized to that antigen, (2) central processing, in which immunocompetent cells participate in the differentiation and development of specific antibodies and mature effector cells, and (3) the efferent arc, in which an immune response is mounted against the specific antigens by the specific antibodies and the mature effector cells.

Innate and adaptive immune systems may interact at many levels. Antibodies (IgG and IgM), produced by B lymphocytes, activate complement. Antibodies and complement help neutrophils and macrophages to eliminate antigen. Macrophages transport the antigen to lymph nodes and present it to lymphocytes in a form they can recognize; they also synthesize and secrete a variety of powerful biological molecules, including collagenase, lysozyme, interferon (α and β), interleukin 6, tumor necrosis factor, fibronectin, several growth and stimulating factors, arachidonic acid derivatives, and oxygen metabolites. Lymphocytes produce lymphokines, which stimulate neutrophils and macrophages to attack the antigen

more effectively. The immune system also interacts with other systems such as the clotting, fibrinolytic, and kinin systems, in the protection of the body from an antigen.[1] It is the combined responses of both natural and acquired immune systems that provide protection against harmful agents. These responses may be appropriate, in which case the individual is protected, or may be inappropriate, that is, either insufficient or excessive (hypersensitivity and autoimmune reactions), in which case the individual is harmed.

2.1.1. Components of the Immune Response

The use of monoclonal antibodies that recognize selected cell surface glycoproteins has made it possible to characterize the cells involved in the immune response. The list of current (as of the Fourth International Workshop on Human Leukocyte Differentiation Antigens) clusters of differentiation (CD) and the cell types expressing these CD antigens is shown in Table 2.1. All these cells arise from pluripotential stem cells through two main lines of differentiation: (1) the lymphoid line, producing lymphocytes, and (2) the myeloid line, producing monocytes/macrophages and polymorphonuclear granulocytes (neutrophils, eosinophils, and basophils/mast cells); this myeloid line also gives rise to megakaryocytes, which eventually produce platelets.[6]

2.1.1.1. Lymphocytes

Lymphocytes are mononuclear cells produced in primary lymphoid organs (thymus and adult bone marrow) that migrate secondarily into the secondary lymphoid tissues (lymph node, spleen, gut-associated lymphoid tissue, mammary-associated lymphoid tissue, and conjunctival-associated lymphoid tissue) and in blood. They compose approximately 30% of the total peripheral white blood cell count. Lymphocytes may be classified as T lymphocytes, B lymphocytes, and non-T non-B (third population) lymphocytes.

TABLE 2.1. Components of the immune response detected by monoclonal antibodies.

Antigen designation[a]	Cell specificity	Function
CD1	Thymocytes, Langerhans' cells	
CD14	Macrophages	
CD13	Monocytes and granulocytes	
CD33	Monocytes and myeloid stem cells	
CD11b	Monocytes, granulocytes, some TPCs[b]	α chain of complement receptor CR3
CD16	Granulocytes, TPCs, and macrophages	Fc receptor IgG (Fc$_\gamma$RIII)
CD2	T lymphocytes, some TPCs	Sheep erythrocyte receptor
CD5	T lymphocytes, B lymphocyte subset	
CD3	T lymphocytes	Part of T cell antigen receptor
CD7	T lymphocytes, NK[b] cells	Fc receptor IgM (?)
CD4	T helper-inducer lymphocytes	MHC[b] class II immune recognition
CD8	T cytotoxic-suppressor lymphocytes, some TPCs	MHC class I immune recognition
CD28	T cytotoxic-suppressor lymphocyte subset	
CD10	Pre-B lymphocytes	
CD19	B lymphocytes	
CD20	B lymphocytes	
CD21	B lymphocytes	Complement receptor CR2
CD22	B lymphocytes	
CD25	Activated T lymphocytes, B lymphocytes, and macrophages	IL-2[b] receptor
CD35	B lymphocytes, erythrocytes, granulocytes, T lymphocytes, plasma cells, macrophages	Complement receptor CR1
CDw32	B lymphocytes, granulocytes, macrophages, platelets	Fc receptor IgG (Fc$_\gamma$RII)
CD45	All leukocytes	Leukocyte common antigen
CD11a	All leukocytes	α chain of LFA-1 (adhesion molecule)
CD41	Megakaryocytes, platelets	Gp11b/111a
CD42	Megakaryocytes, platelets	Gp1b

[a] CD, Cluster designation (based on Fourth International Workshop on Human Leukocyte Differentiation Antigens).
[b] TPC, Third population cells (natural killer and killer cells); NK, natural killer cell; MHC, major histocompatibility complex; IL-2, interleukin 2.

2.1.1.1.1. T Lymphocytes

T lymphocytes, or thymus-derived cells, possess surface histocompatibility products (HLA-DR) and cell surface receptors for antigen (TCR-CD3), for sheep erythrocytes (CD2), and for the plant-derived mitogens (concanavalin A and phytohemagglutinin); they also possess CD5 and CD7 surface molecules. The T lymphocyte has an important role in recognition of foreign material, in specific effector responses, in helping B lymphocytes to synthesize antibody, in immunoregulatory functions, and in immunological memory. They also may participate in abnormal reactions such as the type IV hypersensitivity or cell-mediated diseases. T lymphocytes can be further subdivided

into subsets: T helper lymphocytes (CD4) and T cytotoxic/suppressor lymphocytes (CD8).[7] T helper lymphocytes (CD4) participate in the recognition of foreign material, proliferation, and generation of antibodies and other specialized T lymphocytes. On the other hand, CD8 T cytotoxic lymphocytes (CD8) are involved in cell killing, and T suppressor lymphocytes (CD8) are responsible for modulating immune responses, preventing uncontrolled, host-damaging inflammatory responses.

CD4 lymphocytes may be subdivided into subsubsets. For example, there are two separate populations of CD4 lymphocytes (T helper 1 and T helper 2), based on the production of different lymphokines. T helper 1 lymphocytes secrete interleukin 2 (IL-2) and interferon γ, but do not secrete IL-4 or IL-5; they can be cytolytic and can provide B lymphocyte help for IgG, IgM, and IgA synthesis, but not for IgE synthesis. T helper 2 lymphocytes secrete IL-4 and IL-5, but not IL-2 or interferon γ; they are not cytolytic and can provide B lymphocyte help for IgE, IgG, IgM, and IgA synthesis. Studies suggest that T helper 1 lymphocytes participate in inflammatory reactions associated with delayed-type hypersensitivity reactions and low antibody production (e.g., contact dermatitis and *Mycobacterium tuberculosis* infection), whereas T helper 2 lymphocytes participate in inflammatory reactions associated with persistent antibody production (e.g., allergic diseases, including vernal conjuntivitis).[8]

CD8 lymphocytes also may be subdivided into subsubsets. For example, evidence exists that there are at least three subpopulations of T suppressor lymphocytes.

2.1.1.1.2. B Lymphocytes

B lymphocytes, or bone marrow-derived cells,[9,10] possess on their surfaces immunoglobulin, class II histocompatibility glycoproteins (HLA-DR), and receptors for the Fc portion of antibody (CDw32) and for complement components, including CR1 (CD35) and CR2 (CD21). They also possess surface receptors for Epstein–Barr virus, for the plant mitogen known as pokeweed mitogen, for the purified protein derivative of *M. tuberculosis*, and for lipopolysaccharide. B lymphocytes, assisted by T helper lymphocytes, respond to specific antigenic stimulation by blastogenic transformation, antibody synthesis, and eventual evolution to end-stage plasma cells and memory cells. B lymphocytes are further subdivided into five separate classes synthesizing five different immunoglobulins: IgG, IgA, IgM, IgD, and IgE. In addition to the subsets depending on antibody class synthesis, B lymphocytes also differentiate into other subsets. There is a subpopulation of B lymphocytes characterized by the presence of the surface membrane glycoprotein CD5 (a surface glycoprotein ordinarily present on T lymphocytes)[11]; this subpopulation appears to be associated with autoantibody

production.[6,12] There is another subpopulation of B lymphocytes with suppressor activity.

Antibodies bind to antigens to form antigen–antibody complexes. These immune complexes, if not cleared by normal mechanisms, may result in vessel and surrounding tissue damage through activation of complement components and subsequent neutrophil and macrophage granule release.

2.1.1.1.3. Third Population Lymphocytes or Null Lymphocytes

Third population cells (TPCs), including natural killer cells and killer cells, are lymphoid cells that do not carry the conventional cell surface glycoproteins characteristic of T or B lymphocytes, that is, TCR or immunoglobulin. Most TPC surface antigens detectable by monoclonal antibodies are shared with T lymphocytes and cells of the myelomonocytic series (Table 2.1). Natural killer cells are small, nonadherent, and have granulocytes containing perforin, an enzyme responsible for cytolysis. Natural killer (NK) cells compose an important component of the early, natural response part of the immune system; without prior antigenic contact, natural killer cells spontaneously kill transformed (malignant) cells and virus-infected cells without major histocompatibility complex restriction. Killer (K) cells do have surface receptors for the Fc portion of immunoglobulin. They participate in type II Gell and Coombs hypersensitivity reactions through the so-called antibody-dependent cell-mediated cytotoxicity (ADCC) reaction. They also are involved in removal of cellular antigens when the target cell is too large to be phagocytized.

2.1.1.2. Monocytes/Macrophages

Bone marrow-derived stem cells give rise to promonocytes, which subsequently differentiate into blood monocytes. Blood monocytes migrate into tissues to become macrophages. Aside from class II MHC glycoprotein on their cell surfaces (HLA-DR), monocytes/macrophages possess receptors for complement components, including CR1 (CD35) and CR3 (CD11b), as well as for the Fc por-

TABLE 2.2. Secretory products of macrophages.[a]

Enzymes	Coagulation factors
Lysozyme	Factors X, IX, VII, V
Neutral proteases (collagenase and elastase)	Protein kinase
	Thromboplastin
Acid proteases (cathepsins)	Prothrombin
Acid lipases	Fibrinolysis inhibitor
Acid nucleases	Components of complement cascade
Acid phosphatases	C1, C4, C2, C3, C5
Acid glycosidases	Factors B and D
Acid sulfatases	Properdin
Arginase	C3b inactivator
Plasminogen activator	β IH[b]
Lipoprotein lipase	Other proteins
Phospholipase A_2	Transcobalamin II
Cytolytic proteinase	Transferrin
Angiotensin convertase	Fibronectin
Inhibitors of enzymes	Interferons α and β
α_2-Macroglobulin	Tumor necrosis factor α
α_1-Antiprotease	Interleukins 1 and 6
Lipocortin	Macrophage colony-stimulating factor
α_1-Antichymotrypsin	Granulocyte macrophage colony-stimulating factor
Reactive oxygen intermediates	
O_2, H_2O_2, OH, hypohalous acids	Haptoglobin
Lipids	Platelet-derived growth factor
PGE_2[b]	Transforming growth factor β
$PGF_{2\alpha}$[b]	Erythropoietin
Prostacyclin	Thymosin B_4
Thromboxane A_2	Apolipoprotein E
Leukotrienes B, C, D, and E	Serum amyloid A
Mono-HETES[b]	Serum amyloid P
Di-HETES	Small molecules
Platelet-activating factor	Purines
	Pyrimidines

[a] Adapted from Refs. 13 to 15.
[b] PGE_2, prostaglandin E_2; $PGF_{2\alpha}$, prostaglandin $F_{2\alpha}$; HETES, hydroxyeicosatetraenoic acids.

tion of immunoglobulin G molecules (CD16), fibronectin, interferons (α, β, and γ), IL-1, tumor necrosis factor, and macrophage colony-stimulating factor. Monocytes/macrophages may be subdivided depending on two different functions, that is, phagocytosis and antigen presentation to lymphocytes.

2.1.1.2.1. Phagocytosis

The human blood monocyte possesses a horseshoe-shaped nucleus with faint azurophilic granules, ruffled membrane, a well-developed Golgi complex, and many intracytoplasmic lysosomes. Monocytes/macrophages are members of the natural immune system and they play a central role in host defense through phagocytosis. The phagocytic macrophages form a network, the reticuloendothelial system, found in many organs of the body. The reticuloendothelial system includes Kupffer cells in the liver, intraglomerular mesangial cells in the kidney, alveolar macrophages in the lung, microglial cells in the brain, spleen sinus cells, and lymph node sinus cells.

However, monocytes/macrophages can also participate in abnormal reactions: They can be attracted by complement components in type III hypersensitivity or immune complex-mediated diseases; furthermore, they can participate in granuloma formation as epithelioid cells (modified macrophages) or multinucleated giant cells (fusion of several epithelioid cells) in type IV hypersensitivity or cell-mediated diseases. Monocytes/macrophages secrete a variety of powerful biological molecules that are important (Table 2.2).[13–15] Among these molecules, the enzymes collagenase and elastase participate in connective tissue degradation.

2.1.1.2.2. Antigen-Presenting Cells

Macrophages are the preeminent antigen-presenting cells. They phagocytose the antigen, partially degrade it, and transport the fragments to the cell surface. The combination of these degraded fragments in close juxtaposition to class II MHC glycoproteins forms the recognition unit for the helper T cell receptors (TCRs) specific for the epitope of the antigen.[16–18] Antigen-presenting cells produce a variety of soluble factors during the presentation of the antigen to T helper lymphocytes, including IL-1, which promotes the differentiation of both T and B lymphocytes.

Langerhans' cells are also important antigen-presenting cells,[19] particularly for the eye. They are derived from bone marrow macrophage precursors and, like macrophages, they also possess a high density of class II MHC glycoproteins on their cell surfaces (HLA-DR), along with receptors for complement component (CR1/CD35) and the Fc portion of immunoglobulin G (CD16). Unlike macrophages, Langerhans' cells have a racket-shaped cytoplasmic granule (the Birbeck granule), are not phagocytic, and have the characteristic surface marker CD1.

Other cells that do not arise from the monocyte/macrophage lineage may also be important in processing and presenting antigen; B lymphocytes, constitutively rich in class II MHC glycoproteins, are functionally important as antigen-presenting cells, particularly when the B lymphocyte is specific for the antigen being presented.

Cells other than macrophages, Langerhans' cells, or B lymphocytes can acquire the ability to "present" antigens through the induction of class II MHC glycoproteins on their cell surface under the influence of cytokines (interferon γ and tumor necrosis factor); these cells include connective tissue fibroblasts, corneal endothelial cells, or vascular endothelial cells.[20,21] It has been suggested that such induction of expression of "inappropriate" class II MHC glycoproteins might contribute to the pathogenesis of a variety of autoimmune diseases.[22]

2.1.1.3. Polymorphonuclear Granulocytes

Polymorphonuclear granulocytes are leukocytes that form part of the natural immune system. They play a central role in host defense through phagocytosis, but if they accumulate in excessive numbers, persist, and are activated in an uncontrolled manner, the result may be deleterious to host tissues. As the name suggests, they contain a multilobed nucleus and many granules. Polymorphonuclear leukocytes are classified as neutrophils, basophils, or eosinophils, depending on the differential staining of their granules.

2.1.1.3.1. Neutrophils

Neutrophils represent over 90% of the circulating granulocytes. They possess surface receptors for the Fc portion of IgG (CD16) and for complement components, including C5a (important in chemotaxis), and CR1 (CD35) and CR3 (CD11b) (important in adhesion and phagocytosis). When appropriately stimulated by chemotactic agents (complement components, fibrinolytic and kinin system components, and products from other leukocytes, platelets, and certain bacteria), neutrophils move from blood to tissues through margination (adhesion through endothelial cells) and diapedesis (movement through the capillary wall). Neutrophils release the contents of their primary (azurophilic) granules (lysosomes) and secondary (specific) granules (Table 2.3) into an endocytic vacuole, resulting in phagocytosis of a microorganism or in tissue injury (type III hypersensitivity reactions or immune complex-mediated diseases).[23,24] Secondary granules release collagenase, which participates in connective tissue degradation. Aside from the products secreted by the granules, neutrophils also release lipids, such as arachidonic acid derivatives, as well as reactive oxygen derivates.[24]

TABLE 2.3. Secretory products of neutrophils.[a]

Azurophil granules	Specific granules	Other granules
Myeloperoxidase	Alkaline phosphatase	Acid phosphatase
Acid phosphatase	Histaminase	Heparitinase
5'-Nucleotidase	Collagenase	β-Glucosaminidase
Lysozyme	Lysozyme	α-Mannosidase
Elastase	Vitamine B_{12}-binding	Acid proteinase
Cathepsin G	proteins	Elastase (?)
Cathepsin B	Plasminogen activator	Gelatinase (?)
Cathepsin D	Lactoferrin	Laminin receptor
Proteinase 3	Receptors	Glycosaminoglycans
β-Glycerophosphatase	Laminin	
β-Glucuronidase	C3bi	
N-Acetyl-β-glucosaminidase	fMet-Leu-Phe	
α-Mannosidase	Cytochrome b	
Arylsulfatase	Flavoproteins	
α-Fucosidase		
Esterase		
Histonase		
Cationic proteins		
Defensins		
Bactericidal permeability increasing protein (BPI)		
Glycosaminoglycans		
Azurophil-derived bactericidal factors (ADBFs)		

[a] Adapted from Refs. 23 and 24.

2.1.1.3.2. Eosinophils

Eosinophils represent 3 to 5% of the circulating granulocytes. They possess surface receptors for the Fc portion of IgE (low affinity) and IgG (CD16) and for complement components. Eosinophils play a specialized role in allergic and parasitic conditions. Although less important, they also participate in type III hypersensitivity reactions or immune complex-mediated diseases following attraction to the inflammatory area by products from mast cells, basophils (eosinophil chemotactic factor of anaphylaxis; ECF-A), and complement. Eosinophils release the contents of their granules to the outside of the cell after fusion of the intracellular granules with the plasma membrane (degranulation). Table 2.4 shows the known secretory products of eosinophils.

2.1.1.3.3. Basophils/Mast Cells

Basophils represent less than 0.2% of the circulating granulocytes. They possess surface

TABLE 2.4. Secretory products of eosinophils.[a]

Peptides and enzymes
  Lysosomal hydrolases
    Arylsulfatase
    β-Glucuronidase
    Acid phosphatase
    Alkaline phosphatase
    β-Glycerophosphatase
    Ribonuclease
  Proteinases
    Collagenase
    Cathepsin
  Histaminase
  Peroxisomes
  Major basic protein
  Eosinophil cationic protein
  Eosinophil peroxidases
  Phospholipases
  Lysophospholipases
Lipids
Reactive oxygen intermediates

[a] Adapted from Ref. 24.

TABLE 2.5. Differences between mast cell subtypes.[a]

Property	Mucosal mast cell (MMC)	Connective tissue mast cell (CTMC)
Staining (Alcian blue/safranin)	Blue	Red-blue
Protease type	Tryptase	Tryptase and chymase
T lymphocyte dependency	Yes	No
Migration	Migratory	Nonmigratory
Life span	Short	Long
Half-life	<40 days	>6 months
Proteoglycan	Chondroitin sulfate	Heparin

[a] Adapted from Ref. 25.

receptors for the Fc portion of IgE (high affinity) and IgG (CD16) and for complement components, including C5a, CR1 (CD35) and CR3 (CD11b). The mast cell is often indistinguishable from the basophil in a number of properties. There are at least two classes of mast cells, distinguished on the basis of their neutral protease composition, T lymphocyte dependency, and ultrastructural characteristics (Table 2.5)[25–28]: one consists of the mucosa-associated mast cells (MMCs), and the other includes connective tissue-associated mast cells (CTMCs). Basophils and mast cells play a specialized role in allergic reactions. They also can participate in type III hypersensitivity or immune complex-mediated diseases. IgE antibody induced by the antigen binds to circulating basophils or to tissue mast cells, which then release histamine, platelet-activating factor,

and other biological molecules when antigen binds to two adjacent IgE molecules on the mast cell surface (Table 2.6).[25] Histamine and other vasoactive amines cause an increase in vascular permeability, allowing the immune complexes to become trapped in the vessel wall.

2.1.1.4. Platelets

Blood platelets, cells highly adapted for blood clotting, also are involved in the immune response to injury, reflecting their evolutionary heritage as myeloid (inflammatory) cells. They possess surface receptors for the Fc portion of IgG (CD16) and IgE (low affinity), for class I histocompatibility glycoproteins (HLA-A, -B, or -C), and for factor VIII. They also carry molecules such as Gp11b/111a (CDw41), which binds fibrinogen, and Gp1b (CDw42), which binds von Willebrand's factor.

Following endothelial injury, platelets adhere to and aggregate at the endothelial surface, releasing from their granules permeability-increasing molecules (Table 2.7).[29] Endothelial injury may be caused by type III hypersensitivity or immune complex-mediated reactions. Platelet-activating factor released by basophils/mast cells after antigen–IgE antibody complex formation induces platelets to aggregate and release their vasoactive amines. These amines separate endothelial cells and allow the immune complexes to enter the vessel wall. Once the immune complexes are deposited, they initiate an inflammatory reaction through activation of complement components and polymorphonuclear granulocyte lysosomal enzyme release.

TABLE 2.6. Secretory products of mast cells and basophils.[a]

Histamine
Serotonin
Rat mast cell protease I and II
Heparin
Chondroitin sulfate
β-Hexosaminidase
β-Glucuronidase
β-D-Galactosidase
Arylsulfatase
Eosinophil chemotactic factor of anaphylaxis (ECF-A)
Slow reactive substance of anaphylaxis (SRS-A)
High molecular weight neutrophil chemotactic factor
Arachidonic acid derivatives
Platelet-activating factor

[a] Adapted from Ref. 25.

TABLE 2.7. Secretory products of platelets.[a]

Alpha granules	Dense granules
Fibronectin	Serotonin
Fibrinogen	Adenosine diphosphate (ADP)
Plasminogen	Others
Thrombospondin	Arachidonic acid derivatives
von Willebrand's factor	
α_2-Plasmin inhibitor	
Platelet-derived growth factor (PDGF)	
Platelet factor 4 (PF4)	
Transforming growth factors (TGFs) α and β	
Thrombospondin	
β-Lysin	
Permeability factor	
Factors D and H	
Decay-accelerating factor	

[a] Adapted from Ref. 29.

2.1.2. Immunoregulation

The integrity of the immune response is crucially dependent of a complex series of interactions of the cells involved in the immune response and their secretory products (Tables 2.1–2.7). Obviously, these interactions must be tightly regulated. Abnormalities in this regulation lead to expression of inflammatory diseases.

2.1.2.1. The Major Histocompatibility Complex

Immunological recognition, including interaction between antigen-presenting cells and lymphocytes, as well as between different lymphocytes, results in a complex network, the primary conductor of which is the genetic material located in humans on the short arm of chromosome 6, a region known as the major histocompatibility complex (MHC). This genetic material is divided into three distinct families: class I, II, and III MHC genes. Class I MHC genes encode the human leukocyte antigens HLA-A, HLA-B, and HLA-C, present on the surface of all nucleated cells. Class I antigens consist of one glycosylated polypeptide heavy chain with three globular domains, $\alpha 1$, $\alpha 2$, and $\alpha 3$, noncovalently associated by its $\alpha 3$ domain with a nonglycosylated peptide light chain, a β_2-microglobulin encoded outside of the MHC on chromosome 15. Class II MHC genes encode the human leukocyte antigens HLA-DP, HLA-DQ, and HLA-DR, present on the surface of a small number of cell types (macrophages, monocytes, Langerhans' cells, and T and B lymphocytes), but their synthesis and cell surface expression can be induced by interferon γ on various other cells, including connective tissue fibroblasts, corneal endothelial cells, and vascular endothelial cells.[20,21] Class II antigens consist of two noncovalently associated polypeptide chains, the α chain and the β chain, both with two globular domains. Class III MHC genes encode three proteins of the complement system (C2, factor B, and C4). They have been mapped within a 0.7-centimorgan (cM) region between HLA-B and HLA-DR.[30] The tight linkage of these regions suggests that regulation of class I, II, and III MHC gene expression may occur concomitantly.

The surface MHC glycoproteins are essential for immune recognition of antigen and subsequent activation of the immune response. T helper lymphocytes recognize antigen through the TCR in association with class II MHC glycoproteins on antigen-presenting cells. T helper lymphocytes can cooperate with B lymphocytes in association with class II MHC glycoproteins to induce antibody production. They also can release lymphokines that help macrophages to attack the antigen. Cytotoxic

T lymphocytes, involved in viral infections and in tissue graft rejections, recognize viral antigens and foreign graft tissue antigens in association with class I MHC glycoproteins. The result of these specific interactions will lead to the ultimate response, that is, resistance (strong immune response) or susceptibility (low or no reactivity) to the antigen.[6]

In human beings, certain diseases are associated with unusual frequencies of one or more of these MHC glycoproteins, which may affect host susceptibility to the disease, resistance to it, or both. HLA-B27 is present in 90% of patients with ankylosing spondylitis and in 80% of patients with Reiter's disease. HLA-DRw4 is present in 64% of patients with rheumatoid arthritis. Other HLA glycoproteins have been found in association with other disorders.[6]

2.1.2.2. Humoral Mechanisms: Antibodies

The immune response may also be modulated by humoral mechanisms. Circulating antibodies can participate in immunoregulation by three mechanisms.

In the first mechanism, "antigen blocking," high concentrations of circulating antibody compete with receptors on B lymphocytes for circulating antigen, preventing activation of antigen-specific B lymphocytes.

In the second mechanism, "receptor cross-linking," antibody binds to Fc receptors and to antigen receptors (antigen binding region of the antibody) on B lymphocytes, usually resulting in the prevention of B lymphocyte activation; however, this mechanism can sometimes result in B lymphocyte activation, particularly when the ratio of antigen to antibody is high. It appears that the early-formed antibody induces B lymphocyte activation and further antibody synthesis; once the antibody concentration exceeds the antigen concentration, B lymphocyte activation is inhibited. Therefore the ratio of antigen to antibody plays an important role in regulating the immune response.

In the third mechanism, "idiotypic regulation," antibody binds to B lymphocyte antigen receptors. *Idiotype* refers to the antigen receptor present in the variable region of an immunoglobulin, and which is specific for a given antigen. Jerne[31] suggested that idiotypes produced in response to antigen stimulate production of anti-idiotypic antibodies that then regulate production of idiotypes. Anti-idiotypes stimulate production of anti-anti-idiotypes, which then regulate production of anti-idiotypes. Because anti-idiotypes resemble the original antigen, they can bind directly to the B lymphocyte or T lymphocyte antigen receptor and, depending on their concentration, they can either activate or inactivate B or T lymphocytes.[31,32]

2.1.2.3. Cellular Mechanisms

The immune response also may be modulated by cellular mechanisms. T suppressor lymphocytes inhibit T helper lymphocyte or B lymphocyte activation. They can be antigen specific, idiotype specific, and antigen nonspecific. T contrasuppressor lymphocytes inhibit T suppressor lymphocyte functions, allowing T helper activation.[33,34] T lymphocyte lymphokines play an important role in regulating the components of the immune response.

Immunoregulation also may be accomplished by regulatory B lymphocytes and B lymphocyte lymphokines. For example, B lymphocyte-derived enhancing factor (BEF) inhibits T suppressor lymphocyte activation, allowing B lymphocyte functions such as antibody synthesis. On the other hand, B lymphocyte-derived suppressor factors (BSFs) inhibit B lymphocyte activation.

2.1.2.4. Summary

Antigen is presented to T helper lymphocytes (class II MHC) and B lymphocytes (class II MHC) by antigen-presenting cells (class II MHC), which stimulates them (recognition of "nonself" through class II MHC cell surface glycoproteins). Once activated, T helper lymphocytes help specific B lymphocytes to produce antibodies. Antibody production is regulated by blocking or cross-linking. T helper lymphocytes and B lymphocytes are regulated by antiidiotypes, T suppressor lymphocytes (also stimulated by antigen), and T and B lymphocyte-derived lymphokines.

2.1.3. Abnormalities of the Immune Response

2.1.3.1. Hypersensitivity Reactions

If the immune response of an organism to an antigen is excessive or inappropriate, tissue damage may occur. Gell, Coombs, and Lackmann[35] described four types of tissue-damaging hypersensitivity reactions: (1) type I or anaphylactic, (2) type II or cytotoxic, (3) type III or immune complex mediated, and (4) type IV or cell mediated (delayed). Because only type III and type IV hypersensitivity reactions are thought to play a primary role in the pathogenesis of scleral inflammation,[1] we focus our general review on them.

2.1.3.1.1. Type III Hypersensitivity Reactions

Type III hypersensitivity reactions are mediated by immune complexes. The antibody reacts with the antigen whether within the circulation (circulating immune complexes) or at extravascular sites where antigen may have been deposited (in situ immune complexes). The resulting immune complex activates the complement cascade, which attracts neutrophils and macrophages that release proteolytic enzymes capable of causing tissue damage. Tissue damage appears as areas of fibrinoid necrosis. The distribution of tissue injury is determined by the sites of deposition of the immune complexes (vessels, renal glomeruli, joints). Two general types of antigen may cause immune complex deposition: (1) exogenous, such as bacteria, virus, parasites, fungi, or drugs, and (2) endogenous or "self" components, such as nuclear antigens, immunoglobulins, or tumor antigens (resulting in autoimmunity; this is discussed in Section 2.1.3.2).

Immune complex-mediated diseases may be generalized, if immune complexes are formed in the circulation and are deposited in many organs, or localized, if the complexes are formed and deposited locally (local Arthus reaction) to particular organs such as the kidney (glomerulonephritis), joints (arthritis), or the small blood vessels of the skin (purpura).

2.1.3.1.1.1. Systemic Immune Complex Disease. The classic condition ascribed to systemic immune complex disease is acute serum sickness. Rabbits given a single intravenous injection of bovine serum albumin (BSA) develop necrotizing arteritis and glomerulonephritis, similar to the lesions seen in humans with polyarteritis nodosa (PAN).[36,37] These lesions appear at 10 to 14 days, the period when circulating immune complexes are being formed in slight antigen excess.

The process is initiated by the introduction of antigen into the circulation and its interaction with immunocompetent cells, resulting approximately 5 days later in the formation of antibodies. Antibodies react with the antigen still present in the circulation to form antigen–antibody complexes. Antigen–antibody complexes formed in the circulation are deposited in various tissues. The factors that determine whether immune complex formation will result in tissue deposition and disease are diverse, and include the following.

1. *Immune complex size*: The size of an immune complex is determined by the ratio of antigen to antibody. Large immune complexes (great antibody excess) are readily phagocytized by the reticuloendothelial system and small immune complexes (great antigen excess) are too small to localize in tissues. The most pathogenic complexes are of intermediate size (formed in slight antigen or antibody excess) because of their longevity in the circulation.[38]

2. *Antigen and antibody valences*: Monovalent and oligovalent antigens bind only one or a few antibody molecules and form small immune complexes, whereas multivalent antigens bind and cross-link many antibody molecules and form large, lattice-like structures.[39]

3. *Reticuloendothelial system function*: Because the reticuloendothelial system normally phagocytizes the circulating immune complexes, its dysfunction increases the persistence of immune complexes in circulation and tissue deposition.

4. *Local characteristics of vessels*: The focal distribution of vasculitis lesions in animals and humans can be explained partially by structural and hemodynamic differences among various blood vessels and by the tendency of immune complexes to deposit at the branch points of the vessels.[40,41]

Local vasoactive factors increase vascular permeability, which allows immune complexes to leave the circulation and deposit within or outside the vessel wall.[42,43] The increased vascular permeability results from the action of vasoactive amines derived from platelets (platelet-activating factor) and IgE (serotonin and histamine). These amines induce contraction of vascular endothelial cells, disrupting their close apposition and producing interendothelial gaps through which immune complexes travel, becoming trapped in the basement membrane or depositing in the tissues.

Once immune complexes are deposited in or outside the vessel wall, complement components are activated, some of which (1) are chemotactic factors for neutrophils and eosinophils and mononuclear leukocytes (C3a, C5a, and C5b67), (2) increase vascular permeability and cause contraction of smooth muscle (C3a and C5a), or (3) cause cell membrane damage (membrane attack complex, C5 through C9). Antibodies IgG_1, IgG_2, IgG_3, and IgM all activate the classic complement pathway efficiently, whereas IgG_4, IgA, and aggregates of IgE interact with the complement system via the alternative pathway. During the active phase of the disease, consumption of complement components decreases the serum levels.

Neutrophils attracted by complement components cause vessel and surrounding tissue damage through the release of lysosomal enzymes, reactive oxygen metabolites, and proinflammatory substances such as platelet-activating factor, leukotrienes, and prostaglandins. Platelets may adhere to locally damaged endothelium and aggregate, obstruct blood vessels, and release more inflammatory mediators, augmenting vessel and tissue necrosis. The reaction spirals into an amplification cascade, causing damage to vessel walls and other surrounding tissues. The resultant pathological lesion is termed vasculitis if it occurs in blood vessels, glomerulonephritis if it occurs in renal glomeruli, arthritis if it occurs in joints, and so on. The immune complexes can be seen by immunofluorescence microscopy as deposits of immunoglobulin and complement.

A chronic form of serum sickness or immune complex disease results from repeated or prolonged exposure to an antigen. This occurs in systemic vasculitic diseases such as rheumatoid arthritis, systemic lupus erythematosus, and polyarteritis nodosa. However, although immunoglobulins and complement as part of immune complexes can be seen by immunofluorescence techniques, the inciting antigens are unknown.

2.1.3.1.1.2. Local Immune Complex Disease (Arthus Reaction). The classic condition ascribed to local immune complex disease is the Arthus reaction.[44] In this model, necrotizing vasculitis is seen at the site of locally injected antigen in animals preimmunized (having circulating antibodies) with the same antigen. Vessel damage occurs because of the reaction of preformed antibody with locally injected antigen in vessel walls. As the antigen diffuses into the vascular wall, large immune complexes are formed because of the excess of antibodies, which precipitate locally and trigger the inflammatory reaction discussed earlier. The Arthus reaction develops over a few hours and reaches a peak 4 to 10h after injection; the area discloses edema, hemorrhage, and occasionally ulceration as a result of inflammatory reaction, rupture of the vessel wall, or thrombosis of the vessel lumen. The immune complexes precipitated in the vessel walls, usually capillaries and postcapillary venules, can be seen by light microscopy as neutrophilic infiltration of the vessel wall and by immunofluorescence microscopy as deposits of immunoglobulin and complement.

2.1.3.1.2. Type IV Hypersensitivity Reactions

Type IV hypersensitivity reactions are also known as delayed hypersensitivity reactions because they require more than 12h after the antigenic challenge to develop. They are mediated by cells (T lymphocytes) and not by antibodies. After antigen presentation by the antigen-presenting cells, T lymphocytes proliferate and release lymphokines, which may cause direct cytotoxicity or may stimulate neutrophils and macrophages to produce tissue damage.[6] Four kinds of type IV hypersensitivity can be distinguished: (1) Jones–Mote, (2) contact, (3) tuberculin, and (4) granulomatous. The first three reactions develop between 24 and 72 h after antigen challenge, whereas the fourth type requires at least 14 days.[6]

Granulomatous hypersensitivity causes many of the pathological hallmarks of diseases such as tuberculosis, schistosomiasis, or scleral inflammation. Persistence of microbiological agents (*M. tuberculosis*, viruses, parasites, and fungi), foreign body deposition (talc), or immune complexes provides the long-term stimulus for the inflammatory response to produce granulomas.[45] Histologically, granulomas are composed of macrophages and epithelioid cells (modified macrophage) with variable numbers of neutrophils, eosinophils, lymphocytes, and plasma cells. Also seen in this type of reaction is the multinucleated giant cell (Langhans' giant cell), which is derived from fusion of several epithelioid cells; this cell is believed

to be an end stage of differentiation of the monocyte/macrophage line.[46]

2.1.3.2. Autoimmunity

Autoimmunity is an immune response directed against endogenous structures of an organism (autoantigens or self-antigens); the organism escapes from the normal state of tolerance to its own tissue antigens to the abnormal state of responding to self as nonself.[47] The immune response characterized by tissue damage may be exerted by immunoglobulins (autoantibodies) and/or by T lymphocytes. Both type II and type III hypersensitivity reactions have been implicated.

A growing number of diseases have been attributed to autoimmunity, although for many of them the evidence is not firm. Examples of these diseases range from highly organ-specific diseases such as pernicious anemia, insulin-dependent diabetes mellitus, or Hashimoto's thyroiditis to multisystem disorders such as lupus erythematosus or rheumatoid arthritis (Table 2.8). At least three requirements should be met before autoimmunity can be ascribed to a disease: (1) the presence of an immune

TABLE 2.8. Autoimmune diseases.

Organ specific	Nonorgan specific
Probable	Probable
Hashimoto's thyroiditis	Systemic lupus erythematosus
Graves' disease	Rheumatoid arthritis
Primary myxedema	Sjögren's syndrome
Thyrotoxicosis	Reiter's syndrome
Pernicious anemia	Possible
Autoimmune encephalomyelitis	Polyarteritis nodosa
Addison's disease	Polymyositis-dermatomyositis
Goodpasture's syndrome	Systemic sclerosis
Autoimmune thrombocytopenia	Mixed connective tissue disease
Autoimmune hemolytic anemia	
Myasthenia gravis	
Insulin-dependent diabetes mellitus	
Pemphigus vulgaris	
Pemphigoid	
Possible	
Primary biliary cirrhosis	
Chronic active hepatitis	
Ulcerative colitis	
Noninfectious uveitis	
Noninfectious scleritis	

reaction, (2) clinical or experimental evidence that the immune reaction is not secondary to tissue damage but is of primary pathogenetic significance, and (3) the absence of another well-defined cause of the disease.

2.1.3.2.1. Mechanisms of Autoimmunity

Susceptibility to autoimmunity or loss of self-tolerance is genetically controlled by genes within the MHC. A variety of infectious agents, including bacteria, mycoplasmas, and particularly viruses, have been implicated in triggering autoimmunity. The development of an autoimmune disease probably entails the interaction of genetically controlled mechanisms with environmental factors such as infectious agents.[48] Several general mechanisms for autoimmunity have been postulated.

1. *Newly induced class II MHC expression*: Macrophages, Langerhans cells, monocytes, and T and B lymphocytes are the only cells that constitutively express class II MHC glycoproteins. Other cells, such as connective tissue fibroblasts or vascular endothelial cells, may be induced to express class II glycoproteins under inflammatory stimulation (interferon γ). It has been suggested that such aberrant expression of class II MHC glycoproteins could trigger an autoimmune response.[22]

2. *Modification of a self molecule*: If a self molecule is complexed with a new carrier (infectious agent or drug), the carrier part of the complex may be recognized by T lymphocytes as nonself; T lymphocytes help B lymphocytes, resulting in autoantibody production. Another mechanism for self molecule modification is through partial degradation (e.g., by an infectious agent); the degraded self molecule (collagen, gamma globulin) may disclose new antigenic determinants that will trigger an autoimmune response.

3. *Antigen mimicry*: Infectious agents may share regions of amino acid sequence with self molecules; the immune response elicited by the infectious agent also may damage the self molecule.

4. *Allelic variation in MHC genes*: An antigen (e.g., an infectious agent) when presented in association with a particular allelic form of

HLA glycoprotein ("susceptible"), may mimic an autoantigen, eliciting an autoimmune response.

5. *Polyclonal B lymphocyte activation*: Autoreactive B lymphocytes may be activated (antigen nonspecific) by B lymphocyte mitogens such as infectious agents or their products, leading to polyclonal activation. Some of the nonspecific immunoglobulins produced may react with self molecules, resulting in autoantibody production. For example, bacterial lipopolysaccharide may induce mouse B lymphocytes to form autoantibodies in vitro; some viruses (Epstein–Barr virus) are nonspecific, polyclonal B lymphocyte mitogens (human B lymphocytes have surface receptors for Epstein–Barr virus) and may thus induce the production of autoantibodies.

6. *Idiotypic networks*: Abnormalities in the immune response involving the idiotypic network may lead to the production of antibodies (idiotype) against self molecules. Anti-idiotypic antibodies against the idiotype (e.g., anti-thyroid-stimulating hormone [TSH]) resemble the original antigen (e.g., TSH) and may react with the antigen receptor on specialized cells (e.g., TSH receptors on thyroid cells in Graves' disease).[49]

7. *Abnormalities of immunoregulatory T cells*: The normal immune system has the capacity to produce a small amount of autoantibodies without the production of autoimmune reactions; T suppressor lymphocytes normally control this autoantibody production (through preventing T lymphocyte help to B lymphocytes). Loss of T suppressor lymphocyte function (e.g., following viral infection) may allow the production of large amounts of autoantibodies, leading to autoimmunity.

2.2. Connective Tissue and the Immune Response

2.2.1. Fibroblast Functions and the Immune Response

When connective tissue sustains an inflammatory (immunological, mechanical, or chemical) injury, fibroblasts migrate to the involved area to repair the damage. Specific chemoattractants have been identified that direct their migration for subsequent synthesis of new matrix components and eventual scar formation. Lymphocyte-derived chemotactic factor released from T lymphocytes, platelet-derived growth factor released from platelets, and leukotriene B_4 released from leukocytes have been shown to provide chemotactic signals for fibroblasts.[50-53] The C5-derived fragment from serum complement activation by the classic or alternative pathways can also provide chemotactic signals for fibroblasts.[54] Collagen, elastin, and fibronectin, as well as some of their degradation products, can be chemoattractants for fibroblasts.[55-57]

Fibroblast functions such as collagen, collagenase, and hyaluronic acid production can be modulated by components of the immune response. Type I collagen production is stimulated by a lymphokine, the collagen production factor, and by a monokine, interleukin 1, but it is inhibited by another lymphokine, interferon γ.[58-62] Collagenase and hyaluronic acid productions are stimulated by interleukin 1.[59,60,63]

Fibroblasts have been found to synthesize several complement components.[64-66] C1q, the recognition unit of the classic pathway, and collagen have structural similarities because the genes for each share part of their coding region.[67,68] Complement synthesis by fibroblasts can be regulated by several components of the immune response, including interleukin 1, tumor necrosis factor, and interferon γ.[69-71]

Fibroblasts have been shown to express class I HLA glycoproteins constitutively,[72-74] but under certain inflammatory stimuli, including that of interferon γ, they can also express class II HLA glycoproteins.[75-77] Class II HLA expression may allow fibroblasts to be involved in the initiation and perpetuation of an immune inflammatory response.

Following stimulation by interleukin 1, fibroblasts may synthesize and secrete prostaglandins such as PGE_2.[78] Prostaglandin E_2 production provides a regulatory signal in modulating the intensity of the inflammation during the immune response.

2.3. The Sclera and the Immune Response: Scleritis

2.3.1. Immune Characteristics of the Sclera

The sclera is composed of fibroblasts, proteoglycans, collagen, elastin, and glycoproteins. Although the sclera does not have its own capillary network, its nutrition derives from the overlying episclera and underlying choroid. The sclera contains immunoglobulins, albumin, and the classic and alternative pathway components of complement.[79,80] Complement present in the sclera may be activated by immune complexes through the classic pathway or by microorganisms through the alternative pathway. Inflammatory functions of activated complement include increased vascular permeability, mast cell degranulation, opsonization of immune complexes and microorganisms, neutrophil chemotaxis, and cytolysis.[6] IgG, IgA, albumin, and complement components C4, C2, C3, C5, C6, and C7 levels are higher in the posterior than in the anterior sclera, probably because of a greater adjacent vascular supply from the choroid.[80] Conversely, levels of C1, the recognition unit of the classic complement pathway, are higher in the anterior than in the posterior sclera. The preferential activation of complement by immune complexes anteriorly may explain, at least in part, why anterior scleritis is more common than posterior scleritis.[80] Because the diffusion of C1, the largest complement component (M_r 647,000), into the sclera may be restricted, local production may help to explain its presence. Scleral fibroblasts constitutively produce C1.[81] After exposure to an inflammatory stimulus such as human interferon γ, scleral fibroblasts increase production of C1 and are induced to secrete new C2 and C4. No other complement components (C3, C5, C6, and C7) are secreted by scleral fibroblasts.[81]

Scleral fibroblasts constitutively express class I HLA glycoproteins (HLA-A, -B, and -C) but can be induced to express class II HLA glycoproteins (HLA-DR, -DP, and -DQ) under exposure to an inflammatory stimulus such as interferon γ.[81] HLA-DR expression in human scleral specimens has been found to be high in patients with scleritis.[1] These findings suggest that scleral fibroblasts have the ability to participate in immunological diseases. Aberrant expression of HLA-DR has been proposed by Bottazzo et al.[22] to play a pivotal role in the initiation and perpetuation of the immune response leading to autoimmune disorders.

Immune complexes may be important in the pathogenesis of scleritis associated with autoimmune diseases.[1,82] Activation of C1, already present in the sclera, by immune complexes may play a role in some types of scleral inflammation.

Normal human sclera has few or no macrophages, Langerhans' cells, neutrophils, or lymphocytes. After scleral inflammation, there is a marked increase in T helper lymphocytes, with a high T helper-to-T suppressor ratio. These findings suggest that T lymphocytes, as part of cell-mediated immune responses, also play a role in some forms of scleritis.[1]

2.3.2. The Susceptible Host: Immunogenetics

Immunogenetic susceptibility has been found to be important in the development of some of the systemic vasculitic disorders associated with scleritis. For example, in the connective tissue disease most frequently associated with scleritis, rheumatoid arthritis, the class II *MHC* locus is associated with susceptibility to rheumatoid joint disease. A majority of patients with rheumatoid arthritis carry *HLA-DR4*, *HLA-DR1*, or both.[83] *HLA-DR4* can be divided into five subtypes: *Dw4*, *Dw10*, *Dw13*, *Dw14*, and *Dw15*. Only *Dw4* and *Dw14*, present in 50 and 35% of the patients, respectively, promote, independently of each other, susceptibility to rheumatoid arthritis.[84,85] No immunogenetic studies have been performed in patients with scleritis.

2.3.3. Etiology

Scleral inflammation can often be associated with systemic vasculitic diseases, including the connective tissue vascular diseases, polyarteritis nodosa, and Wegener's granulomatosis. The antigen(s) responsible for scleritis associated with systemic vasculitic diseases in an immunogenetically susceptible individual remains unidentified. It is possible that scleritis associated with systemic vasculitic diseases shares the same causative factors of these disorders. It is also possible, indeed likely, that any of these disorders is triggered by more than one etiological factor. For example, current research on rheumatoid arthritis etiology is focused on exogenous infectious agents such as viruses or mycobacteria, and endogenous substances such as connective tissue molecules. Exogenous infectious agents are hypothesized as causative factors because of data showing that a persistent but only weakly cytotoxic virus may generate an immune reaction that becomes self-sustaining. Endogenous substances are considered as possible triggers because of data showing that certain individuals immunogenetically disposed to develop rheumatoid arthritis have abnormal lymphocytes that allow a chronic persistent arthritis to develop in response to connective tissue molecules such as proteoglycans or collagen. Another possibility involves components of the two theories already mentioned: an infection in a susceptible individual could result in production of antibodies that cross-react with connective tissue molecules in the joints.

2.3.3.1. Exogenous Agents

2.3.3.1.1. Viruses

To date, no virus has been proved to cause rheumatoid arthritis, but because of the capacity of viruses to alter immune responses they remain prime candidates for the initiation or propagation of this disease. Viral or subviral components or new virus-induced antigens expressed on the infected cell surface (either virus material or a combination of infected cell and virus material) may act as neoantigens and invoke an immune response.[86] A virus can also invoke an immune response by unmasking a substructure present in the infected cell, by secondary derepression of a gene encoding an infected cell membrane antigen.[87,88] Other possible mechanisms have been implicated in the production of autoimmunity triggered by viruses (see Section 2.1.3.2.1).

Many viruses have been proposed as etiological factors for rheumatoid arthritis.[89,90] Rubella virus, cytomegalovirus, herpes virus type 1, human T cell lymphotropic virus type I, Epstein–Barr virus, and parvovirus are some examples but only the two latter have received sustained scientific support.

1. *Epstein–Barr virus*: Eighty percent of patients with rheumatoid arthritis have circulating antibodies in high titers directed against antigens specific for Epstein–Barr virus (EBV).[91] The EBV receptor on the B lymphocyte, the target cell, is identical to complement receptor type 2 (CR2), which binds C3d, C3bi, and, with less affinity, C3b. Epstein–Barr virus infection of B cells results in polyclonal activation and overproduction of autoantibodies, including rheumatoid factor.[92] Patients with rheumatoid arthritis shed more EBV in throat washings than do control subjects.[93] Support for the hypothesis that EBV does not cause rheumatoid arthritis comes from reports in which increased antibody titers against EBV were not found in early rheumatoid arthritis.[94] However, there has been found an identical amino acid sequence between the viral glycoprotein gp110 and the "susceptibility regions" HLA-Dw4, -Dw14, and -DR1.[95] Patients with serological evidence of a previous EBV infection have serum antibodies that recognize the same peptides from both gp110 and HLA-Dw4.[95,96] Tolerance of self-antigens in these patients could affect the immune response to EBV, leading to a continuous infection that would be manifested as rheumatoid arthritis. Epstein–Barr virus antibody titers in patients with scleritis have not been reported.

2. *Parvoviruses*: Parvoviruses are small DNA viruses that cause disease in humans and in animals such as the Aleutian mink. Parvoviruses can integrate their own DNA into human chromosomes, perhaps leading to expression of antigens that generate an immune response. Two patients with early rheumatoid arthritis have been reported to have had a recent infection with parvovirus B19[97]; two other patients with acute infection with parvovirus B19 were found to be transiently positive for rheumatoid factor and to develop arthritis.[98] After 6 months, the rheumatoid factor reverted to negative and the arthritic symptoms disappeared. No data on parvovirus infections in patients with scleritis have been reported.

The ideal viral pathogen that could cause rheumatoid arthritis or scleritis should be ubiquitous, persistent, and have the capability to alter immune responses in the genetically susceptible individual. It is possible that these characteristics might be distributed among two or more viruses that would work in series or parallel.

2.3.3.1.2. Mycobacteria

Mycobacteria express heat shock proteins on their cell surface in response to various kinds of stress. Heat shock proteins are the arthritogenic factors of adjuvant arthritis in rats.[99] Patients with rheumatoid arthritis have elevated serum levels of IgG and IgA to heat shock proteins from mycobacteria[100] and synovial fluid proliferation of lymphocytes with CD3-associated T cell receptor (the lymphocytes that proliferate in response to mycobacterial antigens).[101] Lymphocytic proliferation in response to mycobacterial antigens could be perpetuated by heat shock proteins on synovial cells and therefore participate in the genesis of rheumatoid arthritis. No data on mycobacterial infections in patients with scleritis have been reported, nor are there reports of studies on antibodies to heat shock proteins.

2.3.3.2. *Endogenous Substances*

There is no doubt that autoimmunity has an important role in the development of rheumatoid arthritis, but data supporting autoimmunity as the initial cause of the disease are less firm. The connective tissue molecules proteoglycans and collagen are the endogenous proteins most often implicated in these hypothesis. Proteoglycans and collagen may provoke cell-mediated and humoral immune responses in experimental rheumatoid arthritis.[102,103] They also may be involved in the generation of autoimmune mechanisms in rheumatoid arthritis in humans.[104–110]

2.3.3.2.1. Glycosaminoglycans

Glycosaminoglycans have been shown to be antigenic in rheumatoid arthritis.[109,111] Cell-mediated and humoral immune responses can derange the molecular structure of glycosaminoglycan. The degraded components can be recognized by the immune cells of the host as a foreign material and create a vicious circle of chronic inflammation.

Immunological cross-reactivity of glycosaminoglycans between sclera and other organs suggest that autoimmunity to these molecules might participate in scleral inflammation.[112–114] Dermatan sulfate, isolated from bovine sclera and bovine cartilage, can, according to the size, be divided into large and small dermatan sulfate. The small dermatan sulfates of both sclera and cartilage tissues have closely related core proteins and display immunological cross-reactivity.[114] Immunological and histochemical studies have revealed that these small proteoglycans are bound to collagen type I.[115,116] Small dermatan sulfates have the ability to inhibit fibrillogenesis of both collagen type I and type II through the core protein of the proteoglycan structure.[117,118] No data on glycosaminoglycan-induced scleritis in animals or antibodies to glycosaminoglycans in patients with scleritis have been reported.

2.3.3.2.2. Collagen

Collagen has also been shown to be antigenic in rheumatoid arthritis.[119–123] Collagen type II-induced arthritis in animals, and cellular and humoral sensitivity to collagen type II in humans with rheumatoid arthritis, have supported the possibility of collagen autoimmunity as a potential etiological factor; however, there are data showing that antibodies against collagen type II do not precede the clinical onset of rheumatoid arthritis.[124] Most of the more recent studies in humans conclude that rheumatoid arthritis is not caused by the devel-

opment of autoantibodies to collagen type II, but that the activated immune system in rheumatoid arthritis develops clonal proliferation of B cells expressing antibody against epitopes of collagen type II normally masked by the native helical conformation of collagen and its coating with proteoglycan and other noncollagenous glycoproteins. Anti-collagen antibodies against the degraded, fragmented type II collagen can amplify the immune response, resulting in synovitis and centripetal polarization of destructive arthritis.[125]

We investigated whether or not immunization with collagen type I or type III participates in the pathogenesis of scleritis. Outbred female Wistar-Lewis rats (150 to 225 g, 7 to 10 weeks old) were injected intradermally in 8 to 10 sites (small blebs) on the back with native collagen type I or type III (1 mg/ml). Native collagen type I and III, previously dissolved in 0.1 M acetic acid, were emulsified with equal volumes of Freund's incomplete adjuvant. Rats were boosted intraperitoneally 1 week following the first immunization and, since then, once a week for 8 weeks. Daily clinical ocular evaluation did not show any area of scleritis. Histopathology studies on sclera following sacrifice and bilateral enucleation of the animals, ranging up to 6 months after primary immunization, did not reveal inflammatory changes. These data suggest that autoimmunity to collagen is not an etiological factor in the pathogenesis of scleritis.

We also investigated whether or not patients with scleritis, particularly necrotizing scleritis, have antibodies to collagen type I. Sera from patients with necrotizing scleritis were examined by enzyme-linked immunosorbent assay (ELISA) for antibodies to native collagen type I. No differences in anti-collagen type I antibodies were found between sera from patients with necrotizing scleritis and sera from normal individuals. These data suggest that autoimmunity to collagen type I is not an etiological factor in the pathogenesis of scleritis.

2.3.4. Pathogenesis

The immunopathological findings of vessel thrombosis and inflammatory infiltration of the vessel walls in scleritis associated with autoimmune diseases suggest that immune complex-mediated inflammatory micro-angiopathy plays a pivotal role in some types of scleral inflammation.[1] Immune complexes, either circulating or formed in the sclera itself, may localize in the episcleral vasculature and scleral perforating vessels.[1] The mechanism of selective localization in the vessel walls is not clear, but the ratio of antigen to antibody in a complex may be important.[126]

Scleral fibroblasts under inflammatory conditions increase production of the complement component C1, which can be activated by immune complexes through the classic pathway.[81] Complement components increase vascular permeability and generate chemotactic factors for neutrophils (e.g., C3a and C5a). Further activation of complement can lead to assembly of the membrane attack complex (C56789), thus effecting cellular damage. Neutrophils release their lysosomal enzymes, reactive oxygen metabolites, and proinflammatory substances such as platelet-activating factor, leukotrienes, and prostaglandins. Platelets may adhere to locally damaged endothelium and aggregate, obstruct blood vessels, and release more inflammatory mediators, augmenting vessel and tissue necrosis.[127,128]

Scleral fibroblasts under inflammatory conditions express class II HLA glycoproteins, which allow them to participate in the afferent arm of the immune response as cells presenting antigen to T helper lymphocytes.[1,81] At the molecular level, class II HLA glycoproteins, antigen, and T cell receptor (TCR) form a trimolecular complex that results in activation of the T helper lymphocytes.[129] T helper lymphocytes, as part of the efferent arm of the immune response, react to the antigen through the action of lymphokines in combination with the same class II HLA glycoproteins.

Scleral fibroblasts as well as other inflammatory cells and lymphokines have the potential to produce matrix-degrading enzymes such as collagenase, elastase, proteoglycanase, and glycoproteinases under inflammatory conditions.[130–134] The components of the degraded matrix released may be recognized by the immune cells of the host as foreign material and trigger a vicious circle of chronic inflammation in which a truly autoimmune component against sclera eventually participates.

Immune complex-mediated vasculitis and cell-mediated immune responses may interact as part of the immune network activated in scleral inflammation. It is not clear whether immune complexes act to trigger the cell-mediated immune response, whether T lymphocyte activation by an unknown antigen results in B lymphocyte activation and production of antibodies that can form immune complexes, or whether both these phenomena occur simultaneously. Whichever the case is, both mechanisms are important in the pathogenesis of some forms of scleritis.[1]

Systemic vasculitic diseases associated with scleritis are frequently associated with circulating immune complexes as well as immune complex deposition in vessel walls in many organs, including the eye.[1,127,135–144] Immune complexes are capable of activating the complement cascade.[127,128,145] T helper lymphocyte activation by antigen bound to class II HLA glycoproteins on antigen-presenting cells in an immunogenetically susceptible individual also participates in the pathogenesis of these diseases.[83,146–149]

Hembry and co-workers[150] produced an animal model of necrotizing scleritis following an Arthus reaction (local immune complex disease). Necrotizing scleritis was seen at the site of scleral injection with ovalbumin in rabbits previously sensitized over a prolonged period with the same antigen by intradermal injection.

We investigated whether or not scleritis can result from circulating immune complexes eventually deposited in the sclera. New Zealand White rabbits underwent right internal carotid artery dissection for catheterization with a permanent cannula. In vitro preformed immune complexes in varying degrees of antigen (ovalbumin) or antibody (anti-ovalbumin antibodies obtained in rabbits after intracardiac injection 7 days following intraperitoneal immunization with ovalbumin) excess were injected once a day for 7 days. Daily clinical ocular evaluation did not show any area of scleritis. Histopathology studies on sclera, following sacrifice and bilateral enucleation of animals 7 days after first intravascular injection, did not reveal inflammatory changes. Further investigations with this model are needed, because the factors that govern the deposition of immune complexes in vessel walls are diverse (immune complex size, antigen and antibody valences, reticuloendothelial system function, local characteristic of vessels, etc.), and the duration of immune complex supply required to produce scleritis is undoubtedly quite long. Both the quantity and quality of the host immune response seem to be responsible for the variable vasculitic manifestations of immune complex disease in animal models and in humans.[151]

Summary

The sclera has the ability to participate in immunological diseases. The normal sclera contains immunoglobulins, albumin, and many of the classic and alternative pathway components of complement, and has few or no macrophages, Langerhans' cells, neutrophils, or lymphocytes.

Under inflammatory conditions, scleral fibroblasts express class II HLA glycoproteins, increase production of the recognition unit of the classic complement pathway, C1, and are induced to secrete new C2 and C4 complement components. Inflammatory functions of activated complement include increased vascular permeability, mast cell degranulation, opsonization of immune complexes and microorganisms, neutrophil chemotaxis, and cytolysis.

Under inflammatory conditions, the sclera shows immune complex vessel deposition and a marked increase of macrophages and T lymphocytes, with a high T helper lymphocyte-to-T suppressor lymphocyte ratio.

The development of scleritis probably entails the interaction of genetically controlled mechanisms with environmental factors, such as infectious agents (e.g., viruses, mycobacteria) or trauma. This interaction gives rise to an autoimmune process that damages the vessels through immune complex vessel deposition, subsequent complement activation, and neutrophil enzyme release (type III hypersensitivity). Persistent immunological injury leads to a chronic granulomatous response (type IV hypersensitivity) mediated by macrophages, epithelioid cells, multinucleated giant cells, and lymphocytes.

References

1. Fong LP, Sainz de la Maza M, Rice BA, Kupferman AE, Foster CS: Immunopathology of scleritis. Ophthalmology 98:472, 1991.
2. Foster CS, Forstot SL, Wilson LA: Mortality rate in rheumatoid arthritis patients developing necrotizing scleritis or peripheral ulcerative keratitis. Ophthalmology 91:1253, 1984.
3. Foster CS: Immunosuppressive therapy for external ocular inflammatory disease. Ophthalmology 87:140, 1980.
4. Hakin KN, Watson PG: Systemic associations of scleritis. Int Ophthalmol Clin 31(3):111, 1991.
5. Foster CS: Basic ocular immunology. In Kaufman HE, Barron BA, McDonald MB, Waltman SR (Eds): *The Cornea*. Churchill Livingstone, New York, 1988, pp 85–122.
6. Roitt IM, Brostoff J, Male DK: *Immunology*, 2nd ed. Gower Medical Publishing, London, 1989, pp 2.1–2.18.
7. Parnes JR: Molecular biology and function of CD4 and CD8. Adv Immunol 44:265, 1989.
8. Romagnani. S: Human TH1 and TH2 subsets: regulation of differentiation and role in protection of differentiation and role in protection and immunopathology. Int Arch Allergy Immunol 98:279, 1992.
9. Hermans MJA, Hartsuiker H, Opstaelten D: An insight to study of B-lymphocytopoiesis in rat bone marrow. Topographical arrangement of terminal deoxynucleotidyl transferase-positive cells and pre-B cells. J Immunol 44:67, 1989.
10. Osmond DG: Population dynamics of bone marrow. B lymphocytes Imm Rev 93:103, 1986.
11. Hardy RR, Hayakawa K, Parks DR, Herzenberg LA: Murine B cell differentiation lineages. J Exp Med 1959:1169, 1984.
12. Hardy RR, Hayakawa K, Schimizu M, Herzenberg LA: Rheumatoid factor secretion from human Leu-1 B cells. Science 236:81, 1987.

13. Adams DO, Hamilton TA: The cell biology of macrophage activation. Annu Rev Immunol 2:283, 1984.

14. Nathan CF, Cohn ZA: Cellular components of inflammation: monocytes and macrophages. In Kelley W, Harris E Jr, Ruddy S, Sledge CB (Eds): *Textbook of Rheumatology*. W.B. Saunders, Philadelphia, 1985, pp 144–169.

15. Adam DO, Hamilton TA: Phagocytic cells: cytotoxic activities of macrophages. In Gallin JI, Goldstein IM, Snyderman R (Eds): *Inflammation: Basic Principles and Clinical Correlates*. Raven, New York, 1988, pp 471–492.

16. Davis MM, Bjorkman PJ: T-cell receptor genes and T-cell recognition. Nature (London) 334:395, 1988.

17. Terhorst C, Alarcon B, deVries J, Spits H: T lymphocyte recognition and activation. In Hames BD, Glover DM (Eds): *Molecular Immunology*. IRC Press, Oxford, 1988, pp 145–188.

18. Weiss A, Imboden JB: Cell surface molecules and early events involved in human T lymphocyte activation. Adv Immunol 41:1, 1987.

19. Murphy GF: Cell membrane glycoproteins and Langerhans cells. Hum Pathol 16:103, 1985.

20. Collins T, Korman AJ, Wake CT, Boss JM, Kappes DJ, Fiers W, Ault KA, Gimbrone MA, Strominger JL, Pober JS: Immune interferon activates multiple class II major histocompatibility complex genes and the associated invariant chain gene in human endothelial cells and dermal fibroblasts. Proc Natl Acad Sci USA 81:4917, 1984.

21. Maurer DH, Hanke JH, Michelson E, Rich RR, Pollack MS: Differential presentation of HLA-DR, DQ, and DP restriction elements by interferon-gamma-treated dermal fibroblasts. J Immunol 139:715, 1987.

22. Bottazzo GF, Pujol-Borrell R, Hanafusa T: Role of aberrant HLA-DR expression and antigen presentation in induction of endocrine immunity. Lancet 2:1115, 1983.

23. Baggiolini M: The neutrophil. In Weissman G (Ed): *The Cell Biology of Inflammation*. North Holland/Elsevier, New York, 1980, pp 163–187.

24. Henson PM, Henson JE, Fittschen C: Phagocytic cells: degranulation and secretion. In Gallin JI, Goldstein IM, Snyderman R (Eds): *Inflammation: Basic Principles and Clinical Correlates*. Raven, New York, 1988, pp 363–390.

25. Siraganian RP: Mast cells and basophils. In Gallin JI, Goldstein IM, Snyderman R (Eds): *Inflammation: Basic Principles and Clinical Correlates*. Raven, New York, 1988, pp 513–542.

26. Pearce FL: Functional differences between mast cells from various locations. In Befus AD, Beinenstock J, Denburg JA (Eds): *Mast Cell Differentiation and Heterogeneity*. Raven, New York, 1986, pp 215–222.

27. Befus D, Goodacre R, Dyck N, Bienenstock J: Mast cell heterogeneity in man. I. Histologic studies of the intestine. Int Arch Allergy Appl Immunol 76:232, 1985.

28. Irani AA, Schechter NM, Craig SS, DeBlois G, Schwartz LB: Two types of human mast cells that have distinct neutral protease compositions (tryptase/chymotryptic protease). Proc Natl Acad Sci USA 83:4464, 1986.

29. Weksler BB: Platelets. In Gallin JI, Goldstein IM, Snyderman R (Eds): *Inflammation: Basic Principles and Clinical Correlates*. Raven, New York, 1988, pp 543–557.

30. Whitehead AS, Colten HR, Chang CC, Demars R: Localization of MHC-linked complement genes between HLA-B and HLA-DR by using HLA mutant cell lines. J Immunol 134:641, 1985.

31. Jerne N: Towards a network theory of the immune system. Ann Inst Pasteur Immunol 125:373, 1974.

32. Herzenberg LA, Black SJ: Regulatory circuits and antibody responses. Eur J Immunol 10:1, 1980.

33. Asherson GL, Collizi V, Zembala M: An overview of T-suppressor cell circuits. Annu Rev Immunol 4:37, 1986.

34. Lehner T: Antigen-presenting, contrasuppressor human T-cells. Immunol Today 7:87, 1986.

35. Gell PGH, Coombs RA, Lackmann P: *Clinical Aspects of Immunology*, 3rd ed. Blackwell Scientific Publications, Oxford, 1974.

36. Germuth FG: A comparative histologic and immunologic study in rabbits of induced hypersensitivity of the serum sickness type. J Exp Med 97:257, 1953.

37. Hawn C, Janeway C: Histological and serological sequences in experimental hypersensitivity. J Exp Med 85:571, 1947.

38. Knutsen D, Van Es L, Kayser B, Glassock R: Soluble oligovalent antigen–antibody complexes. II. The effect of various selective forces upon relative stability of isolated complexes. Immunology 37:495, 1979.

39. Barnett E, Knutsen D, Abrass C, Chia D, Young L, Liebling M: Circulating immune

complexes: their immunochemistry, detection, and importance. Ann Intern Med 91:430, 1979.

40. Giacomelli F, Wiener J: Regional variation in the permeability of rat thoracic aorta. Am J Pathol 75:513, 1974.

41. Huttner I, More R, Rona G: Fine structural evidence of specific mechanism for increased endothelial permeability in experimental hypertension. Am J Pathol 61:395, 1970.

42. Cochrane CG: Studies on the localization of circulating antigen–antibody complexes and other macromolecules in vessels. I. Structural studies. J Exp Med 118:489, 1963.

43. Cochrane CG: Studies on the localization of circulating antigen–antibody complexes and other macromolecules in vessels. II. Pathogenic and pharmacodynamic studies. J Exp Med 118:503, 1963.

44. Cochrane CG, Janoff A: The Arthus reaction: a model of neutrophil and complement mediated injury. In Zweifach B, Grant L, McCluskey R (Eds): *The Inflammatory Process*, Academic Press, New York, 1974, pp 85–162.

45. Meltzer MS, Nacy CA: Delayed-type hypersensitivity and the induction of activated, cytotoxic macrophages. In Paul WE (Ed): *Fundamental Immunology*, 2nd ed. Raven, New York, 1989, pp 765–780.

46. Poulter LW, Seymour GJ, Duke O, Janossy G, Panayi G: Immunohistological analysis of delayed-type hypersensitivity in man. Cell Immunol 74:358, 1982.

47. Todd JA, Steinman L: Autoimmunity. Curr Op Ophthalmol 4:699, 1992.

48. Lee M, Sarvetnick N: Transgenes in autoimmunity. Curr Op Ophthalmol 4:723, 1992.

49. Bauman GP, Hurtubise P: Anti-idiotypes and autoimmune disease. Clin Lab Med 8:399, 1988.

50. Postlethwaite AE, Snyderman R, Kang AH: The chemotactic attraction of human fibroblasts to a lymphocyte-derived factor. J Exp Med 144:1188, 1976.

51. Postlethwaite AE, Kang AH: Characterization of guinea pig lymphocyte-derived chemotactic factor for fibroblasts. J Immunol 124:1462, 1980.

52. Seppa H, Seppa S, Yamada KM: The cell binding fragment of fibronectin and platelet-derived growth factor are chemoattractants for fibroblasts. J Cell Biol 87:323, 1980.

53. Mensing H, Czarnetozki BM: Leukotriene B$_4$ induces *in vitro* fibroblast chemotaxis. J Invest Dermatol 82:9, 1984.

54. Postlethwaite AE, Snyderman R, Kang AH: Generation of a fibroblast chemotactic factor in serum by activation of complement. J Clin Invest 64:1379, 1979.

55. Postlethwaite AE, Seyer JM, Kang AH: Chemotactic attraction of human fibroblasts to type I, II, and III collagens and collagen-derived peptides. Proc Natl Acad Sci USA 75:871, 1978.

56. Senior RM, Griffin GL, Mecham RP, Wrenn DS, Prasad KU, Urry DW: Val-Gly-Val-Ala-Pro-Gly, a repeating peptide in elastin, is chemotactic for fibroblasts and monocytes. J Cell Biol 99:870, 1984.

57. Postlethwaite AE, Keski-Oja J, Kang AH: Induction of fibroblast chemotaxis by fibronectin. Localization of the chemotactic region to a 140,000 molecular weight. J Exp Med 153:494, 1981.

58. Postlethwaite AE, Smith GN, Mainardi CL, Seyer JM, Kang AH: Lymphocyte modulation of fibroblast functions *in vitro*: stimulation and inhibition of collagen production by different effector molecules. J Immunol 132:2470, 1984.

59. Postlethwaite AE, Raghow R, Stricklin GP, Poppleton H, Seyer JM, Kang AH: Modulation of fibroblast functions by human recombinant interleukin 1: increased steady-state accumulation of type I procollagen messenger RNAs and stimulation of other functions but not chemotaxis by human recombinant interleukin 1 α and β. J Cell Biol 106:311, 1988.

60. Schmidt JA, Mizel SB, Cohen D, Green I: Interleukin 1, a potential regulator of fibroblast proliferation. J Immunol 128:2177, 1982.

61. Duncan MR, Berman D: Gamma interferon is the lymphokine and beta interferon the monokine responsible for inhibition of fibroblast collagen production and late but not early fibroblast proliferation. J Exp Med 162:516, 1985.

62. Jimenez SA, Freundlich B, Rosenbloom J: Selective inhibition of human diploid fibroblast collagen synthesis by interferons. J Clin Invest 74:1112, 1984.

63. Postlethwaite AE, Lachman L, Mainardi CL, Kang AH: Stimulation of fibroblast collagenase production by human interleukin 1. J Exp Med 157:801, 1983.

64. Al-Adnani MS, McGee JOD: C1q production and secretion by fibroblasts. Nature (London) 263:145, 1976.

65. Reid KBM, Solomon E: Biosynthesis of the first component of complement by human fibroblasts. Biochem J 167:647, 1977.

66. Rothman BL, Merrow M, Despins A, Kennedy T, Kreutzer DL: Effect of lipopolysaccharide on C3 and C5 production by human lung cells. J Immunol 143:196, 1989.

67. Reid JBM, Porter RR: Subunit composition and structure of subcomponent C1q of the first component of human complement. Biochem J 155:19, 1976.

68. Chu ML, DeWet W, Bernard M, Ding JF, Mosabito LM, Meyers J, Williams C, Ramirez F: Human pro-α_1(I) collagen gene structure reveals evolutionary conservation of a pattern of introns and exons. Nature (London) 310:337, 1984.

69. Katz Y, Strunk RC: IL-1 and tumor necrosis factor: similarities and differences in stimulation of expression of alternate pathway of complement and IFN-β2/IL-6 genes in human fibroblasts. J Immunol 142:3862, 1989.

70. Katz Y, Strunk RC: Synthesis and regulation of C1 inhibitor in human skin fibroblasts. J Immunol 142:2041, 1989.

71. Katz Y, Cole FS, Struck RC: Synergism between gamma-interferon and lipopolysaccharide for synthesis of Factor B, but not C2, in human fibroblasts. J Exp Med 167:1, 1988.

72. Fujikawa LS, Colvin RB, Bhan AK, Fuller TC, Foster CS: Expression of HLA-A/B/C and -DR locus antigens on epithelial, stromal, and endothelial cells of the human cornea. Cornea 1:213, 1982.

73. William KA, Ash JK, Coster DJ: Histocompatibility antigen and passenger cell content of normal and diseased human cornea. Transplantation 39:265, 1985.

74. Whitsett CF, Stulting RD: The distribution of HLA antigens on human corneal tissue. Invest Ophthalmol Vis Sci 25:519, 1984.

75. Young E, Stark WJ, Prendergast RA: Immunology of corneal allograft rejection: HLA-DR antigens on human corneal cells. Invest Ophthalmol Vis Sci 26:571, 1985.

76. Dreizen NG, Whitsett CF, Stulting RD: Modulation of HLA antigen expression on corneal epithelial and stromal cells. Invest Ophthalmol Vis Sci 29:933, 1988.

77. Harrison SA, Mondino BJ, Kagan JM: Modulation of HLA antigen expression on conjunctival fibroblasts by gamma-interferon. Invest Ophthalmol Vis Sci 31:163, 1990.

78. Zucali JR, Dinarello JA, Oblon DJ, Gross MA, Anderson L, Weiner RS: Interleukin 1 stimulates fibroblasts to produce granulocyte–macrophage colony stimulating activity and prostaglandin E$_2$. J Clin Invest 77:1857, 1986.

79. Brawman-Mintzer O, Mondino BJ, Mayer FJ: The complement system in sclera. Invest Ophthalmol Vis Sci 29:1756, 1988.

80. Brawman-Mintzer O, Mondino BJ, Mayer FJ: Distribution of complement in the sclera. Invest Ophthalmol Vis Sci 30:2240, 1989.

81. Harrison SA, Mondino BJ, Mayer FJ: Scleral fibroblasts. Invest Ophthalmol Vis Sci 31:2412, 1990.

82. Rao NA, Marak GE, Hidayat AA: Necrotizing scleritis: a clinicopathologic study of 41 cases. Ophthalmology 92:1542, 1985.

83. Pitzalis C, Kingsley G, Lanchbury JS, Murphy J, Panayi G: Expression of HLA-DR, DQ and DP antigens and interleukin-2 receptor on synovial fluid T lymphocyte subsets in rheumatoid arthritis: evidence for "frustrated" activation. J Rheumatol 14:662, 1987.

84. Zoschke D, Segall M: Dw subtypes of DR4 in rheumatoid arthritis: evidence for a preferential association with Dw4. Hum Immunol 15:118, 1986.

85. Nepom GT, Byers P, Seyfried C, Healey LA, Wilske KR, Stage D, Nepom BS: HLA genes associated with rheumatoid arthritis: identification of susceptibility alleles using specific oligonucleotide probes. Arthritis Rheum 32:15, 1989.

86. Robb JA: Virus–cell interactions: a classification of viruses causing human disease. Prog Med Virol 23:51, 1977.

87. Wheelcock EE, Toy ST: Participation of lymphocytes in viral infections. Adv Immunol 16:123, 1973.

88. Woodruff JF, Woodruff JJ: Lymphocyte interaction with viruses and virus-infected tissues. Prog Med Virol 19:120, 1975.

89. Venables PJW: Infection and rheumatoid arthritis. Curr Opin Rheumatol 1:15, 1989.

90. Phillips PE: Evidence implicating infectious agents in rheumatoid arthritis and juvenile rheumatoid arthritis. Clin Exp Rheumatol 6:87, 1988.

91. Alspaugh MA, Henle G, Lennette ET, Henle W: Elevated levels of antibodies to Epstein–Barr virus antigens in sera and synovial fluids of patients with rheumatoid arthritis. J Clin Invest 67:1134, 1981.

92. Slaughter L, Carson DA, Jensen FC, Holbrook TL, Vaughn JH: *In vitro* effects of Epstein–Barr virus on peripheral blood mononuclear cells from patients with rheumatoid arthritis and normal subjects. J Exp Med 148:1429, 1978.

93. Yao QY, Rickinson AB, Gaston JS, Epstein MA: Disturbance of the Epstein–Barr virus–host balance in rheumatoid arthritis patients: a quantitative study. Clin Exp Immunol 64:302, 1986.

94. Silverman SL, Schumacher HR: Antibodies to Epstein–Barr viral antigens in early rheumatoid arthritis. Arthritis Rheum 24:1465, 1981.

95. Roudier J, Petersen J, Rhodes GH, Luka J, Carson DA: Susceptibility to rheumatoid arthritis maps to a T-cell epitope shared by the HLA-Dw4 DR β-1 chain and the Epstein–Barr virus glycoprotein gp110. Proc Natl Acad Sci USA 86:5104, 1989.

96. Roudier J, Rhodes GH, Petersen J, Vaughan JH, Carson DA: The Epstein–Barr virus glycoprotein gp110, a molecular link between HLA-DR4, HLA-DR1, and rheumatoid arthritis. Scand J Immunol 27:367, 1988.

97. Cohen BJ, Buckley MM, Clewley JP, Jones VE, Puttick AH, Jacoby RK: Human parvovirus infection in early rheumatoid and inflammatory arthritis. Ann Rheum Dis 45:832, 1986.

98. Naides SJ, Field EH: Transient rheumatoid factor positivity in acute human parvovirus B19 infection. Arch Intern Med 148:2587, 1988.

99. van Eden W, Thole JE, van der Zee R, Noordzij A, van Embden JDA, Hensen EJ, Cohen IR: Cloning of the mycobacterial epitope recognized by T lymphocytes in adjuvant arthritis. Nature (London) 331:171, 1988.

100. Tsoulfa G, Rook GA, van-Embden JDA, Young DB, Mehlert A, Isenberg DA, Hay FC, Lydyard AP: Raised serum IgG and IgA antibodies to mycobacterial antigens in rheumatoid arthritis. Ann Rheum Dis 48:118, 1989.

101. Holoshitz J, Koning F, Coligan JE, DeBruyn J, Strober S: Isolation of CD4-CD8-mycobacteria-reactive T lymphocyte clones from rheumatoid arthritis synovial fluid. Nature (London) 339:226, 1989.

102. Trentham DE, Townes AS, Kang AH, David JR: Humoral and cellular sensitivity to collagen in type II collagen-induced arthritis in rats. J Clin Invest 61:89, 1978.

103. Eguro H, Goldner JL: Antigenic properties of chondromucoprotein and inducibility of experimental arthritis antichondromucoprotein immune globulin. J Bone Jt Surg 56A:129, 1974.

104. Keiser H, Sandson JI: Immunodiffusion and gel-electrophoretic studies of human articular cartilage proteoglycan. Arthritis Rheum 17:219, 1974.

105. Glant T, Hadas E, Nagy M: Cell-mediated and humoral immune responses to cartilage antigenic components. Scand J Immunol 9:39, 1979.

106. Endler AT, Zielinski CH, Menzel EJ, Smolen JS, Schwägerl W, Endler M, Eberl R, Frank O, Steffen C: Leucocyte migration inhibition with collagen type I and collagen type III in rheumatoid arthritis and degenerative joint diseases. Z Rheumatol 37:87, 1978.

107. Trentham DE, Dynesius RA, Rocklin RE, David JR: Cellular sensitivity to collagen in rheumatoid arthritis. N Engl J Med 299:327, 1978.

108. Mestecky J, Miller EJ: Presence of antibodies specific to cartilage-type collagen in rheumatoid synovial tissue. Clin Exp Immunol 22:453, 1975.

109. Glant T, Csongor, Szücs T: Immunopathologic role of proteoglycan antigens in rheumatoid joint disease. Scand J Immunol 11:247, 1980.

110. van der Eerden JJJM, Broekhuyse RM: Ocular antigens. III. Localization of immunogenic determinants of structural glycoproteins from lens capsule, corneal stroma and sclera in connective tissues of the eye. Ophthal Res 5:47, 1973.

111. Glant T, Hadhazy CS, Csernyanszky H: Species-common antigen of connective tissues. Acta Biol Acad Sci Hung 26:197, 1975.

112. Perkins ES: The antigenic relationships of ocular and other tissues. Trans Ophthalmol Soc UK 83:271, 1963.

113. van der Eerden JJJM, Brokhuyse RM: Ocular antigens. IV. A comparative study of the localization of immunogenic determinants of ocular structural glycoproteins in connective tissues of various organs. Ophthal Res 5:65, 1973.

114. Coster L, Rosenberg LC, van der Rest M, Poole AR: The dermatan sulfate proteoglycans of bovine sclera and their relationship to those of articular cartilage. J Biol Chem 262:3809, 1987.

115. Scott JE: Collagen–proteoglycan interactions. Biochem J 187:887, 1980.

116. Scott JE, Oxford CR: Dermatan sulphate-rich proteoglycan associates with rat tail-tendon collagen at the d band in the gap region. Biochem J 197:213, 1981.

117. Birk DE, Lande MA: Corneal and scleral collagen fiber formation in vitro. Biochim Biophys Acta 670:362, 1981.

118. Vogel KG, Paulsson M, Heinegard D: Specific inhibition of type I and type II collagen fibrillogenesis by the small proteoglycan of tendon. Biochem J 223:587, 1984.

119. Trentham DE, Townes AS, Kang AH: Autoimmunity to type II collagen: an experimental model of arthritis. J Exp Med 146:857, 1977.

120. Trentham DE, Dynesius RA, David JR: Passive transfer by cells of type II collagen-induced arthritis in rats. J Clin Invest 62:359, 1978.

121. Trentham DE, Dynesius RA, Rocklin RE, David JR: Cellular sensitivity to collagen in rheumatoid arthritis. New Engl J Med 299:327, 1978.

122. Trentham DE, Townes AS, Kang AH, David JR: Humoral and cellular sensitivity to collagen in type II collagen-induced arthritis in rats. J Clin Invest 61:89, 1978.

123. Trentham DE: Collagen arthritis as a relevant model for rheumatoid arthritis: Evidence pro and con. Arthritis Rheum 25:911, 1982.

124. Möttönen T, Hannonen P, Oka M, Rautiainen J, Jokinen I, Arvilommi H, Palosuo T, Aho K: Antibodies against native type II collagen do not precede the clinical onset of rheumatoid arthritis. Arthritis Rheum 31:776, 1988.

125. Jasin HE: Autoantibody specificities of immune complexes sequestered in articular cartilage of patients with rheumatoid arthritis and osteoarthritis. Arthritis Rheum 28:241, 1985.

126. Hylkema HA, Kijlstra A: Ocular localization of preformed immune complexes. In O'Connor GR, Chandler JW (Eds): *Advances in Immunology and Immunopathology of the Eye.* Masson, New York, 1985.

127. Fauci A, Haynes B, Katz P: The spectrum of vasculitis: clinical, pathological, immunologic, and therapeutic considerations. Ann Intern Med 89:660, 1978.

128. van Es LA, Dana MR, Valentijn RM, Kaufman RH: The pathogenic significance of circulating immune complexes. Neth J Med 27:350, 1984.

129. Weiss A, Imboden J, Hardy K, Manger B, Terhorst C, Stobo J: The role of the T3/antigen receptor complex in T-cell activation. Annu Rev Immunol 4:593, 1986.

130. Wooley DE: Mammalian collagenases. In Piez KA, Reddi AH (Eds): *Extracellular Matrix Biochemistry.* Elsevier, New York, 1984.

131. Gosline JM, Rosenbloom J: Elastin. In Piez KA, Reddi AH (Eds): *Extracellular Matrix Biochemistry.* Elsevier, New York, 1984.

132. Sandy JD, Brown HLG, Lowther DA: Degradation of proteoglycan in articular cartilage. Biochim Biophys Acta 543:536, 1978.

133. Hakomori S, Fukuda M, Sekiguchi K, Carter WB: Fibronectin, laminin, and other extracellular glycoproteins. In Piez KA, Reddi AH (Eds): *Extracellular Matrix Biochemistry.* Elsevier, New York, 1984.

134. Herman JH, Wiltse DW, Dennis MV: Immunopathologic significance of cartilage antigenic components in rheumatoid arthritis. Arthritis Rheum 16:287, 1973.

135. Inman RD, Hamilton NC, Redecha PB, Hochhauser DM: Electrophoretic transfer blotting analysis of immune complexes in rheumatoid arthritis. Clin Exp Immunol 63:32, 1986.

136. Rapoport R, Kozin F, Mackel S, Jordon R: Cutaneous vascular immunofluorescence in rheumatoid arthritis. Am J Med 68:325, 1980.

137. Jasin HE: Mechanism of trapping of immune complexes in joint collagenous tissues. Clin Exp Immunol 22:473, 1975.

138. Theofilopoulos A: Evaluation and clinical significance of circulating immune complexes. Prog Clin Immunol 4:63, 1980.

139. Gocke D, Hsu K, Morgan C, Bombarieri S, Lochshin M, Christain C: Association between polyarteritis and Australia antigen. Lancet 2:1149, 1970.

140. Ronco P, Verrous T, Mignon F, Kourilsly D, Van Hille P, Meyrier A, Mery J, Morel-Maroger L: Immunopathological studies of polyarteritis nodosa and Wegener's granulomatosis. A report of 43 patients with renal biopsies. Q J Med 52:121, 1983.

141. Howell S, Epstein W: Circulating immune complexes in Wegener's granulomatosis. Am J Med 60:259, 1976.

142. Horn R, Fauci A, Rosenthal A, Wolff S: Renal biopsy pathology in Wegener's granulomatosis. Am J Pathol 74:423, 1974.

143. Pinching A, Lokckwood C, Pussell BA, Rees A, Swaney P, Evans D, Bowley N, Peters D: Wegener's granulomatosis: observations on 18 patients with severe renal disease. Q J Med 208:435, 1983.

144. Shasby D, Schwarz M, Forstot J: Pulmonary immune complex deposition in Wegener's granulomatosis. Chest 81:338, 1982.

145. Pope RM, Teller DC, Mannik M: The molecular basis of self-association of antibodies to IgG (rheumatoid factor) in rheumatoid

arthritis. Proc Natl Acad Sci USA 71:517, 1974.

146. Pitzalis C, Kingsley G, Haskard D, Panayi G: The preferential accumulation of helper-inducer T lymphocytes in inflammatory lesions: evidence for regulation by selective endothelial and homotypic adhesion. Eur J Immunol 18:1397, 1988.

147. van Boxel JA, Paget SA: Predominantly T-cell infiltrate in rheumatoid synovial membranes. N Engl J Med 293:517, 1975.

148. Pitzalis C, Kingsley G, Lanchbury JS, Murphy J, Panayi G: Abnormal distribution of the helper-inducer and suppressor-induced T-lymphocyte subsets in the rheumatoid joint. Clin Immunol Immunopathol 45:252, 1987.

149. Lasky HP, Bauer K, Pope RM: Increased helper inducer and decreased suppressor inducer phenotypes in the rheumatoid joint. Arthritis Rheum 31:52, 1988.

150. Hembry RM, Playfair J, Watson PG, Dingle JT: Experimental model for scleritis. Arch Ophthalmol 97:1337, 1979.

151. Christian C, Sargent J: Vasculitis syndromes: clinical and experimental models. Am J Med 61:385, 1976.

3
Diagnostic Approach to Episcleritis and Scleritis

Scleral inflammation gives rise to a spectrum of conditions, ranging from a trivial, self-limiting episode to a vision-threatening necrotizing process. Clinical differentiation of these conditions is important because they follow different courses and have different prognostic significance. Several classifications have been proposed on the basis of clinical, clinicopathological, and etiological aspects. The most frequently used is based on the anatomical site of the inflammation and on the clinical appearance of the disease at presentation (Table 3.1). This classification, proposed by Watson and Hayreh,[1] has proved to be satisfactory because it enables one to assign most patients to a particular category and subcategory at the initial clinical examination, with almost no changes over the course of the disease. Two main groups can be differentiated: episcleritis and scleritis (Figs. 3.1 and 3.2; see color insert). Episcleritis is a benign recurrent disease with little systemic disease association, whereas scleritis not only can cause great pain, loss of vision, and in some cases destruction of the eye, but also may portend an underlying, potentially lethal systemic disease (Table 3.2). There are distinct clinical patterns that help to distinguish episcleritis from scleritis. There are also distinguishing features that may help uncover the underlying systemic diseases. Early detection and characterization of the scleral and systemic disease leads to early treatment, which can improve both ocular and systemic prognoses. This chapter provides specific guidelines for a diagnostic approach in patients with episcleritis and scleritis.

Although the process of clinical reasoning in medicine is based on several subjective factors such as interpretation of evidence, deductive reasoning, experience, and intuition, attempts at specific sequential analysis of the process can improve the ways in which the problems of individual patients are approached and solved. In a simplified model, the specific approach in clinical problem solving that can be applied to scleritis includes five phases (Table 3.3). The first phase includes investigation of the illness through the interview and physical examination of the patient. Constructing a diagnostic hypothesis generates more questions, answers to which determine which possibilities best fit the illness. As the ophthalmologist completes this phase, possible diagnoses come to mind. The second phase consists of selection of diagnostic tests, each with its own level of accuracy and usefulness for investigating the possibilities raised in the former phase. Because relatively few tests can be used to effectively establish the diagnosis of the underlying systemic disease associated with episcleritis and scleritis, the ophthalmologist can be selective and parsimonious in the request for tests. The third phase includes the decision as to whether a tissue biopsy should be performed. Biopsies can be costly, time consuming, and entail some discomfort; it is important, therefore, to consider whether or not the results are likely to add useful information to the diagnosis solving

TABLE 3.1. Clinical classification of episcleral and scleral inflammation.[a]

Episcleritis
  Simple
  Nodular
Scleritis
  Anterior scleritis
    Diffuse scleritis
    Nodular scleritis
    Necrotizing scleritis
      With inflammation
      Without inflammation (scleromalacia perforans)
  Posterior scleritis

[a] Adapted from Ref. 1.

process. In the fourth phase, the clinical data must be integrated with test and biopsy results to confirm or discard the preliminary diagnoses. In the fifth and final phase, the comparative risks and benefits of therapeutic possibilities for the particular diagnosis is presented to the patient and, after appropiate discussion of the

options, a therapeutic plan is initiated and the response to therapy observed. Each step in this simplified model of the clinical approach to scleral disease can be analyzed individually.

3.1. Investigation of the Illness

The first phase consists of the interview and the physical examination of the patient. During the interview the ophthalmologist evaluates the major complaint, characteristics of the present illness, past and family diseases, and past and present therapies; a review of systems is made as well. The physical examination is made not only of the eye, but also of the head and extremities.

3.1.1. Major Complaint and History of Present Illness

The major complaint is the main problem that motivated the patient to seek medical help.

TABLE 3.2. Diseases associated with episcleritis and scleritis.

Noninfectious
  Connective tissue diseases and other inflammatory conditions
    Rheumatoid arthritis
    Systemic lupus erythematosus
    Ankylosing spondylitis
    Reiter's syndrome
    Psoriatic arthritis
    Arthritis and inflammatory bowel disease
    Relapsing polychondritis
  Vasculitic diseases
    Polyarteritis nodosa
    Allergic granulomatous angiitis (Churg–Strauss syndrome)
    Wegener's granulomatosis
    Behçet's disease
    Giant cell arteritis
    Cogan's syndrome
    Vasculitic diseases associated with connective tissue diseases and other
      inflammatory conditions
  Miscellaneous
    Atopy
    Rosacea
    Gout
    Foreign body granuloma
    Chemical injury
Infectious
  Bacterial
  Fungal
  Viral
  Parasitical

TABLE 3.3. Phases of clinical approach to episcleritis and scleritis.

---

1. Investigation of the illness
   Interview
     Major complaint
     History of present illness
     Past history
     Family history
     Past and present therapy history
     Review of systems
   Physical examination
     Systemic examination
       Head
       Extremities
     Ocular examination
       Episclera and sclera
       Other ocular structures
2. Diagnostic tests
   Blood and urine tests
   Imaging studies
3. Tissue biopsy
4. Integration of clinical findings with test and biopsy results
5. Therapeutic plan
   Assessment of different therapeutic possibilities
   Discussion of risks and benefits with patient

The ophthalmologist must begin with an open-ended question to allow the patient to freely describe the major complaint and the history of the present illness. Even though this may result in a disjointed and incomplete story, inflections of voice, facial expression, descriptive efforts with hands, and attitude may betray important clues to the meaning of what the patient has been experiencing. The ophthalmologist should actively guide the interview in order to develop organization and content, to clarify terms the patient uses, and to evaluate symptoms as of little or considerable importance. Severity of symptoms may be estimated by the extent to which they interfere with sleep or work patterns. The patient soon learns that events must be dated, sequences established, and onset and characteristics of symptoms precisely described. The main symptoms present in scleral diseases are the following.

1. *Pain* is the most common symptom for which patients with scleral disorders seek medical assistance, and is the best indicator of the presence of active inflammation. It is due to both direct stimulation and stretching of the nerve endings by the inflammation. Important issues to consider in pain evaluation are the patient's age, cultural background, environment, and psychological circumstances such as depression, anxiety, and tension. Inquiry should be made concerning character, location, radiation, timing, and analgesic response. No pain, mild discomfort, or occasional pain localized to the eye, is characteristic of episcleritis. Severe, penetrating pain that radiates to the forehead, the brow, the jaw, or the sinuses, awakens the patient during the night, and is only temporarily relieved by analgesics, is characteristic of scleritis. Differential diagnoses of other painful eye diseases, including corneal surface problems, angle-closure glaucoma, and acute anterior uveitis, are easily excluded by ocular examination. Differential diagnoses of other painful periocular diseases, including migraine, sinusitis, herpes zoster ophthalmicus, and orbital tumors, are excluded by careful ocular and periocular examination, and additional imaging studies.

2. *Redness*, although not a symptom, can be detected by the patient's family or friends, or by the patient while looking in the mirror. Almost all patients with episcleritis and scleritis present to the physician with redness as a clinical manifestation. Clinically obvious redness may be absent in scleromalacia perforans (necrotizing scleritis without inflammation) and in posterior scleritis.

3. *Tearing* or *photophobia* without mucopurulent discharge occurs in approximately one-fourth of patients with episcleral and scleral inflammation, but is usually mild or moderate.

4. *Tenderness* to palpation may be described by the patient. In general, ocular tenderness will be localized to the site of inflammation in episcleritis or will be diffuse with possible radiation to other parts of the head in true scleritis.

5. *Decreased visual acuity* is almost never a symptom of episcleritis but is a common finding in scleritis. The extension of the scleral inflammation to the adjacent structures may cause keratitis, uveitis, glaucoma, papillitis, macular edema, annular ciliochoroidal detachment, and

serous retinal detachment; these abnormalities may impair visual acuity.

3.1.2. Past History

The past medical and ocular history elicitation serves primarily to discover already known systemic diseases that can be causing the presence of scleritis (Table 3.2). Past ocular surgical procedures, especially within a year prior to the onset of scleritis, can have potential diagnostic importance. Determination of past medical history is also important for discovering certain conditions, such as gastric ulceration, diabetes, liver or renal disease, or hypertension, that might eventually modify future therapy.

3.1.3. Family History

The family history can be important in several respects. The growing field of immunogenetics has demonstrated that diseases frequently associated with scleritis, such as rheumatoid arthritis, systemic lupus erythematosus, ankylosing spondylitis, Reiter's syndrome, Behçet's disease, atopy, and gout, have a genetic basis. This information may give clues for specific systemic diagnoses that can be pursued with additional studies. Also, psychological factors such as attitudes toward illness, fears, and expectations can be assessed from previous illnesses within the family.

3.1.4. Past and Present Therapy History

The history of past and present therapies and response to them is extremely important. Type of therapy, route of administration, dosage, response, side effects, complications, concomitant treatments for other conditions, and reasons for discontinuation often provide insight about the nature of the illness and for future therapeutic decision making. Careful attention to detail may often reveal simple, correctable mistakes, such as inadequate dosage; poor compliance, too short a trial of a slow-acting medication; medications given for other conditions; or foods that interfere with medications prescribed for the scleritis.

There is a great variability in patient response to nonsteroidal antiinflammatory drugs. Sometimes one nonsteroidal antiinflammatory drug may be better than another for a particular patient; therefore, inadequate response to one nonsteroidal antiinflammatory drug does not indicate probable unresponsiveness to other nonsteroidal antiinflammatory drugs. Furthermore, at least 2 to 4 weeks is required for full evaluation of a particular nonsteroidal antiinflammatory agent. Therefore caution is indicated in drawing conclusions from the therapeutic response to only one type of nonsteroidal antiinflammatory drug or from responses to nonsteroidal antiinflammatory drugs used for brief periods.

The most important features of the steroid therapy history include the length of therapy, the route of administration, the maximal and average doses, the side effects, and whether periodic attempts to decrease the dose were made (and if so, the size of the decrements). This historical information may be essential in deciding whether to initiate immunosuppressive therapy.

The patient should be asked whether he or she has ever used immunosuppressive drugs; type, dosage, response, and side effects are extremely important to future treatment planning.

3.1.5. Review of Systems

Because episcleritis and especially scleritis can be associated with systemic disorders, a routine inquiry covering the different systems of the body should be made. Systemic manifestations may lead the ophthalmologist to suspect certain types of disorders, such as connective tissue diseases with or without vasculitis, atopy, rosacea, gout, and infectious diseases. Our review of systems questionnaire for episcleritis and scleritis, with the corresponding associated systemic diseases, is shown in Table 3.4.

Constitutional symptoms such as chills, fever, poor appetite, recent weight loss, and fatigue may suggest a systemic process. Skin lesions, including rashes, vesicles, and ulcers, may be manifestations of connective tissue, vasculitic, and infectious diseases; they also may be present in atopy and rosacea. Hair abnormalities

TABLE 3.4. Review of systems questionnaire for episcleritis and scleritis.

Manifestations	Associated systemic diseases[a]
Skin, hair, and nails	
Rash/vesicles/ulcers	Connective tissue, vasculitic, and infectious diseases, atopy, Ros
Sunburn easily	SLE
Hyper/depigmentation	SLE, leprosy
Loss of hair	SLE, leprosy
Painfully cold fingers	RA, SLE, GCA
Scaling	Reit, PA, atopy
Nail lesions	Reit, PA, vasculitic diseases
Respiratory	
Constant coughing	RA, SLE, AS, RP, Ch-S, Weg, TB, Lyme
Coughing blood	RA, SLE, AS, Weg, TB
Shortness of breath	RA, SLE, AS, RP, Ch-S, Weg, Atopy, TB
Asthma attacks	Ch-S, atopy
Pneumonia	SLE, AS, RP, Ch-S, Weg, atopy, TB
Cardiac	
Anginal chest pain	RA, SLE, PAN, GCA
Genitourinary	
Blood in urine	SLE, Reit, RP, PAN, Ch-S, Weg, TB
Urinary discharge	Reit
Pain during urination	Reit
Prostate trouble	AS, Reit, IBD, Ch-S, TB
Testicular pain	PAN, mumps, Lyme
Genital lesions	Reit, Behçet, mumps, TB, Syph
Kidney stones	Gout, IBD
Rheumatological	
Painful joints	Connective tissue and vasculitic diseases, gout, TB, Lyme
Morning stiffness	RA, SLE, AS
Muscle aches	RA, SLE, AS, PAN, GCA, Lyme
Back pain	AS, Reit, PA, IBD
Heel pain	AS, Reit, gout
Big toe pain	Gout, PA
Gastrointestinal	
Abdominal pain	SLE, Reit, IBD, PAN, Ch-S, Behçet
Nausea, vomiting	SLE, IBD, RP, PAN, Cogan
Difficult swallowing	RA, SLE
Blood in stool	IBD, PAN, Ch-S, Behçet
Diarrhea	SLE, Reit, IBD, PAN
Constipation	IBD
Anal lesions	IBD
Neurological	
Headaches	SLE, RP, GCA, mumps, Lyme
Numbness/tingling	Connective tissue, vasculitic, and infectious diseases
Paralysis	Connective tissue, vasculitic, and infectious diseases
Seizures	SLE, RP, PAN, Ch-S, mumps, Lyme
Psychiatric	SLE, Reit, Ch-S, Behçet, GCA, mumps, Lyme
Neuralgia	Leprosy, VZV
Ear	
Deafness	RP, Weg, GCA, Cogan, mumps, Syph
Swollen ear lobes	RP
Ear infections	RP, Weg
Vertigo	RP, Cogan
Noises in ears	RP, Cogan

TABLE 3.4. *Continued*

Manifestations	Associated systemic diseases[a]
Nose/sinus	
Nasal mucosal ulcers	SLE, Weg
Rhinitis/nosebleeds	Weg, atopy, leprosy, Syph
Swollen nasal bridge	RP, leprosy, Syph
Sinus trouble	Weg
Mouth/throat	
Oral mucosal ulcers	SLE, Reit, IBD, Behçet
Persistent hoarseness	RA, SLE, RP, leprosy
Jaw claudication	GCA

[a] SLE, Systemic lupus erythematosus; RA, rheumatoid arthritis; RP, relapsing polychondritis; PAN, polyarteritis nodosa; Weg, Wegener's granulomatosis; Ch-S, allergic granulomatous angiitis (Churg–Strauss syndrome); GCA, giant cell arteritis; Reit, Reiter's syndrome, PA, psoriatic arthritis; AS, ankylosing spondilitis; IBD, arthritis associated with inflammatory bowel disease; VZV, varicella-zoster virus (herpes zoster); Syph, syphilis; TB, tuberculosis; Ros, rosacea; Lyme, Lyme disease; Behçet, Behçet's disease; Cogan, Cogan's syndrome.

TABLE 3.5. General examination of the head and extremities in episcleritis and scleritis.

Clinical finding	Associated systemic disease[a]
Saddle nose deformity	RP, Weg, leprosy, Syph
Auricular pinna deformity	RP, leprosy
Nasal mucosal ulcers	Weg
Oral/lip/tongue mucosal ulcers	SLE, Reit, IBD, Behçet
Facial butterfly rash	SLE
Alopecia	SLE, Syph
Facial telangiectasias	SLE, Ros
Rhinophyma	Ros
Temporal artery erythema	GCA
Parotid enlargement	Mumps
Teeth abnormalities	Syph
Lymphadenopathy	RA, SLE, infectious disease
Skin hypopigmentation	RP, leprosy
Skin rashes	Connective tissue and vasculitic disease, Syph, atopy
Skin vesicles	VZV
Skin ulcers	Vasculitic disease
Skin scaling	SLE, Reit, PA, Syph
Ear/arms/legs tophi	Gout
Ulcers in fingertips	Vasculitic disease
Nail lesions	SLE, Reit, PA
Subcutaneous nodules	PA, SLE, PAN, Weg, Ch-S gout
Arthritis	Connective tissue, vasculitic, and infectious systemic diseases
Tendinitis	AS, Reit
Erythema nodosum	IBD, Behçet, TB

[a] SLE, Systemic lupus erythematosus; RA, rheumatoid arthritis; RP, relapsing polychondritis; PAN, polyarteritis nodosa; Weg, Wegener's granulomatosis; Ch-S, allergic granulomatous angiitis (Churg–Strauss syndrome); GCA, giant cell arteritis; Ros, rosacea; Reit, Reiter's syndrome; PA, psoriatic arthritis; IBD, arthritis associated with inflammatory bowel disease; VZV, varicella-zoster virus (herpes zoster); Syph, syphilis; TB, tuberculosis; Behçet, Behçet's disease; AS, ankylosing spondylitis.

such as hair loss may be found in systemic lupus erythematosus, and nail findings may be associated with Reiter's syndrome, psoriatic arthritis, and vasculitic diseases. Respiratory manifestations are most commonly present in allergic granulomatous angiitis (Churg–Strauss syndrome), Wegener's granulomatosis, systemic lupus erythematosus, atopy, and tuberculosis. Cardiac symptoms such as anginal chest pain may be found in some vasculitic diseases. Genitourinary lesions may suggest Reiter's syndrome, Wegener's granulomatosis, and polyarteritis nodosa. Rheumatological abnormalities may be present in any connective tissue or vasculitic disease and in many of the infectious diseases that may cause episcleritis or scleritis. Gastrointestinal symptoms are frequently found in systemic lupus erythematosus, polyarteritis nodosa, Reiter's syndrome, and inflammatory bowel disease. Neurological manifestations may be associated with connective tissue, vasculitic, and infectious diseases. Ear and nose abnormalities are commonly associated with relapsing polychondritis, Wegener's granulomatosis, and Cogan's syndrome. Mouth lesions such as oral ulcers are characteristically present in Behçet's disease.

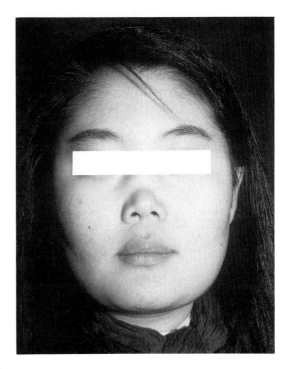

FIGURE 3.3. Loss of cartilage in both the nose (saddle nose deformity) and the ears ("floppy ears") is an important clue for diagnosis of relapsing polychondritis.

3.1.6. Systemic Examination

Physical signs are the objective marks of the disease and represent indisputable facts. Their significance is enhanced when they confirm a functional or structural change already suggested by the patient's history or review of systems. Sometimes, the physical signs may be the only evidence of disease, especially when the history has been inconsistent or confusing and the review of systems meaningless. Skill in physical diagnosis reflects a way of thinking more than a way of doing.

In a patient with a scleral disease, the examination of the head and extremities, including the nose, the mouth, the external ear, the skin, and the joints may reveal significant signs either ignored by the patient or considered as of little importance (Table 3.5).

3.1.6.1. Head

The detection of a "saddle nose" deformity and/or auricular pinna deformity can be important for the diagnosis of relapsing polychondritis (Fig. 3.3) or leprosy; a saddle nose deformity and/or nasal mucosal ulcers can be manifestations of Wegener's granulomatosis. Ulcers in the mouth, even if minimal, may guide one to the suspicion of systemic lupus erythematosus, Reiter's syndrome, arthritis associated with inflammatory bowel disease, or Behçet's disease (Fig. 3.4). A "butterfly" rash extending across the bridge of the nose to the malar areas and/or alopecia obligate one to consider systemic lupus erythematosus. Alopecia also can be a sign of syphilis. Erythema, telangiectasias, papules, or pustules on the forehead,

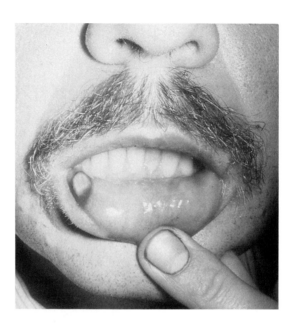

FIGURE 3.4. Classic aphthous ulcers can be important clues in the diagnosis of Behçet's disease.

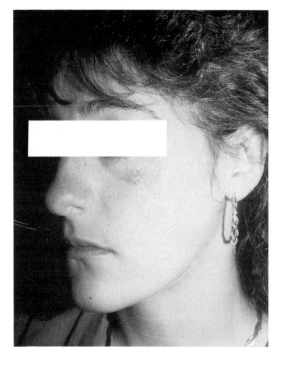

FIGURE 3.5. Rash on left lower lid and cheek suggested systemic lupus erythematosus, which was confirmed by a review of systems, blood tests, and biopsy.

cheek, nose, and chin with or without the presence of rhinophyma can establish the diagnosis of acne rosacea. The detection of a temporal artery tenderness obligates one to consider giant cell arteritis. The finding of parotid enlargement can lead to the diagnosis of mumps infection or sarcoidosis. 'Peg top' teeth and/or deafness and/or saddle nose deformity can be signs of congenital syphilis. Lymphadenopathy may be present in rheumatoid arthritis, systemic lupus erythematosus, or any infectious disease. The finding of hypopigmented areas may lead to the consideration of relapsing polychondritis or leprosy. A rash can be a manifestation of any vasculitic disease (Fig. 3.5), atopy, or syphilis. Vesicles in periocular areas, the forehead, or the tip of the nose may confirm a herpes zoster infection. Skin purpuric lesions or ulcers can be important clues for the diagnosis of any of the vasculitic diseases.

3.1.6.2. Extremities

The finding of nailbed thrombi (Fig. 3.6), small infarcts of the fingers, or purpuric lesions is suggestive of any vasculitic disease. Skin scaling may lead to the consideration of systemic lupus erythematosus, Reiter's syndrome, psoriatic arthritis, or syphilis. The presence of tophi in cartilage is an important clue for the diagnosis of gout. Nail abnormalities can be manifestations of Reiter's syndrome or psoriatic arthritis. The detection of subcutaneous nodules obliges one consider rheumatoid arthritis, systemic lupus erythematosus, polyarteritis nodosa, allergic granulomatous angiitis (Churg–Strauss syndrome), Wegener's granulomatosis, or gout (Fig. 3.7). The finding of articular abnormalities can be compatible with any of the systemic noninfectious or infectious diseases (Fig. 3.8). Erythema nodosum would make one consider inflammatory bowel disease, Behçet's disease, or tuberculosis.

3.1.7. Ocular Examination

Examination of the eye enables one to detect and characterize scleral disease. It is important to distinguish the benign, self-limiting, and frequently symptomless episcleritis from the much more severe, destructive, and often painful scleritis, which can lead to loss of vision and portend serious systemic disease. Early diagnosis may lead to early treatment of the ocular and general condition. Differentiation between the two entities and further characterization of each can be accomplished if the eye is

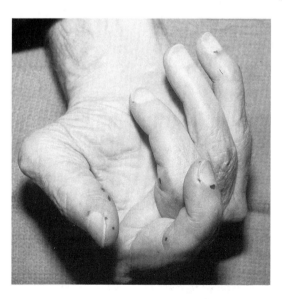

FIGURE 3.6. Vasculitic lesions on fingers and periungual infarcts in a patient with rheumatoid vasculitis and necrotizing scleritis.

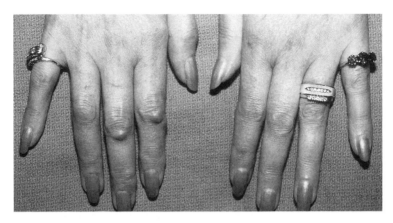

FIGURE 3.7. Subcutaneous nodules (right second and third digits) in a patient with rheumatoid arthritis.

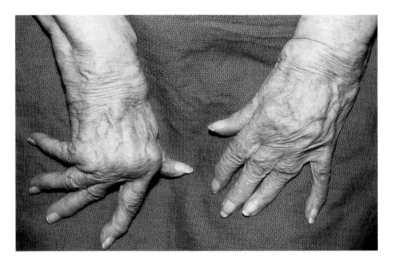

FIGURE 3.8. Characteristic rheumatoid joint disease with the "Z" deformity of wrist and metacarpal joints.

examined methodically and thoroughly, following a strict routine of examination.

3.1.7.1. Episcleral and Scleral Examination

Three vascular networks can be distinguished in the anterior segment of the eye: a conjunctival network, a superficial episcleral network, and a deep episcleral network (Fig. 3.9). In episcleritis, maximum congestion is in the superficial episcleral vascular network, with no changes in the deep episcleral network. The edema is localized to the episcleral tissue; the superficial episcleral network is displaced forward because of underlying episcleral edema, and the deep episcleral network remains flat (Fig. 3.10). In scleritis, maximum congestion is in the deep episcleral network, although there is also some congestion in the superficial episcleral network. The edema is localized to the scleral and episcleral tissue; the deep epi-

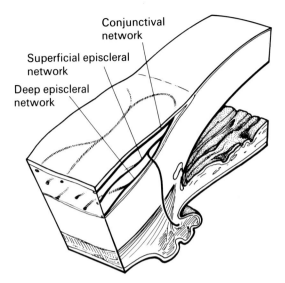

FIGURE 3.9. Three vascular networks can be distinguished in the anterior segment of the eye: the conjunctival network, the superficial episcleral network, and the deep episcleral network.

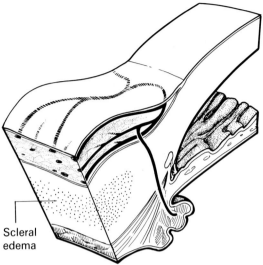

FIGURE 3.11. Scleritis. The edema is localized to the scleral and episcleral tissue; the deep and superficial episcleral networks are displaced forward because of underlying scleral and episcleral edema.

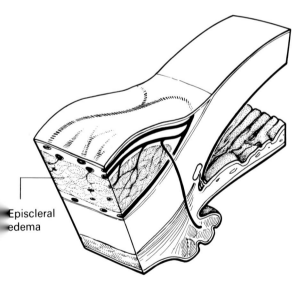

FIGURE 3.10. Episcleritis. The edema is localized to the episcleral tissue; the superficial episcleral network is displaced forward because of underlying episcleral edema, and the deep episcleral network remains flat.

scleral network is displaced forward because of underlying scleral edema and the superficial episcleral network is also displaced forward because of underlying episcleral and scleral edema (Fig. 3.11).

3.1.7.1.1. External Examination of the Eye in Daylight

External evaluation of the eye in daylight is sometimes the only way to distinguish episcleritis from scleritis, because tungsten and fluorescent lights do not disclose subtle color differences. In episcleritis, the eye appears bright red. In deep scleritis, the eye has a diffuse, grayish blue tinge; this is because after several attacks of scleral inflammation, the sclera may become more translucent and sometimes thinner, allowing the dark uvea to show through (Fig. 3.2).

A dark brown or black-tinged area surrounded by active scleral inflammation indicates that a necrotic process is taking place (Fig. 3.12). If tissue necrosis progresses, the scleral area can become avascular, producing a

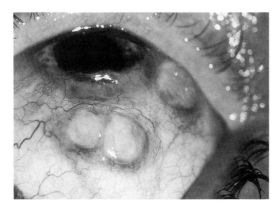

FIGURE 3.12. External examination in daylight may show an obvious diffuse, grayish blue tinge of the eye with scleritis; the presence of brownish areas indicates a necrotizing process.

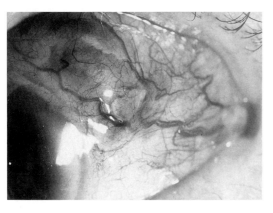

FIGURE 3.13. Necrotizing scleritis. Note the dark area surrounded by active inflammation, characteristic of a necrotizing process.

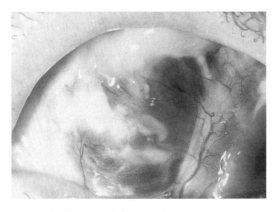

FIGURE 3.14. Necrotizing scleritis. The sequestrum is partially removed.

white sequestrum in the center surrounded by a well-defined dark brown or black circle (Fig. 3.13). The slough may be gradually removed by granulation tissue, leaving the underlying uvea bare or covered by a thin layer of conjunctiva (Fig. 3.14). The same necrotic process without surrounding inflammation is typical of scleromalacia perforans (Fig. 3.15).

The sclera in the elderly becomes thinner and more translucent because of a decrease in water content and proteoglycan content. This is accompanied by subconjunctival deposition of lipids, giving the sclera a yellowish color.[2] Calcium phosphate may be deposited in small rectangular areas just anterior to the insertions of medial and lateral rectus muscles in individuals over 70 years of age. These areas, called senile scleral plaques, may become translucent, showing a bluish or brownish color due to the underlying uvea (Fig. 3.16). This increase in translucency is clearly distinguished from that seen in scleral disease, after or without inflammation, because in scleritis the areas are less generalized, can have sequestra, and do not usually localize only on the insertions of the horizontal rectus muscles.

Color or black-and-white photography of the upper face, including both eyes, may show subtle color or shadow changes. This is an important way of documenting the condition for further evaluation of disease progression.

3.1.7.1.2. Slit-Lamp Examination

The slit-lamp examination serves mainly to reveal the depth of inflammation, determining which network of vessels is predominantly affected. Because episcleritis never involves sclera, the main object of slit-lamp illumination is to determine whether or not there is scleral edema.

3.1.7.1.2.1. Diffuse Illumination. Diffuse illumination by the slit-lamp confirms the macroscopic impression of avascular areas with sequestra and/or uveal show (Figs. 3.2 and 3.12–3.15). It also helps to differentiate the configuration of the vessels; in episcleritis congested vessels follow the usual radial pattern whereas in scleritis this pattern is altered and new, abnormal vessels are formed. This neovascularization usually takes place around the avascular areas (Fig. 3.17).

3.1.7.1.2.2. Slit-Lamp Illumination. Slit-lamp white illumination detects the depth of maximum vascular congestion and scleral edema. Because in episcleritis the vascular congestion is in the superficial episcleral network, the anterior edge of the slit-lamp is displaced forward because of underlying episcleral edema; the posterior edge of the slit-lamp beam is flat [Figs. 3.10 and 3.18 (see color insert)]. In scleritis the maximum vascular congestion is in the deep episcleral network; the posterior edge of the slit-lamp beam is displaced forward because of underlying scleral edema [Figs. 3.11 and 3.19 (see color insert)]. There is also some congestion in the superficial episcleral network; the anterior edge of the slit-lamp beam is displaced forward because of underlying episcleral and scleral edema. The topical application of a vasoconstrictor such as 10% phenylephrine makes detection of the congested episcleral network easier; because the vasoconstrictor blanches the superficial network without significant effect on the deep network, the eye will appear white in episcleritis but will remain congested in scleritis.

Slit-lamp illumination is also important in evaluating the depth and nature of associated corneal pathology (Fig. 3.20), the presence and degree of cells in the anterior chamber or vitreous, and the existence of synechiae.

3.1.7.1.2.3. Red-Free Illumination. Red-free illumination with a green filter in the slit-lamp helps determine with certainty the areas of maximum vascular congestion, the areas with new vascular channels, and the areas that are totally avascular.

Red-free illumination is also useful for further study of the areas of lymphocytic infiltration of the episcleral tissue, manifested as yellow spots; because these areas are found in episcleritis, their detection makes the differentiating between episcleritis and scleritis easier.

3.1.7.2. General Eye Examination

Episcleritis and scleritis can appear as isolated lesions or can be accompanied by other

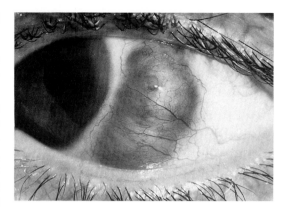

FIGURE 3.15. Necrotizing scleritis in same patient shown in Fig. 3.14; 1 year later, scleral loss has increased, leaving the underlying uvea covered by a thin layer of conjunctiva.

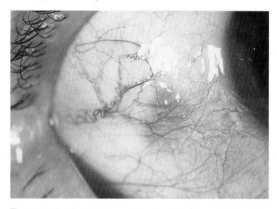

FIGURE 3.16. Senile scleral plaques. Note the brownish appearance anterior to the insertion of the lateral rectus muscle, due to scleral translucency secondary to calcium deposition.

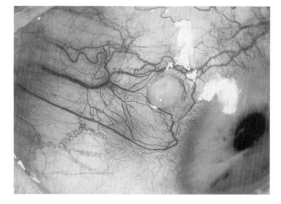

FIGURE 3.17. Diffuse illumination from a slit-lamp can show the altered pattern of congested vessels in scleritis; new vessel formation around the avascular areas may appear in necrotizing scleritis.

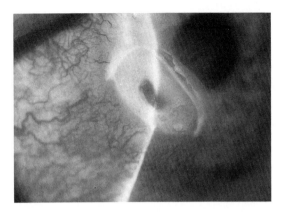

FIGURE 3.20. Slit-lamp illumination may help to evaluate the depth of corneal involvement; this patient had peripheral ulcerative keratitis and necrotizing scleritis associated with rheumatoid arthritis.

ment, keratitis, uveitis, cataract, glaucoma, disk edema, and macular edema. Concomitant manifestations of episcleritis and scleritis include any other ocular abnormalities present as part of the same systemic inflammatory disease that can also affect the sclera. In fact, many of the episcleritis- and scleritis-associated systemic diseases may involve other ocular structures such as the extraocular muscles, eyelids, conjunctiva, cornea, anterior and posterior uvea, retina, and optic nerve (Table 3.6). Because involvement of some of these structures in episcleritis and scleritis is an important reason for loss of vision and destruction of the eye, a complete general eye examination must never be omitted.

3.1.7.2.1. Visual Acuity

Visual acuity may be reduced in patients with scleritis, but almost never is in patients with episcleritis. The whole object of early diagnosis is early, appropriate treatment to prevent impaired vision. A further reduction in vision

ocular manifestations. These manifestations can appear as a complication of the inflammatory process itself or concomitantly with the scleral disease. Complications of episcleritis and scleritis include extraocular muscle involve-

TABLE 3.6. Other ocular manifestations in episcleritis- and scleritis-associated systemic disease.[a]

Associated disease	EOM	E	C	K	AU	PU	R	ON
Rheumatoid arthritis	−	−	−	+	−	−	−	−
Systemic lupus erythematosus	+	+	−	+	−	−	+	+
Ankylosing spondylitis	−	−	−	−	+	−	−	−
Reiter's syndrome	−	−	+	+	+	+	−	−
Psoriatic arthritis	−	+	+	+	+	−	+	−
Arthritis/inflammatory bowel disease	−	−	+	+	+	+	+	+
Relapsing polychondritis	+	+	+	+	+	+	+	+
Polyarteritis nodosa	+	+	+	+	+	−	+	+
Allergic granulomatous angiitis (Churg–Strauss syndrome)	−	−	−	+	−	−	−	−
Wegener's granulomatosis	+	+	+	+	−	+	+	+
Cogan's syndrome	−	−	−	+	+	+	+	+
Behçet's disease	−	−	−	−	+	+	+	+
Giant cell arteritis	+	+	+	+	+	−	−	+
Gout	−	−	+	+	−	−	−	−
Rosacea	−	+	+	+	−	−	−	−
Atopy	−	+	+	+	−	+	+	−
Tuberculosis	+	+	+	+	+	+	+	+
Leprosy	+	+	+	+	+	+	−	−
Syphilis	+	+	+	+	+	+	+	+
Herpes zoster	+	+	+	+	+	+	+	+
Herpes simplex	+	+	+	+	+	+	+	+
Mumps	+	+	+	+	+	+	+	+
Lyme disease	+	+	+	+	+	+	+	+

[a] EOM, Extraocular muscle palsies; E, eyelids; C, conjunctiva; K, cornea; AU, anterior uveitis; PU, posterior uveitis; R, retina; ON, optic nerve.

most frequently will be due to the extension of the scleral inflammation to adjacent structures leading to keratitis, anterior uveitis, cataract, posterior uveitis, retinal detachment, optic neuritis, or glaucoma. The most common method of visual acuity measurement is the Snellen eye chart. The Snellen eye chart tests the ability of the eye to resolve high-contrast targets. The best corrected visual acuity, tested either by refraction or at least by pinhole, must be documented. Improvement or worsening of the patient's vision without evidence of other ocular complications can be critically useful in monitoring the effect of medical therapy.

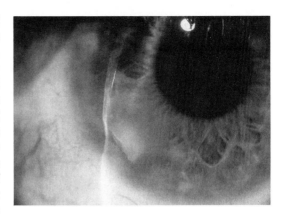

FIGURE 3.21. Corneal examination may disclose peripheral stromal infiltration associated with scleritis.

3.1.7.2.2. Pupils and Extraocular Muscles

The standard measurements of the direct and consensual pupillary reaction to light, and the swinging flashlight test to detect a Marcus Gunn or reverse Marcus Gunn pupil can be helpful in assessing the status of the optic nerve. The optic nerve can be affected by sustained high intraocular pressure, by direct spread of posterior scleral inflammation by long-standing posterior uveitis, or by the same systemic diseases that may affect the sclera. For example, detection of an Argyll Robertson pupil, that is, a pupil that does not react to light but does react to convergence, in the presence of scleral inflammation, obligates one to consider syphilis.

Reduction of extraocular muscle function may occur because of inflammatory infiltration or edema of a muscle secondary to surrounding scleral inflammation or because of III, IV, or VI cranial nerve palsies due to direct involvement of the nerve supply in the orbit by some systemic diseases that may also affect the sclera.

3.1.7.2.3. Cornea

Careful slit-lamp examination of the cornea should always be performed, because corneal involvement may occur in almost one-third of the patients who develop scleritis. Corneal changes are primarily peripheral and adjacent to areas of scleral inflammation; therefore they are usually more extensive in diffuse than in no-

dular scleritis. Infiltrates (Fig. 3.21), thinning, edema, neovascularization, and ulceration (Fig. 3.22; see color insert) may result from the spread of the adjacent scleral inflammation. Several characteristic patterns of keratitis-associated scleritis have been described, ranging from a relatively benign thinning to a progressive, destructive peripheral ulcerative keratitis that can lead to perforation and eventual loss of the eye. Early detection of corneal involvement may lead to adequate treatment, which may improve the ocular prognosis. Because many scleritis-associated systemic diseases may also involve the peripheral cornea, scleral and corneal changes may be caused by the same immunological mechanisms.

Mild corneal changes occur in a small minority of patients with episcleritis, but they do not become permanent.

3.1.7.2.4. Anterior Uvea

Anterior chamber examination with the slit-lamp beam may reveal an anterior uveitis characterized by a mild to moderate amount of flare and cells in the aqueous and anterior vitreous with a few small endothelial keratic precipitates. Mild anterior uveitis may be found in a small percentage of cases of episcleritis. Scleritis-associated anterior uveitis tends to increase in frequency and severity as the scleral inflammation progresses and, if the uveitis is uncontrolled, visual loss is guaranteed. Anterior uveitis may result from the spread of the adjacent scleral inflammation or from the same process which also affects the sclera. Because a variety of scleritis-associated systemic diseases may involve the anterior uvea, immunologic mechanisms responsible for the scleral and uveal reactions may be interrelated.

3.1.7.2.5. Lens

Cataract formation can be caused by long-standing anterior uveitis-associated scleritis and is one of the primary causes of visual loss in patients with scleritis. The detection of a cataract in a young patient with scleritis may, in the absence of other etiologies, be an indication of the severity of the disease. Rapid lens opacification may occur in some eyes with circumferential scleral inflammation. Posterior subcapsular cataracts can appear in patients receiving local or systemic steroids. It has been reported that the risk of developing a posterior subcapsular cataract in a patient with anterior scleritis receiving steroid therapy is three times higher than the same risk in a patient receiving steroid therapy for any other reason.

3.1.7.2.6. Fundus

Direct and indirect ophthalmoscopy and fundus examination, with the 90-, 78-, and 60-diopter lenses, may reveal inflammation of the choroid, ciliochoroidal effusions, choroidal detachments, retinal vasculitis, retinal detachment, macular edema, or optic nerve pathology in association with scleral inflammation. Posterior uveal involvement is always present in posterior scleritis, but only rarely in anterior scleritis. Therefore the detection of posterior uveitis in association with anterior scleritis mandates a search for the presence of posterior scleritis. The posterior uveal involvement is believed to be caused by inflamed sclera overlying the choroid or by the same processes responsible for some scleritis-associated systemic diseases.

3.1.7.2.7. Intraocular Pressure

Tonometry, either by Schiøtz tonometer, applanation tonometer, or pneumotonometer,

should always be performed, because the onset of glaucoma during the course of scleritis, as with the onset of uveitis, may be an ominous sign of further complications and progressive visual loss. High intraocular pressure is believed to be caused primarily by overlying scleral inflammation, by damage to the trabecular meshwork secondary to anterior uveitis, or by peripheral anterior synechiae secondary to anterior uveitis. Glaucoma, particularly in combination with uveitis, is the most common reason for enucleation in uncontrolled scleritis.

3.2. Diagnostic Tests

Once the history of the present illness, review of systems, and physical examination have been completed, diagnosis of the type of scleral disease has been reached, and some preliminary systemic diagnoses have emerged as the most likely causes. The second phase of the approach to scleral diseases includes the selection of diagnostic tests for confirming or rejecting the possibilities suspected in the former phase (Table 3.7). It is important to emphasize that, unless the cause of scleritis is infectious, blood and urine laboratory tests alone will rarely establish a systemic disorder diagnosis; rather they will confirm it in the context of the clinical characteristics discovered in the first phase. Therefore "blanket" testing in scleritis is both expensive and wasteful.

Once the diagnosis has been established, selected laboratory testing is helpful in monitoring the effect of therapy on disease activity.

3.2.1. Blood Tests

3.2.1.1. Rheumatoid Factor

Rheumatoid factor (RF) is generally defined as an autoantibody specific for epitopes in the Fc fragment of immunoglobulin G (IgG). Rheumatoid factor was discovered by E. Waaler[3] in 1937 while he was working with a complement test using sheep erythrocytes (srbc) coated with anti-srbc rabbit antibodies. Waaler noted that serum from rheumatoid arthritis (RA) patients contained a factor that

TABLE 3.7. Laboratory tests for suspected systemic disease.[a]

Systemic disease	Laboratory test[b]
Noninfectious	
Rheumatoid arthritis	RF, ANA (anti-DNA–histone), CIC, C, Cryog, limb joint X rays, HLA typing
Systemic lupus erythematosus	ANA (anti-dsDNA, anti-Sm), CIC, IgG, C, Cryog, UA
Ankylosing spondylitis	CIC, sacroiliac X ray, HLA typing
Reiter's syndrome	CIC, sacroiliac X ray, UA, HLA typing
Psoriatic arthritis	Limb and sacroiliac X rays
Arthritis and IBD	Limb, sacroiliac, and abdominal X rays
Relapsing polychondritis	CIC, C
Polyarteritis nodosa	HBsAg, Cryog, C, CIC, angiography, UA
Churg–Strauss syndrome	WBC/eosinophil count, IgE, CIC, chest X ray
Wegener's granulomatosis	IgA, IgE, RF, ANCA, CIC, sinus and chest X ray BUN, Creat clearance, UA
Behçet's disease	CIC, C, HLA typing
Giant cell arteritis	ESR, CIC, IgG
Cogan's syndrome	CIC, C
Atopy	Eosinophil count, IgE, chest X ray
Gout	Uric acid, limb X ray
Infectious	Serologies

[a] Blood, urine, and X-ray-based tests.
[b] ESR, Erythrocyte sedimentation rate; ANA, anti-nuclear antibodies; anti-dsDNA, antibody to double-stranded DNA; anti-Sm, antibodies to small nuclear ribonucleoproteins—Sm; anti-RNP, antibodies to small nuclear ribonucleoproteins—RNP; CIC, circulating immune complex; IgG, IgA, and IgE, immunoglobulins; C, complement (C3 and C4, as tested by CH50); Cryog, cryoglobulins; RF, rheumatoid factor; HBsAg, hepatitis B surface antigen; WBC, white blood count; ANCA, anti-neutrophil cytoplasmic antibodies; immunofluorescence method; UA, urinalysis; BUN, blood urea nitrogen; Creat, creatinine.

could agglutinate the antibody-coated erythrocytes, and the antibodies were necessary to obtain agglutination.[2] Later, in 1948, Rose et al.[4] also noted, while working with a complement test for rickettsia, agglutination induced by the sera of RA patients.

Approximately 80% of the patients with RA exhibit RF positivity (seropositive RA).[5] However, RF is not specific for RA. Rather, it is found in the sera of a variable portion of patients with other rheumatic diseases and with nonrheumatic diseases (Table 3.8)[6–8]; many of these conditions are associated with the presence of IgM RF. Rheumatoid factor is also found in some apparently normal individuals and in 10 to 20% of nonrheumatic individuals over 65 years old who will not develop RA. Rheumatoid factor positivity frequently precedes the onset of RA.[9,10] The specificity of the RF for RA increases with the titer of serum RF[11] and with positivity on two or more consecutive occasions.

The presence of RF in RA is associated with more rapid radiographic deterioration of involved joints, greater functional impairment, and more frequent appearance of extra-

TABLE 3.8. Disease commonly associated with rheumatoid factor.

Connective tissue disease
  Rheumatoid arthritis
  Systemic lupus erythematosus
  Scleroderma
  Sjögren's syndrome
  Polymyositis–dermatomyositis
Acute viral infections
  Rubella
  Cytomegalovirus
  Hepatitis
  Infectious mononucleosis
  Influenza
Chronic bacterial infections
  Tuberculosis
  Leprosy
  Syphilis
  Brucellosis
  Salmonellosis
  Subacute bacterial endocarditis
Parasitic infections
  Malaria
  Trypanosomiasis
  Filariasis
Chronic inflammatory disease
  Sarcoidosis
  Chronic pulmonary disease
  Chronic liver disease
Mixed cryoglobulinemia
Hypergammaglobulinemic purpura

articular manifestations (e.g., subcutaneous nodules, vasculitis, neuropathy, ulcers, Felty's syndrome, Sjögren's syndrome).[5,12-16]

Rheumatoid factor can be IgG, IgM or IgA antibody class. Most procedures used to detect RF activity are based on the agglutination of carrier particles (polystyrene latex or red blood cells) passively coated with human or rabbit IgG preparations. These techniques are modifications of the originally described sensitized sheep cell agglutination test (Waaler–Rose) or latex fixation tests and detect primarily IgM RF. IgM RF is not specific of RA because it is found in a wide variety of acute and chronic inflammatory diseases, and even in some normal individuals. Interest in improving sensitivity, quantitative accuracy, and detection of other isotypes of RF has led to the development of specific radioimmunoassays (RIAs) and enzyme-linked immunoabsorbant assays (ELISAs) capable of measuring nanogram quantities of IgA and IgG RF.[17,18] The detection of IgG RF presents special problems in that both the RF activity and the antigenic sites are located in the IgG molecule. Furthermore, non-RF IgG present as antigen bound to IgM RF can contribute to false-positive results. Thus, most immunoassays for IgG RF require tubes or microtest wells coated with rabbit IgG and often incorporate procedures to remove or destroy IgM RF.[19,20] The specificity of the RF for RA increases when IgM RF, IgA RF, and IgG RF are positive.

3.2.1.2. Anti-Nuclear Antibodies

In 1948, Hardgraves and colleagues initiated the study of antibodies to nuclei with the description of the lupus erythematosus (LE) phenomenon,[21] which demonstrates the ingestion of traumatized cells from systemic lupus erythematosus (SLE) patients by neutrophils.[22] The phenomenon is now known to be caused by the reaction of antibodies against nucleoprotein (DNA–histone) with cell nuclei and the subsequent phagocytosis of such "sensitized" nuclei. The LE test has been replaced by a more sensitive and specific test, the indirect immunofluorescent assay (IFA) for the detection of anti-nuclear antibodies (ANAs).[23-25]

The finding of ANAs indicates, in the majority of cases, an ongoing or latent inflammatory condition within the broad classification of connective tissue diseases.[26] However, infections such as chronic active hepatitis, infectious mononucleosis, and lepromatous leprosy, and other autoimmune diseases such as primary biliary cirrhosis and chronic glomerulonephritis, also are characterized by this serological abnormality.[27] Anti-nuclear antibodies may occasionally be found in normal subjects, although usually in low titers; the frequency increases with age.

Anti-nuclear antibodies actually compose a family of autoantibodies directed against components of the cell nucleus; they are important markers of SLE and related syndromes (Table 3.9). Among the ANAs, antibodies to DNA–histone, double-stranded DNA (dsDNA), single-stranded DNA (ssDNA), RNA, histone, nuclear ribunucleo protein (nRNP), and Small RNP (Sm) all occur in SLE, whereas antibodies to Ro/SSA and La/SSB/Ha occur in SLE and Sjögren's syndrome; antibodies to nRNP also can be detected in patients with mixed connective tissue disease, an entity whose features overlap those of SLE, scleroderma, and poly-

TABLE 3.9. Antibodies to nuclear or cytoplasmic antigens.[a]

Antibody	Disease	Pattern
Anti-DNA–histone	SLE, RA	H, P
Anti-dsDNA	SLE	H, P
Anti-ssDNA	SLE, other disease	Negative
Anti-histone	SLE	S
Anti-nRNP	SLE, MCTD	S
Anti-Sm	SLE	S
Anti-Ro/SSA	SLE, Sjögren	Negative
Anti-La/SSB/Ha	SLE, Sjögren	S
Anti-PM-Scl	PM	S
Anti-Mi$_1$, Mi$_2$	PM	?
Anti-Jo$_2$	PM	CYT (?)
Anti-Ku	PM	?
Anti-Scl$_{70}$	PSS	S
Anti-centromere	PSS	N

[a]SLE, Systemic lupus erythematosus; MCTD, mixed connective tissue disease; PM, polymyositis; PSS, progressive systemic sclerosis; RA, rheumatoid arthritis; H, homogeneous; P, peripheral; S, speckled; N, nucleolar; CYT, cytoplasmic; Sjögren, Sjögren's syndrome.

myositis; antibodies to PM-Scl, Mi_1, Mi_2, Jo_2, and Ku all are found in patients with polymyositis; antibodies to Scl_{70} and centromere occur in patients with progressive systemic sclerosis, whereas antibodies to anti-DNA–histone occur in patients with rheumatoid arthritis.[27] Some of these entities are not associated with episcleritis or scleritis; however, they are important in the differential diagnosis of other connective tissue diseases that may be associated with episcleritis and scleritis (Table 3.2). The pattern of immunofluorescence positivity revealed by an ANA test is of considerable diagnostic significance. Major fluorescence patterns include homogeneous, peripheral (rim), speckled and nucleolar. The ANA pattern is relatively valuable but is much less important than the identification of a specific ANA or anti-cytoplasmic antibody (ACA) (e.g., anti-nRNP, anti-La/SSB, and anti-PM-Scl). The homogeneous pattern can be produced by anti-DNA–histone and dsDNA antibodies associated with the LE phenomenon; the peripheral pattern also can be caused by antibodies to DNA–histone and dsDNA; the speckled pattern correlates with anti-Sm, anti-nRNP, anti-La/SSB, and anti-Scl_{70} antibodies; the nucleolar pattern can be produced by anti-centromere antibodies. Disease associations with typical staining patterns are shown in Table 3.9.[28-34]

The ANA test is an indirect fluorescence reaction in which a droplet of patient serum is reacted with substrate cells fixed with acetone or methanol on a slide. As many as 20 or 30 different sera can be examined on the same slide. After a certain reaction period has elapsed, all excess serum is washed off to remove other serum components except bound ANA. In the next step the preparation is then covered with fluorescein-tagged anti-human IgG. This anti-immunoglobulin probe binds to any human IgG ANA on the slide. The slide is washed again to remove unbound anti-immunoglobulin. Fluorescence of the nuclear structures of the leukocytes indicates an adherence of patient antibodies to nuclear proteins.[27]

Anti-nuclear antibody titers and patterns acquired from different laboratories vary greatly. The factors that lead to variable results include the use of different substrate cells (such as mouse liver, mouse kidney, monkey kidney [Vero cells]), or human tissue culture lines (WIL-2, KB, or Hep-2 cells), the use of different fluoresceinated antibodies, microscopes of different powers and sensitivities, and varying levels of technical skill. Within the active, untreated SLE patients, positive ANAs will be detected in 95% of the tests performed with mouse liver or kidney cells and in 98% of the tests performed with human tissue culture lines. The difference between the two substrates is due, at least in part, to the relative absence of the Ro/SSA antigen in mouse liver or kidney cells and its presence in the tissue culture lines. We advocate ANA testing on two cell lines: one on mouse liver, mouse kidney, or monkey kidney cells, and the other on WIL-2, KB, or Hep-2 cells.

Absence of a positive ANA in tissue culture lines makes the diagnosis of SLE unlikely. A negative ANA in a patient with clinical evidence for a specific connective tissue disease suggests the test should be repeated for confirmation, because the result could be due to faulty testing; in case of confirmed negative ANA, sequential testing is advocated.

A positive ANA in a patient with clinical evidence for a specific connective tissue disease requires specific ANA testing. A positive ANA in a patient with limited or nonspecific clinical findings requires continued observation until disease expression is more complete.

3.2.1.3. Anti-Neutrophil Cytoplasmic Antibodies

Autoantibodies (IgG) directed against a cytoplasmic antigen of human neutrophils—the anti-neutrophil cytoplasmic antibodies (ANCAs; synonym, anti-cytoplasmic antibodies or ACPAs)—can be detected in patients with systemic vasculitis such as Wegener's granulomatosis, microscopic polyarteritis nodosa, and segmental necrotizing glomerulonephritis.[35-38] Although still a subject of debate, these diseases are thought to be part of the spectrum of one disease process.

The presence of ANCAs is specific and sensitive for Wegener's granulomatosis, an entity often associated with episcleritis and scleritis;

the specificity is 99% by indirect immuno-fluorescence techniques and 98% by ELISA detection; the sensitivity is 96% for active generalized disease, 67% for active regional disease, and 32% for disease in full remission after initial regional symptoms.[36-38]

Two types of ANCA have been described. A granular cytoplasmic staining pattern—produced by C-ANCA—is directed in at least 95% of cases against proteinase 3 (PR-3), a neutral serine protease of human neutro-phils.[39,40] A perinuclear staining pattern—produced by P-ANCA—is directed against a variety of different antigens (myeloperoxidase, elastase, and lactoferrin).[39] It has been sug-gested that C-ANCA is associated with lung and sinus involvement, whereas P-ANCA oc-curs most frequently with renal disease.[41]

The discovery of ANCAs has provided an invaluable tool in the evaluation of patients with ocular or orbital inflammation suggestive of systemic vasculitis.[42] At the Massachusetts Eye and Ear Infirmary, we have found elevated ANCA titers to be highly specific and sensitive for Wegener's granulomatosis in patients with scleritis.[43] Either type of ANCA can be found in patients with limited or generalized Wege-ner's granulomatosis with ocular or orbital inflammation.[42,43]

Because of its high specificity, a positive ANCA is suggestive of Wegener's granu-lomatosis; however, because ANCA is positive only in 67% of patients with active limited disease and in 32% of patients in full remission after limited disease, one or even repeatedly negative ANCA testing does not exclude the diagnosis, especially in patients with limited clinical features and characteristic histological findings.

3.2.1.4. Circulating Immune Complexes

The formation of circulating immune com-plexes, (CICs) by binding of antigens to their corresponding antibodies is a physiological process usually of benefit to the host because it allows the neutralization or the elimination of exogenous antigens. Circulating immune com-plexes primarily involve antigens from exogen-ous sources (food, drugs, or microbes) and endogenous sources (autoantigens and tumor antigens). Deposition of CICs seems to be dependent on a variety of factors, including size of complex, nature of antigen, immuno-globulin class, antibody affinity, ability to fix complement, interaction with RFs, and the clearance capacity of the reticuloendothelial system.[44] Circulating immune complexes usu-ally are eliminated efficiently by the mononu-clear phagocytic system, particularly by Kupffer cells in the liver[45]; therefore, CICs can be detected for only a short period of time after a specific antigenic challenge. However, CICs may persist in the blood circulation of patients with autoimmune disorders such as polyar-teritis nodosa, allergic granulomatous angiitis (Churg–Strauss syndrome), Wegener's granu-lomatosis, and some connective tissue diseases; CICs may deposit in renal glomeruli, synovial tissue, or vessel walls, participating in the development or persistence of major inflam-matory lesions.

Although CIC detection is not essential for the diagnosis of any condition, their presence helps support a specific disorder under the following conditions: (1) CICs may be detected in early arthritis several months prior to the definitive diagnosis of RA[46]; (2) CICs may help to distinguish seronegative RA from other arthropathies such as ankylosing spondylitis or Reiter's syndrome, because CICs are found in 70% of patients with seronegative RA and they are found only rarely in patients with an-kylosing spondylitis or Reiter's syndrome.[47,48] Circulating immune complex detection may also be useful to monitor disease activity[49-51]; patients with rheumatoid vasculitis have high levels of CICs.[52] Significant decreases in CIC level may be interpreted as a favorable re-sponse to therapy; conversely, significant in-creases in CIC level may signify the need for more aggressive therapy.

Because of the enormous diversity of anti-gens involved in CICs, it is doubtful that antigen-specific assays will ever find widespread use in clinical immunological studies. Therefore the techniques available for detection of CICs are antigen nonspecific. The sensitivity of each method for detecting CIC varies according to the nature of the CIC involved and the influence of various interfering factors. Only a limited number of procedures are suitable for routine laboratory investigation. Some of the most widely used methods are described in the following sections.

3.2.1.4.1. Fluid-Phase Binding Assays

Fluid-phase binding assays are based on the fact that precipitation of radiolabeled C1q receptor (a subcomponent of the first component of complement that binds CIC) differs from precipitation of radiolabeled C1q receptor bound to CIC.

3.2.1.4.1.1. C1q-Binding Assay. In the C1q-binding assay, CICs are allowed to bind C1q in liquid phase. Radiolabeled C1q is added to ethylenediaminetetraacetic acid (EDTA)-treated serum in the presence of polyethylene glycol, which precipitates CICs bound to C1q.[53] After 1 h, free C1q is separated from the precipitated bound C1q by centrifugation. The percentage of radioactivity precipitated corresponds to the C1q-binding activity of the sample and indicates the level of CICs. This test is particularly sensitive for CICs containing IgM, therefore explaining the high level of positivity usually observed in rheumatoid arthritis. Circulating immune complexes containing IgG_4, IgA, IgD, and IgE are not detected. The technique is reasonably reliable but C1q needs to be radiolabeled, a procedure that can inactivate the delicate complement molecule if harshly executed.

3.2.1.4.2. Cell-Binding Assays

These assays try to quantify the binding of CICs to cells.

3.2.1.4.2.1. Raji Cell-Binding Assay. The basis of the Raji cell-binding assay is the binding of CICs to C3b and C3bi receptors on a continuous lymphoblastoid cell line originally derived from a patient with Burkitt's lymphoma (Raji cells).[54] Raji cells are characterized by a lack of surface immunoglobulins, by few or low-affinity receptors for IgG Fc, and by a large number of receptors for complement. Circulating immune complexes bound to cells are quantitated with a labeled anti-IgG antibody. This test is particularly sensitive for CICs containing IgG. The technique is reasonably reliable but Raji cell lines cultured in different laboratories are quite different and express different levels of C3 receptors. Therefore data from different sources cannot be compared directly; for the same reason, longitudinal studies in a specific laboratory can be done only if the line is continuously subcloned.

3.2.1.5. Complement

The complement cascade consists of a group of serum proteins that participate in inflammation through the actions of increased vascular permeability, chemotaxis, opsonization, and cell lysis.[55,56] Once the first component is activated, each component is activated by its predecessor. C4 can be activated by the classic pathway, which can be initiated by antigen–antibody reactions. C3 can be activated by the classic pathway and by the alternative pathway, which can be activated by microorganisms. Because the levels of complement components in various body fluids may be decreased during complement activation, their measurements can give a rough index of disease activity under conditions in which complement activation is prominent.

Any disease that gives rise to CICs may show a hypocomplementemia, provided the CICs contain IgG or IgM antibodies capable of activating complement. Serial serum complement levels may be depressed in rheumatoid arthritis with vasculitis[52,57,58]; they also may be depressed in systemic lupus erythematosus exacerbations, particularly when there is renal involvement.[59,60] Conversely, as the disease activity declines, there may be a parallel return of the complement level toward normal.

There are primarily two types of clinical assays for complement components: (1) tests that detect and quantify the presence of complement components (immunochemical assays) and (2) tests that determine functional or total hemolytic activity of the complete complement cascade (CH50, or complement hemolytic 50%).

3.2.1.5.1. Quantitation Tests

The basis of immunochemical assays is the reaction of complement proteins with specific antibodies.[61] The most widely used immunochemical assay is radial immunodiffusion. In this technique, monospecific antibody directed against a complement protein is incorporated into an agarose gel, holes are punched in the gel, and test samples or known standards are placed in the holes. As the antigenic complement protein diffuses into the gel and encounters its specific antibody, a precipitin ring forms, which is proportional to the concentration of complement placed in the hole. A standard curve is constructed from the size of the rings produced by samples of known concentration, and the concentration of complement in the test sample is determined. A more rapid and slightly more sensitive technique is electroimmunodiffusion. In this technique, the sample is unidirectionally electrophoresed into an antibody-containing gel, yielding a set of "rockets" whose height is proportional to concentration. Quantitation tests for complement components include measurements of C3 and C4 complement proteins.

3.2.1.5.2. Functional Tests

The CH50 is a reliable and sensitive test for assessment of the classic complement pathway as a whole.[62] The CH50 represents the concentration of sample serum that lyses 50% of a standard cell suspension. Dilutions of the sample are incubated with a standard suspension of sheep erythrocytes in the presence of rabbit antibodies against sheep erythrocytes. The antibody solution has a standard concentration that lyses half of the cells in a given time in the presence of 1 ml of standard guinea pig complement (1 hemolytic or CH50 unit). If any of the classic pathway or terminal components are absent, the CH50 value will be 0 or extremely low.

A useful routine complement screen must include measurements of C3, C4 by immunochemical assays, and total hemolytic activity by CH50 assay.

3.2.1.6. HLA Typing

Histocompatibility leukocyte antigen (HLA) testing is of significance in a patient with episcleritis or scleritis and manifestations compatible with diseases that have shown specific HLA association; these diseases include ankylosing spondylitis (HLA-B27), Reiter's syndrome (HLA-B27), Behçet's disease (HLA-B51), and rheumatoid arthritis (HLA-DR4). Specific HLA positivity plays little or no role in the diagnosis of a disease because many HLA-B27, -B51, and -DR4 individuals in the general population remain unaffected, and these diseases may occasionally occur in individuals negative for HLA-B27, -B51, and -DR4.[63,64] Diagnosis is based on suspicion, history, clinical evaluation, or radiological confirmation. For example, a patient with symptoms suggesting ankylosing spondylitis but with normal spinal radiographs does not have ankylosing spondylitis even if he is HLA-B27 positive (6% of normal Caucasians are HLA-B27 positive). In contrast, a HLA-B27-negative individual with sacroiliitis does have the disease (5 to 10% of Caucasians with ankylosing spondylitis are HLA-B27 negative). However, the presence of HLA-B27, -B51, and -DR4 increases the probability that the presumptive diagnosis is correct, particularly when clinical and radiological findings are difficult to recognize with certainty.

3.2.1.7. Antibody Titers against Infectious Organisms

The fluorescent treponemal antibody-absorption test (FTA-ABS) and the microhemagglutination test for *Treponema pallidum* (MHA-TP) are sensitive for all stages of syphilis except primary, early secondary, and early congenital forms. The FTA-ABS test is 98% sensitive and the MHA-TP test is 98 to 100% sensitive in tertiary syphilis.[65–68] The MHA-TP test is more specific than the FTA-ABS test, with only 1% or less of positive reactions in rheumatoid arthritis, systemic lupus erythematosus, leprosy, relapsing fever, or yaws.[68] However, FTA-ABS and MHA-TP do not indicate active, as opposed to previous, disease.

The ELISA for *Borrelia burgdorferi* antibodies is the most sensitive and specific test for the diagnosis of Lyme disease; this ELISA is usually negative in stage 1, but is positive in 90% of patients in stage 2 and in almost 100% of patients in stage 3.[69] The IFA method is also a reliable test.

Herpes zoster is readily diagnosed clinically in most instances. Occasionally, other diseases that can mimic herpes zoster may increase the possibility of misdiagnosis; in these cases, anti-VZV titers may be helpful. Initial varicella-zoster virus (VZV) infection (chickenpox) produces cellular immune responses and IgG, IgM, and IgA anti-VZV antibodies[70]; high levels of IgG anti-VZV persist throughout childhood. Recurrent VZV infection (herpes zoster) produces a rapid increase in antibodies to viral-associated membrane antigen, detectable by complement fixation, ELISA, or IFA. Anti-VZV titers in herpes zoster are meaningful only when drawn as acute and convalescent sera about 1 month apart and demonstrate at least a two- to fourfold rise in titer. A single positive test for virus does not indicate whether a viral infection took place recently or not.

The ELISA test is the blood test most commonly used for the diagnosis of toxoplasmosis and toxocariasis. The presence of high IgM anti-*Toxoplasma* and anti-*Toxocara* titers indicates a recent infection.

3.2.2. Skin Testing

The intracutaneous tuberculin purified protein derivative (PPD) is a reliable method for recognizing prior mycobacterial infection unless the patient was vaccinated with BCG previously. The usual tuberculin test is of intermediate-strength PPD (5 tuberculin units) and is applied in the forearm. Reactions should be read by measuring the transverse diameter of induration as detected by gentle palpation at 48 to 72 h.[71] Patients with tuberculosis have reactions with a mean of 17 mm; patients infected but with no active disease have similar reactions. Therefore a positive test means a prior mycobacterial infection and does not rule out other etiological factors, as it may be a coincidental finding. Repeated skin testing with PPD does not lead to positive reactions in uninfected persons.

Every individual is normally exposed and sensitized to many antigens. Modern prophylactic immunization results in the purposeful exposure to antigens from microorganisms responsible for diphtheria, tetanus, mumps, influenza, and other virus infections. In addition, natural exposure results in sensitization to antigens prepared from streptococci, staphylococci, certain common fungi, and other ubiquitous antigens. Skin tests elicit delayed cutaneous hypersensitivity reactions to these antigens in most healthy subjects. Impairment of delayed hypersensitivity reaction to an antigen in an adequately exposed subject is called *anergy*. Anergy or hyporeactivity to skin testing is typical although not diagnostic of lepromatous leprosy, herpes zoster, or sarcoidosis. Systemic steroid therapy may reverse anergy, whereas immunosuppressive therapy such as cyclosporine may suppress a positive skin test.

Skin testing can also help detect allergies such as pollen, animal dander, mold, dust, and many other environmental allergens. Direct reproduction of an immediate allergic reaction by introducing a small amount of extract of suspected allergen into the skin is a good method with which to diagnose atopy. Two procedures, the intradermal test and the prick test, are the most consistent and interpretable.

3.2.3. Radiological Studies

All techniques of X-ray imaging rely on two basic properties of tissues to produce their images: the ability to absorb X-ray photons and the ability to scatter them.

1. Chest X rays are of diagnostic significance in tuberculosis, Wegener's granulomatosis, allergic granulomatous angiitis (Churg–Strauss syndrome), and atopy.
2. Sinus films showing mucosal thickening and/or destruction of bony walls can be helpful in the diagnosis of Wegener's granulomatosis.
3. Sacroiliac X rays are of diagnostic significance in ankylosing spondylitis, Reiter's

syndrome, psoriatic arthritis, and arthritis associated with inflammatory bowel disease.

4. Limb joint X rays, such as hand, wrist, foot, and knee joint X rays, can show the arthritic changes characteristic of rheumatoid arthritis, juvenile rheumatoid arthritis, gout, psoriatic arthritis, and arthritis associated with inflammatory bowel disease.

3.2.4. Anterior Segment Fluorescein Angiography

The information that can be obtained from anterior segment fluorescein angiography may be a valuable adjunct to the diagnosis of scleritis. For example, although most forms of anterior scleral disease can be diagnosed clinically, difficulties sometimes arise in distinguishing between severe episcleritis and diffuse anterior scleritis, or between the relatively benign diffuse or nodular anterior scleritis and the early changes of the more severe necrotizing scleritis. Early detection of the most severe forms of scleritis is crucial if one is to institute correct treatment before more destructive changes occur. Because the adequate therapy of scleritis depends on an accurate diagnosis, it is important to find objective methods to evaluate the different clinical conditions. Anterior segment fluorescein angiography has been found to show characteristic patterns in the various forms of episcleritis and scleritis, providing considerable information in guiding subsequent therapy.[72]

Corneal involvement can be found in 29% of patients with scleritis and 15% of patients with episcleritis. Although most of the different forms of keratitis associated with scleral disease can be diagnosed clinically, differentiation between the early changes of the relatively benign peripheral corneal opacification with or without neovascularization and the early changes of the more serious corneal thinning, either with limbal guttering or with peripheral corneal ulceration, can sometimes be difficult. Early detection of the most severe forms of keratitis associated with scleritis is important if one is to institute adequate treatment before visual acuity becomes affected. Because the accurate diagnosis of keratitis as-

sociated with scleritis can add valuable information to the choice of therapy, it is important to find objective methods to evaluate early keratitis. Anterior segment fluorescein angiography can sometimes help in this regard.[73]

Adequate medical treatment for scleral inflammation with or without corneal involvement frequently results in halting the process, either through new vessel formation to cover the defect or through recanalization of existing vessels.[74] Although most of the individual responses to treatment can be easily monitored by clinical examination, difficulties sometimes arise in being certain if the scleral disease with or without corneal involvement is completely under control. Anterior segment fluorescein angiography can sometimes be of assistance in monitoring the effect of medical therapy.[75]

If in spite of intensive medical therapy no new vessels are formed or no preexisting vessels are recanalized, progressive thinning of the sclera and/or cornea with possible eventual perforation may occur. In these cases, tectonic surgery such as scleral or corneal or sclerocorneal grafting must be considered to maintain the integrity of the eye.[76] Although the site and extent of the surgical procedure can be frequently decided by clinical examination, determination of the amount of necrotic tissue to be removed and replaced surgically can sometimes be difficult. Anterior segment fluorescein angiography can sometimes be useful in deciding the extent of appropriate surgical intervention.[75]

3.2.4.1. Anterior Segment Fluorescein Angiography Techniques

Conventional photographic fluorescein angiography,[72,77–83] low-dose photographic fluorescein angiography,[84] low-dose fluorescein videoangiography,[85] and scanning angiographic microscopic fluorescein videoangiography[86] are different techniques used to describe the circulatory dynamics of the anterior segment of the eye, such as the direction of flow, the distinction between arteries and veins, and the integrity of the circulation.

Fluorescein angiography has been available for examining the retinal microcirculation since

1961,[87] when venous injection of low molecular weight sodium fluorescein was used to demonstrate abnormalities in the retinal capillaries, in the retinal pigment epithelial cells, and in Bruch's membrane. The tight apposition of contiguous retinal capillary endothelial cells may explain, at least in part, why normal retinal vessels do not leak fluorescein.[88] Iris capillary endothelial cells also are joined by tight junctions, and anterior segment fluorescein angiography was introduced in 1968[89,90] with the primarily purpose of diagnosing iris lesions. Conventional anterior segment fluorescein angiography has not, however, been widely used for conjunctival and scleral abnormalities because normal conjunctival and episcleral vessels leak molecules smaller than serum albumin, such as fluorescein. Low molecular weight molecules may escape from the conjunctival and episcleral vessel lumens by crossing the interendothelial clefts, the endothelial cells through pinocytotic vesicles, or both.[91] Interestingly, the limbal vessels never leak fluorescein, suggesting that their endothelial cells are united by tight junctions.[92] Five milliliters of 10% sodium fluorescein via antecubital vein injection rapidly extravasates from conjunctival and episcleral vessels, restricting the diagnostic value of this technique to the demonstration of either early leakage or gross hypoperfusion.[72] If leakage is to be avoided, the fluorescein must be bound to large molecules. Fluorescein-labeled isothiocyanate (FITC)–dextran conjugates are molecules of high molecular weight that do not leak from anterior segment vessels. FITC–dextrans have been shown to enhance the diagnostic value of the angiograms in retinal vessels of rats, cats, and monkeys[93–95] and in episcleral vessels of rabbits.[84] Their application for human use is still pending approval. Meanwhile, low-dose fluorescein angiogram techniques have been shown to give better quality anterior segment angiograms than does conventional dose fluorescein.[84] Approximately 90% of injected fluorescein is bound to serum albumin and 10% remains unbound.[96] It is known that the unbound fluorescein leaks from the vessels[95]; because the time for binding to serum albumin is directly proportional to the dose given, by reducing the dose of injected fluorescein, leakage from the episcleral vessels can be minimized. Intravenous injection of six-tenths of a milliliter of 20% sodium fluorescein, followed by film photography, provides better dynamic studies in normal and diseased conjunctival and episcleral vessels.[84] But although photographic low-dose anterior segment fluorescein angiography gives high spatial resolution, the slow recycling rate of most flash units (one frame per second) restricts the temporal resolution of flow characteristics and direction. Low-dose anterior segment fluorescein videoangiography with an image capture rate of 25 frames per second, associated with an image intensifier that enhances sensitivity in spite of high luminescence, improves temporal resolution and magnification for flow dynamic studies in the anterior segment of the human eye.[85] The use of a microcomputer program in conjunction with low-dose anterior segment videoangiography provides complete control of the angiogram, allowing immediate access to any frame, comparison between different frames, and subtraction of any sequence of the study from the remaining ones.[9] Anterior segment fluorescein videoangiography with a scanning angiographic microscope shows advantages over the photographic and videocamera methods through longer depth of focus, larger field of view, lower light levels, coaxial illumination, and real-time traverse of conjunctival/episcleral vasculature.[86] Anterior segment fluorescein videoangiography techniques with fluorescein-labeled dextrans may become the probes of choice for the study of the anterior segment vasculature of the human eye.

3.2.4.2.1. Arterial Phase

The first vessels to fill in an angiography of the bulbar conjunctiva and episclera are the anterior ciliary arteries. These run radially within the episclera toward the limbus, following variable courses (Fig. 3.23). Between 2 and 5 mm posterior to the limbus the anterior ciliary arteries divide into two branches, which run circumferentially to meet other branches from adjacent anterior ciliary arteries. These

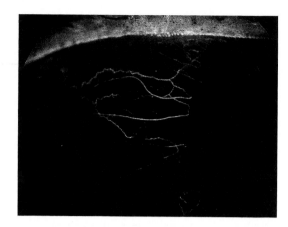

FIGURE 3.23. Anterior segment fluorescein angiogram: arterial phase. Note the extraordinary radiality of the anterior ciliary tributaries, culminating in the formation of loops and anastamoses at the corneoscleral limbus.

anastomoses form the anterior episcleral arterial circle, which broadly resolves into five distinct vascular networks: (1) anterior conjunctival, (2) superficial episcleral, (3) deep episcleral, (4) limbal, and (5) iris. Because the anterior episcleral arterial circle is a variable anatomical entity, it may take between 1.5 and 14s to fill.

The arteries from the anterior episcleral circle run forward to the limbus, curve backward radially, and divide to form the anterior conjunctival arteriolar plexus. The anterior conjunctival arterioles fill approximately 1.5s after the segment of the anterior episcleral segment that supplies them. The anterior conjunctival circulation, supplied by the anterior ciliary arteries, fluoresce approximately 4s before the posterior conjunctival circulation, supplied by the peripheral palpebral arch, which is itself formed by terminal vessels derived from the ophthalmic artery. This explains the watershed zone between anterior and posterior conjunctival circulation, which can fill late.

Branches from the anterior episcleral arterial circle run posteriorly and divide to form the anterior episcleral arteriolar plexus. Neither superficial nor deep vascular layers can be detected. These vessels fill shortly after the anterior episcleral arterial circle.

The limbal vessels often share their origins with the anterior conjunctival vessels. Unlike conjunctival and episcleral vessels, they do not leak fluorescein, probably because they have thicker endothelium and fewer fenestrations.[92] They may fill late.

Radial arterioles of the iris begin to fill, either coinciding with filling of the anterior ciliary arteries or 1 to 2s later, implying that the iris receives arterial supply from the anterior ciliary circulation.

3.2.4.2. Normal Anterior Segment Fluorescein Angiography

Anterior segment fluorescein angiography occurs in three phases: an arterial phase, a capillary phase, and a venous phase.[84] Vessels that fill early with high fluorescence and high tortuosity, thick walls, and pulsatile flow, are considered arteries. Vessels that fill after arteries, with lower fluorescence, lower tortuosity, thinner walls, and no pulsatile flow are considered veins. Furthermore, arteries never show streaming of blood and branch rarely, whereas veins often show laminar flow and branch a good deal. However, because veins fill gradually and diffusely, subsequent to artery filling, the moment of their first perfusion is difficult to evaluate.

Despite excellent anatomical descriptions[98-101] and modern videoangiographic techniques,[85,86] controversy still exists regarding the flow patterns within the vessels of the anterior segment of the eye. Whereas some studies support the view that the anterior ciliary arterial flow is from the region of the rectus muscles toward the inside of the eye through perforating vessels, that is, centripetal,[86,102-106] others suggest that the anterior ciliary arterial flow is primarily supplied by retrograde flow from the intraocular medial and lateral long posterior ciliary arteries, that is, centrifugal.[72,78,83,85,107] Some investigators who favor the centripetal distribution theory believe that other interpretations of the dynamic events result from deficiencies in photographic and conventional videocamera techniques.[86] Resolution of this controversy will require additional studies. Because the main applicabi-

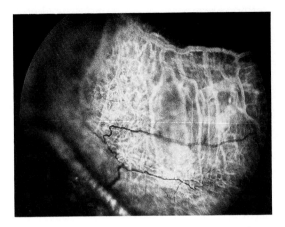

FIGURE 3.24. Anterior segment fluorescein angiogram: capillary phase. Note the rich abundance of the capillary vascular supply in the episclera. Note also the tiny capillary twigs extending into the far corneal periphery.

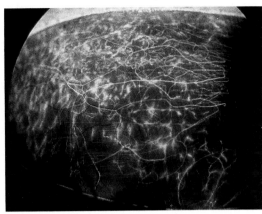

FIGURE 3.25. Anterior segment fluorescein angiogram: venous phase. Filling of venous collectors is shown. Note the scattered "bright spots" residual from the capillary phase. Leakage from capillaries is normal.

lity of anterior segment fluorescein angiography in scleral diseases is to detect areas of vascular closure in the episcleral or conjunctival circulation, the issue of direction of flow is not critical for patient management.

The different phases of the angiography presented below assume the conventional centripetal distribution of the anterior segment circulation of the eye.

3.2.4.2.2. Capillary Phase

Episcleral and conjunctival capillaries are difficult to differentiate at this stage but both emerge from the anterior episcleral arterial circle and from branches of the anterior ciliary arteries. Usually, all the capillaries are filled between 6 and 30 s after fluorescein injection; episcleral capillaries and limbal arcades are the latest to fill (Fig. 3.24).

3.2.4.2.3. Venous Phase

Anterior conjunctival venules and limbal arcades drain into the limbal venous circle, which is a circle of fine venules behind the limbal arcades and medial to the anterior episcleral arterial circle (Fig. 3.25). The limbal venous circle drains into episcleral collecting venules that run toward the rectus muscles.

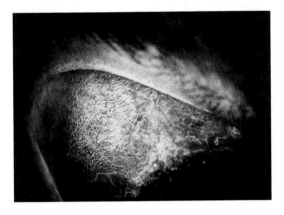

FIGURE 3.26. Anterior segment fluorescein angiogram: capillary phase. Note the total lack of perfusion of the inferior one-fourth of the vascular plexuses in the scleral/episcleral field (below the bright area of normal capillary filling).

These collecting venules meet anterior episcleral venules and perforating scleral venules before they leave the globe over the rectus muscles as anterior ciliary veins.[84,106]

Although leakage from conjunctiva and episcleral capillaries in low-dose fluorescein angiography can first be seen at 4 to 10 s, there is not much masking of anatomical structures before 30 s after fluorescein injection.[84] Limbal arcades are the latest to leak (always after

30 s); it is thought that this leakage may be the result of diffusion from the surrounding sub-conjunctival space.

In the interpretation of an anterior fluorescein angiogram particular attention must to be paid to areas of vascular hypoperfusion or occlusion (Fig. 3.26). Other important considerations are transit time or time between arteriole and venule first filling (early, normal, or delayed), type of arteriolar or venular filling (early, normal, delayed, or absent), and type of capillary leakage (early, normal, or delayed).

3.2.5. Other Imaging Studies

3.2.5.1. Ultrasonography

Diagnostic ultrasonography consists of the propagation of high-frequency sound waves reflected by interfaces between tissues. The reflected waves create echoes that are displayed on an oscilloscope screen. Ultrasonography is a useful test to detect changes in and around the eye. The main advantages of this method are that it is relatively inexpensive, rapid, produces images in real time, can obtain images in different planes (changing rapidly from one plane to another), and it produces no biological hazards. The main disadvantages are the need for direct contact with the globe or eyelid, the dependence on operator skills, and the inferior spatial resolution and resolving power compared to those of computerized tomography scanning or magnetic resonance imaging.[108]

Ultrasonography is the most helpful ancillary test in detecting posterior inflammation of the sclera, and therefore should always be performed before computerized tomography or magnetic resonance techniques are used. Flattening of the posterior aspect of the globe, thickening of the posterior coats of the eye (choroid and sclera), and retrobulbar edema are the main findings in posterior scleritis (Fig. 3.27).[109–112] Occasionally, retinal or choroidal detachment also may be detected (Fig. 3.28). The combination of both A scan and B scan techniques simultaneously produces the most useful results in distinguishing posterior scleritis from orbital, choroidal, and retinal

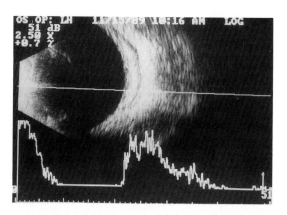

FIGURE 3.27. B scan ultrasonagram of a patient with posterior scleritis. Note the marked thickening of the retinochoroid later and the collection of edema fluid in Tenon's space.

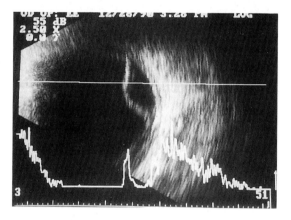

FIGURE 3.28. B scan ultrasonagram with associated A scan tracing. Note the obvious retinal detachment in this patient in whom the fundus could not be seen because of dense cataract.

diseases, which clinically may mimic posterior scleritis.[110]

3.2.5.1.1. A Scan Ultrasonography

The A scan technique shows one-dimensional time-amplitude representations of echoes received along the beam path. The echoes appear as vertical deflections rising from a horizontal zero line. In the axial A echogram of the normal eye, high echoes are produced by the two corneal surfaces, by the two lens surfaces, and by the vitreoretinal interface. The vitreoretinal interface echo is followed by a complex

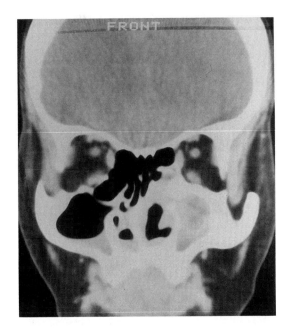

FIGURE 3.29. Computrized tomogram demonstrating opacification of the left maxillary sinus in this patient with Wegener's granulomatosis.

of echoes representing retina, choroid, sclera, and retrobulbar fat. Posterior scleral thickening due to inflammation can be detected by high-amplitude continuous spikes.

3.2.5.1.2. B Scan Ultrasonography

The B scan technique combines transducer scanning and electronic processing to produce two-dimensional cross-section images of the eye along any desired scan plane. The echoes are presented as dots instead of spikes. In the axial B echogram of the normal eye, echoes are produced by the anterior and posterior surface of the cornea separated by a sonolucent interval representing the corneal stroma, by the anterior surface of the iris, by the posterior surface of the iris merging with the anterior lens surface, and by the vitreoretinal interface. In the normal eye, echoes from the retina cannot be separated from echoes from the choroid and the sclera. Posterior scleral thickening due to inflammation can be detected by multiple reflections of the sound beam. The echoes remain after sound beam attenuation, indicating high internal reflectivity caused by

multiple, relatively flat interfaces. If retrobulbar edema surrounds the optic nerve, the "T" sign, which consists of squaring off of the normally rounded optic nerve shadow with extension of the edema along the adjacent sclera, is seen.

3.2.5.2. Computerized Tomography Scanning

Routine ocular computerized tomography (CT) scans consist of multiple axial "cuts" at different levels of the orbit. Eye, orbital walls, extraocular muscles, and paranasal sinuses are, therefore, sectioned longitudinally in the horizontal plane.[113] The ability of the X-ray CT to delineate small, soft tissues of different densities makes it a useful diagnostic tool to detect extraocular muscle or lacrimal gland enlargement, sinus tissue involvement (Fig. 3.29), or posterior scleral thickening,[110,114] which are important features for the differential diagnosis of posterior scleritis from orbital inflammatory diseases and orbital neoplasms.[114–116] Radiopaque medium may be injected during the scan to enhance the scleral thickening. The primary disadvantages of CT scanning are poor contrast between some soft tissues, radiation hazard (orbital CT scan: 2 to 3 rads, depending on the slice thickness and the number of cuts made; this is similar to an orbital series of skull X rays), and lack of scanning in the sagittal plane.

3.2.5.3. Magnetic Resonance Imaging

The most frequent atomic nucleus in living tissue is the hydrogen nucleus. The hydrogen nucleus is composed of a single proton, which has a positive electrical charge and spins on its axis. A magnetic field is generated around this rotating electrical charge. The magnetic resonance imaging (MRI) technique is based on two different tissue properties: the density of hydrogen nuclei present in the tissue and the spin-relaxation rates.[113] Magnetic resonance imaging provides superior soft tissue contrast compared to CT scanning.

Differentiation of localized inflammatory pseudotumor from posterior scleritis in pro-

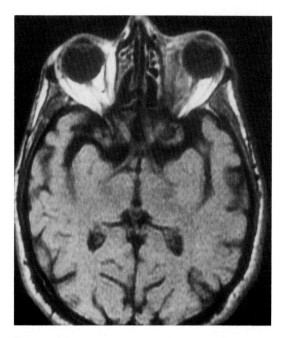

FIGURE 3.30. Magnetic resonance imaging (MRI) scan demonstrating retrobulbar "bright zones" characteristic of inflammatory pseudotumor.

ptosis (Fig. 3.30), or of choroidal tumors from posterior scleritis in subretinal mass, is easily accomplished with MRI. In addition, some orbital tumors causing choroidal folds and retinal striae, also signs of posterior scleritis, can be successfully detected by MRI. Magnetic resonance imaging does not use ionizing radiation and although intravenous injection of gadolinium is useful, there is often less need to rely on injectable agents to provide soft tissue detail. Other advantages of MRI over CT include its ability of visualize planes other than the axial plane with no loss of spatial resolution, its ability to detect areas of demyelinating activity in multiple sclerosis, and its ability to detect microinfarcts in patients with vasculitic diseases (Fig. 3.31). On the other hand, MRI is much more expensive than CT and it is a relatively slow process compared to CT; MRI cannot be performed in the presence of a metallic foreign body because it can harm vital orbital structures; patients with cardiac pacemakers should not be imaged with MRI because of the possibility of pacemaker malfunctions.

3.3. Biopsy

The third phase of the approach to scleritis includes the decision as to whether a tissue biopsy should be performed. Ocular tissue biopsy may be indicated in some cases of diffuse, nodular, or necrotizing scleritis that may be associated with a systemic vasculitic disease or with a local or systemic infection (see Chapter 5).

3.3.1. Biopsy for Suspected Systemic Vasculitic Disease

Episcleral and perforating scleral vessels consist of capillary and postcapillary venules; because capillaries do not have tunica media, a purely classic, histopathological definition of vasculitis cannot be applied to them. The term *inflammatory microangiopathy* has been adopted by us to define histopathological neutrophilic infiltration in and around the

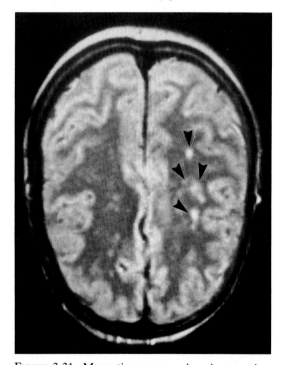

FIGURE 3.31. Magnetic resonance imaging scan in a patient ultimately shown to have systemic lupus erythematosus. Note the T2 bright spots indicative of microinfarcts compatible with a microangiitis.

vessel wall of capillary and postcapillary venules. Inflammatory microangiopathy may also be defined as immunoreactant deposition in the vessel wall, as detected by immunofluorescence studies (Fig. 3.32; see color insert).

Detection of inflammatory microangiopathy in conjunctival and/or scleral tissues from patients with recurrent nodular or diffuse scleritis may be helpful in supporting a diagnosis of suspected systemic vasculitic disease. However, because inflammatory microangiopathy in conjunctival and/or scleral tissues is nearly always present in necrotizing scleritis,[117] tissue biopsy in these cases is not required.

Conjunctival and/or scleral inflammatory microangiopathy can be associated with inflammation of small- and medium-sized vessels elsewhere in the body as part of systemic vasculitic syndromes. Vasculitis of small- and medium-sized vessels may appear in skin or other involved organs in patients with rheumatoid arthritis, systemic lupus erythematosus, relapsing polychondritis, arthritis associated with inflammatory bowel disease, psoriatic arthritis, polyarteritis nodosa, Behçet's disease, Cogan's syndrome, Wegener's granulomatosis, and allergic granulomatous angiitis (Churg–Strauss syndrome). Although in ankylosing spondylitis, Reiter's syndrome, and giant cell arteritis the presence of vasculitis is mostly found in large-sized vessels, small- and medium-sized vessels may also be affected.

The presence of inflammatory microangiopathy in conjunctival and/or scleral tissue can be helpful in making the decision to institute immunosuppressive therapy. In patients with systemic vasculitic disease and recurrent nodular or diffuse scleritis, the demonstration of inflammatory microangiopathy in conjunctival and/or scleral tissue implies systemic involvement of the same vasculitic process. Immunosuppressive therapy can be life saving for this group of patients. In patients with suspected (no definitive diagnosis) systemic vasculitic disease and recurrent nodular or diffuse scleritis, the demonstration of inflammatory microangiopathy in conjunctival and/or scleral tissue provides additional justification for the institution of immunosuppressive therapy.

3.3.2. Biopsy for Suspected Local or Systemic Infectious Disease

Detection of an infectious agent in conjunctival and/or scleral tissues is essential in confirming a suspected infectious scleritis. Bacteria, fungi, viruses, and parasites may be isolated from conjunctiva and/or scleral tissues of patients with diffuse, nodular, or necrotizing scleritis, as a result of direct invasion either from local or systemic infections. Infectious agent isolation in conjunctival and/or scleral tissue allows the institution of specific local or systemic treatment that may improve the ocular and systemic prognoses.

3.4. Data Integration: Diagnosis

In the fourth phase of the clinical approach to patients with scleritis, the clinical data are integrated with test and biopsy results to confirm or discard the preliminary diagnosis. Although clinical data, test results, and biopsy findings may not be diagnostic when each is considered independently, the combination of the three can lead to better diagnostic predictions.

3.5. Therapeutic Plan

In the fifth and final phase, therapeutic possibilities for the particular diagnosis are discussed with the patient. Whether considering medical or surgical procedures, the proper role of the doctor is to educate the patient, apprising him or her of the relative risks and benefits of possible strategies, and providing an opinion of what probability this ratio favors a specific strategy. The therapeutic plan should reflect an agreement between a well-informed patient and an ophthalmologist who, by virtue of education and training, is an expert in the type of therapy selected, and in the early recognition and management of drug-induced complications.

Summary

The approach to the patient with scleritis should include five phases. The first phase includes the investigation of the illness through the interview and physical examination of the patient. Because scleritis often portends an underlying, potentially lethal systemic disease, this phase cannot be overemphasized. The interview consists of an analysis of the major complaint and history of the present illness; episcleritis presents as an uncomfortable, watery, red eye with absence of severe pain and scleral swelling, whereas scleritis presents with deep, severe, periorbital pain radiating to the head, temple, and jaw, often preventing the patient from sleep. The history continues with the past and family history, and an exhaustive review of systems. Within the latter, constitutional symptoms such as chills, fever, poor appetite, recent weight loss, and fatigue may suggest a systemic process; skin and hair, respiratory, genitourinary, rheumatological, gastrointestinal, neurological, and ear, nose, and throat manifestations should lead the ophthalmologist to suspect certain types of systemic disorders such as connective tissue diseases with or without vasculitis, infectious diseases, gout, rosacea, or atopy. Physical examination includes not only the eye but also the head and extremities; scleral examination includes an external examination in daylight and a slit-lamp examination with white and red-free light. As the ophthalmologist completes this phase, possible diagnoses should come to mind.

The second phase consists of selection of the blood, urine, and imaging studies that are needed to investigate the possibilities raised in the first phase. In the third phase, the decision is made as to whether a tissue biopsy is likely to add useful information to the diagnosis or to the therapy. The fourth phase integrates the clinical findings with tests and biopsy results, leading to a specific diagnosis. In the fifth phase, a therapeutic plan is initiated and the response is observed.

References

1. Watson PG, Hayreh SS: Scleritis and episcleritis. Br J Ophthalmol 60:163, 1976.
2. Spencer WH: Sclera. In Spencer WH (Ed): *Ophthalmic Pathology*, 3rd ed. W.B. Saunders, Philadelphia, 1985, pp 389–422.
3. Waaler E: On the occurrence of a factor in human serum activating the specific agglutination of sheep blood corpuscles. Acta Pathol Microbiol Scand 17:172, 1940.
4. Rose HM, Ragan C, Pearce E, *et al.*: Differential agglutination of normal and sensitized sheep erythrocytes by sera of patients with rheumatoid arthritis. Proc Soc Exp Biol Med 68:1, 1948.
5. Carson DA: Rheumatoid factor. In Kelley WN, Harris ED Jr, Ruddy S, Sledge CB (Eds): *Textbook of Rheumatology*, 3rd ed. W.B. Saunders, Philadelphia, 1989, pp 664–679.
6. Dresner E, Trombly P: The latex-fixation reaction in nonrheumatic diseases. N Engl J Med 261:981, 1959.
7. Howell DS, Malcolm JM, Pike H: The FII agglutinating factors in the serum of patients with nonrheumatic diseases. Am J Med 29:662, 1960.
8. Kunkel HG, Simon HJ, Fudenberg H: Observations concerning positive serologic reactions for rheumatoid factor in certain patients with sarcoidosis and other hyperglobulinemic states. Arthritis Rheum 1:289, 1958.
9. Aho K, Palosuo T, Raunio V, Puska P, Aromaa A, Salonen JT: When does rheumatoid disease start? Arthritis Rheum 28:485, 1985.
10. Ball J, Lawrence JS: The relationship of rheumatoid serum factor to rheumatoid arthritis. Ann Rheum Dis 22:311, 1963.
11. Del Puente A, Knowler WC, Pettitt DJ, Bennett PH: The incidence of rheumatoid arthritis is predicted by rheumatoid factor titer in a longitudinal population study. Arthritis Rheum 31:1239, 1988.
12. Bland JH, Brown EW: Seronegative and seropositive rheumatoid arthritis. Clinical, radiological, and biochemical differences. Ann Intern Med 60:88, 1964.
13. Mongan ES, Cass RM, Jacox RF, Vaugher JH: A study of the relation of seronegative and seropositive rheumatoid arthritis to each other and to necrotizing vasculitis. Am J Med 47:33, 1969.
14. Sharp JT, Calkins E, Cohen AS, *et al.*: Observations on the clinical, chemical, and serologi-

cal manifestations of rheumatoid arthritis based on the course of 154 cases. Medicine 43:41, 1964.

15. Sievers K: The rheumatoid factor in definite rheumatoid arthritis: an analysis of 1279 adult patients, with a follow-up study. Acta Rheum Scand Suppl 9:1, 1965.

16. Koopman WJ, Schrohenloher RE: Rheumatoid factor. In Utsinger PD, Zvaifler NJ, Ehrlich GE (Eds): *Rheumatoid Arthritis.* Lippincott, Philadelphia, 1985, pp 217–241.

17. Koopman WJ, Schrohenloher RE: A sensitive radioimmunoassay for quantitation of IgM rheumatoid factor. Arthritis Rheum 23:302, 1980.

18. Koopman WJ, Schrohenloher RE, Solomon A: A quantitative assay for IgA rheumatoid factor. J Immunol Methods 50:89, 1982.

19. Hay FC, Nineham LJ, Roitt IM: Routine assay for detection of IgG and IgM antiglobulins in seronegative and seropositive rheumatoid arthritis. Br Med J 3:203, 1975.

20. Wernick R, LoSpalluto JJ, Fink CW, Ziff M: Serum IgG and IgM rheumatoid factors by solid phase radioimmunoassay: a comparison between adult and juvenile rheumatoid arthritis. Arthritis Rheum 24:1501, 1981.

21. Hardgraves MM, Richmond H, Morton R: Presentation of two bone marrow elements: the "tart" cell and "LE" cell. Proc Staff Meet Mayo Clin 23:25, 1948.

22. Haserick JR, Sunderberg RD: The bone marrow as a diagnosis aid in acute disseminated lupus erythematosus. J Invest Dermatol 11:209, 1948.

23. Friou GJ: Clinical application of lupus serum-nucleoprotein reaction using fluorescent antibody technique. J Clin Invest 36:890, 1957.

24. Holman HR, Kunkel HG: Affinity between the lupus erythematosus serum factor and cell nuclei and nucleoprotein. Science 126:162, 1957.

25. Holborow EJ, Weir DM, Johnson GD: A serum factor in lupus erythematosus with affinity for tissue nuclei. Br Med J 2:732, 1957.

26. Fries JF: *Systemic Lupus Erythematosus: A Clinical Analysis.* W.B. Saunders, Philadelphia, 1975.

27. Reichlin M: Antinuclear antibodies. In Kelley WN, Harris ED Jr, Ruddy S, Sledge CB (Eds): *Textbook of Rheumatology,* 3rd ed. W.B. Saunders, Philadelphia, 1989, pp 690–706.

28. Notman DD, Kurata N, Tan EM: Profiles of antinuclear antibodies in systemic rheumatic disease. Ann Intern Med 83:464, 1975.

29. Ballou SP, Kushner I: Anti-native DNA detection by the crithidia luciliae method: an improved guide to the diagnosis and management of systemic lupus erythematosus. Arthritis Rheum 22:321, 1979.

30. Munves EF, Schur PH: Antibodies to Sm and RNP: prognosticators of disease involvement. Arthritis Rheum 26:848, 1983.

31. Tan EM, Rodnan GP, Garcia I, Moroi Y, Fritzler MJ, Peebles C: Diversity of antinuclear antibodies in progressive systemic sclerosis. Arthritis Rheum 23:617, 1980.

32. Fritzler MJ, Kinsella TD, Garbutt E: The CREST syndrome: a distinct serologic entity with anticentromere antibodies. Am J Med 65:520, 1980.

33. Bresnihan B, Bunn C, Snaith ML, Hughes GR: Antiribonucleoprotein antibodies in connective tissue diseases: examination by counterimmunoelectrophoresis. Br J Med 1:610, 1977.

34. Martinez-Lavin M, Vaughn JH, Tan EM: Autoantibodies and the spectrum of Sjögren's syndrome. Ann Intern Med 91:185, 1979.

35. van der Woude FJ, Rasmussen N, Lobatto S, Wiik A, Permin H, van Es LA, van der Giessen M, van der Hem GK, The TH: Autoantibodies against neutrophils and monocytes; tool for diagnosis and marker of disease activity in Wegener's granulomatosis. Lancet 1:425, 1985.

36. Ludemann G, Gross WL. Autoantibodies against cytoplasmic structures of neutrophil granulocytes in Wegener's granulomatosis. Clin Exp Immunol 69:350, 1987.

37. Savage CS, Winearls CG, Jones S, *et al.*: Prospective study of radioimmunoassay for antibodies against neutrophil cytoplasm in diagnosis of systemic vasculitis. Lancet 1:1389, 1987.

38. Nölle B, Specks U, Lüdemann J, *et al.*: Anticytoplasmic autoantibodies: their immunodiagnostic value in Wegener's granulomatosis. Ann Intern Med 111:28, 1989.

39. Falk RJ, Jennette JC: Antineutrophil cytoplasmic autoantibodies with specificity for myeloperoxidase in patients with systemic vasculitis and idiopathic necrotizing and crescentic glomerulonephritis. N Engl J Med 318:1651, 1988.

40. Bullen CL, Liesegang TJ, McDonald TJ, DeRemee RA: Ocular complications of Wegener's granulomatosis. Ophthalmology 90:279, 1983.

41. Jennette JC, Wilkman AS, Falk RJ: Antineutrophil cytoplasmic autoantibody-

associated glomerulonephritis and vasculitis. Am J Pathol 135:921, 1989.

42. Pulido JS, Goeken JA, Nerad JA, *et al.*: Ocular manifestations of patients with circulating antineutrophil cytoplasmic antibodies. Arch Ophthalmol 108:845, 1990.

43. Soukiasian SH, Foster CS, Niles JL, Raizman MB: Diagnostic value of anti-neutrophil cytoplasmic antibodies (ANCA) in scleritis associated with Wegener's granulomatosis. Ophthalmology 99(1):125, 1992.

44. Cochrane C, Hawkins D: Studies on circulating immune complexes. III. Factors governing the ability of circulating complexes to localize in blood vessels. J Exp Med 127:137, 1968.

45. Nydegger UE, Kazatchkine MD, Lambert PH: Immune complexes. In Fougereau M, Dausset J (Eds): *Progress in Immunology IV.* Academic Press, New York, 1980.

46. Jones VE, Jacoby RK, Wallington T, Holt P: Immune complexes in early arthritis. I. Detection of immune complexes before rheumatoid arthritis is definite. Clin Exp Immunol 44:512, 1981.

47. Zubler RH, Nydegger UE, Perrin LH, Fehr K, McCormick J, Lambert PH, Miescher PA: Circulating and intraarticular immune complexes in patients with rheumatoid arthritis. J Clin Invest 57:1308, 1976.

48. Gabay R, Zubler RH, Nydegger UE, Lambert PH: Immune complexes and complement catabolism in ankylosing spondylitis. Arthritis Rheum 20:913, 1977.

49. Lessard J, Nunnery E, Cecere F, McDuffy S, Pope RM: Relationship between the articular manifestations of rheumatoid arthritis and circulating immune complexes detected by three methods and specific classes of rheumatoid factors. J Rheumatol 10:411, 1983.

50. Hamburger MI, Lawley TJ, Kimberly RP, Plotz PH, Frank MM: A serial study of systemic reticuloendothelial system Fc receptor functional activity in systemic lupus erythematosus. Arthritis Rheum 25:1, 1982.

51. LLoyd W, Schur PH: Immune complexes, complement, and antiDNA in exacerbations of systemic lupus erythematosus (SLE). Medicine 60:208, 1981.

52. Scott DG, Bacon PA, Tribe CR: Systemic rheumatoid vasculitis: a clinical and laboratory study of 50 cases. Medicine (Baltimore) 60(4):288, 1981.

53. Zubler RH, Lange G, Lambert PH, Miescher PA: Detection of immune complexes in unheated sera by a modified ^{125}I-C1q binding test. Effect of heating on the binding of C1q by immune complexes and application of the test to systemic lupus erythematosus. J Immunol 116:232, 1976.

54. Theofilopoulos AN, Wilson CB, Dixon FJ: The Raji cell radioimmune assay for detecting immune complexes in human sera. J Clin Invest 57:169, 1976.

55. Hugli TE: The structural basis for anaphylatoxin and chemotactic function of C3a, C4a, and C5a. CRC Crit Rev Immunol 2:321, 1981.

56. Hugli TE, Muller-Eberhard HJ: Anaphylatoxins: C3a and C5a. Adv Immunol 26:1, 1987.

57. Scott DGI, Bacon PA, Allen C, Elson CJ, Wallington T: IgG rheumatoid factor, complement, and immune complexes in rheumatoid synovitis and vasculitis: comparative and serial studies during cytotoxic therapy. Clin Exp Immunol 43:54, 1981.

58. Hunder GG, McDuffie FC: Hypocomplementinemia in rheumatoid arthritis. Am J Med 54:461, 1973.

59. Shur PH: Complement studies of sera and other biologic fluids. Hum Pathol 14:338, 1983.

60. Ruddy S, Everson LK, Shur PH, Austen KF: Hemolytic assay of the ninth complement component: elevation and depletion in rheumatic diseases. J Exp Med 134:259S, 1971.

61. Ruddy S, Carpenter CB, Müller-Eberhard HJ, *et al.*: Complement component levels in hereditary angioneurotic edema and isolated C'2 deficiency in man. In Miescher PA, Grabar P (Eds): *Mechanisms of Inflammation Induced by Immune Reactions.* Vth International Immunopathology Symposium. Schwabe, Basel, 1968, p 231.

62. Mayer MM: Complement and complement fixation. In Kabat EA, Mayer MM (Eds): *Experimental Immunochemistry.* Charles C Thomas, Springfield IL, 1961, p 133.

63. Calin A: HLA-B27: to type or not to type? Ann Intern Med 92:208, 1980.

64. Calin A: HLA-B27 in 1982. Reappraisal of a clinical test. Ann Intern Med 96:114, 1982.

65. Holmes KK, Lukehart SA: Syphilis. In Braunwald E, Isselbacher KJ, Petersdorf RG, Wilson JA, Martin JB, Fauci As (Eds): *Harrison's Principles of Internal Medicine,* 11th ed, Vol 1. McGraw-Hill, New York, 1987, pp 639–649.

66. Spoor TC, Wynn P, Hartel WC, Bryan CS: Ocular syphilis: acute and chronic. J Clin Neurol Ophthalmol 3:197, 1983.

67. Harner RE, Smith JL, Israel CW: The FTA-ABS in late syphilis. A serological study in 1985 cases. JAMA 203:545, 1968.

68. Hart G: Syphilis tests in diagnostic and therapeutic decision making. Ann Intern Med 104:368, 1986.

69. Lesser RL, Kornmehl EW, Pachner AR, Kattah J, Hedges TR, Newman NM, Ecker PA, Glassman MI: Neuroophthalmologic manifestations of Lyme disease. Ophthalmology 97:699, 1990.

70. Harper DR, Grose C: IgM and IgG responses to varicella-zoster virus p32/p36 complex after chickenpox and zoster, congenital and subclinical infectios, and vaccination. J Infect Dis 159:444, 1989.

71. Jones HE, Miller SD, Greenburg HH: Measurement of tuberculin reactions. N Engl J Med 287:721, 1972.

72. Watson PG, Bovey E: Anterior segment fluorescein angiography in the diagnosis of scleral inflammation. Ophthalmology 92:1, 1985.

73. Watson PG, Booth-Mason S: Fluorescein angiography in the differential diagnosis of sclerokeratitis. Br J Ophthalmol 71:145, 1987.

74. Bron AJ, Easty DL: Fluorescein angiography of the globe and anterior segment. Trans Ophthalmol Soc UK 90:339, 1970.

75. Watson PG: Anterior segment fluorescein angiography in the surgery of immunologically induced corneal and scleral destructive disorders. Ophthalmology 94:1452, 1987.

76. Raizman MB, Sainz de la Maza M, Foster CS: Tectonic keratoplasty for peripheral ulcerative keratitis. Cornea 10(4):312, 1991.

77. Amalric P, Rebière P, Jourdes JC: Nouvelles indications de l'angiographie fluoresceinique du segment anterieur de l'oeil. Ann Ocul 204:455, 1971.

78. Ikegami M: Fluorescein angiography of the anterior ocular segment. 1. Hemodynamics in the anterior ciliary vessels. Nippon Ganka Gakkai Zasshi 78:371, 1974.

79. Matsui M, Justice J Jr: Anterior segment fluorescein angiography. Int Ophthalmol Clin 16:189, 1976.

80. Kottow MH: *Anterior Segment Fluorescein Angiography*. Williams & Wilkins, Baltimore, 1978.

81. Saari KM: Anterior segment fluorescein angiography in inflammatory diseases of the cornea. Acta Ophthalmol 57:781, 1979.

82. Marsh RJ, Ford SM: Blood flow in the anterior segment of the eye. Trans Ophthalmol Soc UK 100:388, 1980.

83. Talusan ED, Schwartz B: Fluorescein angiography: demonstration of flow pattern of anterior ciliary arteries. Arch Ophthalmol 99:1074, 1981.

84. Meyer PA, Watson PG: Low dose fluorescein angiography of the conjunctiva and episclera. Br J Ophthalmol 71:2, 1987.

85. Meyer PA: Pattern of blood flow in episcleral vessels studied by low-dose fluorescein videoangiography. Eye 2:533, 1988.

86. Ormerod LD, Fariza E, Hughes GW, Doane MG, Webb RH: Ophthalmology 97:745, 1990.

87. Novotny HR, Alvis DL: A method of photographing fluorescence in circulating blood in the human retina. Circulation 24:82, 1961.

88. Ashton N: The blood retinal barrier and vasoglial relationship in retinal disease. Trans Ophthalmol Soc UK 85:199, 1965.

89. Jensen VA, Lundback K: Fluorescence angiography of the iris in recent and long-term diabetes: preliminary communication (XVII Scandinavian Ophthalmological Congress, Copenhagen 1967). Acta Ophthalmol (Copenhagen) 46:584, 1968.

90. Cobb B: Vascular tufts at the pupillary margin. Trans Ophthalmol Soc UK 88:211, 1968.

91. Raviola G: Conjunctival and episcleral blood vessels are permeable to blood-borne horseradish peroxidase. Invest Ophthalmol Vis Sci 24:725, 1983.

92. Iwamoto T, Smelser GK: Electron microscopic studies of corneal capillaries. Invest Ophthalmol Vis Sci 4:815, 1965.

93. Rabkin MD, Bellhorn MB, Bellhorn R: Selected molecular weight dextrans for in vivo permeability studies of rat retinal vascular disease. Exp Eye Res 24:607, 1977.

94. Bellhorn R: Permeability of blood-ocular barriers of neonatal and adult cats to fluorescein-labelled dextrans of selected molecular size. Invest Ophthalmol Vis Sci 21:282, 1981.

95. Lightman SL, Caspers-Velu LE, Hirose S, Nussenblatt RB, Palestine AG: Angiography with fluorescein-labeled dextrans in a primate model of uveitis. Arch Ophthalmol 105:844, 1987.

96. Palestine AG, Brubaker RF: Plasma binding of fluorescein in normal subjects and in diabetic patients. Arch Ophthalmol 100:1160, 1982.

97. Meyer PA, Fitzke FW: Computer assisted analysis of fluorescein videoangiograms. Br J Ophthalmol 74:275, 1990.

98. Risco JM, Nopanitaya W: Ocular microcirculation; scanning electron microscopic study.
Invest Ophthalmol Vis Sci 19:5, 1980.

99. Ashton N: Anatomical study of Schlemm's
canal and aqueous veins by means of neoprene
casts. Br J Ophthalmol 35:291, 1951.

100. Ashton N: Anatomical study of Schlemm's
canal and aqueous veins by means of neoprene
casts. II. Aqueous veins. Br J Ophthalmol
36:265, 1952.

101. Morrison JC, Van Buskirk EM: Anterior
collateral circulation in the primate eye.
Ophthalmology 90:707, 1983.

102. Brancato R, Frosini R, Boshi M: L'Angiografia
superficiale a fluorescein del bulbo oculare.
Ann Ottal Clin Ocul 95:433, 1969.

103. Laatikainen L: Perilimbal vasculature in
glaucomatous   eyes.   Acta   Ophthalmol
111(suppl):54, 1971.

104. Raitta C, Vannas S: Fluorescein angiographic
features of the limbus and perilimbal vessels.
Ear Nose Throat J 50:58, 1971.

105. Shimizu K, Ujie K: [*Structure of Ocular
Vessels*] Igaku-Shoin, Tokyo, 1978.

106. Bron AJ, Easty DL: Fluorescein angiography
of the globe and anterior segment. Trans
Ophthalmol Soc UK 90:339, 1970.

107. Meyer PA: The circulation of the human
limbus. Eye 3:121, 1989.

108. Smith ME, Haik BG, Coleman DJ: Diagnostic
ocular ultrasonography. In Masters BR (Ed):
Noninvasive   Diagnostic   Techniques   in

Ophthalmology. Springer-Verlag, New York,
1990, pp 47–60.

109. Benson WE, Shields JA, Tasman W, Crandall
AS: Posterior scleritis. A cause of diagnostic confusion. Arch Ophthalmol 97:1482,
1979.

110. Benson   WE: Posterior   scleritis.   Surv
Ophthalmol 32:297, 1988.

111. Cappaert WE, Purnell EW, Frank KE: Use of
B-sector scan ultrasound in the diagnosis of
benign choroidal folds. Am J Ophthalmol
84:375, 1977.

112. Rochels R, Reis G: Echography in posterior
scleritis. Klin Monatsbl Augenheilk 177:611,
1980.

113. Taveras JL, Haik BG: Magnetic resonance
imaging in ophthalmology. In Masters BR
(Ed): *Noninvasive Diagnostic Techniques in
Ophthalmology*. Springer-Verlag, New York,
1990, pp 32–46.

114. Mauriello JA, Flanagan JC: Management of
orbital inflammatory disease. A protocol. Surv
Ophthalmol 29:104, 1984.

115. Trokel SL, Hilal SK: Submillimeter resolution
CT scanning of orbital diseases. Ophthalmology 87:412, 1980.

116. Trokel SL: Computed tomographic scanning
of orbital inflammations. Int Ophthalmol Clin
22(4):81, 1982.

117. Fong LP, Sainz de la Maza M, Rice BA,
Foster CS: Immunopathology of scleritis.
Ophthalmology 98:472, 1991.

4
Clinical Considerations of Episcleritis and Scleritis: The Massachusetts Eye and Ear Infirmary Experience

Because episcleritis and scleritis are entities encountered infrequently in general ophthalmic practice, the diagnosis and subsequent treatment may be missed or delayed because of the relative lack of experience in their detection and management. Fraunfelder and Watson[1] reported that in a series of 30 enucleated eyes (sent from hospitals from all parts of Great Britain) with a primary histological diagnosis of scleritis, the clinical diagnosis of scleritis had been missed in 12 (40%), often because the scleritis was masked by multiple complications such as uveitis, glaucoma, and keratolysis. Many of these 12 eyes had not received antiinflammatory treatment and many of the 18 eyes affected by clinical scleritis had received insufficient antiinflammatory treatment. The main reason for enucleation was pain with loss of vision. Many of these patients had had the ocular inflammation for up to 30 years before the enucleation.

Inflammation of the wall of the eyeball ranges from innocent and harmless self-limiting episcleritis, requiring little or no antiinflammatory therapy, to painful, sight-threatening, necrotizing scleritis requiring intensive antiinflammatory and/or immunosuppressive therapy if the globe is to be preserved; moreover, scleritis may often be the presenting manifestation of many potentially lethal systemic diseases. It is therefore vital that the correct diagnosis is made and that subsequent adequate treatment be given as early as possible in the course of the disease.

Because of the comparative rarity of scleritis, general considerations on the symptoms, signs, pathological findings, prognoses, and treatments, are difficult to obtain. The excellent episcleritis and scleritis survey[2] and treatise,[3] performed by Watson and co-workers at Moorfields Eye Hospital in London in 1976, have provided us with an exceptional perspective of the spectrum of episcleritis and scleritis. The Scleritis Clinic at Moorfields Eye Hospital in London was established in 1963 and since then has been receiving highly selected patients with inflammatory conditions of sclera or episclera. All the patients are referred, because of difficulties in diagnosis, difficulties in treatment, or both. Subsequent reports by Watson and co-workers on different aspects of diagnosis and management have also been helpful and have served as the foundation on which contemporary studies of smaller patient populations rests.[4–13]

In an attempt to contribute to the study of the intricacies of scleral disease, we have analyzed our experience with patients with episcleritis and scleritis seen at the Massachusetts Eye and Ear Infirmary in Boston. The Immunology Service at the Massachusetts Eye and Ear Infirmary in Boston was established in 1975. The patients referred to this service, primarily from the northeastern United States, typically have destructive, progressive inflammation of the conjunctiva, cornea, sclera, uvea, or retina. Patients with episcleritis and scleritis are referred mainly because of difficulties with diagnosis and management. Our study is based on a review of those patients with episcleritis and scleritis treated during the 11-year period from May 1980 to May 1991 and about whom we have adequate follow-up information. This study group is composed of 266 patients (358 eyes), 94 with episcleritis (127 eyes) and 172 with scleritis (231 eyes). The mean follow-up time for patients with episcleritis was 11 months (range, 1 month to 10 years) and for patients with scleritis was 15 months (range, 1 month to 11 years).

Objective data on the prevalance of scleritis are difficult to obtain because they can vary greatly depending on the type of institution in which the studies are performed. Data on the prevalance of episcleritis are even more difficult to estimate because patients may not seek medical advice because of rapid resolution or they may be treated by general physicians. They may go to an ophthalmology department only if the condition is persistent and/or recurrent. Examples of the prevalance variability depending on the type of institution are the following: of 9600 new patient referrals to the Department of Ophthalmology of Southern General Hospital and Victoria Infirmary in Glasgow during an 8-year period, 8 cases of scleral inflammation were diagnosed (0.08%).[14] Of 6600 new patient referrals to the Immunology Service at the Massachusetts Eye and Ear Infirmary Hospital in Boston during an 11-year period (May 1980 to May 1991), 266 cases of episcleritis and scleritis were diagnosed (4%), including 94 cases with episcleritis (1.4%) and 172 cases with scleritis (2.6%).

Data from highly selected patients of ophthalmology services will be biased to higher numbers of patients with scleritis with respect to patients with episcleritis, to higher numbers of patients with episcleritis and scleritis with respect to the total number of new patient referrals, and to higher numbers of patients with more severe subcategories with respect to patients with more benign subcategories. Recognizing this, the prevalance of the different types of episcleritis and scleritis in our series is shown in Table 4.1.

This chapter focuses on the clinical considerations of episcleritis and scleritis and their subcategories.

4.1. Episcleritis

4.1.1. Introduction

Episcleritis is a benign inflammatory disease that is characterized by edema and cellular infiltration of the episcleral tissue. Whether treated or not, the condition is self-limited after a few days, and although it may recur over a period of many years it rarely leaves any residual ocular damage. In two-thirds of the cases the disease is considered idiopathic.

4.1.2. Patient Characteristics

Episcleritis occurs in young adults, usually women, with a peak incidence in the fourth decade.[3] In our series of patients with episcleritis, the mean age of onset of the first episode was 43 years (Table 4.2). Episcleritis was three times as common in women as in men (Table 4.3). Although episcleritis may affect individuals of all races, there are no studies on the

TABLE 4.1. Episcleritis and scleritis classification.

Diagnosis	No. (%) of patients	Eyes	Type	No. (%) of patients	Eyes
Episcleritis	94 (35.34)	127	Simple	78 (82.98)	108
			Nodular	16 (17.02)	19
Scleritis	172 (64.66)	231	Diffuse	77 (44.77)	107
Total:	266	358	Nodular	39 (22.67)	50
			Necrotizing	39 (22.67)	48
			Scleromalacia	6 (3.49)	11
			Posterior	11 (6.40)	15

TABLE 4.2. Age distribution among patients with episcleritis and scleritis.

Diagnosis	Mean age of onset (years)	Age range (years)
Episcleritis	43.39	14–79
Simple	42.09	14–79
Nodular	49.75	20–78
Scleritis	51.59	11–87
Diffuse	46.82	11–78
Nodular	49.80	18–82
Necrotizing	61.92	34–87
Scleromalacia	61.67	38–75
Posterior	49.10	26–67
Mean age (entire population):	48.83	11–87

incidence and prevalence within racial groups. Some early reports suggested that the condition had a Mendelian dominant transmission[15,16]; our experience shows that episcleritis is not per se a hereditary condition, although some of the episcleritis-associated systemic diseases, such as rheumatoid arthritis, systemic lupus erythematosus, ankylosing spondylitis, Reiter's syndrome, Behçet's disease, gout, and atopy, have a genetic basis.

4.1.3. Clinical Manifestations

Episcleritis is usually characterized by recurrences involving different eyes at different times and affecting one area after another. Sometimes, however, the patient develops the inflammation in both eyes at the same time.

Over 60% of patients with episcleritis may have recurrences for 3 to 6 years after the onset of the disease, but the episodes become less frequent after the first 3 to 4 years, until the problem no longer recurs.[2,3] In our series of patients with episcleritis, the duration ranged from 1 month to 38 years. Bilaterality was found in 35% of our patients (Table 4.4). The main symptom is mild discomfort, which can be described as a feeling of heat, sharpness, or irritation, and the main sign is redness, which can be localized in one sector or can involve the whole episclera. Pain, if any, is usually described as a slight ache localized to the eye. On rare occasions severe pain radiating to the forehead and tenderness to the touch may be present but these symptoms are more commonly characteristic of scleritis; if marked pain and/or tenderness to touch exist in a patient who appears clinically to have episcleritis, the likelihood is considerable that in fact the patient has some component of occult scleritis. Redness, best examined in daylight, may range in intensity from a mild red flush to fiery red, but it is not accompanied by the bluish tinge present in scleritis. In a severe attack of episcleritis, lid swelling and associated spasm of the sphincter of the iris and ciliary muscle, resulting in miosis and temporary myopia, may occur, but this is a rare occurrence. Other symptoms include tearing (never true discharge) and mild photophobia.

Clinical examination with the slit-lamp, particularly with red-free light, discloses that the

TABLE 4.3. Sex distribution among patients with episcleritis and scleritis.

Diagnosis	Sex		Total
	No. (%) male	No. (%) female	
Episcleritis	**24 (25.53)**	**70 (74.47)**	**94**
Simple	21 (26.92)	57 (73.08)	78
Nodular	3 (18.75)	13 (81.25)	16
Scleritis	**67 (38.95)**	**105 (61.05)**	**172**
Diffuse	33 (42.86)	44 (57.14)	77
Nodular	13 (33.33)	26 (66.67)	39
Necrotizing	17 (43.59)	22 (56.41)	39
Scleromalacia	1 (16.67)	5 (83.33)	6
Posterior	3 (27.27)	8 (72.73)	11
Total:	91 (34.21)	Total: 175 (65.79)	

TABLE 4.4. Bilaterality among patients with episcleritis and scleritis.

Diagnosis	Bilaterality[a]	Total
Episcleritis	**33 (35.11)**	**94**
Simple	31 (39.74)	78
Nodular	2 (12.50)	16
Scleritis	**59 (34.30)**	**172**
Diffuse	30 (38.96)	77
Nodular	11 (28.21)	39
Necrotizing	9 (23.08)	39
Scleromalacia	5 (83.33)	6
Posterior	4 (36.36)	11
Total:	92 (34.59)	

[a] Number (%) of patients with bilateral involvement at some point during the course of the disease.

TABLE 4.5. Decrease in visual acuity among patients with episcleritis and scleritis.[a]

Diagnosis	No. (%) of eyes affected	Total
Episcleritis	**2 (2.13)**	**94**
Simple	2 (2.56)	78
Nodular	0	16
Scleritis	**64 (37.21)**	**172**
Diffuse	20 (25.97)	77
Nodular	5 (12.82)	39
Necrotizing	32 (82.05)	39
Scleromalacia	2 (33.33)	6
Posterior	5 (45.45)	11

[a] Decrease in visual acuity greater than or equal to two lines (on the Snellen eye chart) at the end of the follow-up period or a visual acuity of 20/80 or worse at presentation (worse of the two eyes). Mean follow-up period for episcleritis, 11 months (range, 1 month to 10 years); mean follow-up period for scleritis, 15 months (range, 1 month to 11 years).

inflammation is entirely localized within the episcleral tissue. The underlying sclera is never involved. The superficial edge of the narrow beam of the slit lamp is displaced forward, showing the episcleral edema. The deep edge of the narrow beam of the slit lamp remains flat against the sclera, showing no displacement forward by underlying scleral edema. The distribution of inflammation is more commonly in the interpalpebral area (Fig. 3.1 in Chapter 3).[17,18] The superficial episcleral vessels, following the usual radial pattern, appear congested with little coexisting congestion of the over-

lying conjunctival vessels and the underlying deep episcleral vessels, and without coexisting congestion of the scleral vessels. Topical phenylephrine (10%) or epinephrine (1:1000) instilled in the cul-de-sac has a greater vasoconstrictor effect on the episcleral vessels than on the scleral vessels. This is a useful method by which to distinguish episcleritis (where redness should diminish greatly) (Figs. 4.1 and 4.2; see color insert) from scleritis (where redness should be minimally affected by these drugs).[3] The edema of the episcleral tissue is diffusely distributed and sometimes manifests itself as subconjunctival grayish infiltrates that appear yellow when viewed with a red-free light. These infiltrates have been shown to be composed of inflammatory cells, particularly lymphocytes.

Although episcleritis does not develop into scleritis, scleritis will produce an overlying episcleritis. None of our patients with episcleritis developed scleritis, even after many recurrences and a long duration of the disease. Episcleritis rarely causes loss of vision because the associated complications, such as corneal involvement or uveitis, are uncommon and are never severe. In our series of patients with episcleritis, only 2.4% (of eyes) had loss of vision (defined as loss of two or more lines on the Snellen eye chart at the end of the follow-up period or visual acuity of 20/80 or less at presentation) (Table 4.5). This fall in visual acuity was attributed to cataracts in all of the patients. Mild peripheral corneal changes such as superficial and midstromal inflammatory cell infiltration can be observed occasionally in patients with episcleritis in the area adjacent to the conjunctival and episcleral edema, but these infiltrates never progress to corneal ulceration. They rarely are permanent unless the attacks are recurrent in the same area. None of our patients with episcleritis had peripheral ulcerative keratitis. Intraocular structures are almost never involved. In a small minority of cases, cells in the anterior chamber and aqueous flare may appear, but these are never severe. Eleven percent of our patients with episcleritis developed a mild anterior uveitis (Table 4.6). Glaucoma and cataract are not directly attributed to the episcleral inflammation unless they are induced by steroid treatment (Tables 4.7 and 4.8).[2,18] Although transient diplopia has been reported in patients with episcleritis, there is no clear association between extraocular muscle imbalance and episcleral inflammation.[18]

Anterior segment fluorescein angiogram shows a rapid filling of all the vascular networks, but the vascular pattern itself remains normal. Leakage from all vessels is rapid but remains similar to that usually seen in normal conjunctiva or episclera.

4.1.4. Classification of Episcleritis

Episcleritis may be divided into subcategories of simple episcleritis and nodular episcleritis. Both have the same characteristics described above but they differ in onset of the signs and symptoms, in localization of the inflammation, and in clinical course.

4.1.4.1. Simple Episcleritis

Simple episcleritis is more common than nodular episcleritis (Table 4.1). The involved area appears diffusely congested and edematous (Figs. 3.1, 3.2, 3.18, 3.19, 3.22, and 4.1). The onset of redness is usually rapid after the symptoms appear, reaching its peak in a few hours and gradually subsiding over a period varying from 5 to 60 days. In a study performed by Watson and co-workers,[19] in which they assessed the efficacy of two different topical antiinflammatory drugs, the majority of the attacks in patients of the control group (placebo) lasted between 5 and 10 days.[19] Each attack is self-limited and usually clears without the need for treatment. Recurrence in the same or opposite eye, involving the same or different areas, may occur within a period of 2 months. Over 60% of patients with simple episcleritis have recurrences for 3 to 6 years after the onset of the disease, but the episodes become less frequent after the first 3 to 4 years until the disease no longer recurs.[2,3]

There is a less defined group of patients who, instead of having numerous evanescent attacks, have a few prolonged ones. These patients are predominantly the ones who have

TABLE 4.6. Anterior uveitis associated with episcleritis and scleritis.

Diagnosis	No. (%) of anterior uveitis patients	Total
Episcleritis	**10 (10.64)**	**94**
Simple	9 (11.54)	78
Nodular	1 (6.25)	16
Scleritis	**73 (42.44)**	**172**
Diffuse	28 (36.36)	77
Nodular	11 (28.21)	39
Necrotizing	27 (69.23)	39
Scleromalacia	2 (33.33)	6
Posterior	5 (45.45)	11
	Total: 83 (31.20)	

TABLE 4.7. Glaucoma in episcleritis and scleritis patients.

Diagnosis	No. (%) of glaucoma patients	Total
Episcleritis	**4 (4.25)**	**94**
Simple	3 (3.85)	78
Nodular	1 (6.25)	16
Scleritis	**22 (12.79)**	**172**
Diffuse	7 (9.09)	77
Nodular	4 (10.26)	39
Necrotizing	9 (23.08)	39
Scleromalacia	1 (16.67)	6
Posterior	1 (9.09)	11
	Total: 26 (9.77)	

TABLE 4.8. Cataract in episcleritis and scleritis patients.

Diagnosis	No. (%) of cataract patients	Total
Episcleritis	**2 (2.13)**	**94**
Simple	2 (2.56)	78
Nodular	0	16
Scleritis	**29 (16.86)**	**172**
Diffuse	7 (9.09)	77
Nodular	4 (10.26)	39
Necrotizing	16 (41.02)	39
Scleromalacia	1 (16.67)	6
Posterior	1 (9.09)	11
	Total: 31 (11.65)	

some associated disease. Most of our patients with infectious etiologies had one long episode that resolved completely after appropriate treatment.

4.1.4.2. Nodular Episcleritis

In nodular episcleritis the onset of redness gradually increases over a period of 2 to 3 days. As simple episcleritis, the inflammation of nodular episcleritis is localized to the episclera; unlike simple episcleritis, however, the inflammation of nodular episcleritis is confined to a well-defined area, forming a slightly tender, dark red nodule with little surrounding congestion (Fig. 4.3; see color insert). The nodule, usually round or oval, enlarges rapidly and varies from 2 to 6 mm or larger in size.[20,21] The overlying conjunctiva can be moved over the nodule, but the nodule cannot be moved over the underlying sclera. The episcleral nodule evolves over a chronic course of inflammation, becoming paler and flatter, usually after 4 to 6 weeks, and then disappears entirely. When the episcleral nodule disappears, the underlying sclera appears normal. If there is increased residual scleral translucency, scleral inflammation instead of episcleral inflammation should be suspected; however, repeated attacks of nodular episcleritis localized at the same site for many years may increase scleral translucency. Recurrences in the same site on the same eye, at a different site on the same eye, or on the other eye, may occur, sometimes with more than one nodule at a time. The episcleral nodule can be differentiated from a conjunctival phlyctenule because the overlying conjunctiva can be moved over the episcleral nodule.[21] The episcleral nodule can be differentiated from a scleral nodule by slit-lamp examination, particularly with a red-free light; the deep edge of the narrow beam of the slit-lamp remains flat against the sclera in episcleritis and is displaced forward in scleritis.

4.1.5. Associated Diseases

Connective tissue diseases, herpes zoster, rosacea, gout, syphilis, and atopy are the diseases most commonly associated with episcleritis.[2,5,17] Thirty-two percent of our patients with episcleritis had an associated disease (Table 4.9), including 13% with a connective tissue disease or a vasculitic disease, 7% with rosacea, and 7% with atopy. Diagnoses of her-

TABLE 4.9. Disease associated with episcleritis and scleritis.

Diagnosis	No. (%) of patients with associated disease	Total
Episcleritis	**30 (31.91)**	**94**
Simple	22 (28.21)	78
Nodular	8 (50.00)	16
Scleritis	**98 (56.98)**	**172**
Diffuse	35 (45.45)	77
Nodular	17 (43.59)	39
Necrotizing	37 (94.87)	39
Scleromalacia	4 (66.67)	6
Posterior	5 (45.45)	11
Total:	128 (48.12)	

pes zoster and herpes simplex infections were ascribed to one patient each (1%). A chemical injury and gout were associated with one case each (1%) (Table 4.10). No associated diseases were found in the remaining patients.

Although gout and syphillis have been considered to be possible causes of episcleritis, the reported incidence varies between 0[17] and 7%[3] for gout and between 0[18] and 3%[3] for syphilis. Only one case of gout and no cases of syphilis were detected in our series. Erythema nodosum is considered a hypersensitivity reaction to a variety of antigenic stimuli, and thus may be seen in the course of several diseases of both known and idiopathic cause, some of which also can be associated with episcleritis: bacterial (streptococcal), mycobacterial (tuberculosis), and chlamydial (psittacosis) infections, sarcoidosis, arthritis associated with inflammatory bowel disease, and Behçet's disease. However, erythema nodosum may occur without any identifiable systemic illness.[22,23] Episcleritis can appear at the same time as the painful subcutaneous nodules of erythema nodosum appear on the legs and usually resolves as the nodules disappear.[3,18,24,25] Because erythema nodosum is a sign of other potential underlying diseases, whether identifiable or not, we have not considered it as a separate diagnostic entity. Two of our patients with episcleritis had erythema nodosum; in neither of them was a specific associated disease found. Although some patients with episcleritis give a past history of rheumatic heart disease, the conditions

TABLE 4.10. Diseases associated with episcleritis.

Associated disease	Type of episcleritis		No. of patients affected
	Simple	Nodular	
Noninfectious			
Connective tissue diseases and other inflammatory conditions			
Rheumatoid arthritis	1	2	3
Systemic lupus erythematosus	1	0	1
Ankylosing spondylitis	0	0	0
Reiter's syndrome	1	0	1
Psoriatic arthritis	2	0	2
Arthritis and IBD[a]	3	0	3
Relapsing polychondritis	0	0	0
Vasculitic diseases			
Polyarteritis nodosa	0	0	0
Allergic granulomatous angiitis (Churg–Strauss syndrome)	0	0	0
Wegener's granulomatosis	0	0	0
Behçet's disease	1	0	1
Giant cell arteritis	0	0	0
Cogan's syndrome	1	0	1
Miscellaneous			
Atopy	3	4	7
Rosacea	6	1	7
Gout	1	0	1
Foreign body granuloma	0	0	0
Chemical injury	1	0	1
Infectious			
Bacteria			
Gram-positive cocci	0	0	0
Gram-negative rods	0	0	0
Mycobacteria			
Atypical mycobacterial disease	0	0	0
Tuberculosis	0	0	0
Leprosy	0	0	0
Spirochaetes			
Syphilis	0	0	0
Lyme disease	0	0	0
Chlamydia	0	0	0
Actinomyces			
Nocardiosis	0	0	0
Fungi			
Filamentous	0	0	0
Dimorphic fungi	0	0	0
Viruses			
Herpes zoster	1	0	1
Herpes simplex	0	1	1
Mumps	0	0	0
Parasites			
Protozoa			
Acanthamoeba	0	0	0
Toxoplasmosis	0	0	0
Helminths			
Toxocariasis	0	0	0
Total:	22	8	30

[a] IBD, Inflammatory bowel disease.

have not been described as occurring at the same time.[3] Two of our patients with episcleritis had had rheumatic fever in the past; however, we did not consider the conditions associated because they had not been concomitant.

4.1.6. Precipitating Factors

There are several factors that have been described as putative triggers of recurrent episcleritis, but the reports come from sporadic anecdotes without any statistical basis. Emotional stress has been related to recurrent attacks, as in the case of the physician who had episodes of active episcleritis associated with the medical board examination, professional paper presentations, and job interviews.[26] In many instances our patients experienced the onset of some recurrent attacks during stressful life periods. The influence of emotions on physical illness has also been described for ulcerative colitis, systemic lupus erythematosus, peptic ulcer disease, and various forms of cutaneous diseases (dyshidrosis, alopecia areata, and neurodermatitis).[27–31] Studies designed to investigate the relationship between stress and inflammation do not allow any definitive conclusion (indeed, design and execution of such studies are difficult because of the variables involved and the subjective nature of the data), but insights gained from the emerging, embryonic field of neuroimmunology lend scientific support to such a relationship. Various neurochemicals, released during various emotional states such as anger, anxiety, and depression affect various types and subtypes of white blood cells through specific cell surface receptors.[32] It is even possible, through operant conditioning techniques, to develop in experimental animals a state of immunosuppression in response to a nonimmunosuppressive stimulus.[33]

Ovulation and/or menstruation also have been associated with recurrent attacks,[34–38] as in the case of a woman who, for 5 years, regularly had episodes of active episcleritis a few days prior to her menstrual period,[36] or as in the case of another woman who, for 7 years, had recurrent episcleritis during her ovulation period.[38] Once again, the field of neuroen-docrine immunology may potentially provide logical explanations for such an association.[39] No clear association between the onset of episcleritis and a specific moment of the menstrual cycle was evident in any of our female patients.

Exposure to airborne allergens, either occupational (e.g., vapor of printing inks), seasonal (e.g., pollen), or perennial (e.g., house dust mite), has also been found to trigger recurrent attacks, as in the case of the patient who had active episcleritis after contact with printer's inks.[3,18,21] Although several of our patients had positive skin tests to multiple allergens, only seven (7%) (Table 4.10) had a clear history of atopy with allergic asthma, hay fever, perennial allergic rhinitis, or atopic dermatitis (eczema). Skin testing was investigated by McGavin et al.[18] in 17 patients with episcleritis. Of the eight patients who had a positive reaction to some allergen (three with mild reaction to one antigen, usually house dust or house dust mite), only three of them gave a clear history of either hay fever or asthma. Twelve percent of the patients with episcleritis in Watson and Hayreh's series[2] had a history of asthma and hay fever. Allergy to food products has also been reported as a potential trigger of active episcleritis; recurrent attacks or stable periods have been described, depending on the ingestion or avoidance of the specific products in the diet.[40–42] None of our patients had a clear association between the onset of the disease and the ingestion of specific food products, but this area of dietary allergy has been an especially difficult one to study, historically and experimentally, and so we cannot exclude the possibility that sensitivity to one or another products consumed by some of our patients might be a provocative factor for recurrent episcleritis.

4.2. Scleritis

4.2.1. Introduction

Unlike episcleritis, scleritis is a severe inflammatory condition that is characterized by edema and inflammatory cell infiltration of the sclera. Without treatment, the condition may be progressively destructive, sometimes leading to loss of vision or loss of the eye. Furthermore, scleritis may be the presenting manifestation of a potentially lethal systemic vasculitic disorder or may herald the onset of an occult systemic vasculitis in a patient with an already diagnosed systemic disease that is apparently in remission. Because medical intervention can halt the relentless progression of both ocular and systemic destructive processes, early detection may not only prevent devastating ocular complications but also may prolong survival and improve the quality of life.

4.2.2. Patient Characteristics

Scleritis is most common in the fourth to sixth decades of life, with a peak incidence in the fifth decade,[5,13,18] and affects women more frequently than men (1.6:1).[5] In our series of patients, the condition had a mean age at onset of the first episode of 52 years (range, 11 to 87 years) (Table 4.2) and it was 50% more common among women than men (Table 4.3). Our experience shows that scleritis may occur in patients of all races, but there are no studies on its incidence and prevalence within racial groups. Scleritis is not a familial condition, although some of the scleritis-associated systemic diseases (rheumatoid arthritis, systemic lupus erythematosus, ankylosing spondylitis, Reiter's syndrome, Behçet's disease, gout, and atopy) have a genetic basis.

4.2.3. Clinical Manifestations

Scleritis, like episcleritis, is characterized by recurrences involving the same or different eyes at different times, or both eyes at the same time. Recurrences may appear for many years, especially if the initial attack has not been successfully treated. More than 69% of patients may have recurrences for 3 to 6 years after the onset of the disease; however, after this period the episodes become less frequent until the disease no longer recurs.[2,3] In our series of patients with scleritis, the duration of the disease ranged from 1 month to 30 years. The condition was bilateral in 34% of our patients

(Table 4.4). The symptoms and signs of scleritis, when present, are much more severe than in episcleritis. The main symptom is pain, which may be insidious in onset, severe in intensity, penetrating in character, and only temporarily relieved by analgesics. Pain was present in 65% of our patients. The pain is sometimes localized to the eye, but it more frequently radiates to the forehead, the jaw, and the sinuses. In these cases, the patient may be erroneously diagnosed as having migraine, temporomandibular joint arthritis, sinusitis, herpes zoster, or orbital tumor. Although the pain may always be present, it can recrudesce with violent paroxysms, sometimes triggered by touching the temple or the eye, preventing the patient from laying his head on the affected side. These paroxysms may occur more frequently at night, causing anxiety, depression, and lack of sleep. The pain is probably caused either by distention or destruction of the sensory nerve fibers in the sclera as a result of edema, inflammatory mediators, or necrosis.[3] Pain is, therefore, a good indicator of the presence of active scleritis; it always vanishes with adequate medical treatment of the inflammatory condition.

The primary sign of scleritis is redness, which is gradual in onset, increasing over a period of several days. This redness has a bluish-red tinge in appearance, best seen when the examination is performed in natural light (Fig. 4.4; see color insert). Redness is present in almost all eyes with scleritis. It may be localized to one sector, most frequently in the interpalpebral area (followed by the superior quadrants),[18] or may involve the whole sclera. After recurrent attacks of scleral inflammation, the sclera becomes translucent due to postedema rearrangement of the collagen fibers; because the underlying choroidal pigment becomes visible, the translucent sclera shows a blue-gray color best seen when viewed in daylight (Fig. 4.5; see color insert). These areas may be invisible by slit-lamp examination.

Other symptoms include tearing (which is rarely severe and never accompanied by discharge), and mild to moderate photophobia. If the inflammatory process is severe, an associated spasm of the sphincter of the iris and ciliary muscle may appear, resulting in miosis and temporary myopia.

Clinical examination with the slit-lamp, particularly with a red-free light, shows that the inflammation is localized within the scleral and episcleral tissue. The deep edge of the narrow beam of the slit lamp is displaced forward, showing the underlying scleral edema. The superficial edge of the narrow beam of the slit lamp also is displaced forward, showing the underlying episcleral edema. The deep episcleral vessels are more congested than the superficial episcleral vessels, without coexisting congestion of the conjunctival network. The use of a topical vasoconstrictor (topical phenylephrine [10%] or epinephrine [1:1000]) makes the differentiation between episcleritis and scleritis easier, because the drug constricts the congested superficial episcleral network with minimal effect on the congested deep episcleral network (Figs. 4.6 and 4.7; see color insert).

Scleritis may cause loss of vision through the complications it produces. The main causes of vision loss in patients with scleritis are keratitis, uveitis, glaucoma, cataract, exudative retinal detachment, and macular edema. In our series of patients with scleritis, 37% (of affected eyes) had a loss of vision at the end of the follow-up period (Table 4.5), revealing the permanent changes in visual acuity, even after treatment.

4.2.4. Classification

Scleritis can be divided in anterior and posterior forms. Even recognizing that posterior scleritis is underdiagnosed, anterior scleritis is much more frequent.[2] In a series of 30 enucleated eyes with the primary histological diagnosis of scleritis, Fraunfelder and Watson[1] found that anterior scleritis was present histologically in 100% of eyes; 43% of them also had posterior scleritis. None of these eyes in this series was found to be affected by posterior scleritis alone. In our own series of patients, 94% of the patients had an anterior scleritis (Table 4.1). Anterior scleritis may be further classified, depending on clinical appearance, into diffuse, nodular, necrotizing with inflammation (necrotizing), and necrotizing without inflammation (scleromalacia perforans).[2] This classification

has been shown to be useful, because only 8% of Tuft and Watson's patients progressed from one subcategory to another during the course of their scleral inflammation.[13] Diffuse anterior scleritis is the most common subcategory, followed by nodular anterior scleritis, necrotizing anterior scleritis, scleromalacia perforans anterior scleritis, and posterior scleritis (Table 4.1).[2,13,43] Although any of these types can be associated with any disease, they serve as an indicator of severity and, therefore, as a guide to therapy. In our series, the association between age and type of scleritis was significant. The mean age of patients with diffuse anterior scleritis (46.8 years) was lower than the mean age of patients with the nodular type (49.8 years), which was in turn lower than the mean age of patients with necrotizing varieties (61.9 years for necrotizing and 61.6 years for scleromalacia perforans). The mean age of patients with posterior scleritis was 49.1 years (Table 4.2). The sex distribution within each subcategory always maintained the female predominancy (Table 4.3), and bilaterality was more frequently linked with scleromalacia perforans anterior scleritis and diffuse anterior scleritis, as opposed to posterior scleritis, nodular anterior scleritis, and necrotizing anterior scleritis (Table 4.4). In our series, the associations between type of scleritis and loss of vision (Table 4.5), anterior uveitis (Table 4.6), associated disease (Table 4.9), and peripheral ulcerative keratitis (Table 4.9) were striking.

4.2.4.1. Diffuse Anterior Scleritis

The inflammation of diffuse anterior scleritis is generalized, involving either some small area or the whole anterior segment (Fig. 4.8). The onset is insidious, gradually increasing in signs and symptoms for 5 to 10 days. Without treatment it may last several months. It is a form that may be misdiagnosed as simple episcleritis and therefore sometimes is undertreated. On slit-lamp examination the superficial and deep episcleral plexuses are not only congested but also distorted and tortuous, losing the normal radial pattern of the vessels. When the inflammation disappears, the sclera may show a bluish color due to the rearrangement of the collagen

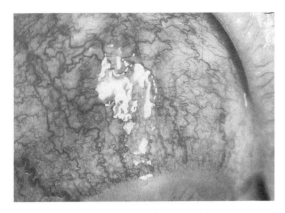

FIGURE 4.8. Diffuse anterior scleritis. The globe is tender to the touch and the inflammation has affected the entire anterior hemisphere of the sclera.

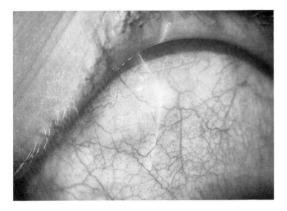

FIGURE 4.9. Slit-lamp photomicrograph illustrating the presence of a true scleral nodule in a patient with nodular scleritis. This patient's initial presentation was with diffuse anterior scleritis.

fibers. This increased translucency is not accompanied by scleral thinning or loss of tissue.

Although many of the patients initially diagnosed with diffuse scleritis maintain this category throughout the course of their scleral inflammation, attention must be paid to the possibility of progression to another clinical category during subsequent exacerbations of the disease (Fig. 4.9). Of 30 patients with recurrent diffuse scleritis analyzed by Tuft and Watson,[13] 12 patients progressed from the diffuse to the nodular variety and 3 patients from the diffuse to the necrotizing variety.

Although permanent loss of visual acuity secondary to keratitis, uveitis, glaucoma, cat-

aract, and macular edema may be present in diffuse anterior scleritis, it is always less severe than in the necrotizing variety. Similarly, although associated diseases may be found in diffuse anterior scleritis, the incidence is smaller than in the necrotizing subcategories. In our series of patients, a loss of visual acuity was recorded in 26% of the patients with diffuse anterior scleritis (Table 4.5). Disease association was found in 45% of the patients with diffuse anterior scleritis (Table 4.9); the connective tissue diseases, especially rheumatoid arthritis, were the most common diagnoses (Table 4.11). Patients with diffuse anterior scleritis and connective tissue diseases may progress to necrotizing anterior scleritis if a vasculitic process appears during the course of the connective tissue disease; therefore the presence of avascular areas in patients with diffuse anterior scleritis must be looked for during a careful follow-up (Fig. 4.10). The finding of a diffuse anterior scleritis in association with a connective tissue disease requires an early and adequate treatment of the ocular and systemic diseases to avoid the development of a vasculitic process.

The fluorescein angiogram usually shows a rapid although structurally normal flow pattern, with a decreased transit time for the dye; however, in some patients the flow pattern is distorted, with the appearance of abnormal

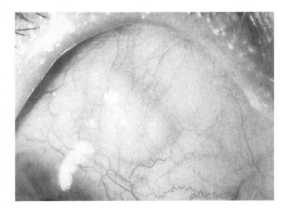

FIGURE 4.10. Residua of nodular scleritis following successful abolition of active inflammation with systemic therapy. Note that the residua of the previous scleral nodule is now white, with an avascular appearance. This area ultimately "melted," leaving an area of scleral thinning and uveal "show."

TABLE 4.11. Diseases associated with scleritis.

Associated disease	Type of scleritis[a]					No. of patients affected
	D	N	NE	SC	P	
Noninfectious						
Connective tissue diseases and other inflammatory conditions						
Rheumatoid arthritis	11	5	11	4	1	32
Systemic lupus erythematosus	4	2	0	0	1	7
Ankylosing spondylitis	1	0	0	0	0	1
Reiter's syndrome	2	1	0	0	0	3
Psoriatic arthritis	0	0	1	0	1	2
Arthritis and IBD[b]	2	3	2	0	0	7
Relapsing polychondritis	6	2	3	0	0	11
Vasculitic diseases						
Polyarteritis nodosa	1	0	1	0	0	2
Churg–Strauss syndrome	0	0	0	0	0	0
Wegener's granulomatosis	2	1	11	0	0	14
Behçet's disease	0	1	0	0	0	1
Giant cell arteritis	0	0	0	0	1	1
Cogan's syndrome	1	0	0	0	0	1
Miscellaneous						
Atopy	1	0	0	0	0	1
Rosacea	1	0	0	0	0	1
Gout	0	0	0	0	1	1
Foreign body granuloma	0	0	1	0	0	1
Chemical injury	0	0	0	0	0	0
Infectious						
Bacteria						
Gram-positive cocci	0	0	1	0	0	1
Gram-negative rods	0	0	1	0	0	1
Mycobacteria						
Atypical mycobacterial disease	0	0	0	0	0	0
Tuberculosis	1	0	0	0	0	1
Leprosy	0	0	0	0	0	0
Spirochaetes						
Syphilis	0	1	0	0	0	1
Lyme disease	1	0	0	0	0	1
Chlamydia	0	0	0	0	0	0
Actinomyces						
Nocardiosis	0	0	0	0	0	0
Fungi						
Filamentous fungi	0	0	1	0	0	1
Dimorphic fungi	0	0	0	0	0	0
Viruses						
Herpes zoster	0	0	2	0	0	2
Herpes simplex	1	0	1	0	0	2
Mumps	0	0	0	0	0	0
Parasites						
Protozoa						
Acanthamoeba	0	0	1	0	0	1
Toxoplasmosis	0	0	0	0	0	0
Helminths						
Toxocariasis	0	1	0	0	0	1
Total:	35	17	37	4	5	98

[a]D, Diffuse anterior scleritis; N, nodular anterior scleritis; NE, necrotizing anterior scleritis; SC, scleromalacia perforans anterior scleritis; P, posterior scleritis.
[b]IBD, Inflammatory bowel disease.

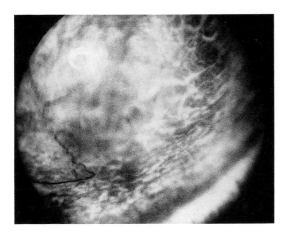

FIGURE 4.11. Anterior segment fluorescein angiography: early venous phase. Note the leakage of fluorescein dye as well as the two areas of relative capillary nonprofusion.

distorted, with the appearance of abnormal anastomoses between the larger vessels in the superficial or deep episcleral networks, which may show rapid early leakage (Fig. 4.11). These anastomoses may persist and remain permeable for a prolonged period, even though the eye is uninflamed.

4.2.4.2. Nodular Anterior Scleritis

The inflammation of nodular anterior scleritis is localized to a scleral nodule (or nodules), which is immobile and firm to the touch (Fig. 4.12; see color insert). Signs and symptoms gradually reach a peak in 5 to 10 days, and without treatment they may last for several months. Although it can be misdiagnosed as nodular episcleritis, detailed slit-lamp examination reveals the congestion and tortuosity of the superficial and deep episcleral plexuses overlying the nodule. The nodule has a violaceous color due to the vascular congestion and has abnormal anastomosis due to the bypass from the arterial channels to the venous channels. It is usually localized in the interpalpebral region close to the limbus. When the inflammation disappears, the sclera involved may show a bluish color due to the increased translucency secondary to the rearrangement of the collagen fibers, without scleral thinning or loss of tissue. Sometimes a mild depression remains in the area where the nodule was.

Although many of the patients initially diagnosed with nodular scleritis maintain this category throughout the course of their scleral inflammation, they must be carefully watched for the possibility of progression to another clinical category during subsequent exacerbations of the disease. Of 54 patients with recurrent nodular scleritis analyzed by Tuft and Watson,[13] 10 patients progressed from the nodular to the necrotizing variety and 2 patients from the nodular to the diffuse variety.

The incidence of patients with either loss of visual acuity or with associated diseases is always smaller in those with nodular anterior scleritis than in those with necrotizing anterior scleritis with inflammation. In our series of patients, a loss of visual acuity was recorded in 13% of the patients with nodular anterior scleritis (Table 4.5). Disease association was found in 44% of the patients with nodular anterior scleritis (Table 4.9); the most common diagnoses were of the connective tissue diseases, especially rheumatoid arthritis (Table 4.11). Patients with nodular anterior scleritis and connective tissue diseases may progress to necrotizing anterior scleritis if a vasculitic process appears during the course of the connective tissue disease. The main changes that indicate the development of a necrotizing process are the presence of avascular areas in the nodule or nodules (Fig. 4.13), which can

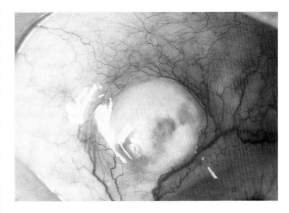

FIGURE 4.13. Nodular scleritis evolving into necrotizing scleritis. The area of scleral necrosis is clearly apparent at the 10 to 11 o'clock position in the anterior sclera adjacent to the corneoscleral limbus. This is an area of previous nodular scleritis.

separate from the remaining sclera (leaving the underlying choroid bare or covered only by a thin layer of conjunctiva), and the progression of the nodular scleritis around the circumference of the globe. The finding of a nodular anterior scleritis in association with a connective tissue disease requires an early and adequate treatment of the ocular and systemic disease to avoid the development of a vasculitic process.

The fluorescein angiogram is similar to that of diffuse anterior scleritis. It shows a rapid although structurally normal flow pattern, although in some patients the flow pattern is characterized by the appearance of abnormal anastomotic vascular channels that may persist for a long time, even without inflammation. These anastomoses may show rapid early leakage of the dye.

4.2.4.3. Necrotizing Anterior Scleritis with Inflammation (Necrotizing Scleritis)

Necrotizing scleritis is the most severe and destructive form of scleritis, sometimes leading to the loss of the eye from multiple complications, severe pain, or even occasionally perforation of the globe. The onset of redness and pain usually is insidious, gradually increasing over 3 to 4 days, although occasionally it can be more acute, reaching the peak after 2 days. The pain, always present without adequate medication, may be so intense and provoked by minimal touch to the scalp that it sometimes seems out of proportion to the ocular findings. It usually worsens at night, keeping the patient awake and leading to severe distress and anxiety.

The main characteristic determined by ocular examination is the presence of white avascular areas surrounded by swelling of the sclera and acute congestion of the abnormal vascular episcleral channels (Fig. 4.14; see color insert). The damaged sclera becomes translucent and shows the brown color of the underlying choroid. The inflammation may start in one small patch and remain there with no spreading; without adequate treatment the inflammation leaves an area of avascular necrotic sclera or sequestrum, which may slough away, leaving

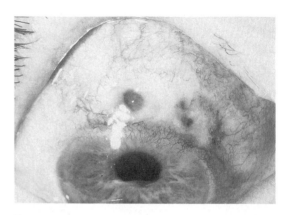

FIGURE 4.15. Necrotizing scleritis. Note the area of full thickness scleral loss with uveal prolapse. This uvea is covered by a thin layer of conjunctival epithelium.

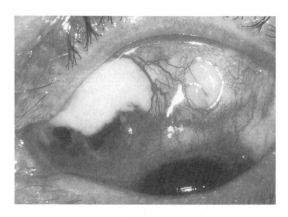

FIGURE 4.16. Necrotizing scleritis. Note that even the conjunctival covering in this patient has broken down, leaving necrotic sclera and uvea exposed.

the choroid covered only by conjunctiva (Fig. 4.15). More frequently, the inflammation starts in one small area that eventually becomes avascular and spreads around the circumference of the globe, often joining other avascular areas that have subsequently appeared (Fig. 4.16), until the whole anterior segment becomes involved. The progression around the globe, leading to loss of tissue, may appear within a few weeks if the inflammation is severe or within several months if the inflammation is moderate. The choroid usually does not protrude through the necrotic areas unless the intraocular pressure rises, but spontaneous or accidental perforation may occasionally occur. If the defect is small, replacement by thin

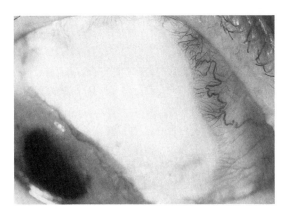

FIGURE 4.17. Scleral allograft in a patient with scleral perforation secondary to progressive necrotizing scleritis.

fibrous tissue may occur, but if the defect is large, scleral allograft should be performed to maintain the integrity of the globe (Fig. 4.17); scleral grafting must always be associated with systemic immunosuppressive therapy, which may halt the progression of the destructive process.[44]

Extension of the inflammatory process may cause keratitis, uveitis, glaucoma, cataract, and macular edema, which may lead to loss of visual acuity. Eighty-two percent of our patients with necrotizing anterior scleritis had loss of visual acuity (Table 4.5).

Necrotizing scleritis is not only a destructive ocular disease; its presence is also considered an ominous sign of potentially lethal systemic vasculitic disease. Watson and Hayreh[2] reported that 29% of the patients with necrotizing scleritis died within 5 years of the onset of the scleritis; many of these deaths were caused by systemic vasculitic lesions. In another study performed by Foster et al.,[45] 7 of 20 patients with necrotizing scleritis died within 8 years of the onset of the scleritis; none of the 7 patients had been treated with immunosuppressive therapy. Many of these deaths had been caused by vascular-related events. Eleven of the 13 patients who remained alive had received immunosuppressive therapy. The presence of a necrotizing scleritis may coincide with the onset of vasculitic lesions in a patient with an already known connective tissue disease that is apparently in remission, worsening consider-

ably the ocular and systemic prognoses. A clear example is necrotizing scleritis appearing at the time when systemic vasculitis complicates rheumatoid arthritis. These rheumatoid patients have more destructive joint disease, rheumatoid subcutaneous nodules, cutaneous vascular lesions, more elevated levels of circulating immune complexes, higher titers of rheumatoid factor, more profound hypocomplementemia, and immunoglobulin and complement deposition in vessels of perineural tissue, rheumatoid nodules, synovium, skin, and conjunctiva and/or sclera.[18,46–55] Necrotizing scleritis also may appear during the course of a systemic vasculitic disease such as polyarteritis nodosa or Wegener's granulomatosis, demonstrating further evidence of the severity of the disease. Interestingly, necrotizing scleritis may be the first manifestation whose study leads to the diagnosis of a vasculitic disease. Necrotizing scleritis also may be a manifestation of an infectious process that destroys the sclera either through direct microbial damage or through an autoimmune process. In our series, 95% of patients with necrotizing scleritis had an associated disease (Table 4.9); of those in whom an etiology was found, 81% had a systemic connective tissue and/or vasculitic disease and 19% had an infectious disease (Table 4.11). The most common diagnoses were Wegener's granulomatosis, rheumatoid arthritis, and relapsing polychondritis. Necrotizing scleritis was the manifestation whose diagnostic study led to the discovery of a noninfectious associated disease in 9% of the patients (Table 4.12). Infectious etiologies included bacterial infections, fungal infections, viral infections, and parasitic infections (Table 4.11).

The finding of an avascular area either at some point during the course of a recurrent diffuse or nodular scleritis or during an initial presentation of a scleritis is a highly significant indication of the presence of a necrotizing scleritis. Early treatment of the ocular condition may prevent the extension of the necrotic process before further tissue loss occurs and intraocular complications appear (Figs. 4.18 and 4.19). Early treatment of the associated disease may prevent the extension of the vasculitic

TABLE 4.12. Scleritis as first manifestation of associated disease.

Associated disease	Type of scleritis[a]					No. of patients affected
	D	N	NE	SC	P	
Wegener's granulomatosis	2	2	10	0	0	14
Relapsing polychondritis	2	1	3	0	0	6
Rheumatoid arthritis	0	1	1	0	0	2
Reiter's syndrome	0	1	0	0	0	1
Polyarteritis nodosa	0	0	1	0	0	1
Systemic lupus erythematosus	0	1	0	0	0	1
Behçet's disease	0	1	0	0	0	1
Total (%):	4	7	15	0	0	26 (15.12%)

[a]D, Diffuse anterior scleritis; N, nodular anterior scleritis; NE, necrotizing anterior scleritis; SC, scleromalacia perforans anterior scleritis; P, posterior scleritis.

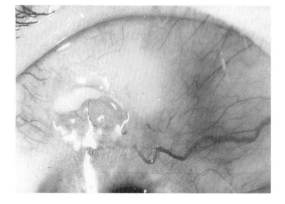

FIGURE 4.18. Necrotizing scleritis and peripheral ulcerative keratitis in a patient with positive antineutrophil cytoplasmic antibody staining and abnormal sinus X rays; Wegener's granolomatosis.

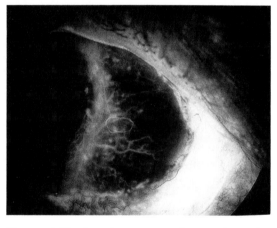

FIGURE 4.20. Anterior segment fluorescein angiogram of a patient with necrotizing scleritis affecting the temporal hemisphere of the sclera. Note the vast expanse of avascularity.

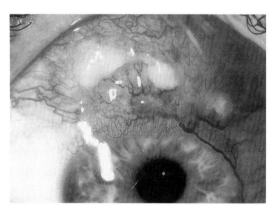

FIGURE 4.19. Same patient as in Fig. 4.18, 4 weeks into therapy with systemic cyclophosphamide. The inflammatory process is beginning to resolve.

process before systemic complications appear.

The fluorescein angiogram in necrotizing scleritis shows hypoperfusion in the venous site of the capillary network, which may lead to nonperfusion if the venules become thrombosed and permanently occluded (Fig. 4.20). Because these venules rarely open, they are replaced by newly formed vessels that produce persistent leakage. Unlike in episcleritis and diffuse or nodular anterior scleritis, the transit time of the dye in necrotizing scleritis is markedly increased even when the eye is congested. If the inflammation is severe, vaso-occlusive changes in the conjunctival vessels also may occur.

4.2.4.4. Necrotizing Anterior Scleritis without Inflammation (Scleromalacia Perforans)

Scleromalacia perforans, a term coined by van der Hoeve in 1931,[56] is characterized by the appearance of yellow or grayish anterior scleral nodules that gradually develop a necrotic slough or sequestrum without surrounding inflammation; this sequestrum eventually separates from the underlying sclera, leaving the choroid bare or covered only by a thin layer of conjunctiva (Fig. 4.21).[56] The choroid does not bulge through these areas unless the intraocular pressure rises. Although spontaneous perforation is rare, traumatic perforation may easily occur.[1,3,57] If the perforation is not repaired, phthisis bulbi will occur.[57] Because the condition presents with an insidious onset, slow progress, and with lack of pain or tenderness to the touch, it is detected by the patient's family, by the patient while looking in the mirror, or by the rheumatologist by chance; they notice the yellow or grayish patch or patches on the sclera, anywhere between the corneal limbus and the equator.

One of the first characteristic findings which can be seen on slit-lamp examination is a reduction in the number and size of vessels in the episclera surrounding the sequestrum, giving a porcelain-like appearance. These vessels anastomose with each other and sometimes cross the abnormal area to join with perilimbal ves-

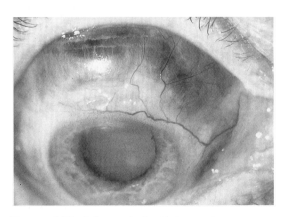

FIGURE 4.21. Scleromalacia perforans in a patient with rheumatoid arthritis. Note the extraordinary degree of scleral loss, with uveal bulge under the stretched conjunctiva.

sels. As the necrotic process progresses, the sequestrum is gradually removed. Fluorescein angiography shows that the necrotic process in scleromalacia perforans appears to be caused by arteriolar obliteration, unlike in necrotizing scleritis, in which the necrotic process appears to be caused by venular obliteration.[4,5]

van der Hoeve originally noticed[56,58] and other authors subsequently confirmed[2,59–67] the association of these ocular changes with severe, progressive, long-standing rheumatoid arthritis with extraarticular manifestations. In our series, 67% of patients with scleromalacia perforans had an associated disease (Table 4.9) that was, in all cases, long-standing rheumatoid arthritis (Table 4.11). The characteristic sufferer of this condition is a woman (Table 4.3) with an age range from 38 to 75 years, most commonly in the sixth decade (Table 4.2), and with bilateral involvement (Table 4.4).

Keratitis, uveitis, glaucoma, cataract, and macular edema may appear and may lead to loss of vision. In our series, 33% of the patients with scleromalacia perforans had loss of vision (Table 4.5).

4.2.4.4.1. Differential Diagnosis

Differential diagnosis of scleromalacia perforans includes necrotizing scleritis with inflammation, and scleral degenerations such as paralimbic (or intercalary) scleromalacia and senile hyaline plaques (Table 4.13).

4.2.4.4.1.1. Necrotizing Scleritis with Inflammation. The presence of pain and active inflammation helps to differentiate this entity from scleromalacia perforans. Furthermore, in necrotizing scleritis with inflammation, the involvement is most frequently unilateral and the association with rheumatoid arthritis is variable.

4.2.4.4.1.2. Paralimbic Scleromalacia. Paralimbic scleromalacia appears to be a degenerative process that occurs at the corneoscleral limbus of either one or both eyes, and is characterized by a slowly progressive, noninflammatory, painless scleral thinning that leads to a spontaneous small perforation with iris prolapse.[5,21,63,67–71] On slit-lamp examination, a small hole in the limbal sclera can be seen

TABLE 4.13. Differential diagnosis of scleral loss.

Parameter	Scleromalacia perforans	Necrotizing scleritis	Paralimbic scleromalacia	Hyaline plaques
Age predilection (years)	50–75	50–75	25–50	50–75
Sex predilection	Females	Females	—	Either
Inflammation	–	+	–	–
Unilateral/bilateral	Bilateral	Either	Either	Bilateral
Number of areas	Multiple	Variable	Single	Single
Pain	–	+	–	–
Pathology	Necrosis	Inflammation and necrosis	Degeneration	Degeneration
Rheumatoid arthritis	+	Variable	–	–
Progression	+	+	–	–
Prognosis without treatment	Bad	Poor	Good	Good

with incarceration of iris covered by conjunctiva; the appearance resembles the filtering bleb of an Elliot trephining operation. Sometimes the pupil may be peaking toward the area of iris incarceration, but because the hole is small there is no need for surgical closure. A small perforating scleral vessel may run through the defect to anastomose with the posterior ciliary circulation.[5] The intraocular pressure may be low when the perforation occurs but rises rapidly to normal as soon as the iris incarcerates. Paralimbic scleromalacia is a rare condition affecting individuals of either sex between the ages of 25 and 50 years, without evidence of systemic disease or previous ocular inflammation. If there is association with rheumatoid arthritis, the condition should probably be regarded as necrotizing scleritis without inflammation or as scleromalacia perforans. Paralimbic scleromalacia has a good prognosis without treatment.

4.2.4.4.1.3. Senile Scleral Hyaline Plaques.
Senile scleral hyaline plaques also can be mistaken for scleromalacia perforans, because both lesions involve loss of scleral substance, lack of inflammatory reaction, and painless development.[58,69–70] The scleral plaque, which occurs in individuals of either sex between the ages of 60 to 75 years, appears as a dark, oval, nonprogressive patch with a size ranging from 1 to 2 mm in width and from 2 to 6 mm in length.[5,21,63,72–79] The lesion, usually bilateral and symmetrical, is localized to the interpalpebral region, between the insertion of the

lateral or medial rectus muscles and the limbus (Chapter 3, Fig. 3.16). On slit-lamp examination the plaque appears as a translucent area through which the underlying uvea can be seen, surrounded by a calcareous yellowish ring, and covered by atrophic episclera and normal conjunctiva. The central translucent area can be transilluminated by directing the light through the pupil, but although the sclera is thinned (from 0.6 to 0.3 mm)[78] the wall is resistant, with no tendency to perforation. Histologically it is considered a degenerative lesion with a lack of cellular elements, replacement of the superficial layers of the sclera by large masses of hyaline degeneration, and calcification. The collagen fibers in the area adjacent to the plaque are fragmented and swollen, making the sclera weak. The location of the plaque therefore may be determined by the maximal stresses of the muscles. Senile scleral plaque has a good prognosis without treatment, because there is no evidence of systemic disease or previous ocular inflammation associated with this condition.

4.2.4.5. Posterior Scleritis

Posterior scleritis accounts for the inflammation of the sclera posterior to the ora serrata, which may spread to the posterior segment of the eye, involving choroid, retina, and optic nerve. Thus, because a fundus mass, choroidal folds, retinal striae, choroidal or retinal detachments, and disk or macular edema may appear, posterior scleritis may be confused with many

TABLE 4.14. Posterior scleritis: Initial symptoms, external signs, and initial site.

Patient no./ sex/age (years)	Eye[a]	Initial symptoms	External signs	Initial site of scleritis
1/F/66	OU	Visual loss, pain	Redness	Anterior + posterior
2/F/44	OS	Visual loss, pain, flashes	Proptosis, redness	Anterior + posterior
3/F/56	OU	Visual loss, pain, tenderness	Redness	Anterior + posterior
4/F/29	OD	Visual loss, pain	—	Posterior
5/F/34	OS	Visual loss, pain	Redness	Anterior + posterior
6/M/49	OD	Visual loss, pain	Chemosis, ptosis, redness	Anterior
7/F/26	OD	Pain	—	Posterior
8/M/51	OD	Visual loss, pain, diplopia	Proptosis, redness, lid swelling, ptosis, chemosis	Anterior + posterior
9/M/67	OU	Visual loss	—	Posterior
10/F/58	OU	Visual loss, pain, tenderness	Redness	Anterior
11/F/60	OD	Visual loss, pain, diplopia	Exotropia, redness	Anterior

[a] OU, Both eyes; OS, left eye; OD, right eye.

other diseases such as primary or secondary choroidal tumors, uveal effusion syndrome, rhegmatogenous retinal detachments, Vogt-Koyanagi–Harada syndrome, central serous retinal detachments, and optic neuritis.[4,80–86] Because posterior scleritis also may extend outward, involving extraocular muscles and orbital tissues, it also may be confused with orbital tumors or orbital inflammatory diseases.[84,87,88] Furthermore, posterior scleritis is often associated with anterior scleritis; but it also may occur alone, in which case the absence of anterior scleral involvement makes the diagnosis difficult.[1,2,7,8,84] And if the concomitant anterior scleritis is severe, posterior scleritis may be overlooked. Therefore posterior scleritis is a more common condition than is realized, and the diagnosis is often missed or delayed.[1,3–5,7] Recognition of the protean clinical manifestations and confirmation by ancillary testing are important to reach a correct diagnosis of posterior scleritis. Early diagnosis leads to early therapy and prevention of complications that could cause permanent loss of vision.

Posterior scleritis may be a posterior extension of either nodular or diffuse anterior scleritis. In our series, anterior scleritis was present or had occurred in 8 of 11 patients (73%) with posterior scleritis (Table 4.14); 5 patients presented with anterior and posterior involvement and 3 patients with only anterior involvement. The three patients presenting with anterior scleritis developed posterior scleritis at a mean interval of 12 months (range, 4 to 18 months). Posterior scleritis may present alone, in which case anterior involvement may or not appear later.[3] None of our three patients presenting with posterior scleritis had anterior involvement during the follow-up period. Evidence of posterior scleritis must, therefore, be searched for during the course of an anterior scleritis, although the absence of anterior scleritis does not exclude the possibility of posterior scleritis.

4.2.4.5.1. Symptoms and Signs

Symptoms and signs at presentation are variable because they depend on the degree and site of inflammation. The most common presenting symptoms are loss of vision and pain, although diplopia, flashes, and tenderness may also be present[3,7,86] (Table 4.14). The most common presenting sign is redness, related to anterior scleritis; conjunctival chemosis, proptosis, lid swelling, lid retraction, and limitation of ocular movements may also be detected[3,7,86] (Table 4.14).

Some decrease of visual acuity is almost always present and its severity depends on the site, type, and degree of the complications associated. The reduction in vision may reflect a transient hyperopia, which is caused by a decrease in the axial length of the globe secondary to posterior scleral thickening.[85,89,90] In these

TABLE 4.15. Posterior scleritis: Effect on visual acuity.

Patient no.	VA at presentation[a]	Final VA	Follow-up (months)	Fundus findings[b]
1	20/40	20/30	15	Macular edema OU + disk edema OU
	20/50	20/30		
2	20/40	20/20	3	Choroidal folds + retinal striae + subretinal mass
3	20/300	20/25	70	Macular edema OU + disk edema OU + choroidal detachment OS
	CF[c]	20/40		+ serous retinal detachment OS
4	CF[c]	20/20	8	Choroidal folds + subretinal mass + macular edema + disk edema
5	20/40	20/25	2	Choroidal folds + retinal striae + subretinal mass + macular edema
6	20/50	20/30	65	Choroidal folds + subretinal mass + retinal deposits + disk edema
7	20/30	20/30	7	Choroidal folds
8	20/200	20/50	13	Choroidal folds + subretinal mass + disk edema
9	20/40	20/60	1	Choroidal folds OU + retinal deposits OU
	20/40	20/60		
10	20/50	20/25	6	Choroidal folds OD + subretinal mass OD + choroidal detachment
	20/30	20/20		OD
11	20/200	HM[d]	4	Choroidal detachment + serous retinal detachment

[a] Visual acuity (VA) at presentation of posterior scleritis.
[b] OU, Both eyes; OS, left eye; OD, right eye.
[c] Counting fingers.
[d] Hand movements.

cases, patients complain of mild visual loss and asthenopia, which can be corrected with the addition of convex lenses. In other cases, the reduction in vision is not correctable because it is caused by severe complications such as choroidal or retinal detachments, distortion of the macula by an area of scleral inflammation, cystoid macular edema, and optic neuritis.[7,8,84–86,91,92] These complications are frequently reversible, with a good visual outcome if adequate treatment for posterior scleritis is initiated shortly after its onset. If diagnosis and treatment are delayed, permanent damage may cause irreversible visual loss.[7] In our series, visual loss as the initial symptom was noted by 10 of the 11 patients (91%) with posterior scleritis (Table 4.14). Eight of the 15 eyes (53%) had a visual acuity of 20/50 or worse at presentation of posterior scleritis but only 4 of 15 eyes (27%) had a visual acuity of 20/50 or worse at the end of the follow-up period (Table 4.15).

The pain varies from mild to severe and often is referred to the brow, temple, face, or jaw. In our series, pain was present in 10 of the 11 patients (91%) with posterior scleritis; of these, 2 patients described pain as severe, 6 as moderate, and 2 as mild. Five of the 11 patients

referred the pain to other surrounding structures. The pain is often correlated with the severity of the anterior involvement, and therefore patients with posterior scleritis alone have either no pain or pain of a mild degree.[7,84] Mild pain may result from stretching of Tenon's capsule by edema, from stretching of scleral sensory nerve endings by edema, from optic nerve sheath swelling, or from orbital or extraocular muscle swelling.[85] All 8 patients with posterior scleritis who described the pain as severe or moderate also had anterior involvement.

Photopsia may occur secondary to retinal striae or retinal detachment.

The sclera and Tenon's capsule are closely connected, especially around the optic nerve and behind the limbus. Similarly, the connective tissue of the orbit and the connective tissue of the muscle sheaths form a direct continuation of Tenon's capsule. Extension of posterior scleral inflammation to the orbit explains the signs of proptosis, chemosis, lid swelling, and lower lid retraction with upgaze. Extension of posterior scleral inflammation to the extraocular muscles causes myositis, which may lead to diplopia and ptosis due to ocular movement impairment.[92]

4.2.4.5.2. Fundus Findings

The most common fundus findings in posterior scleritis are choroidal folds, subretinal mass, disk edema, and macular edema. Annular ciliochoroidal detachment, serous retinal detachment, intraretinal deposits, and retinal striae may also appear. Because enucleation has been a consequence of misdiagnosis, posterior scleritis must be considered in the differential diagnosis of all these entities.[1,93,94] In our series of 11 patients (15 eyes) with posterior scleritis, 9 eyes had choroidal folds, 6 eyes had subretinal mass, 7 eyes had disk edema, and 6 eyes had macular edema. Annular ciliochoroidal detachments were present in three eyes, two of which also had bullous serous retinal detachments. Intraretinal deposits were found in three eyes. Retinal striae were detected in two eyes (Table 4.15).

4.2.4.5.2.1. Choroidal Folds. Choroidal folds are a series of alternating light and dark lines confined to the posterior pole, often temporal, and rarely extending beyond the equator (Fig. 4.22; see color insert). Although they are usually arranged in a horizontal and parallel pattern, surrounding a subretinal mass, they may be vertical, oblique, or irregular. Increased scleral and choroidal thickening, forcing Bruch's membrane and retinal pigment epithelium into folds, has been proposed as a possible mechanism.[95–98] Because choroidal folds result in reduction of the anteroposterior diameter of the eye, they induce a relative hyperopia. Prompt recognition and treatment of the underlying cause restores visual acuity; however, prolonged choroidal folding may cause mechanical distortion of the neuroreceptors of the retina, leading to permanent loss of vision. Choroidal folds may be the only abnormal fundus finding in a relatively moderate posterior scleritis.

4.2.4.5.2.2. Subretinal Mass. A subretinal mass caused by a circumscribed area of scleral thickening may be detected in posterior scleritis.[7,8,84,86,94] The scleral mass has the same orange color as the adjacent normal pigment epithelium, preserves the overlying normal choroidal vascular pattern, and is frequently surrounded by choroidal folds or by retinal striae.[84,86,94] In some cases, the surface of the mass may show scattered, yellowish-white, circumscribed lesions.

4.2.4.5.2.3. Disk Edema and Macular Edema. Extension of the scleral and choroidal inflammation to the optic nerve may account for an optic neuritis.[93] Disk edema may cause an afferent pupillary defect or visual field changes, but the visual acuity is usually preserved. Extension of the scleral and choroidal inflammation with or without uveitis may cause cystoid macular edema.[8] Untreated disk edema or macular edema will usually result in permanent structural damage and loss of vision. Prompt treatment of posterior scleritis may prevent this.

4.2.4.5.2.4. Annular Ciliochoroidal Detachment and Serous Retinal Detachment. Extension of the scleral inflammation into the choroid allows exudation of fluid, which may account for an annular ciliochoroidal detachment and/ or multiple retinal pigment epithelial detachments (Figs. 4.23 and 4.24) and/or a serous retinal detachment.[93,99] Detachment of the peripheral choroid and ciliary body may push the lens–iris diaphragm forward and precipitate an acute angle-closure glaucoma attack.[100] Subretinal fluid in serous retinal detachment originates from choroid through multiple leaking spots in the retinal pigment epithelium.

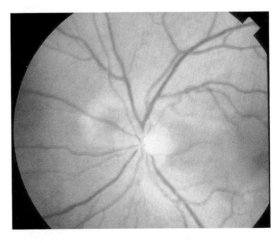

FIGURE 4.23. Posterior scleritis with annular retinochoroidal and serous retinal detachment.

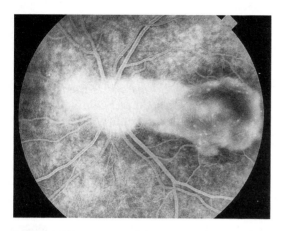

FIGURE 4.24. Same eye as shown in Fig. 4.23: fluorescein angiogram, confirming the findings described in Fig. 4.23.

Serous retinal detachment may be confined to the posterior pole as a serous macular detachment, or may extend or localize more peripherally as a bullous retinal detachment with shifting subretinal fluid. In the latter, the fluid pools inferiorly when the patient is upright and superiorly when the patient is positioned with head down; despite a cloudy subretinal fluid, a pale gray subretinal mass with a surrounding dark gray line and an overlying normal choroidal vascular pattern may sometimes be visible through the poorly mobile bullous serous retinal detachment. The bullous serous retinal detachments do not have retinal holes or fixed retinal folds. The ciliochoroidal or retinal detachments usually resolve completely with prompt and aggressive treatment of the scleritis. Although they may disappear within hours, they are often absorbed slowly over a period of several weeks or months, leaving only a diffuse pigmentation in the affected area; however, if the macular area has been involved, loss of vision will remain as a permanent sequela.[5]

4.2.4.5.3. Associated Diseases

Disease association in posterior scleritis is less common than in anterior scleritis.[2,7] In our series of 11 patients with posterior scleritis, 5 (45%) were found to have an associated systemic disease (Table 4.9). This is in contrast

to the 54% disease association found in our patients with anterior scleritis. Diagnoses of rheumatoid arthritis, systemic lupus erythematosus, psoriatic arthritis, gout, and giant cell arteritis were ascribed to one patient each (Table 4.11). All of these diagnoses had been established before the onset of the posterior scleritis (Table 4.12).

4.2.4.5.4. Complications

Posterior uveitis is universally present in posterior scleral inflammation, because the choroid is always involved by the adjacent posterior scleral inflammation[2,6]; anterior uveitis may also appear, but it is often associated with concomitant anterior scleritis. Glaucoma, particularly in combination with uveitis, is considered to be an ominous sign in the course of scleritis, because its presence indicates a more diffuse and severe process.[3] Whether caused by anterior uveitis, ciliochoroidal detachment, angle neovascularization, or chronic use of steroids, increased intraocular pressure in posterior scleritis may result in the development of irreversible optic nerve damage.[9,100]

4.2.4.5.5. Ancillary Tests

4.2.4.5.5.1. Ultrasonography. Ultrasonography is the most useful test in the diagnosis of posterior scleritis, because it shows the flattening and thickening of the posterior coats of the eye (choroid and sclera) associated with retrobulbar edema[84,86,89,101] (Fig. 4.25). Occasionally, retinal and choroidal detachments may also be detected. B scan ultrasonography shows multiple internal echoes in the area of the scleral thickening and lack of echoes in the area of retrobulbar edema; the multiple echoes remain after sound beam attenuation, indicating high internal reflectivity of the scleral mass (Fig. 4.26). On the other hand, in choroidal thickening without scleral thickening, the echoes do not remain after sound beam attenuation (low internal reflectivity) (Fig. 4.27). When retrobulbar edema surrounds the optic nerve, the "T" sign may appear, which consists of a lack of echoes in the edematous Tenon's space and adjacent optic nerve (Fig. 4.28). A scan ultrasonography shows high-

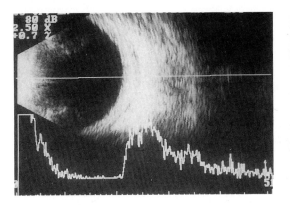

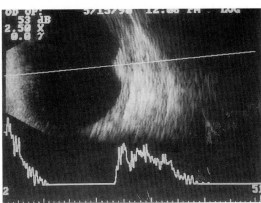

FIGURE 4.25. B scan ultrasonogram with superimposed A scan profile. Note the thickening of the retinal choroid layer and the edema in Tenon's space.

FIGURE 4.27. Ultrasonogram of choroidal thickening in a patient with chronic uveitis without scleritis. Note particularly the A scan tracing showing a lack of high internal reflectivity in the area of the sclera with sound beam attenuation.

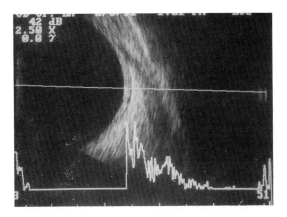

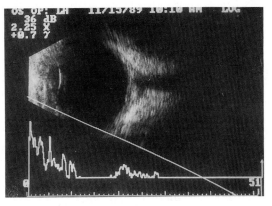

FIGURE 4.26. Ultrasonogram of a patient with posterior scleritis. Note particularly the A scan tracing showing the multiple retrobulbar echoes. The multiple echoes in the area of the sclera indicate high internal reflectivity of the sclera.

FIGURE 4.28. Ultrasonogram "T" sign formed by the sonagraphically, empty space occupied by the optic nerve and the edematous Tenon's space adjacent to the optic nerve.

amplitude internal spikes in the area of the scleral thickening and low-amplitude internal spikes in the area of retrobulbar edema. The combination of both A scan and B scan techniques gives the most useful results in distinguishing posterior scleritis from orbital, choroidal, and retinal entities that clinically may mimic it (Tables 4.16 to 4.18).[86]

4.2.4.5.5.2. Computerized Tomography (CT) Scanning. Computerized tomography also shows scleral thickening, the image of which can be enhanced by radiopaque medium injection.[86,102] Retrobulbar edema may also be seen. The ability of computerized tomography to delineate extraocular muscles, lacrimal glands, optic nerves, scleral coats, orbital walls, and paranasal tissues helps to detect extraocular muscle or lacrimal gland enlargement, optic nerve or scleral inflammation, bone erosion, and sinus involvement, which are important findings for the differential diagnosis of posterior scleritis with orbital inflammatory diseases and orbital tumors.[102–104]

TABLE 4.16. Differential diagnosis of posterior scleritis: Proptosis, chemosis, lid swelling, and limitation of ocular movements.

Parameter	Posterior scleritis	Orbital tumor	Acute diffuse idiopathic orbital inflammation[a]	Thyroid ophthalmopathy[a]
Sex predilection	Female	—	—	Female
Age predilection	Middle aged and elderly	—	—	Middle aged and elderly
Laterality	Unilateral	Unilateral	Unilateral	Bilateral
Onset	Gradual	Gradual	Acute	Gradual
Pain	Variable	+/−	Variable	−
Tenderness	+	−	+	−
Anterior scleritis	+	−	−	−
Visual loss	+	+/−	+/−	Variable
Fundus mass	Variable	+/−	+/−	−
Color of the mass	Orange	Orange	Orange	−
Proptosis	+/−	+	+	+
Motility disturbance	+/−	+	+	+
Conjunctival chemosis	+/−	+	+	−
Lid edema	+/−	+	+	−
Pigment epithelium	Yellowish nodules	Normal	Normal	Normal
Disk edema	+	+/−	+/−	+/−
Uveitis	+	−	+/−	−
Choroidal folds	+	+/−	+/−	+/−
Serous retinal detachment	+	−	+/−	−
Fluorescein angiography (other than choroidal folds)	Multiple small leaks	Normal	Normal	Normal
Ultrasound	Scleral and choroid thickening; retrobulbar edema (high reflectivity)	Orbital mass	Orbital mass (low reflectivity) and/or EOM enlargement	EOM enlargement
CT scan	Scleral and choroid thickening	Orbital mass with sinus involvement/ bone erosion	Orbital mass without sinus involvement or bone erosion. EOM enlargement.	EOM enlargement
Biopsy indication	No biopsy	Biopsy	Biopsy	No biopsy
Response to steroids	Good	Absent	Very good	Variable

[a] EOM, extraocular muscle.

4.2.4.5.5.3. Radioactive Phosphorus (^{32}P) Uptake. The ^{32}P uptake test is of little value in differentiating posterior scleritis from choroidal tumors because the test may be positive or negative in posterior scleritis.[94,105–107] The ^{32}P uptake test also may be positive in a variety of inflammatory, vascular, hemorrhagic, and osseous conditions of the posterior segment.[105]

4.2.4.5.5.4. Fluorescein Angiography. Fluorescein angiography may reveal retinal pigment epithelial detachment (Figs. 4.29 and 4.30), serous retinal detachment, disk edema, or cystoid macular edema. In cases with serous retinal detachment, subretinal fluid shows diffuse choroidal mottling in the early phases, numerous pinpoint spots of hyperfluorescence in the middle phases, and intense staining of the subretinal fluid in the late phases.[84] Choroidal folds are seen as alternating hyperfluorescent and hypofluorescent streaks (Fig. 4.31).[108] The fluorescein pattern confirms their presence in case of clinical doubt. The folds are recognized by the early passage of fluorescein

TABLE 4.17. Differential diagnosis of posterior scleritis: Subretinal mass.

Parameter	Posterior scleritis	Choroidal melanoma	Metastatic uveal carcinoma	Choroidal hemangioma
Sex predilection	Female	—	—	—
Age predilection	Middle aged and elderly	Elderly	Middle aged and elderly	Middle aged and elderly
Laterality	Unilateral	Unilateral	Unilateral	Unilateral
Onset	Gradual	Gradual	Gradual	Gradual
Pain	Variable	—	—	—
Tenderness	+	−	−	−
Anterior scleritis	+	−	−	−
Visual loss	+	Variable	Variable	Variable
Color of the mass	Orange	Hyper- or hypopigmented	Hypopigmented	Pinkish-orange
Overlying retina	Yellow deposits	Orange pigment	Dark mottling	Cystoid edema
Proptosis	+/−	−	−	−
Motility disturbance	+/−	−	−	−
Conjunctival chemosis	+/−	−	−	−
Lid edema	+/−	−	−	−
Disk edema	+	−	−	−
Uveitis	+	−	−	−
Choroidal folds	+	+/−	+/−	−
Serous retinal detachment/subretinal fluid	+/cloudy	+/clear	+/clear	+/clear
Fluorescein angiography (other than choroidal folds)	Small leaks; intrinsic vasculature	Small leaks	Small leaks	Small leaks. Early fluorescence prior to filling retinal vessels.
Ultrasound	Scleral and choroid thickening (high reflectivity); retrobulbar edema	Choroidal mass (low reflectivity); no retrobulbar edema	Choroidal mass (moderate reflectivity); no retrobulbar edema	Choroidal mass (high reflectivity); no retrobulbar edema
Response to steroids	Good	Absent	Absent	Absent

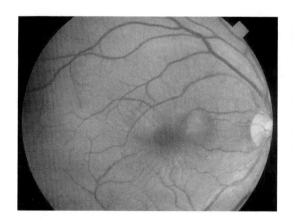

FIGURE 4.29. Fundus photograph, posterior scleritis. Note the detachment of the pigment epithelium supranasal to the fovea, as well as the retinal striae.

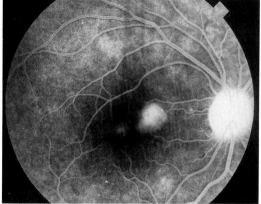

FIGURE 4.30. Fluorescein angiogram of the same patient as in Fig. 4.29. Note the fluorescein accumulation in the area of pigment epithelial detachment.

through the choroid, persisting through the late venous phase without leakage. The light portion of the fold corresponds to the crest and transmits the choroidal fluorescence, whereas the dark portion of the fold corresponds to the valley and does not transmit the choroidal fluorescence. Inclination and subsequent thickness of the retinal pigment epithelium in the valleys, and atrophy of the retinal pigment epithelium in the crests, may be a possible

TABLE 4.18. Differential diagnosis of posterior scleritis: Serous detachment of choroid, ciliary body, and retina.

Parameter	Posterior scleritis	Uveal effusion syndrome	Vogt-Koyanagi–Harada syndrome	Idiopathic central serous chorioretinopathy
Sex predilection	Female	Male	—	Male
Age predilection	Middle aged and elderly	Middle aged	Young and middle aged	Middle aged
Race predilection	—	—	Oriental and pigmented	Caucasian
Laterality	Unilateral	Bilateral	Bilateral	Unilateral
Pain	Variable	—	− (photophobia)	−
Anterior scleritis	+	−	−	−
Uveitis	+	−	+	−
Disk edema	+	+	+	−
Pigment epithelium	Yellowish nodules	"Leopard spots"	Depigmented or hyperpigmented lines	Serous detachments pigment epithelium
Serous retinal detachment	+	+	+	+
Serous ciliochoroidal detachment	+	+	+/−	−
Subretinal fluid	Cloudy	Clear	Cloudy	Clear
Fluorescein angiography	Multiple small leaks	Slow choroidal perfusion; occasional leaks	Multiple small leaks; late-staining subretinal fluid	Serous detachments pigment epithelium
Ultrasound	Scleral and choroidal thickening (high reflectivity); retrobulbar edema; serous ciliochoroid and retinal detachment	Choroid thickened; serous ciliochoroid and retinal detachment	Choroid thickened (low internal reflectivity); serous retinal detachment	Serous retinal detachment
Miscellaneous	Collagen vascular disease association	High protein level in CSF (50% of cases)	Headaches, fever, dysacousis, vitiligo, meningism (50% of cases)	Anxiety

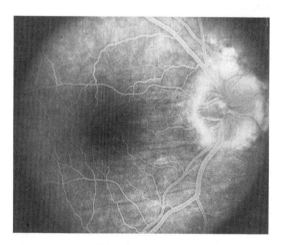

FIGURE 4.31. Fluorescein angiogram: posterior scleritis. Note the choroidal and retinal striae as well as the retinal pigment epithelial window defects.

explanation for the hypofluorescent and hyperfluorescent areas, respectively.[95,108,109] Retinal striae are not seen on fluorescein angiography; this helps to differentiate them from choroidal folds.[95] Because all these findings may also be seen in many other choroidal, retinal, and orbital conditions, fluorescein angiography results should be analyzed in the context of clinical, ultrasonographic, and CT scanning results.

4.2.4.5.6. Differential Diagnosis

Differential diagnosis of posterior scleritis includes the orbital entities that can present with the external signs of proptosis, chemosis, lid swelling, and limitation of ocular movements and the orbital, choroidal, and retinal entities that can present with the fundus signs of subretinal mass, choroidal folds, and serous detachments of the choroid, ciliary body, and retina, and disk and macular edemas.

4.2.4.5.6.1. Proptosis, Chemosis, Lid Swelling, and Limitation of Ocular Movements.

Posterior scleritis, acute diffuse idiopathic orbital inflammations ("pseudotumor"), orbital neoplasms, and thyroid ophthalmopathy, may all present with proptosis, conjunctival chemosis, lid swelling, and limitation of ocular movements (Table 4.16). They also may present with conjunctival injection, choroidal folds, and disk edema.

Idiopathic orbital inflammatory syndromes may be defined as nonspecific idiopathic inflammatory conditions for which no identifiable cause (e.g., ruptured dermoid cyst, infected mucocele, and retained foreign body) or systemic disease (e.g., Graves' disease, Wegener's granulomatosis, and periarteritis nodosa) can be found.[102,110] They have traditionally been termed "pseudotumors" because of a mass like effect simulating a primary orbital neoplasm.[111-115] Because ultrasonography and computerized tomography have made possible the differentiation between diffuse orbital inflammation and localized orbital inflammation, many authors prefer to avoid the generic term "pseudotumor" and describe the idiopathic orbital inflammation either as diffuse (acute or chronic) or as localized to a specific target structure such as occurs in myositis, dacryoadenitis, and perineuritis.[103,104,116] The localized forms of idiopathic orbital inflammation are usually not difficult to differentiate from posterior scleritis, using ultrasonography or computed tomography; isolated findings of inflammatory infiltration of extraocular muscles (myositis), lacrimal gland (dacryoadenitis), or tissue surrounding the optic nerve (perineuritis) are different in appearance from scleral thickening and retrobulbar edema (posterior scleritis). However, the diffuse form of idiopathic orbital inflammation, especially the acute variety, may sometimes show similarities to posterior scleritis. The diagnosis depends mostly on the demonstration of an orbital mass by ultrasonography or computerized tomography but sometimes the definitive orbital mass cannot be found. In both idiopathic orbital inflammation and posterior scleritis, ultrasonography and computerized tomography may show scleral thickening, retrobulbar edema, extraocular muscle enlargement, and diffuse orbital infiltrate; in both conditions, computerized tomography does not show sinus involvement or bone erosion.[88,101,102-104,115,116] Because there are no strong anatomical barriers between sclera and orbit, it is sometimes difficult to know if the inflammation begins in the sclera and spreads to the orbit, as in the case of posterior scleritis, or if the inflammation begins in the orbit and spreads to the sclera, as in the case of diffuse idiopathic orbital inflammation.[92] The main difference in these patients is that, in posterior scleritis, intraocular findings such as anterior scleral, uveal, retinal, and optic nerve involvement are frequent and extraocular findings such as conjunctival chemosis, proptosis, eyelid edema, and decreased ocular motility are less common[84]; in diffuse idiopathic orbital inflammatory disease, extraocular involvement is common and intraocular involvement is relatively rare. Still, in some patients similarities outnumber differences, in which case the entity is considered a diffuse idiopathic orbital inflammatory disease.

Orbital tumors may share some clinical similarities with posterior scleritis, but the finding of an orbital mass by ultrasonography or computerized tomography, and the detection of

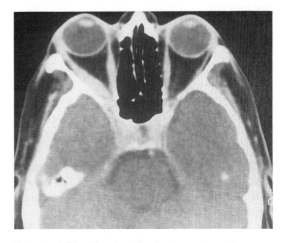

FIGURE 4.32. Computerized tomogram. Note the thickening of the lateral and medial rectus muscles (left eye) in a patient with thyroid opthalmopathy.

sinus involvement and/or bone erosion by computerized tomography, are exclusively characteristic of the former; subsequent biopsy of the mass will categorize the type of tumor.[102–104]

Thyroid ophthalmopathy and posterior scleritis may also have similar symptoms and signs. In both, ultrasonography and computerized tomography may show extraocular muscle enlargement (Fig. 4.32); however, thyroid disease does not show scleral thickening with retrobulbar edema. Aside from the symptoms of thyroid disease and upper lid retraction and lid lag when looking downward, the most definite differential point of thyroid ophthalmopathy is the thyroid-releasing hormone (TRH) infusion test; screening tests, including triiodothyronine (T_3) and thyroxine (T_4) by radioimmunoassay, and T_3 resin uptake, may be normal.[102,103,117,118]

4.2.4.5.6.2. Subretinal Mass.
Aside from posterior scleritis, a subretinal mass may be caused by several choroidal (Table 4.17) and orbital entities (Table 4.16).

Differential diagnosis from choroidal melanoma is important, because many cases of posterior scleritis have been enucleated as a consequence of this mistaken diagnosis.[1,80,81,93,94,106] Choroidal melanoma and posterior scleritis may present with a unilateral subretinal mass with or without serous retinal detachment.[119,120] In both, fluorescein angiography may show multiple point-source leakages. However, hyperpigmentation or hypopigmentation of the choroidal mass with occasional overlying orange lipofuscin pigment contrasts with the uniform normal color of the retinal pigment epithelium over the scleral mass.[119,121] Furthermore, although a choroidal melanoma may also be surrounded by choroidal folds, the finding is not frequent.[95] Ultrasonography may show the choroidal mass with the characteristic findings of low internal reflectivity, acoustic quiet zone, choroidal excavation, and orbital shadowing without retrobulbar edema.[119,122] (Fig. 4.33). It is important to stress that intraocular inflammation does not exclude the possibility of choroidal melanoma. A small percentage of patients, usually with a large, necrotic choroidal melanoma, can

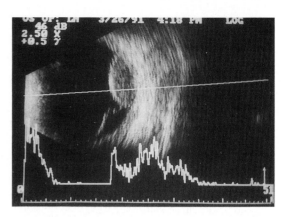

FIGURE 4.33. Ultrasonogram: choroidal melanoma. Note the A scan low internal reflectivity characteristics, the well-defined choroidal mass, and the lack of edema in Tenon's space.

have intraocular inflammation as the presenting sign.[123]

Metastatic uveal carcinomas from breast, lung, kidney, gastrointestinal, or genitourinary tumors may present as a unilateral subretinal mass with or without overlying subretinal fluid, occasionally surrounded by choroidal folds; but they are usually amelanotic with hyperplastic pigmentation (mottling) of the overlying retinal pigmented epithelium.[119,124,125] Differential diagnosis is important, because metastatic uveal carcinoma may be the first sign of a systemic malignancy in as many as 50% of the cases.[124] Ultrasonography shows a solid choroidal tumor with medium to high reflectivity without retrobulbar edema; there is no acoustic quiet zone, choroidal excavation, or orbital shadowing characteristic of choroidal melanomas.[119,122]

Choroidal hemangiomas may also present as a unilateral subretinal mass with or without overlying subretinal fluid. However, they are usually pinkish-orange in color, they are frequently associated with Sturge–Weber syndrome, and they are not surrounded by choroidal folds.[119,126,127] Although fluorescein angiography may show multiple small leaks, as in the case of posterior scleritis, the early filling of the choroidal vessels in the area of the tumor prior to the filling of the retinal vessels is typical of a choroidal hemangioma.[128] Ultrasonography shows a solid tumor with uniform high reflectivity without retrobulbar edema; there is no acoustic quiet zone, choroidal excavation, or orbital shadowing typical of choroidal melanomas.[119,122]

Orbital tumors and diffuse idiopathic orbital inflammatory diseases may also present with a subretinal mass that has the same color as the adjacent normal retinal pigment epithelium, preserved choroidal vascular pattern, and surrounding choroidal folds as in the case of posterior scleritis. However, clinical findings and imaging studies may help to differentiate the different entities (Table 4.16).

4.2.4.5.6.3. Choroidal Folds. Choroidal folds can be caused by multiple entities such as orbital tumors, idiopathic orbital inflammation, thyroid ophthalmopathy (Table 4.16), and primary or secondary choroidal tumors (Table 4.17); they may also be present in macular degeneration with choroidal neovascularization, papilledema, hypotony, and following scleral buckling retinal detachment surgery.[87,95,96,108,109]

Choroidal neovascularization in senile macular degeneration may produce chorioretinal folds. Contraction of a subpigmented epithelial fibrovascular membrane adherent to Bruch's membrane may cause a series of chorioretinal folds radiating outward from the periphery of the contracted membrane.[129] Differential diagnosis is straightforward because of the typical radiating pattern of the chorioretinal folds, the presence of drusen in Bruch's membrane, and the detection of the neovascular membrane. Fluorescein angiography shows a seafan pattern of subretinal vessels, a nonfluorescent halo around the area of staining, and a serous detachment of the retinal pigment epithelium.

Papilledema may also produce choroidal folds. Increased intracranial pressure, most commonly due to intracranial tumors, causes increased cerebrospinal fluid pressure within the optic nerve sheath. The distended sheath may act as a space-occupying lesion causing the formation of the choroidal folds.[130,131] Although bilateral papilledema and choroidal folds may be present in posterior scleritis, the ultrasonographic findings of scleral thickening and retrobulbar edema make the differentiation straightforward.

Chorioretinal folds may appear as a result of the redundancy of the choroid and the retina when the scleral wall shrinks or collapses inward during hypotony.[132,133] The normal ultrasonography and the past ocular history of intraocular surgery or intraocular trauma as causes of hypotony, help to differentiate this entity from posterior scleritis.

Scleral buckle procedures for retinal detachment, causing scleral shrinkage and secondary choroidal folding, can be recognized and differentiated from posterior scleritis.[108]

4.2.4.5.6.4. Annular Ciliochoroidal Detachment and/or Serous Retinal Detachment. Aside from posterior scleritis, serous detachments of the choroid, ciliary body, and retina, may be caused by the uveal effusion syndrome, by intraocular surgery, and by rhegmatogenous retinal detachment with uveal detachment (Table 4.18). Bullous serous detachment of the retina and, less commonly, serous ciliochoroidal detachment, may also be seen in choroidal melanoma, metastatic uveal carcinoma (Table 4.17), and Vogt-Koyanagi–Harada syndrome.[120,134,135] Bullous serous retinal detachment or serous macular detachment without ciliochoroidal detachment can be found in the idiopathic central serous choroidopathy.

Uveal effusion syndrome and posterior scleritis may both present with annular ciliochoroidal detachments, and/or bullous serous retinal detachments, and/or serous macular detachments[136,137]; however, in uveal effusion syndrome there is minimal or no pain, there may be dilated episcleral vessels but no scleritis, and there is usually bilaterality. Furthermore, there is minimal or no uveitis (some vitreous cells); there are hyperpigmented spots in the retinal pigmented epithelium ("leopard spots"), and there is a clear subretinal fluid. Fluorescein angiography in uveal effusion syndrome shows slow perfusion of the choroid and prolonged choroidal hyperfluorescence.[138] Occasionally, there are some focal leaks in the pigment epithelium but this finding is much less common than in posterior scleritis.[137] Ultrasonography shows choroidal thickening and serous ciliochoroid and/or retinal detachments in both entities; however, the detection in some cases of an eye smaller than normal (nanophthalmos), or the finding of retrobulbar edema, may be helpful for establishing the diagnosis of uveal effusion syndrome or posterior scleritis, respectively. Unlike posterior scleritis, the response to steroids in uveal effusion syndrome is poor.

A history of recent intraocular surgery is helpful in differentiating a postoperative serous ciliochoroidal detachment from one appearing in posterior scleritis.

The finding of a retinal break with folds in a retinal detachment with serous ciliochoroidal detachment is characteristic of a rhegmatogenous retinal detachment.

Vogt-Koyanagi–Harada syndrome should also be considered in the differential diagnosis of posterior scleritis, because both may present with bullous serous retinal detachments, serous macular detachments, and, although infrequently in the former, serous ciliochoroidal detachments.[139–142] In both, fluorescein angiography may show multifocal subretinal leaks. Furthermore, in both there may be anterior and/ or posterior uveitis, disk edema, and cloudy subretinal fluid. However, Vogt-Koyanagi–Harada syndrome also presents with signs of integumentary (vitiligo, poliosis, and alopecia) auditory (dysacusis and tinnitus), and neurological (meningeal inflammation) involvement. Patients with Vogt-Koyanagi–Harada syndrome are often orientals or have dark skin pigmentation, and they have bilateral involvement. As in posterior scleritis, ultrasonography in Vogt-Koyanagi–Harada syndrome shows choroidal thickening and serous retinal detachment; however, unlike in posterior scleritis, the choroidal thickening shows a low internal reflectivity, and there is no retrobulbar edema.

Idiopathic central serous chorioretinopathy and posterior scleritis may have serous macular detachments and/or bullous serous retinal detachments, but in the former there are neither the ocular findings of uveitis, anterior scleritis, and disk edema, nor the ultrasonographic findings of sclerochoroidal thickening and retrobulbar edema.[137]

4.2.4.5.6.5. Disk and Macular Edema. Disk and macular edema may occur in posterior scleritis, in many inflammatory conditions of the uveal tract, and after intraocular surgery.[8]

Past and present history, review of systems, ocular examination, laboratory tests, and imaging studies may be helpful in distinguishing these conditions from posterior scleritis.

4.2.5. Associated Diseases

Connective tissue diseases, vasculitic diseases, herpes zoster, herpes simplex, rosacea, gout, tuberculosis, and syphilis are the diseases most commonly associated with scleritis.[2,5,17] In our series, an associated systemic disease was found in 57% of the patients with scleritis (Table 4.9), including 48% with connective tissue or vasculitic diseases and 7% with infectious diseases; rosacea, atopy, and a foreign body were associated with one case each (0.6%) (Table 4.11). Within the connective tissue diseases and vasculitic diseases, rheumatoid arthritis was the most common entity, followed by Wegener's granulomatosis, relapsing polychondritis, systemic lupus erythematosus, and inflammatory bowel disease. Scleritis may be the problem whose diagnostic study leads to the discovery and subsequent treatment of a connective tissue disease or a vasculitic disease. When scleritis is the only presenting complaint, diagnosis and therapy of the potentially lethal systemic disease are often delayed. In our series, scleritis was the first manifestation of connective tissue disease or vasculitic disease in 26 patients (15.12%) (Table 4.12). Mean duration of scleritis signs or symptoms prior to diagnosis was 37 months (range, 1–264 months). The most common diagnosis eventually discovered was Wegener's granulomatosis followed by relapsing polychondritis. Meticulous review of systems (with subsequent studies to pursue leads) was the most fruitful diagnostic endeavor for establishing a diagnosis. Evaluation of biopsied tissue, and laboratory or X-ray studies in the context of review of system findings, confirmed the initial diagnostic impressions.

Systemic disease association was found to be most common in the necrotizing anterior types of scleritis, either with inflammation (95%) and without inflammation (67%), followed by the diffuse anterior (45%), the posterior (45%), and the nodular anterior (44%) types.

Necrotizing anterior scleritis with inflammation was found to be the most frequent subcategory in patients whose scleritis appeared as a first manifestation of a systemic disease (58%) (see Table 4.12).

Although gout has been reported with scleritis, the association in most cases is vague and indefinite.[18,21] One case with gout was detected in our series. Because erythema nodosum is a sign of other underlying diseases, such as bacterial (streptococcal), mycobacterial (tuberculosis), and chlamydial (psittacosis) infections, sarcoidosis, arthritis associated to inflammatory bowel disease, and Behçet's disease, we have not considered it as a separate diagnostic entity, unlike other authors.[2,5] Two of our patients with scleritis (nodular type) had erythema nodosum: One of them had Behçet's disease; no associated disease could be found in the other. Likewise, Raynaud's phenomenon is a vascular manifestation present in several connective tissue and vasculitic diseases, such as systemic lupus erythematosus, rheumatoid arthritis, and giant cell arteritis. Raynaud's phenomenon was present in four of our patients with scleritis, but we, unlike other authors,[13] considered it as part of the primary systemic disease. Some patients with scleritis may give a past history of rheumatic heart disease but the conditions have not been described as occurring at the same time.[3] None of our patients had had rheumatic fever in the past. Hypertension was present in 34 patients with scleritis (20%), either as a part of a connective tissue or vasculitic disease, or as an independent manifestation.

4.2.6. Complications of Scleritis

4.2.6.1. Keratopathy

Because corneal changes in scleritis appear as an extension of the adjacent scleral inflammation, the area most frequently involved is the corneal periphery. Peripheral corneal involvement may precede the onset of scleritis.[143,144] The different patterns of corneal involvement are related to the severity and type of scleral inflammation and they can be classified, depending on whether or not

thinning, infiltration, or ulceration of the peripheral cornea occurs.

4.2.6.1.1. Peripheral Corneal Thinning

Peripheral corneal thinning is the most benign form of corneal involvement associated with scleritis. It is frequently associated with diffuse anterior scleritis and, although it may occur in young patients without any systemic condition, it is often found in middle-aged and elderly individuals with long-standing rheumatoid arthritis.[2] The peripheral cornea becomes grayish and thinned in one or more areas over a period of several years, eventually extending through the full circumference of the eye (Fig. 4.34; see color insert). The gutter, usually about one-third thinner than the normal central cornea, does not extend more than 2 mm centrally and is not necessarily located in the same quadrant as the area of scleral inflammation. Because the central area remains unaffected, there is little effect on visual acuity. The epithelium remains intact throughout the thinning process but vascularization, lipid deposition, and further opacification and thinning may eventually involve the edematous stroma. Deepening of the gutter may result in a progressive astigmatism that interferes with visual acuity. If some pain occurs, it is due to the scleral inflammation rather than to the peripheral corneal thinning. Sometimes the thinned cornea may progress to an area of ectasia. Spontaneous perforation is rare, although trauma can rupture the thin cornea. Peripheral corneal thinning may also occur without scleritis in patients with long-standing rheumatoid arthritis[145–148]; circumferential thinning with a well-demarcated central edge without lipid deposition and minimal vascularization resembles the appearance of an eye wearing a hard contact lens ("contact lens" cornea).[149]

The differential diagnosis of peripheral corneal thinning associated with scleritis includes Terrien's marginal degeneration (Fig. 4.35), pellucid marginal degeneration, and senile furrow degeneration (Table 4.19). All of these are slowly progressive, bilateral, and painless peripheral stromal thinning with intact epithelium. In all of these, there is rare loss of vision or central cornea involvement. Furthermore,

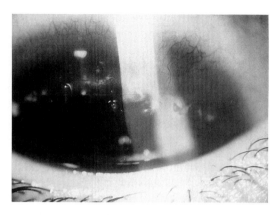

FIGURE 4.35. Terrien's marginal degeneration. Note the quiet eye, the area of corneal thinning in the superior 160° of the corneal periphery, and the lipid/protein deposits in the corneal stroma at the anterior border of the area of active thinning.

in peripheral corneal thinning associated with scleritis and in Terrien's marginal degeneration the peripheral gutter may have lipid deposition and vascularization. However, Terrien's marginal degeneration usually occurs superiorly and, although an atypical pterygium may be present in 20% of the cases, it is not associated with true scleritis.[150,151] Peripheral corneal thinning associated with scleritis may account for some cases considered to be "inflammatory Terrien's marginal corneal disease."[152] Unlike peripheral corneal thinning associated with scleritis, pellucid marginal degeneration is a noninflammatory condition that affects only the inferior cornea and is not accompanied by lipid deposition or vascularization.[153,154] Finally, in senile furrow degeneration, a peripheral corneal thinning of the clear interval between an arcus senilis and the limbus, there is neither vascularization and lipid infiltration in the narrow gutter (0.5 mm or less in width), nor adjacent scleral inflammation.[155,156] Unlike peripheral corneal thinning associated with scleritis, Terrien's marginal degeneration, pellucid marginal degeneration, and senile furrow degeneration are not associated with any systemic disease.

Suppression of the scleral inflammation usually allows regression but in some patients the defect remains. Lubrication or therapeutic soft contact lens may prove effective in some patients. In cases of astigmatic error, spectacles

TABLE 4.19. Differential diagnosis of peripheral corneal thinning associated with scleritis.

Parameter	Peripheral corneal thinning–scleritis	Terrien's marginal degeneration	Pellucid marginal degeneration	Senile furrow degeneration
Age predilection	Middle aged and elderly	Young and middle aged	Young and middle aged	Elderly
Sex predilection	Female	Male	—	—
Laterality	Bilateral	Bilateral	Bilateral	Bilateral
Pain	—	—	—	—
Visual loss	+/−	+/−	+/−	−
Epithelial defect	—	—	—	—
Stromal thinning	+	+	+	+
Progression	Slow	Slow	Slow	Slow
Location	Circumferential	Superior	Inferior	Circumferential
Width	1–2 mm	1–2 mm	1–2 mm	0.5 mm or less
Central edge	Eventually lipids	Gray-white line	Protruding	Arcus senilis (lipid)
Gutter lipids	Eventually develop	+	−	− (lucid interval)
Gutter vessels	Eventually develop	+	−	−
Scleral/conjunctival inflammation	+ (mild to moderate)	+/− (occasional atypical pterygium)	−	−
Perforation	+/−	+/−	+/−	−
Associated disease	Systemic disease (rheumatoid arthritis)	—	—	—
Treatment	Scleritis treatment Contact lenses Tectonic keratoplasty Conjunctival flap	Contact lenses Tectonic keratoplasty	Contact lenses Tectonic keratoplasty	—

or rigid contact lens may be used, depending on the severity. Progression to a thinned, ectatic cornea may be treated by cyanoacrylate glue application with or without conjunctival resection, or by excising the ectatic tissue and replacing it with an annular lamellar keratoplasty or with a conjunctival flap.

4.2.6.1.2. Stromal Keratitis

Extension of the diffuse, nodular, or necrotizing scleral inflammation into the cornea may appear as isolated or multiple white or gray nummular midstromal opacities, which usually are in the periphery, although they can involve the central cornea. The opacities are usually in the same quadrant as the scleral inflammation; therefore the corneal involvement in the diffuse type of scleritis is usually more extensive than in the nodular type. If the treatment for the scleritis is delayed, the lesions may expand toward the center of the cornea and eventually coalesce, so that large areas may become opaque and swollen, leading to an appearance resembling that of the sclera ("sclerosing" changes) (Fig. 4.36; see color insert). Vessels may involve the superficial stroma but they are always far behind the advancing edge of the opacity. Lipid deposition in the stromal opacities can be seen as crystalline deposits ("candy floss").[2]

The opacities may disappear completely with early and vigorous treatment of the scleral inflammation; more often, only partial regression occurs, leaving permanent changes that, if central, may require penetrating corneal grafting for visual restoration.

4.2.6.1.3. Peripheral Ulcerative Keratitis

The most severe form of keratitis associated with scleritis is peripheral ulcerative keratitis (PUK), a potentially devastating process in which the layers of the peripheral cornea are progressively destroyed, leaving the cornea so thin it can easily perforate. The destructive process, usually associated with necrotizing scleritis, begins as a gray, swollen, infiltrated area adjacent to a region of scleral inflammation that in few days may break down, leaving only some layers of deep stroma and/or Desce-

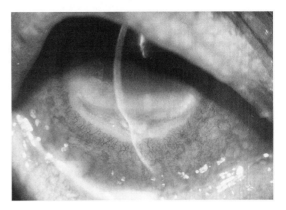

FIGURE 4.37. Peripheral ulcerative keratitis in a patient with rheumatoid arthritis. This slit-lamp photomicrograph illustrates the degree of peripheral corneal ulceration, nearly 80% in depth. The extent, circumferentially, is from 5 to 8 o'clock. The degree of corneal destruction is much greater than is clinically apparent: exploration of the ulcer with a smooth-tipped tying forcep disclosed undermining of this ulcer, leaving an overhanging lip, with active digestion of the corneal stroma extending approximately 5 mm into the cornea from the area of the obvious active peripheral ulcer.

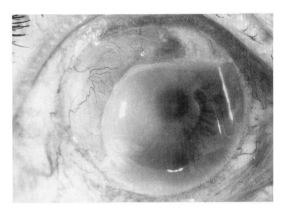

FIGURE 4.38. Peripheral ulcerative keratitis, which has progressed centrally and circumferentially in a patient with anterior scleritis associated with rheumatoid arthritis. Like the ulcer shown in Fig. 4.37, this one has an overhanging lip with undermining of the edge of the ulcer and destruction of stroma far in excess of what one would predict as a result of a simple slit-lamp examination. The digestive process has extended into the pupillary zone in this patient.

met's membrane (Fig. 4.37). An intrastromal yellow-white blood cell infiltrate may easily be seen at the advancing edge of the ulcer, which progresses circumferentially and occasionally centrally (Fig. 4.38), in which case vision will be lost. In some cases, anterior uveitis may also be present. If no treatment is instituted, spontaneous corneal perforation may easily occur.

Fourteen percent of our patients (15% of the eyes) had PUK, and the majority of these were associated with necrotizing scleritis (Table 4.20). Loss of vision was highly associated with the presence of PUK ($p < .05$) (Table 4.20). Peripheral ulcerative keratitis with or without scleritis is frequently an ocular manifestation of a systemic disease.[154-156] Peripheral ulcerative keratitis was highly associated with the presence of a potentially lethal, often occult systemic disease in our patients with scleritis. Most of these cases had the necrotizing variety of scleritis. These data show that the presence of PUK accompanying scleritis should be considered a grave sign: It indicates an extension of the inflammatory process that may cause visual loss and perforation of the eye, and may signal the presence of a potentially lethal systemic disease.

Differentiation from Mooren's ulcer may be difficult because both peripheral ulcerations may be painful and crescent shaped, may follow a circumferential and central progression, and may have an undermined central edge with stromal yellow-white infiltrates. However, in Mooren's ulcer there is neither adjacent scleritis nor systemic disease association.

Treatment for PUK includes cyanoacrylate glue application following keratectomy and

conjunctival resection, while vigorous systemic treatment is directed at controlling the scleral inflammation.[157-160]

4.2.6.2. Uveitis

Uveitis is also caused by extension of the scleral inflammation. Fraunfelder and Watson[1] found that 68% of 30 enucleated eyes with a primary histological diagnosis of scleritis had signs of having had uveitis; scleritis with uveitis and glaucoma was the most common combination of complications leading to enucleation. Wilhelmus et al.,[6] in another series of 100 enucleated eyes with a primary histological diagnosis of scleritis, found that 63% had had anterior uveitis. These findings suggest that scleritis with uveitis, particularly when associated with glaucoma, should be regarded as extremely ominous. The uveitis associated with scleritis is more frequently anterior, mild to moderate in intensity, and appears during the late course of the scleral inflammation.[6]

In our series, 73 of the 172 patients (42%) with scleritis had had at least one episode of anterior uveitis (Table 4.6); of those, 22 patients had bilateral involvement. There was no difference in the sex and age distribution between the patients with scleritis with and without uveitis. The presence of anterior uveitis was highly associated with the presence of necrotizing anterior scleritis (69%) and posterior scleritis (45%); 4 of the 5 patients with posterior scleritis and anterior uveitis also had some degree of anterior scleritis.

Posterior uveitis was present in all cases of posterior scleritis. Because the presence of posterior uveitis in association with anterior scleritis is rare, the detection of posterior uveitis in a patient with anterior scleral inflammation obligates one to search for posterior scleritis.[3]

Loss of visual acuity in patients with scleritis may be caused by complications such as keratitis, uveitis, cataract, glaucoma, or macular edema. Long-standing uveitis may cause cataract, glaucoma, or macular edema. The presence of anterior uveitis with scleritis was highly associated with loss of visual acuity and with the presence of peripheral ulcerative keratitis indicating that uveitis occurs with scleritis cases

TABLE 4.20. Peripheral ulcerative keratitis (PUK) among patients with scleritis.

Diagnosis	Patients		Total
	No. (%) with PUK		
Scleritis	**24 (13.95)**		**172**
Diffuse	5 (6.49)		77
Nodular	3 (7.69)		39
Necrotizing	16 (41.03)		39
Scleromalacia	0		6
Posterior	0		11

undergoing complications that may lead to visual loss.

The presence of anterior uveitis was not more common in patients with associated disease, nor was there any correlation between the presence of anterior uveitis and any particular associated disease.

The presence of uveitis accompanying scleritis should be considered a grave sign, because it indicates not only an extension of the inflammatory process to the intraocular structures but also the presence of complications that may cause progressive visual loss. The detection of uveitis accompanying scleritis requires early and aggressive therapy to control both the uveal and scleral inflammation.

4.2.6.3. Glaucoma

Increased intraocular pressure is caused by the accompanying scleral edema and uveal inflammation. Fraunfelder and Watson[1] found that 46% of 30 enucleated eyes with a primary histological diagnosis of scleritis showed signs of having had glaucoma; scleritis with glaucoma and uveitis was the most common cause of enucleation. Wilhelmus et al.,[9] in another series of 92 enucleated eyes with a primary histological diagnosis of scleritis, found that 49% of them had had glaucoma. These data suggest that the presence of scleritis with glaucoma, particularly when associated with uveitis, should be considered an ominous sign.[1] The reported incidence of increased intraocular pressure in patients with scleritis varies between 12 and 22%.[2,9,18] In our series of 172 patients with scleritis, 22 (13%) had glaucoma. Angle-closure glaucoma, open-angle glaucoma, and neovascular glaucoma are some of the possible mechanisms.

4.2.6.3.1. Angle-Closure Glaucoma

A primary angle-closure attack can appear in scleral inflammation, particularly if the patient has narrow angles. Swelling of the angle structures combined with a mildly dilated pupil may account for the closure of the angle. The therapy includes the standard antiglaucomatous treatment, primarily with hyperosmotic agents, miotics, beta blockers, and laser iridectomy,

combined with antiinflammatory treatment for controlling the scleral inflammation.

Secondary angle closure in patients with scleritis may be caused by anterior synechiae, iridolenticular adhesions, or ciliary body edema secondary to long-standing anterior uveitis.[9] In this case, relief of anterior adhesions (laser iridogonioplasty or filtering procedures) and/or relief of the pupillary block (laser iridectomy), and control of the sclerouveal inflammation may restore the intraocular pressure to normal.

Secondary angle closure may occur in patients with posterior scleritis when a ciliochoroidal effusion displaces the iris–lens diaphragm forward, shallowing the anterior chamber and closing the filtration angle.[100] In this case, treatment with miotics may cause further shallowing of the anterior chamber, whereas treatment of the scleral inflammation with antiinflammatory drugs resolves the inflammatory effusion and allows the angle to reopen.

4.2.6.3.2. Open-Angle Glaucoma

Primary open-angle glaucoma in patients with scleritis may appear because of a preexisting abnormal outflow system that is further impaired by inflammation of the angle structures. Characteristics of these patients are normal angles, cupped disks, and glaucomatous field defects; the increased intraocular pressure returns to normal with antiglaucomatous agents but does not respond to antiinflammatory therapy for the scleritis.[3]

Occlusion of the trabecular meshwork by inflammatory cells in anterior uveitis and scleral inflammation may cause a secondary open-angle glaucoma. Gonioscopically, inflammatory debris may be seen at the angle. Treatment with beta blockers, carbonate dehydratase inhibitors, and antiinflammatory agents may control the intraocular pressure and the sclerouveal inflammation. If these fail to control the intraocular pressure, laser trabeculoplasty or filtering surgery should be performed.

Steroid-induced open-angle glaucoma may appear in patients with scleritis receiving topical steroids or, more rarely, systemic steroids. The increased intraocular pressure may develop within 2 weeks of initiating steroid use or after many months or even years of use. The more potent drugs such as dexamethasone and prednisolone are more likely to induce increased intraocular pressure sooner and to a higher level than weaker agents such as hydrocortisone or fluorometholone. This predisposition is genetically determined. Patients in whom glaucoma has been successfully controlled may develop unacceptable levels of intraocular pressure if steroid therapy is added. Nonsteroidal antiinflammatory drugs and/or immunosuppressive agents may allow a reduction in the steroids. If spontaneous resolution does not occur within 2 to 6 weeks, or if steroids cannot be stopped, or if the pressure is high, therapy for primary open-angle glaucoma may be initiated to prevent progression of optic nerve damage.

4.2.6.3.3. Neovascular Glaucoma

Angle neovascularization has been reported in enucleated eyes with scleral inflammation.[9] Long-standing hypoxic retinopathy such as central retinal artery or vein occlusion may lead to the formation of a fibrovascular membrane that may cover the trabecular meshwork, resulting in total angle closure. A combination of antiinflammatory therapy and panretinal photocoagulation, perhaps supplemented with direct goniophotocoagulation, medical antiglaucomatous treatment, or filtering surgery sometimes succeeds.

The presence of increased intraocular pressure accompanying scleritis indicates an extension of the inflammatory process to the intraocular structures, with the development of complications leading to progressive visual loss. Intraocular pressure should always be measured in patients with scleral inflammation. The detection of glaucoma accompanying scleritis requires early and aggressive therapy to control both the intraocular pressure and the scleral inflammation.

4.2.6.4. Cataract

The presence of long-standing anterior uveitis in patients with severe scleral inflammation, particularly of the necrotizing type, may lead to the formation of a cataract. Another cause of cataract is the use of long-term systemic or local steroid treatment. A comparison between a group of patients without scleritis and a group of patients with scleritis, both receiving long-term systemic or local steroid treatment, showed an increased risk of development of posterior subcapsular cataract in the group of patients with scleritis (36%) as opposed to the group of patients without scleritis (11.5%).[18] In our series of patients with scleritis, 29 (17%) had cataracts.

Although cataract extraction usually is not complicated in patients with scleritis without uveitis, surgery should be attempted only in the absence of scleral inflammation. Cataract removal through a corneal incision is advisable.

Uneventful cataract extraction or any other surgical procedure can, although rarely, precipitate a necrotizing scleritis in patients with autoimmune or infectious diseases.[161-166] In 11 of our patients, necrotizing scleritis developed after ocular surgery (Table 4.21). The interval between surgery and onset of scleritis varied from 2 weeks to 6 months. Ten patients (90.9%) were found to have an underlying autoimmune vasculitic systemic disease. One patient was found to have a local infectious process. Appropriate studies led to the discovery and subsequent treatment of a systemic disease or an infectious process in 6 of the 11 patients; the other 5 had been previously diagnosed. Immune complex-mediated vasculitis and T cell-mediated immune responses can be triggered in patients with underlying systemic autoimmune vasculitic diseases after ocular surgical trauma resulting in necrotizing scleritis. These findings emphasize the need for meticulous diagnostic pursuit of potentially lethal systemic autoimmune vasculitic disease in patients with necrotizing scleritis following intraocular surgery.

Summary

Episcleritis is a benign disease that occurs in young adults, usually women, with a peak incidence in the fourth decade. Although the course is self-limiting, episcleritis is usually characterized by recurrences involving both

TABLE 4.21. Occurrence of necrotizing scleritis after ocular surgery.

Patient no.	Age	Sex	Surgery[a]	Interval[b] (weeks)	Diagnosis	Follow-up (months)
1	75	F	ECCE + PCIOL	12	Rheumatoid arthritis	30
2	67	F	ECCE + PCIOL	24	Rheumatoid arthritis	38
3	82	F	ECCE + PCIOL	4	Rheumatoid arthritis	7
4	68	M	Secondary IOL	24	Rheumatoid arthritis	35
5	66	M	ICCE	4	Wegener's granulomatosis	43
6	69	M	ECCE + PCIOL	20	Wegener's granulomatosis	10
7	78	M	ICCE + ACIOL	20	Wegener's granulomatosis	18
8	69	F	ECCE + PCIOL	24	Wegener's granulomatosis	9
9	68	M	ECCE + PCIOL	3	Ulcerative colitis	10
10	71	F	ICCE	8	Psoriatic arthritis	29
11	70	M	Strabismus	2	*Proteus* infection	2

[a] ECCE, extracapsular cataract extraction; PCIOL, posterior chamber intraocular lens; ICCE, intracapsular cataract extraction; ACIOL, anterior chamber intraocular lens.
[b] Interval between surgery and development of necrotizing scleritis.

eyes at the same time or different eyes at different times. It presents as an uncomfortable, red eye, sometimes with tearing and mild photophobia. Pain, if any, is mild and localized to the eye. Clinical examination with a slit-lamp discloses that the inflammation is entirely localized within the episcleral tissue, never involving the underlying sclera. Redness diminishes greatly after instillation of topical phenylephrine (10%) because this vasoconstrictor has great effect on the superficial episcleral vessels, which are congested in episcleritis. Episcleritis rarely causes loss of vision, corneal involvement, uveitis, or glaucoma. Two types of episcleritis may be distinguished: simple and nodular. In simple episcleritis, in which there is a diffuse vascular congestion, the course lasts between 5 and 10 days without treatment. In nodular episcleritis, in which one or more nodules form, the course lasts between 4 and 6 weeks without treatment. Approximately 32% of patients have an underlying associated disease, including 13% with connective tissue diseases, 7% with rosacea, and 7% with atopy.

Unlike episcleritis, scleritis is a severe inflammatory disease that can be progressively destructive, sometimes leading to loss of vision or loss of the eye. Furthermore, scleritis may be the presenting manifestation of a potentially lethal systemic vasculitic disease or may herald the onset of an occult systemic vasculitis in a patient with an already diagnosed systemic disease that is apparently in remission. Scleritis is most common in the fourth to sixth decades of life, more often in women, with a peak incidence in the fifth decade. Scleritis is also characterized by recurrences involving both eyes at the same time or different eyes at different times. It presents with deep, severe pain, often radiating to the forehead, the jaw, and the sinuses. Other symptoms include tearing and mild photophobia. The main sign is redness that, unlike episcleritis, has a bluish tinge, best seen under natural light. Clinical examination with a slit-lamp discloses that the inflammation is localized within the episcleral and scleral tissue. Redness does not diminish after instillation of topical phenylephrine (10%) because this vasoconstrictor has minimal effect on the deep episcleral vessels, which are congested in scleritis. Scleritis may cause loss of vision, corneal involvement, uveitis, glaucoma, cataract, exudative retinal detachment, and macular edema. Two types of scleritis may be distinguished: anterior and posterior. Anterior scleritis may be further classified into diffuse, nodular, necrotizing with inflammation (necrotizing), and necrotizing without inflammation (scleromalacia perforans). Necrotizing scleritis is the most severe and destructive form because it may lead to the loss of the eye from multiple complications, and because it is highly associated with potentially lethal systemic vasculitic diseases. Aproximately 57% of the patients have an underlying associated disease, including 50% with connective tissue or vasculitic diseases and 7% with infectious diseases. It is therefore extremely important that the correct diagnosis be made and that subsequent adequate treatment be given as early as possible during the course of the disease.

References

1. Fraunfelder FT, Watson PG: Evaluation of eyes enucleated for scleritis. Br J Ophthal 60:227, 1976.
2. Watson PG, Hayreh SS: Scleritis and episcleritis. Br J Ophthalmol 60:163, 1976.
3. Watson PG, Hazleman BL: *The Sclera and Systemic Disorders*. W.B. Saunders, Philadelphia, 1976.
4. Watson PG: Doyne Memorial Lecture, 1982. The nature and the treatment of scleral inflammation. Trans Ophthalmol Soc UK 102:257, 1982.
5. Watson PG: Diseases of the sclera and episclera. In Tasman W, Jaeger EA (Eds): *Duane's Clinical Ophthalmology*, rev ed. Lippincott, Philadelphia, 1992, pp 1–43.
6. Wilhelmus KR, Watson PG, Vasavada AR: Uveitis associated with scleritis. Trans Ophthalmol Soc UK 101:351, 1981.
7. Calthorpe CM, Watson PG, McCartney ACE: Posterior scleritis: a clinical and histopathological survey. Eye 2:267, 1988.
8. Cleary PE, Watson PG: Visual loss due to posterior segment disease in scleritis. Trans Ophthalmol Soc UK 95:297, 1975.
9. Wilhelmus KR, Grierson I, Watson PG: Histopathologic and clinical associations of scleritis and glaucoma. Am J Ophthalmol 91:697, 1981.
10. Lyons CJ, Hakin KN, Watson PG: Topical Flurbiprofen: an effective treatment for episcleritis? Eye 4:521, 1990.
11. Meyer PA, Watson PG, Franks W, Dubord P: "Pulsed" immunosuppressive therapy in the treatment of immunologically induced corneal and scleral disease. Eye 1:487, 1987.
12. Hayreh SS, Watson PG: Prednisolone-21-stearoylglycolate in scleritis. Br J Ophthalmol 54:394, 1970.
13. Tuft SJ, Watson PG: Progression of scleral disease. Ophthalmology 98:467, 1991.
14. Williamson J: Incidence of eye disease in cases of connective tissue disease. Trans Ophthal Soc UK 94:742, 1974.
15. Heinonen O: Über Episcleritis periodica fugax und Erblichkeit. Acta Ophthalmologica 1:166, 1923.
16. Heinonen O: Nachtrag zu meiner Arbeit "Über episcleritis periodica fugax und Erblichkeit." Acta Ophthalmologica, 4:278, 1927.
17. Lyne AJ, Pitkeathley DA: Episcleritis and scleritis. Arch Ophthalmol 80:171, 1968.
18. McGavin DD, Williamson J, Forrester JV, Foulds WS: Episcleritis and scleritis: a study of their clinical manifestations and association with rheumatoid arthritis. Br J Ophthalmol 60:192, 1976.
19. Watson PG, McKay DA, Clemett RS, Wilkinson P: Treatment of episcleritis. A double blind trial comparing betamethasone 0.1%, oxyphenbutazone 10% and placebo eye ointments. Br J Ophthalmol 57:866, 1973.
20. Campbell DM: Episcleritis. Ophthalmic Rec 12:517, 1903.
21. Duke-Elder S, Leigh AG: Diseases of the outer eye. Cornea and sclera. In Duke-Elder S (Ed): *System of Ophthalmology*, Vol 8, Part 2. C.V. Mosby, St. Louis, 1965, p 108.
22. James DG: Erythema nodosum. Br Med J 1:853, 1961.
23. Beerman H: Erythema nodosum. Am J Med Sci 223:433, 1952.
24. McCarthy JL: Episcleral nodules and erythema nodosum. Am J Ophthalmol 51:60, 1961.
25. Friedman AH, Henkind P: Unusual causes of episcleritis. Trans Am Acad Ophthalmol Otolaryngol 71:303, 1967.
26. Margo CE: Recurrent episcleritis and emotional stress. Arch Ophthalmol 102:821, 1984.
27. Rahe RH: Subjects' recent life changes and their near-future illness susceptibility. Adv Psychosom Med 8:2, 1972.
28. Obermayer M: *Psychocutaneous Medicine*. Charles C Thomas, Springfield IL, 1955.
29. Weiner H, Thaler M, Reiser MF: Etiology of duodenal ulcer. Psychosom Med 19:1, 1957.
30. Engel GL: Studies of ulcerative colitis. III. The nature of the psychology process. Am J Med 19:231, 1955.
31. Rothfield N: Clinical features of systemic lupus erythematosus. In Kelley WN, Harris ED, Ruddy S, Sledge CB (Eds): *Textbook of Rheumatology*, 3rd ed. W.B. Saunders, Philadelphia, 1989, pp 1070–1093.
32. Palmblad J: Stress and immunologic competence: studies in man. In Ader R (Ed): *Psychoneuroimmunology*. Academic Press, New York, 1981, pp 229–257.

33. Ader R: A historical account of conditioned immunobiologic responses. In Ader R (Ed): *Psychoneuroimmunology*. Academic Press, New York, 1981, pp 323–345.

34. Benedict WL: Etiology and treatment of scleritis and episcleritis. Trans Am Acad Ophthalmol Otolaryngol 29:211, 1924.

35. Moench LM: Gynaecologic foci in relation to scleritis and episcleritis and other ocular infections. Am J Med Sci 174:439, 1927.

36. Villard E: Episclérite cataméniale. Arch d'Ophtalmol 47:534, 1930.

37. Paufique L, Etienne R: L'étiologie génitale de quelques affections oculaires chez la femme. Arch d'Ophtalmol 9:157, 1949.

38. Drouet P, Thomas C: Episclérite periodique et système endocrino-vegatif. Bull Soc d'Ophtalmol France 7:682, 1952.

39. Zondek B, Bromberg YM: Endocrine allergy. Clinical reactions of allergy to endogenous hormones and their treatment. J Obstet Gynaecol Br Emp 54:1, 1947.

40. Balyeat RM: Scleritis due to allergy. J Am Med Assoc 98:2054, 1932.

41. Sinskey HL, Levin MB, Sacks B: Episcleritis— a new method of approach. Arch Ophthalmol 50:526, 1921.

42. Shoemaker WA: Episcleritis. Am J Ophthalmol 7:468, 1924.

43. Watson PG: The diagnosis and management of scleritis. Ophthalmology 87:716, 1980.

44. Sainz de la Maza M, Tauber J, Foster CS: Scleral grafting for necrotizing scleritis. Ophthalmology 96:306, 1989.

45. Foster CS, Forstot SL, Wilson LA: Mortality rate in rheumatoid arthritis patients developing necrotizing scleritis or peripheral ulcerative keratitis. Ophthalmology 91:1253, 1984.

46. Scott DGI, Bacon PA, Tribe CR: Systemic rheumatoid vasculitis: a clinical and laboratory study of 50 cases. Medicine 60:288, 1981.

47. Scott DGI, Bacon PA, Allen C, Parker C: IgG rheumatoid factor, complement, and immune complexes in rheumatoid synovitis and vasculitis: comparative and serial studies during cytotoxic therapy. Clin Exp Immunol 43:54, 1981.

48. Sokoloff L, Bunim JJ: Vascular lesions in rheumatoid arthritis. J Chronic Dis 5:668, 1957.

49. Douglas W: The digital artery lesion of rheumatoid arthritis. Ann Rheum Dis 24:40, 1965.

50. Ferguson RH, Slocumb CH: Peripheral neuropathy in rheumatoid arthritis. Bull Rheum Dis 11:251, 1961.

51. Hunder GG, McDuffie FC: Hypocomplementemia in rheumatoid arthritis. Am J Med 54:461, 1973.

52. Collins DH: The subcutaneous nodule of rheumatoid arthritis. J Pathol Bacteriol 45:97, 1937.

53. Bennett GA, Zeller JW, Bauer W: Subcutaneous nodules of rheumatoid arthritis and rheumatic fever: a pathologic study. Arch Pathol 30:70, 1940.

54. Kaye BR, Kaye RL, Bobrove A: Rheumatoid nodules. Review of the spectrum of associated conditions and proposal of a new classification, with a report of four seronegative cases. Am Rheum Dis 23:345, 1964.

55. Fong LP, Sainz de la Maza M, Rice BA, Foster CS: Immunopathology of scleritis. Ophthalmology 98:472, 1991.

56. van der Hoeve J: Scleromalacia perforans. Ned T Geneesk 75:4733, 1931.

57. Roca PD: Necrotising (rheumatoid) disease of the sclera. NY St J Med 74:1982, 1974.

58. van der Hoeve J: Scleromalacia perforans. Arch Ophthalmol 11:111, 1934.

59. Wojno Z: Ein Fall von forschreitender Erweichung der Lederhaut. Klin Oczna 13:778, 1935.

60. Kiehle FA: Scleromalacia. Am J Ophthalmol 20:565, 1937.

61. Urrets Zavalia A, Maldonado AI, Obregon OR: Skeromalazie in Verlauf einer chronischen Prophyrinurie. Klin Monatsbl Augenheilk 99:189, 1937.

62. Verhoeff FH, King MJ: Scleromalacia perforans. Report of a case in which the eye was examined microscopically. Arch Ophthalmol 20:1013, 1938.

63. Franceschetti A, Bischler V: La sclérite nodulaire nécrosante et ses rapports avec la scléromalacie. Ann Ocul 183:737, 1950.

64. François J: Scléromalacie perforante. Bull Soc Belge d'Ophtalmol 96:694, 1950.

65. Ashton N, Hobbs HE: Effect of cortisone on rheumatoid nodules of the sclera (scleromalacia perforans). Br J Ophthalmol 36:373, 1952.

66. Rosenthal JW, Williams GT: Scleromalacia perforans as a complication of rheumatoid arthritis. Am J Ophthalmol 54:862, 1962.

67. Anderson B, Margolis C: Scleromalacia: clinical and pathologic study of a case with consideration of differential diagnosis, relationship of collagen disease, and effect of ACTH and cortisone therapy. Am J Ophthalmol 35:917, 1952.

68. Arkle JS, Ingram HV: Scleromalacia perforans. Trans Ophthalmol Soc UK 55:552, 1935.

69. François J: Scleromalacia perforans, arthritis deformans and pemphigus. Trans Ophthalmol Soc UK 71:61, 1951.

70. Sorensen TB: Paralimbal scleromalacia. Acta Ophthalmol 53:901, 1975.

71. Mader TH, Stulting RD, Crosswell HH: Bilateral paralimbal scleromalacia perforans. Am J Ophthalmol 109:233, 1990.

72. Sena JA, Cereboni FC: Scleral excavations. Arch Oftalmol Buenos Aires, 23:313, 1948.

73. Kyrieleis W: Ueber umschriebenen Lederhautschwund (Sleromalazie) in hoeheren Lebensalter. Klin Monatsbl Augenheilk 103: 441, 1939.

74. Kiss J: Fall von seniler Sklerverdunnung. Klin Monatsbl Augenheilk 92:121, 1934.

75. Roper KL: Senile hyaline scleral plaques. Arch Ophthalmol 34:283, 1945.

76. Graves B: Bilateral mesial superficial deficiency of the sclera: scleral plaques. Br J Ophthalmol 25:35, 1941.

77. Katz D: A localized area of calcareous degeneration in the sclera. Arch Ophthalmol 2:30, 1929.

78. Culler AM: The pathology of scleral plaques; report of 5 cases of degenerative plaques in the sclera mesially, one studied histologically. Br J Ophthalmol 23:44, 1939.

79. Drescher EP, Henderson JW: Senile hyaline scleral plaques; report of 3 cases. Proc Staff Meet Mayo Clin 24:334, 1949.

80. Holloway TB, Fry WE: Unsuspected brawny scleritis in a case of retinal detachment with secondary glaucoma. Arch Ophthalmol 6:36, 1931.

81. Howard GM: Erroneous clinical diagnoses of retinoblastoma and uveal melanoma. Trans Am Acad Ophthalmol Otolaryngol 73:199, 1969.

82. Feldon SE, Singleman J, Albert DM, Smith TR: Clinical manifestations of brawny scleritis. Am J Ophthalmol 85:781, 1978.

83. Yeo JH, Jakobiek FA, Iwamoto T, Brown R, Harrison W: Metastatic carcinoma masquerading as scleritis. Ophthalmology 90:184, 1983.

84. Benson WE, Shields JA, Tasman W, Crandall AS: Posterior scleritis. A cause of diagnostic confusion. Arch Ophthalmol 97:1482, 1979.

85. Singh G, Guthoff R, Foster CS: Observations on longterm follow-up of posterior scleritis. Am J Ophthalmol 101:570, 1986.

86. Benson WE: Posterior scleritis. Surv Ophthalmol 32:297, 1988.

87. Blodi FC, Gass JD: Inflammatory pseudotumor of the orbit. Br J Ophthalmol 52:79, 1968.

88. Rootman J, Nugent R: The classification and management of acute orbital pseudotumors. Ophthalmology 89:1040, 1982.

89. Cappaert WE, Purnell EW, Frank KE: Use of B-sector scan ultrasound in the diagnosis of benign choroidal folds. Am J Ophthalmol 84:375, 1977.

90. Kalina RE, Mills RP: Acquired hyperopia with choroidal folds. Ophthalmology 87:44, 1980.

91. Sears ML: Choroidal and retinal detachments associated with scleritis. Am J Ophthalmol 58:764, 1964.

92. Bertelsen TI: Acute sclerotenonitis and ocular myositis complicated by papillitis, retinal detachment and glaucoma. Acta Ophthalmol 38:136, 1960.

93. Gass JDM: *Differential Diagnosis of Intraocular Tumors.* C.V. Mosby, St. Louis, 1974.

94. Feldon SE, Sigelman J, Albert DM, Smith TR: Clinical manifestations of brawny scleritis. Am J Ophthalmol 85:781, 1978.

95. Cangemi FE, Trempe CL, Walsh JB: Choroidal folds. Am J Ophthalmol 86:380, 1978.

96. Newell FW: Choroidal folds. Am J Ophthalmol 75:930, 1973.

97. Bullock JD, Egbert PR: Experimental choroidal folds. Am J Ophthalmol 78:618, 1972.

98. Hyavarinen L, Walsh FB: Benign chorioretinal folds. Am J Ophthalmol 70:14, 1970.

99. Bellows AR, Chylak LT Jr, Hutchinson BT: Choroidal detachment. Clinical manifestation, therapy and mechanism of formation. Ophthalmology 88:1107, 1981.

100. Quinlan MP, Hitchings RA: Angle-closure glaucoma secondary to posterior scleritis. Br J Ophthalmol 62:330, 1978.

101. Rochels R, Reis G: Echography in posterior scleritis. Klin Monatsbl Augenheilk 177:611, 1980.

102. Mauriello JA, Flanagan JC: Management of orbital inflammatory disease. A protocol. Surv Ophthalmol 29:104, 1984.

103. Trokel SL, Hilal SK: Submillimeter resolution CT scanning of orbital diseases. Ophthalmology 87:412, 1980.

104. Trokel SL: Computed tomographic scanning of orbital inflammations. Int Ophthalmol Clin 22(4):81, 1982.

105. Terner IS, Leopold IH, Eisenberg IJ: The radioactive phosphorus (^{32}P) uptake test in ophthalmology. Arch Ophthalmol 55:52, 1956.

106. Zakov ZN, Smith TR, Albert DM: False-positive ^{32}P uptake tests. Arch Ophthalmol 96:2240, 1978.

107. Shields JA: Accuracy and limitations of the ^{32}P test in the diagnosis of ocular tumors: an analysis of 500 cases. Ophthalmology 85:950, 1978.

108. Norton EWD: A characteristic fluorescein angiographic pattern in choroidal folds. Proc R Soc Med 62:119, 1969.

109. Kroll AJ, Norton EWD: Regression of choroidal folds. Trans Am Acad Ophthalmol Otolaryngol 74:515, 1970.

110. Jakobiec FA, Jones IS: Orbital inflammations. In Duane T (Ed): Clinical Ophthalmology, Vol 2. Harper & Row, Hagerstown MD, 1976, pp 1–75.

111. Birch-Hirschfeld A: Zur Diagnostik und Pathologic der Orbital-tumoren. Ber Dtsch Ophthal Ges 32:127, 1905.

112. Jellinek EH: The orbital pseudotumour syndrome and its differentiation from endocrine exophthalmos. Brain 92:35, 1969.

113. Chavis RM, Garner A, Wright JE: Inflammatory orbital pseudotumor. Arch Ophthalmol 96:1817, 1978.

114. Heersink B, Rodrigues MR, Flanagan JC: Inflammatory pseudotumor of the orbit. Ann Ophthalmol 9:17, 1977.

115. Coleman JD, Jack RL, Jones IS, Frazen LA: Pseudotumors of the orbit. Arch Ophthalmol 88:472, 1972.

116. Kennerdell JS, Dressner SC: The nonspecific orbital inflammatory syndromes. Surv Ophthalmol 29:93, 1984.

117. Sergott RC, Glaser JS: Graves' ophthalmopathy. A clinical and immunologic review. Surv Ophthalmol 26:1, 1981.

118. Trokel SL, Jakobiec FA: Correlation of CT scanning and pathologic features of ophthalmic Graves' disease. Ophthalmology 88:553, 1981.

119. Char DH: Clinical Ocular Oncology. Churchill Livingstone, New York, 1989, pp 97–108.

120. Hallden U: Malignant melanoma of the choroid clinically simulating scleritis attended by amotio retinae. Acta Ophthalmol 33:489, 1955.

121. Smith LT, Irvine AR: Diagnostic significance of orange pigment accumulation over choroidal tumors. Am J Ophthalmol 76:212, 1973.

122. Chang S, Dallow RL, Coleman DJ: Ultrasonic evaluation of intraocular tumors. In Jakobiec FA (Ed): Ocular and Anexal Tumors. Aesculapius, Birmingham AL, 1978, pp 290–291.

123. Fraser DJ Jr, Font RL: Ocular inflammation and hemorrhage as initial manifestations of uveal malignant melanoma. Incidence and prognosis. Arch Ophthalmol 97:1311, 1979.

124. Ferry AP, Font RL: Carcinoma metastatic to the eye and orbit. I. A clinicopathologic study of 227 cases. Arch Ophthalmol 92:276, 1974.

125. Yeo JH, Jakobiec FA, Iwamoto T, Brown R, Harrison W: Metastatic carcinoma masquerading as scleritis. Ophthalmology 90:184, 1983.

126. Witschel H, Font RL: Hemangioma of the choroid. A clinicopathologic study of 71 cases and a review of the literature. Surv Ophthalmol 20:415, 1976.

127. Augsburger JJ, Shields JA, Moffat KP: Circumscribed choroidal hemangiomas: long-term visual prognosis. Retina 1:56, 1981.

128. Hayreh SS: Choroidal tumors: role of fluorescein fundus angiography in their diagnosis. Curr Concepts Ophthalmol 4:168, 1974.

129. Gass JDM: Radial chorioretinal folds. A sign of choroidal neovascularization. Arch Ophthalmol 99:1016, 1981.

130. Nettleship E: Peculiar lines in the choroid in a case of postpapillitic atrophy. Trans Ophthalmol Soc UK 4:167, 1884.

131. Bird AC, Sanders MD: Choroidal folds in association with papilloedema. Br J Ophthalmol 57:89, 1973.

132. Gass JDM: Hypotony maculopathy. In Bellows JC (Ed): Comtemporary Ophthalmology, Honoring Sir Stewart Duke-Elder. Williams & Wilkins, Baltimore, 1972, pp 343–366.

133. Collins ET: Intra-ocular tension. I. The sequelae of hypotony. Trans Ophthalmol Soc UK 37:281, 1917.

134. Kreiger AE, Meyer D, Smith TR, Riemer K: Metastatic carcinoma to the choroid with choroidal detachment. Arch Ophthalmol 82:209, 1969.

135. Taake WH, Allen RA, Straatsma BR: Metastasis of a hepatoma to the choroid. Am J Ophthalmol 56:208, 1953.

136. Schepens CL, Brockhurst RJ: Uveal effusion. I. Clinical picture. Arch Ophthalmol 70:189, 1963.

137. Gass JDM, Jallow S: Idiopathic serous detachment of the choroid, ciliary body, and retina (uveal effusion syndrome). Ophthalmology 89:1018, 1982.

138. Wilson RS, Hanna C, Morris MD: Idiopathic chorioretinal effusion: an analysis of extracellular fluids. Ann Ophthalmol 9:647, 1977.

139. Ohno S, Char DH, Kimura SJ, O'Connor GR: Vogt-Koyanagi–Harada syndrome. Am J Ophthalmol 83:735, 1977.

140. Perry HD, Font RL: Clinical and histopathologic observations in severe Vogt-Koyanagi–Harada syndrome. Am J Ophthalmol 83:242, 1977.

141. Pattison EM: Uveomeningoencephalitic syndrome (Vogt-Koyanagi–Harada). Arch Neurol 12:197, 1965.

142. Lubin JR, Loewenstein JI, Frederick AR: Vogt-Koyanagi–Harada syndrome with focal neurologic signs. Am J Ophthalmol 91:332, 1981.

143. Holt-Wilson AD, Watson PG: Non-syphilitic deep interstitial keratitis associated with scleritis. Trans Ophthalmol Soc UK 94:52, 1974.

144. Ferry AP, Leopold IH: Marginal (ring) corneal ulcer as a presenting manifestation of Wegener's granuloma. Trans Am Acad Ophthalmol Otolaryngol 74:1276, 1970.

145. Brown SI, Grayson M: Marginal furrows: a characteristic corneal lesion of rheumatoid arthritis. Arch Ophthalmol 79:563, 1968.

146. Eiferman RA, Carothers DJ, Yankeelov JA: Peripheral rheumatoid ulceration and evidence for conjunctival collagenase production. Am J Ophthalmol 87:703, 1979.

147. Jayson MIV, Easty DL: Ulceration of the cornea in rheumatoid arthritis. Ann Rheum Dis 36:428, 1977.

148. Scharf Y, Meyer E, Nahir M, Zonis S: Marginal mottling of cornea in rheumatoid arthritis. Ann Ophthalmol 16:924, 1984.

149. Lyne AJ: "Contact lens" cornea in rheumatoid arthritis. Br J Ophthalmol 54:410, 1970.

150. Goldman KN, Kaufman HE: Atypical pterygium: a clinical feature of Terrien's marginal degeneration. Arch Ophthalmol 96:1027, 1978.

151. Etzine S, Friedmann A: Marginal dystrophy of the cornea with total ectasia. Am J Ophthalmol 55:150, 1963.

152. Austin P, Brown SI: Inflammatory Terrien's marginal corneal disease. Am J Ophthalmol 92:189, 1981.

153. Krachmer JH: Pellucid marginal corneal degeneration. Arch Ophthalmol 96:1217, 1978.

154. Krachmer JH, Feder RS, Belin MW: Keratoconus and related noninflammatory corneal thinning disorders. Surv Ophthalmol 28:293, 1984.

155. Friedlander MH, Smolin G: Corneal degenerations. Ann Ophthalmol 11:1485, 1979.

156. Sugar A: Corneal and conjunctival degenerations. In Kaufman HE, Barron BA, McDonald MB, Waltman SR (Eds): The cornea. Churchill Livingstone, New York, 1988.

157. Tauber J, Sainz de la Maza M, Hoang-Xuan T, Foster CS: An analysis of therapeutic decision making regarding immunosuppressive chemotherapy for peripheral ulcerative keratitis. Cornea 9(1):66, 1990.

158. Foster CS: Immunosuppressive therapy for external ocular inflammatory disease. Ophthalmology 87:140, 1980.

159. Sainz de la Maza M, Foster CS: The diagnosis and treatment of peripheral ulcerative keratitis. Semin Ophthalmol 6(3):133, 1991.

160. Foster CS: Systemic immunosuppressive therapy for progressive bilateral Mooren's ulcer. Ophthalmology 92:1436, 1985.

161. Sainz de la Maza M, Foster CS: Necrotizing scleritis after ocular surgery: a clinicopathologic study. Ophthalmology 98:1720, 1991.

162. Lyne AJ, Lloyd-Jones D: Necrotizing scleritis after ocular surgery. Tran Ophthal Soc UK 99:146, 1979.

163. Salamon SM, Mondino BJ, Zaidman GW: Peripheral corneal ulcers, conjunctival ulcers, and scleritis after cataract surgery. Am J Ophthalmol 93:334, 1982.

164. Kaufman LM, Folk ER, Miller MT, Tessler HH: Necrotizing scleritis following strabismus surgery for thyroid ophthalmopathy. J Pediatr Ophthalmol Strabismus 26:236, 1989.

165. Mamalis N, Johnson MD, Haines JM, Teske MP, Olson RJ: Corneal–scleral melt in association with cataract surgery and intraocular lenses: a report of four cases. J Cataract Refract Surg 16:108, 1990.

166. Bloomfield SE, Becker CG, Christian CL, Nauheim JS: Bilateral necrotising scleritis with marginal corneal ulceration after cataract surgery in a patient with vasculitis. Br J Ophthalmol 64:170, 1980.

5
Pathology in Scleritis: The Massachusetts Eye and Ear Infirmary Experience

The histopathological aspects of scleral inflammation have been studied extensively in the past. Although certain inferences can be drawn from these descriptions, terms such as "chronic nonspecific inflammation," or even "chronic granulomatous inflammation," only camouflaged our ignorance about the possible pathogenic roles that cells might play. Even sophisticated techniques such as electron microscopy provided limited insights into the delineation of the distinctive composition of the cellular infiltrates as well as into the components of the matrix during inflammation. It was not until the relatively recent development of immunohistochemistry, particularly the exploitation of monoclonal antibody technology, that the etiology and pathogenesis of scleral diseases have become less obscure and intimidating. Our ability to characterize cells and determine extracellular matrix changes during inflammatory reactions contributes to the understanding of mechanisms of lesion production and thereby to the development of treatment options most likely to succeed. Thus it is possible to distinguish between T and B lymphocytes, to determine mononuclear subsets (T helper, T cytotoxic/suppressor, natural killer, macrophages, and Langerhans' cells), and to detect HLA-DR glycoproteins in scleral inflammation; it is now possible to identify and further characterize different types of components of extracellular matrix (collagen, glycosaminoglycans, and glycoproteins) during inflammatory reactions; it is also possible to localize specific antigens (herpes simplex virus) in inflamed tissue.

This chapter has as its primary focus a description of the histopathological, immunopathological, and ultrastructural characteristics of sclera affected by inflammation of diverse origins. Although recognizing that a clear understanding of the etiology and pathogenesis of scleritis is not yet available, study of the pathology of scleritis may contribute to insights into the mechanism of inflammation as well as into the search for the most appropriate forms of treatment.

5.1. General Considerations of Connective Tissue Inflammation

Inflammation is best defined as the reaction of tissue to a noxious stimulus. Either acute or chronic, it is characterized by increased vascular exudation of fluid, plasma proteins, and inflammatory cells. Histologically, connective tissue diseases are characterized by the presence of chronic inflammation. Chronic inflammation may arise as a result of a persistent inciting stimulus following acute inflammation or directly, as a smoldering response. Two main forms of chronic inflammation are recognized: nongranulomatous and granulomatous. Chronic granulomatous inflammation surrounds a central area of extracellular matrix degradation known as fibrinoid necrosis; in some instances, vasculitis may result in further necrosis.

5.1.1. Chronic Nongranulomatous Inflammation

The histological hallmarks of chronic nongranulomatous or nonspecific inflammation are infiltration of mononuclear cells, including macrophages, lymphocytes, and plasma cells, proliferation of fibroblasts, and sometimes blood vessels, and degeneration of the tissue affected by the inflammatory process. Macrophages are important components of chronic inflammation because of the great number of biologically active products they can produce.[1,2] Some of these products cause proliferation of fibroblasts and vessels (interleukin 1, and growth-promoting factors for fibroblasts and blood vessels), some are toxic to tissues (acid proteases, collagenase, elastase, and reactive oxygen intermediates), some are chemotactic for other cell types (neutrophils and lymphocytes), and some produce coagulation and fibrin accumulation (factor V and thromboplastin). Lymphocytes participate in both antibody- and cell-mediated hypersensitivity reactions. After contact with antigen, they produce lymphokines that are chemotactic for monocytes; lymphocytes also cause macrophage activation and differentiation (interferon γ).[3,4] Macrophages produce monokines that activate both T and B lymphocytes (interleukin 1). B lymphocytes produce plasma cells that participate in antibody formation. Neutrophils are usually considered the hallmark of acute inflammation but they also participate in many forms of chronic inflammation as well. Because fibroblasts and neutrophils may release collagenase and other proteases, they play prominent roles in tissue damage. Mast cells and eosinophils may also be present but their precise functions in chronic inflammation are not well understood.

5.1.2. Chronic Granulomatous Inflammation

Chronic granulomatous inflammation is characterized by the presence of epithelioid cells,

which are modified macrophages with abundant, pale pink, ill-defined cytoplasm, resembling an epithelial cell. Their function is poorly understood, but the presence of numerous organelles such as endoplasmic reticulum, Golgi apparatus, vesicles, and vacuoles suggests that they are particularly adapted to secretion of the biologically active products explained above, rather than phagocytosis, antigen processing, and antigen presentation.[5,6] As the epithelioid cells coalesce and fuse, amitotic nuclear division may occur, thus forming a multinucleated giant cell containing a row of nuclei arranged along the periphery, the Langhans'-type giant cell.[7] Multinucleated giant cells have been shown in vitro to secrete more collagenase than do cultures of unfused epithelioid cells. Their presence in tissues may be associated with accelerated rates of matrix degradation. Giant cells, lymphocytes, plasma cells, fibroblasts, neutrophils, mast cells, eosinophils, as well as blood vessel proliferation, and destruction of the tissue, can be seen in a granuloma, but the detection of epithelioid cells is the only requirement for the diagnosis of granulomatous inflammation. Macrophages are chemotactically attracted into an area of inflammation in response to complement components (which may have been attracted by immune complexes),[2] and through interleukin 1 production they activate T lymphocytes. T cell activity then potentiates granuloma formation[2,8] because lymphokines such as interferon γ and possibly interleukin 4 enhance the transformation of macrophages to epithelioid cells and multinucleated giant cells.[9,10] If macrophages are intensively stimulated, they secrete acid proteases (cathepsins), neutral proteases (collagenase and elastase), and reactive (free radical) oxygen intermediates, thereby participating in the production of a central area of extracellular matrix degeneration known as fibrinoid necrosis.

5.1.3. Fibrinoid Necrosis

Fibrinoid necrosis is characterized by the histopathological appearance of a "smudgy" material in association with tissue destruction.[11,12] This material, which stains eosinophilic with eosin, is composed of a mixture of fibrin, proteoglycan filaments, collagen fibers in varying stages of degradation, granular debris, and cell membranes. Accumulation of fibrin is probably the result of coagulation factors (factor V and thromboplastin)[2] released by macrophages as well as of impairment of the normal mechanism for debris removal. The necrosis is probably the result of the enormous quantities of proteases produced by macrophages (including modified macrophages such as epithelioid cells and multinucleated giant cells) and fibroblasts. Intracellular digestion by lysosomal acid hydrolases, and extracellular digestion by neutral proteases, are the main mechanisms of proteoglycan, collagen, and glycoprotein degradation. Microinfarctions resulting from thrombosis of terminal vessels may also play a role, through ischemia, in the tissue destruction.

5.1.4. Vascular Inflammation

Connective tissue vessels may show an inflammatory infiltration that leads to endothelial damage and subsequent reparative proliferation responses of the vascular endothelium. Circulating immune complexes may precipitate in a vessel wall and activate the complement system, which is chemotactic for neutrophils and macrophages. Endothelial cell damage exposes the subendothelium or basement membrane, which is composed of collagen, proteoglycans, and glycoproteins; these components can be degraded by proteolytic enzymes secreted by neutrophils, macrophages, and activated endothelial cells. Activated endothelial cells also enhance aggregation of platelets (platelet-activating factor),[13] fibrinogen accumulation (tissue factor and factor V),[14,15] polymerization of fibrin, and fibrin deposition, which in turn promote thrombus formation and infarction of the tissues supplied by the vessel. Because activated endothelial cells also express HLA-DR glycoproteins, they participate in the immune response through their interaction with T lymphocytes.[16–19] Macrophages activate fibroblasts and together participate in extracellular matrix degradation through enzyme release. Further stimulation of macrophages, probably through a T cell-related delayed hypersensitivity response, results in granuloma formation.

Endothelial cells activated by chronic inflammation migrate through the openings of degraded basement membranes and generate new capillary blood vessels through the complex proliferative process of angiogenesis.[20] Vascular inflammation involves vessels usually present in the tissue and newly formed vessels produced as a result of the inflammation.

5.2. Specific Considerations of Scleral Tissue Inflammation

The sclera, the dense connective tissue that covers about five-sixths of the eye, consists of fibroblasts, collagen, proteoglycans, glycoproteins, and few blood vessels. These components are functionally and metabolically interdependent in maintaining tissue homeostasis. In scleral inflammation, normal scleral homeostasis breaks down, resulting in loss of scleral integrity. The destructive events in the sclera are consequent to a complex interaction of many cell types and their soluble products.

Episcleral and scleral vasculature has not been extensively studied and clearly deserves more careful morphological characterization. Unlike elastic arteries (large-sized vessels), muscular arteries (medium-sized vessels), and arterioles (small-sized vessels), these vessels in the episclera and sclera appear to be capillaries and postcapillary venules, which do not possess a tunica media and consist chiefly of smooth muscle cells. Episcleral and perforating scleral vessels appear to possess a simple wall composed of continuous endothelial cells and pericytes, without smooth muscle cells (see Chapter 1, Figs. 1.23–1.25).

Classic vasculitis is a clinicopathological process characterized by inflammation and necrosis of blood vessels; the classically described histopathological hallmarks as defined in vessels containing a tunica media include neutrophilic infiltration of the vessel wall and fibrinoid degeneration leading to necrosis of the tunica media (Figs. 5.1 and 5.2). Vasculitic syndromes comprise a broad spectrum of disorders involving vessels of different types, sizes,

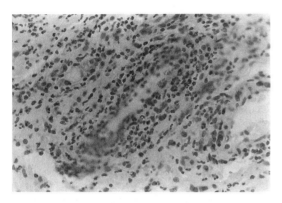

FIGURE 5.1. Vasculitis with neutrophil infiltrate and degeneration of the vascular wall. (Magnification, ×100; hematoxylin–eosin stain.)

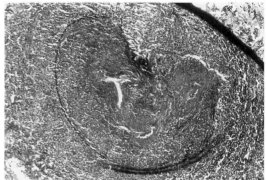

(A)

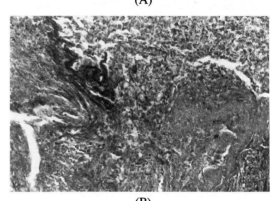

(B)

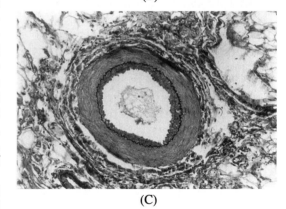

(C)

and locations. Some examples include large-vessel vasculitis in temporal arteritis, medium- and small-vessel vasculitis in polyarteritis nodosa, and small-vessel vasculitis in connective tissue diseases such as rheumatoid arthritis and systemic lupus erythematosus. However, because the types of vessels involved in some conditions vary widely, attempts to classify vasculitic syndromes appropriately have not been satisfactory. The subject is further confused by the fact that clinicopathological classifications do not follow pure histopathological concepts: small-vessel vasculitis (hypersensitivity or leukocytoclastic vasculitis) refers to a heterogeneous group of clinical syndromes that have in common the predominant involvement of arterioles, capillaries, and venules; however, because capillaries do not have a tunica media, a purely classic histopathological definition of vasculitis cannot be applied to them.

We, as ophthalmologists, frequently deal with capillaries and postcapillary venules, and have been frustrated by this confused classification for years; because scleral blood vessel inflammation in scleritis can be associated with inflammation of vessels elsewhere in the body as part of systemic vasculitic syndromes, we have included scleral "vasculitis" as part of our clinicopathological classification. However, we freely admit that this term is histopathologically incomplete and imperfect as regards classic pathology definitions, and have adopted an independent term, "inflammatory microangi-

FIGURE 5.2. (A) Elastin stain (magnification, ×40). Note the large area of vessel wall destruction with fibrinoid necrosis and the absence of elasticum (compare with the normal appearance of the large vessel shown in [C]). (Hematoxylin–eosin stain.) (B) Elastin stain, higher magnification (×100), vividly illustrating the area of vessel wall destruction and vascular lumen obliteration. (Hematoxylin–eosin stain.) (C) Elastin stain, normal artery. Note the continuous black-staining elasticum adjacent to the muscularis. (Magnification, ×40; hematoxylin–eosin stain.)

opathy," to define histopathological neutro-philic infiltration in and around the vessel walls of capillary and postcapillary venules, such as conjunctival, episcleral, and perforating scleral vessels.

Deposition of immune complexes in and around the vessel wall is thought to be an important event in the genesis of vessel damage in systemic vasculitic syndromes often asso-ciated with scleritis. Definitive proof of the presence of immune complexes in vessel wall deposits requires the demonstration of specific antigen and antibody. However, common practice in diagnosing systemic vasculitic syn-dromes (often associated with scleritis) dictates that detection of immunoglobulins and com-plement components in vessel walls provides evidence of immune complex deposition, even if the relevant antigen is unknown, much less detected. This detection can be done by use of immunofluorescence or immunoperoxidase techniques (Fig. 3.32 in Chapter 3). Rec-ognizing the limitations in the interpretation of these findings, we therefore also define inflam-matory microangiopathy as immunoreactant (immunoglobulin and complement component) deposition in capillaries and postcapillary venules such as conjunctival, episcleral, and perforating scleral vessels.

5.2.1. Pathology of Episcleritis

Light and electron microscopic studies of epi-scleral tissue in simple and nodular episcleritis cases show chronic, nongranulomatous inflam-mation with lymphocytes and plasma cells, vas-cular dilatation, and edema.[21,22] Some cases in association with connective tissue diseases may reveal the presence of a granulomatous inflam-mation with epithelioid cells and some multi-nucleated giant cells, with or without central necrosis, resembling the histopathological pic-ture seen in subcutaneous rheumatoid nod-ules.[23-26] Relatively few cases of episcleritis have been studied histologically, probably be-cause there has been little reason to biopsy episcleral tissue: episcleral inflammation is a benign entity with a tendency to disappear spontaneously over the course of several weeks,

and pathological studies are usually noncon-tributory to the diagnosis or to the treatment.

5.2.2. Pathology of Scleritis

5.2.2.1. Noninfectious Scleritis

Light and electron microscopic studies of ocular tissue in patients with noninfectious scleritis may show the same characteristic morpho-logical changes regardless of whether the scleral inflammation is associated with autoimmune systemic diseases, follows surgical or accidental trauma, or is idiopathic.[27-29] Infiltration of the sclera with inflammatory cells may derive from the superficial and deep episcleral vessels, the perforating scleral vessels, and the choroidal vessels. All types of scleritis are histologically similar but vary in severity of morphological changes, necrotizing scleritis having obviously the most destructive lesions.

Because scleral inflammation is always accom-panied by episcleral inflammation and often by conjunctival, uveal tract, and corneal inflam-mation, we describe the morphological changes in sclera, episclera, conjunctiva, uveal tract, and cornea. Occasionally, other ocular struc-tures, including trabecular meshwork, retina, optic nerve, and extraocular muscles, may also be involved in scleritis.

5.2.2.1.1. Sclera

5.2.2.1.1.1. Cells. The sclera in necrotizing scleritis reveals a granulomatous inflammatory reaction, the center of which consists of an area of fibrinoid necrosis surrounded by epithelioid cells, multinucleated giant cells, lymphocytes, plasma cells, and less often neutrophils.[27-31] The involved sclera is diffusely thickened.[32] Mast cells and eosinophils can occasionally be seen throughout the granuloma and around vessels. Fibroblasts within the granuloma either are absent or display degenerative changes, including membrane disruption and loss of organelles; however, in the area outside the granuloma they appear to be metabolically active, containing active cell surfaces with peripheral pseudopodia extending into the sur-rounding matrix, numerous lysosomal granules and mitochondria, and prominent rough endo-

TABLE 5.1. Cellular infiltrates in scleral granulomas.

Cell	Products[a]
Macrophage	Neutral proteases (collagenase, elastase), acid hydrolases, CCs, ROIs, IL-1, factor V, thromboplastin, PDGF, FGF, TGF-β, AAs, PA
T lymphocytes	
Helper/inducer	LDCF, IL-2, IL-3, GM-CSF, FGF, TFG-β, angiogenic factors
Suppressor/cytotoxic	Suppressor factors
Fibroblasts	Extracellular matrix components, collagenase, proteoglycanase, elastase, glycoproteinase, AAs, GM-CSF, IL-1
B lymphocytes/plasma cells	Antibodies
Neutrophils	Neutral proteases (collagenase, elastase), ROIs, AAs
Langerhans' cells	IL-1
Mast cells	Heparin, histamine
Eosinophils	Acid hydrolases, neutral proteases (collagenase)

[a] ROIs, Reactive oxygen intermediates; IL-1, -2, and -3, interleukins 1, 2, and 3; PDGF, platelet-derived growth factor; FGF, fibroblast growth factor; TGF-β, transforming growth factor β; AAs, arachidonic acid metabolites; PA, plasminogen activator; CCs, complement components; LDCF, lymphocyte-derived chemotactic factor; GM-CSF, granulocyte–macrophage colony-stimulating factors.

plasmic reticulum and Golgi apparatus (fibroblastic cells).[27] Cellular infiltrates in scleral granulomas secrete a plethora of enzymes and mediators that interact in a complex pattern to orchestrate the development and perpetuation of the inflammatory process (Table 5.1).

The sclera in diffuse and nodular scleritis shows a nongranulomatous inflammatory reaction characterized by infiltration of mononuclear cells such as macrophages, lymphocytes, and plasma cells. In some cases, however, especially in the most severe ones, mononuclear cells organize into granulomatous lesions. Mast cells, neutrophils, and eosinophils also may be present.

We biopsied the sclera of 26 of 34 (76%) of our patients with noninfectious necrotizing scleritis. Scleral tissue was obtained in many instances at the time of necrotic tissue removal in those cases requiring scleral grafting for structural support (13 patients).[33] Scleral tissue was processed for histopathological studies and stained with hematoxylin–eosin and alkaline Giemsa. Hematoxylin–eosin stains cell nuclei blue and collagen red. Alkaline Giemsa stains mast cell granules metachromatically purple and eosinophil granules red.

The most frequent histopathological finding in sclera consisted of a central focus of fibrinoid necrosis surrounded by granulomatous inflammation with epithelioid cells, lymphocytes, and

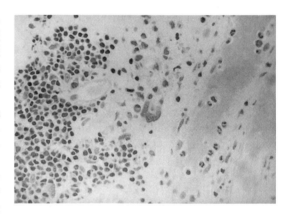

FIGURE 5.3. Scleral biopsy, patient with necrotizing scleritis. Note the granuloma formation with perivasculitis, neutrophil margination in the venule, and the multinucleated giant cell at the edge of the venule.

plasma cells (Fig. 5.3) (Table 5.2). A moderate number of multinucleated giant cells containing a row of nuclei arranged along the periphery were also present in some cases (Fig. 5.4). In addition, scattered numbers of neutrophils, mast cells (Fig. 5.5; see color insert), and eosinophils (Fig. 5.6; see color insert) were dispersed throughout the inflamed tissue and around vessels. Areas outside the granuloma were infiltrated by macrophages, lymphocytes, and plasma cells (Fig. 5.7).

TABLE 5.2. Analysis of histopathology of scleritis.

Cell subset	Necrotizing (%)[a] (n = 26)	Nonnecrotizing (%)[a] (n = 13)
Macrophage	26 (100)	13 (100)
Lymphocyte	26 (100)	13 (100)
Plasma cell	26 (100)	13 (100)
Epithelioid cell	22 (85)	3 (23)
Multinucleated giant cell	7 (27)	0
Neutrophil	13 (50)	3 (23)
Mast cell	8 (31)	4 (31)
Eosinophil	9 (35)	2 (15)

[a] %, Percentage of patients with necrotizing and nonnecrotizing scleritis with the different cell subsets.

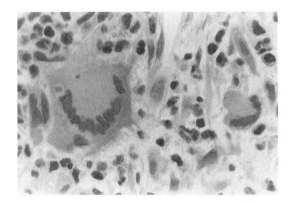

FIGURE 5.4. Same patient as in Fig. 5.3: different field of the specimen, showing many multinucleated giant cells. (Magnification, ×160; hematoxylin–eosin stain.)

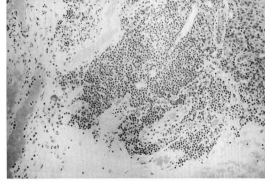

FIGURE 5.7. Granuloma in a scleral biopsy from a patient with necrotizing scleritis. Note the granuloma and the presence of histiocytes, lymphocytes, and plasma cells in areas surrounding the granuloma.

Thirteen of 112 (12%) of our patients with noninfectious diffuse and nodular scleritis underwent scleral biopsy. All patients had had recurrent attacks of active scleritis for at least 6 months. Examination under light microscopy revealed in all cases mononuclear cell infiltration, including macrophages and lymphocytes without fibrinoid necrosis (Table 5.2). In addition, some specimens showed the presence of epithelioid cells characteristic of granulomatous inflammation; none had multinucleated giant cells. Neutrophils and mast cells were scattered in the tissues of some patients.

Identification of cellular subsets and surface glycoproteins in necrotizing scleritis was accomplished with the use of the immunoperoxidase technique, using monoclonal antibodies directed against T lymphocytes (CD3), T helper/inducer lymphocytes (CD4), T cytotoxic/suppressor lymphocytes (CD8), neutrophils (CD16), B lymphocytes (CD22), macrophages (CD14), HLA-DR glycoproteins (anti-HLA-DR) (Becton Dickinson, Inc., Mountain View, CA), and Langerhans' cells (CD1) (Ortho Pharmaceuticals Corp., Raritan, NJ) (Table 5.3). Details of tissue processing and staining have been previously published.[28] A comparison between nine scleral specimens from patients with necrotizing scleritis and four scleral specimens from normal eyes (New England Eye Bank, Boston, MA), revealed a predominance of macrophages (CD14) and T lymphocytes (CD3) in scleral tissue (Table 5.4). Although both T helper/inducer lymphocytes

TABLE 5.3. Mononuclear cell subset antibody panel in immunoperoxidase studies.

Antibody	Specificity
Anti-CD3	T lymphocytes
Anti-CD8	T suppressor/cytotoxic lymphocytes
Anti-CD4	T helper/inducer lymphocytes
Anti-CD16	Neutrophils
Anti-CD22	B lymphocytes
Anti-CD14	Macrophages
Anti-HLA-DR	HLA-DR (class II histocompatibility antigen)
Anti-CD1	Langerhans' cells

(CD4) and T suppressor/cytotoxic (CD8) lymphocytes were increased, a high T helper/T suppressor ratio revealed a predominance of the former. Neutrophils (CD16), Langerhans' cells (CD1), and B lymphocytes (CD22) were present in scleritis but their numbers were not significantly increased when compared with normal tissue. HLA-DR glycoproteins (anti-HLA-DR), present constitutively in macrophages, and after inflammatory stimuli in scleral fibroblasts and endothelial cells, were markedly increased. These findings show the participation of macrophages and T lymphocytes, particularly T helper lymphocytes, in scleritis, and support the idea that macrophages and fibroblasts activate T lymphocytes, which in turn may participate in granuloma formation. Damaged endothelial cells also may play a role as antigen-presenting cells. The T

helper/T suppressor imbalance may contribute to the perpetuation of the highly inflammatory nature of the lesion. In addition to the predominant macrophages and T helper lymphocytes, neutrophils, B lymphocytes, and Langerhans' cells may be present.

5.2.2.1.1.2. Extracellular Matrix. Collagen degradation may take place by two mechanisms, one (intracellular) involving acid proteases of macrophages, and the other (extracellular) involving neutral proteases (collagenase and elastase) of fibroblasts and macrophages.[34]

In intracellular digestion of collagen, the collagen fibrils undergo phagocytosis into phagolysosomes (acid pH) of macrophages, where lysosomal acid proteases lead to tissue breakdown. In extracellular digestion, the collagen fibrils appear swollen and unraveled in areas of scleral stroma (neutral pH) as a result of the release of neutral proteases by fibroblasts and macrophages into the connective tissue matrix. Both intracellular and extracellular mechanisms of collagen degradation may occur simultaneously, distant from the granuloma, suggesting that collagen degradation may precede granuloma formation in scleral inflammation.[35]

Degradation of collagen may be almost total in the center of the granuloma. Fibril fragments may be found in close apposition to the fibroblast plasma membrane or enclosed in invaginations of the fibroblast plasma membrane or vacuole membranes within the

TABLE 5.4. Cell subsets in scleritis.[a]

	Scleral specimen	
Cell subset	Normal (n = 4)	Necrotizing scleritis (n = 9)
Macrophages (CD14)	0.00 ± 0.00^b	43.50 ± 10.91^b
T lymphocytes (CD3)	0.17 ± 0.10^b	145.70 ± 59.46^b
T helper/inducer lymphocytes (CD4)	0.10 ± 0.10^b	192.37 ± 41.24^b
T cytotoxic/suppressor lymphocytes (CD8)	0.19 ± 0.13^b	89.96 ± 38.15^b
Neutrophils (CD16)	0.00 ± 0.00	44.56 ± 34.86
B lymphocytes (CD22)	0.20 ± 0.12	58.56 ± 39.59
HLA-DR glycoproteins (HLA-DR)	1.46 ± 0.22^b	210.00 ± 59.46^b
Langerhans' cells (CD1)	0.00 ± 0.00	6.96 ± 5.47
T helper/T suppressor ratio	1.09 ± 0.06^b	8.20 ± 4.47^b

[a] Mean cell count/mm², ± standard error of the mean.
[b] Significant values, using Student's *t* test ($p < .05$).

TABLE 5.5. Antibody panel used in immunofluorescence studies of scleral specimens.

Antibody	Working dilution	Vendor[a]
Rabbit anti-collagen I	1:20	Biodesign International
Goat anti-collagen II	1:20	Southern Biotechnology Associates
Goat anti-collagen III	1:20	Southern Biotechnology Associates
Goat anti-collagen IV	1:100	Biodesign International
Goat anti-collagen V	1:20	Southern Biotechnology Associates
Mouse anti-collagen VI	1:20	Gift of E. Engvall (La Jolla Cancer Research Foundation, La Jolla, CA)
Mouse anti-collagen VII	1:20	Chemicon International
Mouse anti-heparan sulfate proteoglycan	Undiluted	Chemicon International
Mouse anti-dermatan sulfate proteoglycan	1:50	Seikagaku Kogyo
Mouse anti-hyaluronic acid[b]	Undiluted	Serotec
Mouse anti-chondroitin sulfate	1:50	Serotec
Rabbit anti-fibronectin	1:10	Organon Teknika-Cappel Scientific
Rabbit anti-vitronectin	1:10	Chemicon International
Mouse anti-laminin (200 kDa)	1:10	Chemicon International

[a] Biodesign International (Kennebunkport, ME); Southern Biotechnology Associates (Birmingham, AL); Chemicon International (Temecula, CA); Seikagaku Kogyo (Tokyo, Japan); Organon Teknika-Cappel Scientific (West Chester, PA).
[b] Mouse antibody believed to recognize hyaluronic acid (Serotec, Kidlington, England).

cytoplasm (intracellular mechanism). Derangements of collagen fibril structure such as fibril swelling and unraveling, irregular contour, and increased interfibrillar distance, may also be seen without close apposition to active fibroblasts (extracellular mechanism).[35] In areas distal to the inflammatory focus, collagen appears normal by light microscopy; however, intracellular or extracellular resorptive changes in the absence of inflammatory cells can be seen by electron microscopy.[35,36]

Electron microscopy studies with cuprolinic blue staining show that proteoglycans are reduced or absent in areas of active scleral inflammation before the collagen fibrils undergo resorptive changes; these results suggest that proteoglycan degradation precedes collagen degradation.[37] Our own studies on immunolocalization of extracellular matrix components in two diseased scleral specimens as compared with five normal scleral specimens show similar findings. An indirect immunofluorescence technique was performed in anterior, equatorial, and posterior areas, using monoclonal antibodies against the proteoglycans heparan sulfate, dermatan sulfate, hyaluronic acid, and chondroitin sulfate, collagen types I through VII, and the glycoproteins fibronectin, vitronectin, and laminin (Table 5.5).

1. *Proteoglycans*: The most abundant proteoglycans in normal sclera were dermatan sulfate and chondroitin sulfate; hyaluronic acid and heparan sulfate also were present, although in small amounts. Dermatan sulfate in necrotizing scleritis was frankly decreased when compared to normal sclera. A negative background with scattered areas of mild patchy positivity in diseased sclera contrasted with an intense striped pattern in normal sclera (Figs. 5.8 and 5.9; see color insert). Chondroitin sulfate in necrotizing scleritis also showed a marked reduction in amount of staining, unlike normal sclera, which showed a generalized speckled pattern of intense positivity (Figs. 5.10 and 5.11; see color insert). Because the presence of heparan sulfate and hyaluronic acid was detected in small amounts in normal sclera, comparison of these proteoglycans between normal and diseased sclera did not show obvious differences.

2. *Collagens*: The most abundant types of collagen in normal extravascular sclera were collagens types I and III; type V and type VI also were present. Type II and type VII were not identified. Collagen type IV also was absent except for its dramatic presence in the vessels. Comparison of staining of collagen types I, III, V, and VI between normal and necrotizing scleritis specimens did not show differences in

intensity or pattern. Collagen types I and III showed intense homogeneous fibrillar staining; these two collagen types impart tensile strength (type I) and resilience (type III) to the scleral "skeleton."[38] Collagen type V showed mild, delicate, patchy, granular staining, particularly associated with the edges of the collagen bundles; this pattern leads us to suspect that collagen type V forms a fine network that maintains the structural integrity of the main fibril core (types I and III). Collagen type VI showed an intense, fine, regional, granular staining; this pattern also leads us to suggest that collagen type VI has a role similar to that of type V in maintaining the structural integrity of the collagenous core. The fact that there were no differences in intensity or pattern of the collagen stainings between normal and necrotizing scleritis suggests that proteoglycans are the first extracellular matrix components to be degraded in necrotizing scleritis. Proteoglycan degradation may enhance intracellular and extracellular mechanisms of collagen fibril depletion.

3. *Glycoproteins*: Fibronectin and vitronectin showed subtle, granular, patchy positivity in normal and inflamed sclera. Laminin was absent in extravascular sclera, normal or inflamed, but was dramatically represented in vessel walls.

5.2.2.1.1.3. Vessels. The area of active scleral inflammation shows old and new vessels, many of which display neutrophil and lymphocyte infiltration within and around the vessels, with occasional thrombosis.[28,30,39,40]

Our own studies on scleral vasculature in 26 scleral specimens from patients with noninfectious necrotizing scleritis were accomplished by use of histopathological and direct immunofluorescence techniques. Specimens examined by the direct immunofluorescence technique were incubated with fluorescein- and rhodamine-conjugated goat antibodies directed against human immunoglobulins IgG, IgA, IgM, IgD, and IgE, complement components C3 and C4, and albumin[28] (as a negative control for vascular positivity) (Organon Teknika-Cappel Scientific, West Chester, PA) (Table 5.6). Goat anti-human collagen IV (Biodesign International, Kennebunkport,

TABLE 5.6. Antibody panel used in immunofluorescence studies of scleral specimens.

Antibody	Working dilution
Anti-IgG (fluorescein conjugated)	1:30
Anti-IgA (fluorescein conjugated)	1:16
Anti-IgM (rhodamine conjugated)	1:8
Anti-IgD (fluorescein conjugated)	1:8
Anti-IgE (fluorescein conjugated)	1:8
Anti-C3 (rhodamine conjugated)	1:4
Anti-C4 (fluorescein conjugated)	1:4
Anti-albumin (fluorescein conjugated)	1:30
Anti-collagen IV[a]	1:100

[a] Indirect immunofluorescence technique.

ME) was used as a positive control for vessels. Fluorescence microscopy was performed on a Zeiss (Thornwood, NY) Photomic III fluorescence microscope. All scleral specimens but one (96%) showed an inflammatory microangiopathy characterized by neutrophilic infiltration in and around the vessel wall, as visualized by the histopathological technique (Fig. 5.12), or immunoreactant deposition on the vessel wall, as visualized by the immunofluorescence technique (Fig. 5.13). Inflammatory microangiopathy as detected by the histopathological technique was found in 74% of the scleral specimens; in addition to the neutrophilic infiltration in and around the vessel wall, vessel occlusion was often found within necrotic areas. Inflammatory microangiopathy detected by the immunofluorescence technique was found in 94% of the scleral specimens. These data show

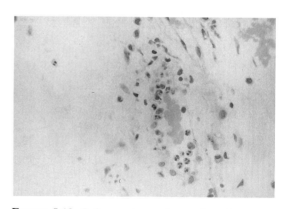

FIGURE 5.12. Inflammatory microangiopathy. Note the neutrophil infiltration in and around the wall of the conjunctival vessel.

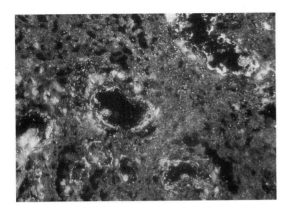

FIGURE 5.13. Inflammatory microangiopathy, as visualized by immunofluorescence microscopy. The antibody used in this specimen is anti-IgG antibody, and the photomicrograph shows the presence of IgG in the vessel walls, with the bright fluorescence in the area of the basement membrane of the vessel wall. (Magnification, ×64.)

that inflammatory microangiopathy is highly associated with the most severe and destructive type of scleritis, necrotizing scleritis; the immunofluorescence technique increases the sensitivity of detection of inflammatory vascular damage in necrotizing scleritis.

Episcleral vessels and perforating intrascleral vessels, as capillaries and postcapillary venules, have a wall that consists of endothelial cells attached to an underlying basement membrane secreted by them, and a discontinuous layer of pericytes. Our studies on immunolocalization of connective tissue components in normal scleral blood vessels showed the presence of collagen types IV, V, and VI, heparan sulfate and chondroitin sulfate, fibronectin, and laminin in endothelial cell basement membranes. Necrotizing scleritis specimens showed marked proliferation of scleral blood vessels with positive stainings for the same connective tissue components as found in normal scleral blood vessels (Fig. 5.14A and 5.14B).

Eight of 13 (61%) scleral specimens from patients with noninfectious recurrent diffuse or nodular scleritis showed inflammatory microangiopathy by histopathological or immunofluorescent techniques. Neutrophilic infiltration in and around the vessel wall was detected in 28% of the scleral specimens; vessel

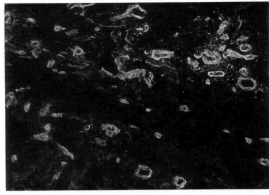

(A)

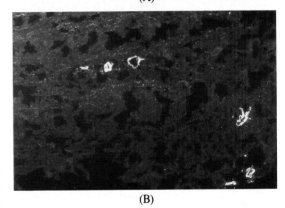

(B)

FIGURE 5.14. (A) Necrotizing scleritis, as visualized by immunofluorescence microscopy. (Magnification, ×40.) The antibody used is anti-collagen type IV. Anti-collagen type IV antibodies stain vascular basement membranes, and this specimen shows, compared with (B), a large number of blood vessels. (B) Normal sclera (same technique and magnification as in [A]). Note the paucity of vessels in this specimen, particularly when compared to that of the patient with necrotizing scleritis (A).

occlusion was not detected in any. Immunoreactant deposition on vessel walls was detected in 80% of the scleral specimens. These data show that inflammatory microangiopathy is less associated with nonnecrotizing scleritis than with necrotizing scleritis and that the immunofluorescence technique increases the sensitivity of detection of inflammatory vascular damage in nonnecrotizing scleritis. Vasculitis/inflammatory microangiopathy may also be detected in the anterior ciliary arteries in enucleation specimens from patients with scleritis (Fig. 5.15; see color insert).

5.2.2.1.2. Episclera

Infiltration of metabolically active fibroblasts, lymphocytes, and plasma cells may involve the episclera in areas overlying active scleral inflammation. In some cases, episcleral necrosis with fibroblast and extracellular matrix degradation may appear as a result of the extension of the scleral necrosis. Zonal granulomatous inflammation around necrotic areas may be seen. Neutrophils, lymphocytes, and plasma cells may localize around episcleral vessels. In some cases, episcleral vessel walls may reveal inflammatory microangiopathy.[23,41]

5.2.2.1.3. Conjunctiva

Destruction of the sclera often involves overlying conjunctiva, which displays an intense stromal inflammatory infiltration and various degrees of epithelial derangements, ranging from squamous changes to epithelial loss. On occasion the substantia propria may show a granulomatous inflammation with epithelioid cells and giant cells. Neutrophils, lymphocytes, eosinophils, plasma cells, and occasionally mast cells may be seen as perivascular accumulations. The walls of some vessels may be extensively infiltrated by neutrophils (Fig. 5.16).[23,41]

5.2.2.1.4. Iris, Ciliary Body, and Choroid

Anterior scleral inflammatory reactions may extend into the underlying uveal tract, sometimes causing perivasculitis and a chronic granulomatous reaction with lymphocytes, plasma cells, giant cells, and epithelioid cells.[11] In posterior scleritis, the underlying choroid is also affected, giving rise to choroidal thickening (granulomatous inflammation) (Fig. 5.17) and less often to choroidal vasculitis.[42,43]

5.2.2.1.5. Cornea

Extension of the scleral inflammation into the cornea causes keratitis, which histologically may appear as an infiltration of the corneal stroma by neutrophils, lymphocytes, and plasma cells. In the case of peripheral ulceration, necrotic epithelium can be seen at the overhanging edge.[44]

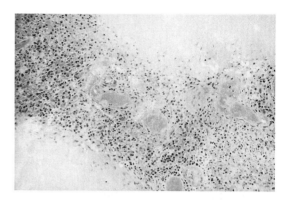

FIGURE 5.16. Conjunctival biopsy, again demonstrating microangiopathy with inflammatory cells in the vessel wall and surrounding dense inflammatory infiltration of the substantia propria.

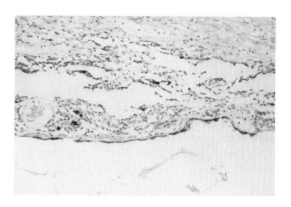

FIGURE 5.17. Enucleation specimen from a patient who had posterior scleritis. Note the inflammatory cell infiltrate in the sclera, but also the granulomatous inflammation of the choroid.

5.2.2.1.6. Other Ocular Structures

Depending on the scleral area involved in scleritis, other ocular structures may also show morphological changes. Occasionally, scleritis is associated with an inflammatory infiltration of the trabecular meshwork and intrascleral outflow channels.[45] Extraocular muscles and periorbital fat may show lymphocyte and plasma cell infiltration.[46] Retinal pigment epithelium can be absent focally with surrounding inflammation in areas underlying choroiditis and scleritis.[42] Retinal and choroidal detachments, intravitreous or subretinal hemorrhages, perivasculitis of the retinal vessels, and central retinal vein occlusion may also appear. Optic nerve and macula may show inflammatory infiltration.[47]

5.2.2.1.7. Clinicopathological Correlates in Noninfectious Scleritis: Association with Systemic Vasculitic Diseases

The clinical spectrum of systemic vasculitis-associated scleritis encompasses diseases thought to be primary vasculitic syndromes (polyarteritis nodosa), diseases that are predominantly granulomatous (Wegener's granulomatosis), and diseases associated with underlying conditions, such as the acquired connective tissue disorders (rheumatoid arthritis) or other inflammatory conditions.[48,49] A classification of vasculitic syndromes that can be associated with scleritis is shown in Table 5.7. In the following sections we review the pathology of some of these conditions.

5.2.2.1.7.1. Polyarteritis Nodosa. The pathology of systemic polyarteritis nodosa (PAN) consists of nongranulomatous focal panmural necrotizing vasculitis of small- and medium-sized muscular arteries, with a predilection for branching points and bifurcations. Polyarteritis nodosa may affect any small- or medium-sized artery of any organ, although there is less involvement of the pulmonary and splenic arteries.[48,50,51] Small- and medium-sized muscular arterial inflammation may extend to arterioles and, sometimes, to contiguous venules and veins. Skin, joints, peripheral nerves, gut, and kidney are the tissues most commonly involved.[52] Episcleritis or scleritis may be manifestations of ocular involvement[52,53]; the latter may range from mild diffuse scleritis to severe necrotizing scleritis.

Histopathologically, systemic vascular lesions of affected organs are characterized by fibrinoid necrosis and neutrophil infiltration, which may extend to involve the full thickness of the arterial wall; less often, eosinophils and lymphocytes are present in and around the vessels. The arterial segment often thromboses or bulges in an aneurysmal fashion. As the

TABLE 5.7. Vasculitic syndromes associated with scleritis.

Noninfectious diseases
    Primarily small- and medium-sized vessel vasculitic diseases
        Primarily vasculitic (and/or granulomatous) diseases
            Polyarteritis nodosa
            Allergic granulomatous angiitis (Churg–Strauss syndrome)
            Wegener's granulomatosis
            Behçet's disease
            Cogan's syndrome
            Schönlein–Henoch purpura
        Connective tissue diseases in which vasculitis may occur
            Adult rheumatoid arthritis
            Systemic lupus erythematosus
            Relapsing polychondritis
            Juvenile rheumatoid arthritis
            Sjögren's syndrome
            Dermatomyositis
        Inflammatory conditions in which vasculitis may occur
            Arthritis and inflammatory bowel disease
            Psoriatic arthritis
    Primarily large-sized vessel vasculitic diseases
        Inflammatory conditions in which vasculitis may occur
            Ankylosing spondylitis
            Reiter's syndrome
        Primarily vasculitic diseases
            Giant cell arteritis
            Takayasu's arteritis
Infectious diseases

lesions heal, there is proliferation of fibrous tissue and endothelial cells of the affected arterial wall, which may lead to further occlusion of the vessel lumen. In any patient different arteries, or even separate branches of the same artery, may be seen in acute, chronic, or healed stages of arteritis.[54] Eosinophil tissue infiltration and granulomas are not characteristically found.[48]

The pathology of scleral involvement demonstrates an inflammatory microangiopathy of scleral vasculature that may lead to occlusion of some vessels. Choroidal vessels may also be involved.[53,55] Unlike lesions elsewhere in the body, ocular involvement in polyarteritis nodosa may show granulomatous changes in and around episcleral and choroidal vessels.[9,55–59]

In our series, polyarteritis nodosa was diagnosed in two patients with scleritis, one with diffuse scleritis and the other with necrotizing scleritis; diagnosis confirmation was obtained after muscle and cutaneous nodule biopsy, respectively. One of the cases is described as follows:

A 56-year-old white woman developed intermittent fever, chills, weight loss, fatigue, and low back pain. Discharge diagnoses after hospitalization at a community hospital were urinary tract infection and lumbar disk disease. Shortly thereafter, she developed cervical pain, dizziness, and progressive lower extremity muscle weakness and, a few weeks later, she experienced pain in her right eye, noises in her right ear, and a grand mal seizure. At the time of the patient's first evaluation by us, she exhibited a profound quadriceps muscle weakness and a heliotropic rash on the skin of the left eyelid. Her temperature was 39.5°C and her pulse was 125 beats/min. Visual acuity was 20/50 OD (right eye) and 20/40 OS (left eye). Slit-lamp ocular examination disclosed a small area of anterior necrotizing scleritis and peripheral ulcerative keratitis (Fig. 5.18). Following admission to the hospital, laboratory tests showed a sedimentation rate of 120 mm/h, normal complete blood count and muscle enzymes, and negative anti-nuclear antibody and rheumatoid factor tests. A few days later, a small nodule below the left elbow was detected (Fig. 5.19); biopsy showed nongranulomatous necrotizing vasculitis compatible with polyarteritis nodosa (Fig. 5.20). Subsequent abdominal angiography disclosed arterial saccular aneurysms in the superior mesenteric artery. Sys-

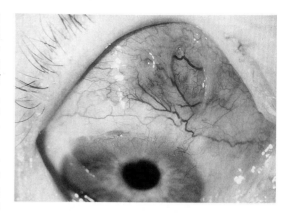

FIGURE 5.18. Fifty-six-year-old woman with necrotizing scleritis and peripheral ulcerative keratitis. Note the intense scleritis and area of necrotizing scleritis, with a loss of approximately 85% of scleral thickness.

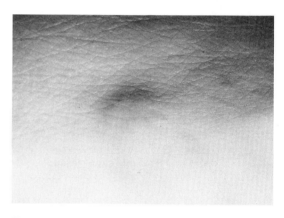

FIGURE 5.19. Subcutaneous nodule below the left elbow (same patient as in Fig. 5.18).

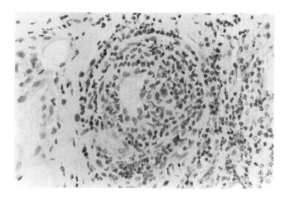

FIGURE 5.20. Polyarteritis nodosa: subcutaneous nodular biopsy of same patient as in Figs. 5.18 and 5.19. Note the enormous mononuclear cell infiltrate in the arteriolar wall. (Magnification, ×40; hematoxylin–eosin stain.)

temic prednisone halted scleral inflammation and cleared systemic symptoms. Cyclophosphamide was instituted and prednisone tapered after 14 months of treatment because of steroid-induced myopathy.

Demonstration of necrotizing vasculitis on biopsy material of involved extraocular tissues confirms the diagnosis of systemic polyarteritis nodosa in a patient with compatible multi-system clinical findings. Inflammatory micro-angiopathy with or without granulomas in conjunctival and/or scleral specimens further strengthens the diagnosis. Biopsy of symptomatic areas such as skin, testes, epididymis, skeletal muscle, and peripheral nerves provides the highest diagnostic yield,[60–62] whereas blind biopsy of asymptomatic organs is often negative. In cases with red cells, red cell casts, or proteinuria, renal biopsy will reveal focal necrotizing glomerulonephritis and, in about half of the cases, a small vessel vasculitis will be demonstrated.

5.2.2.1.7.2. Allergic Granulomatous Angiitis (Churg–Strauss Syndrome). The association of asthma, eosinophilia, pulmonary infiltrations, vasculitis, and extravascular granulomas was termed "allergic angiitis and granulomatosis" by Churg and Strauss in 1951.[63] The pathology of this disease consists of small, necrotizing granulomas and necrotizing vasculitis involving predominantly small arteries, arterioles, venules, and veins rather than small-and medium-sized muscular arteries. Granulomas are composed of a central eosinophilic core surrounded radially by macrophages and giant cells. Inflammatory cells, predominantly eosinophils, are present; neutrophils and lymphocytes also may be found in smaller numbers. Chronic lesions are characterized by macrophages and giant cells and lesser numbers of eosinophils. Necrotizing vasculitis is characterized by segmental fibrinoid necrosis and leukocytic (predominantly eosinophil) infiltration, in and around the vessels; variable numbers of macrophages and giant cells also may be present around the necrotic areas. There may be thrombosis or aneurysmal dilatation at the site of the lesion. Healed areas show proliferation of fibrous tissue and endothelial cells, which may lead to further narrowing of the vessel lumen.[64–66]

Allergic granulomatous angiitis (Churg–Strauss syndrome) may affect any organ in the body; however, unlike classic PAN, lung involvement is predominant, with gastro-intestinal tract, skin, heart, kidney, and peripheral nerves also commonly involved.[67,68] Scleritis may occur as part of the ocular involvement.[69] Scleral tissue from patients with scleritis shows numerous eosinophils, granulomatous proliferation of epithelioid and giant cells, and vascular closure by inflammatory microangiopathy.[69]

Demonstration of necrotizing small vasculitis and eosinophilic necrotizing intra- and extra-vascular granulomas on biopsy material of involved extraocular tissues confirms the diagnosis of Churg–Strauss syndrome in a patient with compatible multisystem clinical findings and laboratory tests.[62–66,69,70] Involved tissues more commonly biopsied for diagnosis are lung, skin, and peripheral nerves. Demonstration of eosinophilic granulomas and inflammatory microangiopathy in conjunctiva and/or scleral specimens further strengthens the diagnosis.

5.2.2.1.7.3. Wegener's Granulomatosis. Complete (classic) Wegener's granulomatosis is characterized by necrotizing granulomatous lesions of the upper and lower respiratory tract (nose, sinuses, and lung), generalized small-vessel vasculitis in the lung and other organs, and focal or diffuse necrotizing glomerulonephritis.[71–76] Less extensive or limited forms of this condition also exist, in which case renal involvement is absent.[77] In highly limited forms of Wegener's granulomatosis, ocular or orbital involvement is present in the absence of systemic manifestations.[78]

In the complete form of Wegener's granulomatosis, ophthalmic involvement may be present in up to 58% of cases.[53,79–82] In the limited form of Wegener's granulomatosis, ocular manifestations, including scleritis, may constitute the major signs and symptoms, or indeed may be the only manifestation of the disease.[81–89] In the highly limited form of Wegener's granulomatosis, ocular or orbital involvement, including scleritis, is the only objective finding of the condition.[78]

Because Wegener's granulomatosis is predominantly a granulomatous disease rather than a form of primary vasculitis,[90] necrotizing granulomas on involved organs are invariably present. Purely granulomatous disease without vasculitis may represent an early manifestation of Wegener's granulomatosis.[91] Granulomas contain a central area of necrosis surrounded by a zone of fibroblastic proliferation with multinucleated giant cells, epithelioid cells, neutrophils, lymphocytes, and plasma cells.[74] Eosinophils are often present.[78] Vasculitis is frequently found. The vascular changes are similar to those of polyarteritis nodosa; acute lesions show fibrinoid necrosis with neutrophil and mononuclear cell infiltration within and often adjacent to the vessel wall, which may lead to lumen narrowing and subsequent obliteration; healed lesions show fibroblastic and endothelial proliferation, which may contribute to further vessel narrowing. Whereas both types of lesions are seen in some areas, only one type of lesion is present in others.[75] Pathologically, lesions of Wegener's granulomatosis differ from extraocular lesions of polyarteritis nodosa in that the former are characterized by granulomas that may be in, around, or clearly separated from the vessel walls. Pathema in Wegener's granulomatosis often differs from that of Churg–Strauss syndrome in that in the former, the disintegrating cells in the center of the granuloma are neutrophils, usually not eosinophils.[92] However, although pathological findings are helpful in differentiating different entities, a specific diagnosis can be confirmed only with the association of characteristic clinical findings.[78]

Pathology of scleral lesions may demonstrate lesions similar to those found in other organs.[9,10,78,84,88,93,94] The constellation of histopathological features on conjunctival and scleral tissues include (1) collagen necrosis, (2) nuclear dust, (3) granulomatous foci with multinucleated giant cells surrounded by epithelioid cells, neutrophils, lymphocytes, and plasma cells, and frequently (4) inflammatory microangiopathy.

The diagnosis of Wegener's granulomatosis is based on the interpretation of clinical features and histological findings. Anti-neutrophil cytoplasmic antibody (ANCA) testing is an important adjunct in the diagnosis of Wegener's granulomatosis because it has been found to be 97% specific and 93% sensitive for the condition.[95] Because of its high specificity, a positive test is suggestive of Wegener's granulomatosis, even in patients without compatible clinical and histopathological findings. The sensitivity of ANCA testing is dependent on disease severity; whereas ANCA testing is positive in 96% of patients with active complete (classic) Wegener's granulomatosis, it is positive only in 67% of patients with active limited disease and in 32% of patients in full remission after limited disease.[96] Therefore, a negative ANCA test does not exclude the diagnosis, especially in patients with limited clinical features and characteristic histological findings.

Pathological detection of necrotizing granulomas with or without vasculitis in involved extraocular tissues confirms the diagnosis of Wegener's granulomatosis in a patient with compatible systemic clinical findings, such as chronic sinusitis, nasal ulceration, chronic cough, or hematuria, with or without positive ANCA testing.[97,98] Pathological detection of necrotizing granulomas with or without inflammatory microangiopathy in conjunctiva and/or scleral specimens in association with complete and, especially, limited clinical features confirms the diagnosis of Wegener's granulomatosis, even if ANCA testing is negative.

Biopsy of involved nasal mucosa, sinus tissue, skin, or sclera offers the best opportunity for obtaining a histological diagnosis.[74,84,92,97,98] Involved lung tissue, preferably through open biopsy, also may be obtained. Because renal involvement ranges from diffuse proliferative glomerulonephritis and interstitial nephritis to hyalinization of glomeruli, results of renal biopsy are rarely distinctive enough from other conditions to be definitive.[49]

Pathological detection of necrotizing granulomas with or without inflammatory microangiopathy in sclera confirms the diagnosis of the highly limited form of Wegener's granulomatosis in a patient with scleritis and positive ANCA testing.[78] In the absence of characteristic ocular histological findings, a positive ANCA test is suggestive of highly limited Wegener's granulomatosis, although not diagnostic. In the absence of a positive ANCA test, the presence of characteristic ocular histological findings without systemic clinical features does not support the diagnosis of Wegener's granulomatosis.

In our series, 13 patients with Wegener's granulomatosis underwent conjunctival and/or scleral biopsies; 1 patient had the complete form, 10 patients had the limited form, and 2 patients had the highly limited form (Table 5.8). In all but one patient the ocular findings were the presenting manifestation that led to the diagnosis of Wegener's granulomatosis. Detection of necrotizing granulomas by histopathology and of inflammatory microangiopathy by histopathology or immunofluorescence confirmed the diagnosis of Wegener's granulomatosis in patients with the compatible

clinical findings and positive ANCA testing. In patients with the highly limited form of Wegener's granulomatosis, characteristic pathological findings confirmed the diagnosis in the context of positive ANCA testing. Prior to the development of ANCA testing, characteristic pathological findings confirmed the condition in patients with compatible clinical features. When clinical findings were nonspecific (e.g., skin ulcer, patient No. 8, Table 5.8), necrotizing granulomas with vasculitis in other tissues (skin) established the diagnosis. One of the cases is described as follows.

A 41-year-old man developed pain, photophobia, and tearing in both eyes 6 months prior to his first examination by us. Nodular scleritis in both eyes

TABLE 5.8. Scleral and conjunctival biopsies in patients with Wegener's granulomatosis.

Patient No. age/sex	Severity[a]	Duration prior to diagnosis (months)[b]	Systemic clinical findings[c]	Abnormal X rays	Biopsy Conjunctivitis	Sclera	ANCA
1/41/M	L	7	Epistaxis, skin lesions, joint swelling, fever, microscopic hematuria	Sinus	NS[d]	G + V[d]	+
2/78/F	HL	4	—	—	NS	G	+
3/65/F	L	5	Epistaxis, tongue blisters, microscopic hematuria, sinusitis	Sinus	NS	G + V	+
4/56/M	HL	2	—	—	G	G	+
5/45/M	L	25	Sinusitis, abnormal LFTs,[d] arthralgias	Sinus	NA[d]	G	+
6/66/M	C	0	Epistaxis, hemoptysis, red blood cell casts, hematuria	Chest/sinus	G + V	G + V	NA
7/69/F	L	24	Sinusitis, cough, hematuria	Chest/sinus	V	G + V	NA
8/45/M	L	5	Skin ulcer	NA	NA	G + V	NA
9/69/M	L	9	Epistaxis, microscopic hematuria	Sinus	G + V	NA	NA
10/78/M	L	24	Cough, arthralgias, sinusitis, microscopic hematuria	Sinus	G + V	NA	NA
11/68/F	L	5	Microscopic hematuria	NA	V	G + V	NA
12/81/M	L	2	Polymyalgia rheumatica	NA	NA	G + V	+
13/68/M	L	36	Cough, arthralgias	Chest	G + V	G + V	NA

[a] C, Complete; L, limited; HL, highly limited.

[b] Duration of scleritis prior to diagnosis (in cases in which scleritis was the first manifestation of the disease).

[c] At the moment of diagnosis.

[d] LFTs, Liver function tests; NS, nonspecific; NA, not available; G, granulomatous foci; V, vasculitis (either by histopathology or by immunofluorescence).

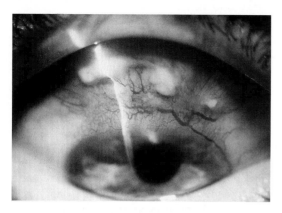

FIGURE 5.21. Forty-one-year-old man with necrotizing scleritis and peripheral ulcerative keratitis: left eye at time of presentation. Note the areas of conjunctival erosion, disclosing loss of sclera underneath the conjunctiva.

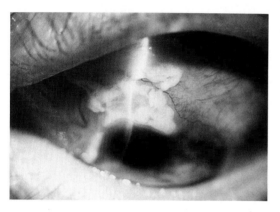

FIGURE 5.22. Left eye (same patient as in Fig. 5.21): Note the extensive ulcerative keratitis and associated necrotizing scleritis.

and marginal corneal thinning in the left eye were diagnosed and topical steroids and systemic nonsteroidal and steroidal antiinflammatory drugs were instituted. Review of systems disclosed an episode of fever and bilateral wrist swelling and pain associated with purpuric rash on his lower extremities 2 months after the beginning of his ocular problem. Efforts to reduce the dosage of prednisone resulted in recurrent ocular pain and inflammation. Laboratory tests revealed an erythrocyte sedimentation rate (ESR) of 64 and red cells in the urinary sediment. The patient was referred to the Immunology Service of the Massachusetts Eye and Ear Infirmary because of an increase in the extent of the marginal corneal thinning. At the time of his first examination

by us, photophobia and tearing were intense and visual acuity was 20/30 in both eyes. Necrotizing scleritis was present superiorly in both eyes and peripheral ulcerative keratitis was present superiorly in the left eye (Figs. 5.21 and 5.22). Review of systems disclosed chronic epistaxis in addition to the aforementioned positive historical features. Diagnostic possibilities considered were polyarteritis nodosa, rheumatoid vasculitis, systemic lupus erythematosus, and Wegener's granulomatosis. Laboratory investigations included complete blood count (CBC), ESR, creatinine, urine analysis (UA) rheumatoid factor (RF), anti-nuclear antibodies (ANA), circulating immune complexes (CICs; C1q binding and Raji cell assay), complement component survey (components C3 and C4, as determined by the complement hemolytic 50% [CHSO] assay), hepatitis B surface antigen (HBsAg), ANCA, sinus and chest X rays, and otorhinolaryngologic consultation. Resection of the conjunctiva overlying the area of scleral inflammation of the left eye was performed as a therapeutic maneuver for the peripheral ulcerative keratitis, and a scleral biopsy was also obtained. Otorhinolaryngologic consultation disclosed inflamed, friable tissue in the nasal mucosa, which was biopsied. Abnormal tests included a CIC (Raji assay) of 228 (0–50), an ESR of 20, microscopic hematuria, and left frontal sinus membrane thickening as revealed by sinus X rays. ANCA testing was still pending. Biopsies of nasal mucosa and conjunctiva revealed nonspecific inflammation with infiltration of neutrophils, lymphocytes, and plasma cells. Biopsy of sclera showed granulomatous in-

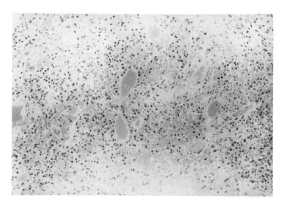

FIGURE 5.23. Biopsied sclera of same patient shown in Figs. 5.21 and 5.22: Note the granulomatous inflammation with epitheloid cells, multinucleated giant cells, and inflammatory microangiopathy. (Hematoxylin–eosin stain.)

flammation with epithelioid cells and scattered giant cells as well as neutrophil infiltration of the vessel walls characteristic of an inflammatory microangiopathy (Fig. 5.23). ANCA testing by indirect immunofluorescence was positive (136; negative, <20). The patient was diagnosed with Wegener's granulomatosis and treatment with cyclophosphamide was instituted. Ocular and systemic manifestations were brought under control and the patient is alive and well 15 months after the initiation of cyclophosphamide therapy.

5.2.2.1.7.4. Connective Tissue Diseases. Scleritis may be an ocular manifestation of several connective tissue diseases. Conjunctival and/or scleral histopathological findings range from nonspecific inflammation with neutrophils, lymphocytes, and plasma cells to a granulomatous reaction with a central area of necrosis rimmed by a corona of epithelioid cells, in turn surrounded by giant cells, lymphocytes, and plasma cells. An inflammatory microangiopathy also may be found. Pathological detection of vascular inflammation in involved tissues, including conjunctiva and/or sclera, in connective tissue diseases should be regarded as an ominous sign, because it may indicate a more severe and widespread destructive process that markedly worsens life prognosis. The two connective tissue diseases in which vasculitis occurs most frequently are rheumatoid arthritis and systemic lupus erythematosus.[48,49]

1. *Rheumatoid arthritis*: Rheumatoid arthritis (RA) is a chronic, inflammatory disease characterized by a polyarthropathy that ranges from mild joint discomfort to severe, symmetric articular involvement. Although the diagnosis of RA is made on the basis of clinical criteria, approximately 70% of patients are positive for rheumatoid factor (RF), as opposed to 1 to 5% of the general population.[99] Patients with a positive RF have a higher incidence of extraarticular manifestations than do patients without a positive RF. Extraarticular manifestations may be related to proliferative granulomas or to vasculitis.

An example of proliferative granuloma in RA is the rheumatoid nodule, which is characterized by a central area of necrosis rimmed by palisading fibroblasts that are surrounded by chronic inflammatory cells with occasional distinct giant cells. Although chronic changes are predominantly granulomatous, small-vessel vasculitis occurs early in the development of the rheumatoid nodule.[100] Immunofluorescent staining of nodules shows small vessel walls containing immunoglobulins.[101] Vessel endothelium, histiocytes, fibroblasts, lymphocytes, and plasma cells proliferate. Fibroblasts may release collagenase and proteoglycanase, resulting in a central necrosis.[102] A similar histology can be found in the sclera: a focus of scleral necrosis surrounded by a wall of epithelioid cells, neutrophils, lymphocytes, plasma cells, and occasional giant cells.[103]

A superimposed systemic vasculitis may complicate RA. The spectrum of rheumatoid vasculitis ranges from a hypersensitivity vasculitis affecting small vessels to a severe, systemic necrotizing vasculitis syndrome similar to that seen in classic polyarteritis nodosa.[104] It is thought that the lesions are related to deposition of circulating antigen–antibody–complement complexes, because there are depressed serum complement levels,[105,106] immunofluorescent staining of IgG, IgM, and C3 in the vessel wall,[107] and large amounts of serum cryoimmunoglobulins.[108] Clinical vasculitis may manifest as cutaneous ulceration, peripheral neuropathy, pericarditis, or arteritis of the viscera (heart, lungs, bowel, kidney, liver, spleen, pancreas, lymph nodes, and testis). Patients with rheumatoid arthritis complicated by systemic vasculitis are more likely to have severe erosive joint disease and rheumatoid subcutaneous nodules than are patients with rheumatoid arthritis without vasculitis.[109,110] Vasculitis may occur in rheumatoid arthritis patients who have had their disease for more than [10] years. Males are afflicted as commonly as females. Patients with rheumatoid arthritis patients who have had their disease for more than 10 years. Males are afflicted as of circulating immune complexes, and lower titers of complement than do patients with rheumatoid arthritis without vasculitis.[109–119] Patients with rheumatoid arthritis and widespread vasculitis have an alarmingly high mortality rate; frequent causes of death are related to mesenteric, coronary, and cerebral artery inflammation.[120,121] Ferguson and Slocumb[115] reported that 8 of 19 (42%) rheumatoid arthritis patients with vascular involvement, manifested by sensorimotor neuropathy in three of four extremities died of vasculitic events.

Pathological detection of inflammatory microangiopathy in conjunctiva and/or sclera in patients with connective tissue diseases and necrotizing scleritis may also indicate a manifestation of widespread vasculitis. Our 10 patients (6 females and 4 males) with RA, necrotizing scleritis, and inflammatory microangiopathy in scleral tissue had had the rheumatoid arthritis for more than 10 years. They had severe, often incapacitating, articular lesions, and had extra-articular manifestations such as rheumatoid nodules, nailfold infarcts (Fig. 5.24), extremity purpuric lesions, peripheral neuropathies, nerve entrapment syndromes, cardiac conduction defects, cardiac valvulopathies, pneumonias, or pleural diseases. Rheumatoid factor titers were high (mean titer, 1:3157; normal, <60), as were circulating immune complexes (mean titer by Raji cell assay, 250; normal, 0–50). All 10 patients required systemic immunosuppressive therapy to halt the progression of scleral destruction; 4 of these also underwent scleral grafting to maintain the integrity of the globe because of the advanced extent of scleral necrosis.[33] Jayson and Jones[122] found systemic vasculitis in 10 of 14 patients with rheumatoid arthritis and necrotizing scleritis; 6 of those patients died of vasculitic complications during the follow-up period.

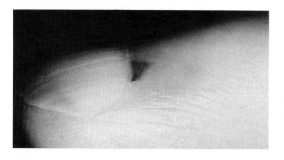

FIGURE 5.24. Periungual nailfold infarct in a patient with rheumatoid arthritis-associated vasculitis.

Foster et al.[123] reported that 7 of 20 patients with rheumatoid arthritis and necrotizing scleritis died of vascular-related events within 8 years of the onset of the scleritis; aggressive treatment with systemic immunosuppressive therapy may favorably alter the ocular and the general outcome. These data suggest that inflammatory microangiopathy in scleral tissue in patients with connective tissue diseases and scleritis indicates a more destructive phase in the patient's clinical systemic course, worsening not only the ocular prognosis, but also the general prognosis as well. Early detection of these clinicopathological changes may lead to early aggressive treatment of both the ocular and the general conditions. One of our cases is described as follows.

A 55-year-old white woman with a 38-year history of rheumatoid arthritis developed pain and redness in both eyes 7 months prior to her first examination by us. She was diagnosed with bilateral nodular scleritis and treated with local and systemic steroidal and nonsteroidal antiinflammatory drugs. As the steroids were tapered, symptoms reappeared and she was sent to our institution for further assessment. Slit-lamp examination revealed necrotizing scleritis with peripheral ulcerative keratitis supratemporally in the right eye and temporal nodular scleritis in the left eye (Figs. 5.25 and 5.26). Visual acuity was 20/50 in the right eye and 20/20 in the left eye. Past history included frequent respiratory infections, pleural effusions, and multiple surgical procedures for her joint disease, including hip replacement and neck fusion. Review of systems confirmed severe crippling arthritis and revealed mitral valve prolapse and rheumatoid nodules. Rheumatoid vasculitis associated with her rheumatoid arthritis was suspected. Investigations disclosed an RF of 10,240, a CIC of 550 (Raji assay; normal, 0–50), and an ANA of 1:16,384. Local measures for her peripheral ulcerative keratitis included keratectomy, cyanoacrylate adhesive application, and soft contact lens fitting; resection of the adjacent conjunctiva overlying the necrotic sclera also was performed, at which time necrotic scleral tissue was biopsied. Histopathological and immunofluorescence studies revealed necrotizing granulomatous inflammation with scattered giant cells in both tissues, with associated inflammatory microangiopathy in the sclera. The patient was diagnosed as having rheumatoid vasculitis, and treatment with cyclophosphamide was instituted. Necrotizing scleritis and peripheral ulcerative kera-

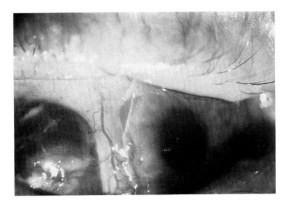

FIGURE 5.25. Fifty-five-year-old patient with rheumatoid arthritis, associated necrotizing scleritis, and peripheral ulcerative keratitis: right eye.

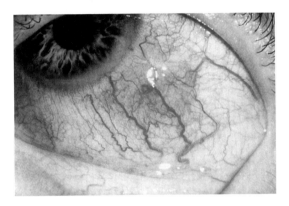

FIGURE 5.26. Same patient as in Fig. 5.25: The left eye shows nodular scleritis.

titis resolved and were quiescent for 18 months, at which time cyclophosphamide was discontinued. Seven months later the patient returned with a recurrence of her necrotizing scleritis with supratemporal bulging uvea in the right eye. Visual acuity had not changed. Review of systems disclosed skin grafts for ulcerative skin lesions in her right leg and foot. A tectonic scleral graft was performed and conjunctival and scleral necrotic tissues were obtained for histopathology and immunofluorescence. Biopsy results showed necrotizing granulomas with giant cells and inflammatory microangiopathy in both tissues. Therapy with cyclophosphamide was resumed and maintained. The scleral graft remained stable and no evidence of additional necrotizing scleritis was seen.

5.2.2.1.8. Clinicopathological Correlates in Infectious Scleritis

Although rare, episcleritis and scleritis may appear in systemic and local infectious diseases, either as a direct invasion by organisms that cause the systemic and local signs, or as a result of the immune response induced by the infectious agent. Improvement in detection of previously unrecognized disease entities and changes in epidemiological trends in the population appear to have played major roles in the decline or emergence of some of the systemic or local diseases that may cause scleritis. The most common systemic infection that may involve the sclera today is herpes zoster[124–126]; occasionally herpes simplex, tuberculosis,[127] and syphilis[128,129] may cause scleritis. The most common cause of local infectious scleritis is *Pseudomonas aeruginosa*.[130–134] Other microorganisms such as *Streptococcus*, *Staphylococcus*, *Proteus*, atypical mycobacteria, *Borrelia*, *Nocardia*, *Aspergillus*, *Acanthamoeba*, *Toxoplasma*, and *Toxocara* have also been implicated.[130,134–138] In the following sections we review the pathology of some of these infections.

5.2.2.1.8.1. Systemic Infections

1. *Herpes zoster*: Herpes zoster episcleral and scleral infections may be the result of a direct viral infection and an autoimmune process induced by the virus, either separately or in combination.[126,139] Varicella-zoster virus (VZV) has been identified by immunofluorescence or electron microscopy and viral culture in some areas of the body, including the skin, central nervous system, sensory ganglia, and corneal epithelium.[136–148] However, in spite of some efforts to try to identify the virus intraocularly,[126] herpes-like particles have been observed only on a few occasions and never in sclera.[149,150] In one of these cases, subsequent culture proved that the herpes-like particles were VZV.[150] Varicella-zoster virus and herpes simplex virus (HSV) are indistinguishable by electron microscopy.[148] However, in contrast to HSV, VZV does not grow in ordinary tissue culture although it does grow in tissue culture containing human embryonic

lung diploid cells,[147] human fetal diploid kidney cells,[148,151] or human foreskin fibroblasts.[152] Also, whereas HSV is a pathogen in some animals (rabbit), VZV is not pathogenic in any animal.[153] Furthermore, HSV and VZV differ in their antigenicity, so that immunofluorescence testing with HSV- and VZV-specific antibody probes may help in the identification.[140] Histopathological studies of scleral and conjunctival specimens from patients with VZV scleritis do not show differences from the specimens from patients with scleritis associated with systemic autoimmune diseases. They reveal a granulomatous infiltration with multinucleated giant cells and epithelioid cells around the necrotic sclera and/or conjunctiva. Neutrophils, lymphocytes, and plasma cells may be seen around the granuloma and around vessels. In some cases, a neutrophilic invasion of the vessel wall can be seen. In our series, one of the two patients with VZV scleritis underwent conjunctival and scleral biopsy. Both tissues showed multiple granulomas with giant cells surrounded by massive infiltration with mononuclear cells and neutrophils; in addition, an inflammatory microangiopathy was also seen. Indirect immunofluorescence techniques were used in an effort to identify the viral antigen in cells infected with VZV. The primary antibody used was mouse anti-human monoclonal antibody directed against VZV (wild strain) (1:30; Chemicon International, Temecula, CA); results were negative. Differences (as determined by light microscopy) between VZV scleritis and scleritis associated with systemic autoimmune diseases may exist, however, if other ocular tissues are available for histopathological study, because the combination of necrosis of iris, ciliary body, choroid, retina, and optic nerve, as well as marked inflammation of the posterior ciliary nerves[126] are not seen in scleritis associated with autoimmune diseases but may be seen in VZV scleritis.

2. *Herpes simplex*: Episcleritis and scleritis are rare entities occurring either as a result of direct viral invasion during the course of a herpes simplex infection, or as a result of an autoimmune response to the virus, months after the initial viral encounter. Conjunctival and scleral specimens in HSV scleritis show granu- lomatous inflammation with multinucleated giant cells and epithelioid cells, perivasculitis, and inflammatory microangiopathy. Herpes simplex virus has a cytopathogenic effect in culture on several cell culture lines (HeLa cells, human amnion cells, and fibroblasts). Herpes simplex virus type 1 can also be directly identified by immunological methods in different tissues of the body, including conjunctiva (indirect immunofluorescence or immunoperoxidase testing).[154–157]

We use immunofluorescence techniques on ocular tissues, including conjunctiva and sclera, to identify viral antigen in cells infected with HSV. The primary antibody used is mouse monoclonal antibody directed against herpes simplex virus type 1 (1:20; Chemicon International). One of our cases is described as follows.

A 49-year-old white male with a history of right maxilla osteosarcoma underwent facial bone surgical removal and replacement with right fibular bone grafting. Several days postoperatively he developed right facial and right leg osteomyelitis, which was treated with systemic antibiotics. Two months later, debridement of the previous right facial graft was performed and replaced with left fibular bone grafting. A new focus of left fibula osteomyelitis prompted his doctors to place a continuous intravenous central line antibiotic pump containing oxacillin and ceftazidime. During this treatment, the patient noticed discomfort and redness in his left eye. Keratitis was diagnosed and treatment with tobramycin drops and gentamicin ointment was instituted. Two weeks later, the eye had deteriorated and the patient was sent to our institution for further studies. At the time of his first examination by us, visual acuity was 20/40 in the right eye and 20/80 in the left eye. Slit-lamp examination revealed blotchy white infiltrates in corneal stroma, extending from 4 to 5 o'clock, 4 to 5 mm from periphery to the center, and without anterior chamber reaction (Fig. 5.27; see color insert). Episcleral and scleral diffuse edema and redness were observed adjacent to the corneal stromal infiltration (Fig. 5.28; see color insert). Infectious keratoscleritis was diagnosed and possible etiological agents considered included fungus, virus (HSV type 1), spirochetes (*Treponema pallidum*), *Acanthamoeba*, and bacteria. Although unlikely, an autoimmune process was not discounted. A corneo–conjunctiva–scleral biopsy was performed and specimens were sent for fungal, bacterial, and *Acanthamoeba* cultures (tissue homogenates) as well as for histopathology and for immunofluorescence (anti-immunoglobulin and anti-complement antibodies, and anti-HSV type 1 antibodies) studies. Conventional blood work included a fluorescent treponemal antibody absorption test (FTA-ABS), which was negative. Gram stain, calcofluor white stain, and appropriate cultures for fungus, bacteria, and *Acanthamoeba* were negative. Histopathology studies revealed a chronic nongranulomatous inflammation, and direct immunofluorescent studies (anti-immunoglobulin and anti-complement antibodies) were negative for detection of vasculitis. Results of immunofluorescent studies, using monoclonal antibodies directed against HSV type 1, were dramatic, revealing positive detection of the viral antigen in cornea, conjunctiva, and sclera, with the appropriate negative controls (Figs. 5.29 and 5.30; see color insert). The patient was diagnosed with HSV type 1 keratoscleritis and treatment with acyclovir and steroids was instituted. Four weeks later the ocular infection had resolved and visual acuity had improved to 20/30.

3. *Tuberculosis*: Episcleritis and scleritis are rarely caused by *Mycobacterium tuberculosis* in developed countries today, but when it occurs it is usually the a consequence of a hematogenous miliary spread of pulmonary tuberculosis.[158–161] More uncommonly, tuberculous scleritis may be the result of a local manifestation of a hypersensitivity reaction to circulating tuberculoproteins, or of an exogenous infection caused either by a direct injury,[162] or by a direct spread of a tuberculous lesion in adjacent ocular tissues.[163–165] Histologically, the classic pattern of tuberculous scleritis in conjunctival and scleral specimens is a granulomatous inflammation surrounding an area of caseation necrosis in which acid-fast bacilli can be demonstrated by Ziehl–Neelsen staining or by fluorescent staining with auramine-rhodamine.[161–169] Perivascular infiltration with chronic inflammatory cells may be seen. Because the histological changes in tuberculous scleritis are similar to the changes present in scleritis associated with systemic autoimmune diseases, identification of the microorganism in conjunctival or scleral tissue is important for ascribing the diagnosis of tuberculosis to scleral inflammation. In some cases, however, identification of the microorganism in ocular tissue cannot be accomplished, in which case the diagnosis of tuberculosis is presumed on the basis of histological ocular granulomatous reaction associated with chest X ray-compatible findings and a positive sputum culture. The diagnosis may be presumed on the basis of histological ocular granulomatous reaction in association with a strongly positive Mantoux test.

4. *Syphilis*: Within 3 weeks of the first encounter with the spirochete *T. pallidum*, usually by sexual contact, primary syphilis occurs, characterized by a chancre of skin or mucous membrane with regional lymphadenopathy. This lesion resolves in 3 weeks. Hematogenous spread of *T. pallidum* underlies the pathogenesis of secondary syphilis, which occurs 2 months to 3 years after the inoculation. In an immunocompetent individual, the humoral and cellular immune responses can suppress the treponemes, resulting in a latent stage. Immune regulation breakdown may occur in about one-third of the affected individuals, leading to tertiary syphilis, in which the treponemes can be detected in certain tissues. Treponeme dissemination through placental invasion followed by hypersensitivity reactions causes congenital syphilis. Episcleritis and scleritis may occur during the course of secondary, tertiary, or congenital syphilis. Histologically, conjunctival and scleral specimens from patients with syphilitic scleritis in any stage of the disease show a plasma cell infiltration with scattered macrophages and lymphocytes. Arterioles in the inflammatory reaction may exhibit swelling and proliferation of endothelial cells to produce concentric "onionskin" layers that markedly narrow the lumen, leading to an obliterative endarteritis.[170,171] Around these vessels there is prominent perivascular cuffing by plasma cells. Tertiary and late congenital syphilis may also show gummas, which consist of granulomas with coagulated necrotic centers surrounded by macrophages and plasma cells, similar to tuberculous lesions.[172] Because treponemes may be scant in sclera, their identification with silver stains (Levaditi's stain or Warthin–Starry stain) or by immunological methods (direct or indirect immunofluorescence or immunoperoxidase testing) may be difficult.[173–176] When scleral treponemes cannot be demonstrated, the presumed diagnosis of syphilitic

scleritis is based on the histological conjunctival or scleral inflammatory reaction with obliterative endarteritis, associated with a positive serological FTA-ABS. We have used indirect immunofluorescence testing in an attempt to demonstrate *T. pallidum* in scleral specimens (rabbit anti-treponemal antibody and fluorescein-labeled sheep anti-rabbit antibody),[162] but our results have been negative.

5.2.2.1.8.2. Local Infections.
Exogenous infectious scleritis is rare, probably because of the tightly bound collagen fibers of the scleral coat. When it occurs, however, it is usually the result of scleral extension of a primary corneal infection. However, primary scleral infections may occur following accidental or surgical injury (pterygium excision with β irradiation or topical thiotepa, retinal detachment repair with diathermy, or strabismus surgery)[134] or as a result of a retained intrascleral foreign body.[13] Cultures of corneal or scleral scrapings may demonstrate the microorganism implicated. Analysis of conjunctival and scleral specimens by light microscopy and appropriate stainings may show the etiological agents,[130,131,136] and subsequent culture of the tissues may help in further identification. Aside from detection of the microorganism, conjunctival and scleral specimens disclose abundant hemorrhage and acute inflammatory, cell infiltration, which may lead to tissue necrosis.[131–133,136]

We use Gram's stain (bacteria and fungus), Gomori methenamine silver (fungus), Warthin–Starry silver stain (spirochete), acid-fast stain (mycobacteria), and calcofluor white stain (*Acanthamoeba*) on histopathological preparations to detect the presence of infectious agents. Alkaline Giemsa can show the presence of viral cytoplasmic or intranuclear inclusion bodies and the morphology of bacteria and fungi. We also use tissue culture techniques for microbe isolation. Scleral specimens are placed in 1 ml of meat broth and homogenized with a tissue grinder (Sage Products, Inc., Cary, IL). One-drop samples are cultured on blood agar (room temperature and 37°C, aerobic and anaerobic), chocolate agar (37°C), Sabouraud dextrose agar (room temperature), and meat broth (37°C) to identify bacteria and fungi. Culture

for *Acanthamoeba* requires placing the sample in Page's saline and transferring it to confluent layers of *Escherichia coli* (25 and 37°C). Homogenates also may be placed on cell culture lines such as HeLa cells, human amnion cells, and human fibroblasts to identify HSV type 1 (cytopathic effect), and human embryonic lung diploid cells, human fetal diploid kidney cells, or human foreskin fibroblasts to identify VZV (cytopathic effect). An illustrative case is described:

A 67-year-old white male, while working on his farm, was struck in the right eye by a cow's tail. Twenty-four hours later, he developed pain and redness with mild discharge in the right eye. A conjunctivitis was diagnosed and erythromycin ointment (Erythromycin) followed by sulfacetamide-prednisolone sodium phosphate (Vasocidin) ointment were instituted. The eye became progressively more red and painful, and a few days later a "scleral/episcleral abscess" was noted. After surgical drainage of the abscess, the contents were cultured but no organisms were recovered. Dexamethasone sodium (Decadron) was injected subconjunctivally, and prednisolone acetate (Pred-Forte) and trimethoprim-polymyxin B (Polytrim) drops were begun. The patient was sent to the Immunology Service of the Massachusetts Eye and Ear Infirmary because of worsening inflammation. At the time of his first examination by us, visual acuities were 20/400 in the right eye and 20/30 in the left eye. The right eye showed a 4+ injection with necrotizing scleritis all around the globe (Fig. 5.31). The left eye was

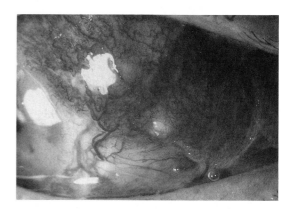

FIGURE 5.31. Right eye of a 67-year-old dairy farmer who was struck in the eye by a cow's tail. Note the intense scleritis, with scleral loss inferior to the area of obvious intense inflammation.

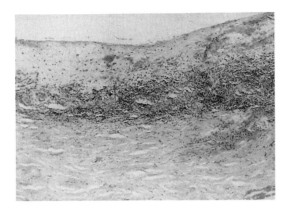

FIGURE 5.32. Scleral biopsy (same patient as in Fig. 5.20): Note the granulomatous inflammation with perivasculitis and collagen necrosis.

normal. Review of systems was negative except for the history of trauma, and laboratory tests, including chest and sinus X rays, and ultrasonography were negative. Excisional scleral biopsy of the affected area was performed as a therapeutic and diagnostic procedure, and specimens were processed for histopathological studies for culture. A chronic granulomatous inflammation with perivasculitis and collagen necrosis was seen (Fig. 5.32). Giemsa and Gomori methenamine silver stain demonstrated the presence of fungal forms with septate hyphae forming acute angles, a morphology consistent with *Aspergillus*. *Aspergillus fumigatus* was later recovered on culture (Fig. 5.33; see color insert). Flucytosine (1%) and amphotericin B (0.15%) (Fungizone) drops, fluconazol (Diflucan) tablets, and polymyxin B-bacitracin (Polysporin) ointment were begun. A small inferior retinal detachment was noted in spite of steady but slow improvement in external ocular inflammation. Six months later, the areas of active necrotizing scleritis had vanished, the small inferior retinal detachment had resolved, and the visual acuity was 20/200. Treatment was discontinued without recrudescence of the inflammatory activity.

5.3. Biopsy

5.3.1. Noninfectious Necrotizing Scleritis

Histopathologically, most cases of noninfectious necrotizing scleritis show inflammatory microangiopathy (96% of scleral specimens and 70% of conjunctival specimens studied) as well as chronic granulomatous inflammation (85% of scleral specimens studied); most of these patients have a potentially lethal underlying systemic vaculitic disease (91% of all noninfectious necrotizing scleritis patients; see Chapter 4). However, scleral and/or conjunctival specimens from noninfectious necrotizing scleritis do not show histopathological findings distinguishing between the different systemic vasculitic diseases.

Because most cases of noninfectious necrotizing scleritis show histopathological evidence of inflammatory microangiopathy (96% of scleral specimens and 70% of conjunctival specimens studied), scleral and/or conjunctival biopsy in noninfectious necrotizing scleritis is not necessary to prove a vasculitic process. Because histopathological changes in noninfectious necrotizing scleritis are similar regardless of the type of associated systemic vasculitic disease, scleral and/or conjunctival biopsy in noninfectious necrotizing scleritis is not helpful in reaching the diagnosis of a specific systemic vasculitic disease. Characteristic histopathological changes in biopsy material of involved extraocular tissues (necrotizing vasculitis with or without granulomas, with or without eosinophils, in small, medium, or large vessels), supplemented by compatible multisystem clinical findings, confirm the diagnosis of a specific systemic vasculitic disease. The clinical detection of necrotizing scleritis confirms a local vasculitic process. The clinical detection of necrotizing scleritis supplemented by compatible multisystem clinical findings is highly suggestive of a specific systemic vasculitic disease. The clinical detection of necrotizing scleritis in patients with already known connective tissue diseases is highly suggestive of a widespread vasculitic process. Either local and systemic vasculitic processes should be treated with a high dosage of corticosteroids or other immunosuppressive drugs.

One exception to this is the need to specifically prove a granulomatous process. Although a chronic granulomatous inflammation may appear in necrotizing scleritis associated with many vasculitic diseases (85% of scleral specimens studied), the presence of granulomas with or without inflammatory microangiopathy in scleral and/or conjunctival specimens confirms the diagnosis of Wegener's granulomatosis in a patient with compatible systemic clinical findings such as chronic sinusitis, nasal ulceration, chronic cough, or hematuria, with or without positive ANCA testing. Histopathological detection of necrotizing granulomas with or without inflammatory microangiopathy in scleral and/or conjunctival specimens confirms the diagnosis of the highly limited form of Wegener's granulomatosis in a patient with necrotizing scleritis and positive ANCA testing. In the absence of positive ANCA testing, the presence of characteristic ocular histopathological findings without systemic clinical features does not support the diagnosis of Wegener's granulomatosis. In the absence of characteristic ocular histopathological findings, a positive ANCA test is suggestive of highly limited Wegener's granulomatosis, although not diagnostic. Wegener's granulomatosis should be treated with cyclophosphamide.

5.3.2. Noninfectious Recurrent Diffuse or Nodular (Nonnecrotizing) Scleritis

Histopathologically, some cases of noninfectious recurrent diffuse or nodular scleritis show inflammatory microangiopathy (61% of scleral specimens and 59% of conjunctival specimens studied) as well as chronic granulomatous inflammation (23% of scleral specimens studied); some of these patients have a potentially lethal underlying systemic vasculitic disease (43% of all noninfectious recurrent diffuse scleritis patients and 41% of all noninfectious recurrent nodular scleritis patients; see Chapter 4). However, scleral and/or conjunctival specimens from noninfectious recurrent diffuse or nodular scleritis do not show histopathological findings distinguishing between the different systemic vasculitic diseases.

Because only some cases of noninfectious recurrent diffuse or nodular scleritis show inflammatory microangiopathy (61% of scleral specimens and 59% of conjunctival specimens studied), scleral and/or conjunctival biopsy in recurrent and severe diffuse or nodular scleritis

may be helpful in detecting an underlying local and probably systemic vasculitic process, which should be treated with a high dosage of corticosteroids or other immunosuppressive drugs; histopathological detection of inflammatory microangiopathy with or without granulomas in scleral and/or conjunctival biopsy in recurrent and severe diffuse or nodular scleritis, supplemented by compatible multisystem clinical findings, is highly suggestive of a specific systemic vasculitic disease. The finding of characteristic histopathological changes in biopsy material of involved extraocular tissues, supplemented by compatible multisystem clinical findings, confirms a specific vasculitic disease.

Scleral and/or conjunctival biopsy in recurrent and severe diffuse or nodular scleritis also may be helpful in detecting a granulomatous process. Although a chronic granulomatous inflammation may appear in diffuse or nodular scleritis associated with many vasculitic diseases (23% of scleral specimens studied), the presence of granulomas with or without inflammatory microangiopathy in scleral and/or conjunctival specimens, in association with complete and, especially, limited clinical features, confirms the diagnosis of Wegener's granulomatosis with or without positive ANCA testing. Histopathological detection of granulomas with or without inflammatory microangiopathy in scleral and/or conjunctival specimens confirms the diagnosis of the highly limited form of Wegener's granulomatosis in a patient with recurrent diffuse or nodular scleritis and positive ANCA testing. In the absence of positive ANCA testing, the presence of characteristic ocular histopathological findings without systemic clinical features does not support the diagnosis of Wegener's granulomatosis. In the absence of characteristic ocular histopathological findings, a positive ANCA test is suggestive of highly limited Wegener's granulomatosis, although not diagnostic.

5.3.3. Infectious Scleritis (Diffuse, Nodular, or Necrotizing Scleritis)

In infectious scleritis, stainings and cultures of scleral scrapings may demonstrate the microorganism implicated. However, when scrapings are negative, analysis of scleral and/or conjunctival specimens by light microscopy and appropriate stainings (Gram's stain, alkaline Giemsa, Gomori methenamine silver, Warthin–Starry silver, acid-fast, and calcofluor white) may reveal the etiological agents, and subsequent culture of the tissues (blood agar, chocolate agar, Sabouraud dextrose agar, meat broth, Page's saline, and transfer to confluent layers of *E. coli*) may help in further identification. Tissue homogenization and subsequent culture on different media or cell culture lines also may be important for microbe isolation. Indirect immunofluorescence techniques may be helpful to identify HSV type 1 or *T. pallidum*.

5.3.4. Biopsy Technique

Scleral biopsy is performed under retrobulbar anesthesia. After careful dissection of the conjunctiva, Tenon's capsule, and episcleral tissue, inflamed or necrotic scleral tissue is removed. This is then bisected, and half is placed on Karnovsky's fixative for histopathological evaluation; the remaining half is placed on saline and then transported to the cryostat, embedded in optimum cutting temperature (OCT) compound, and frozen immediately at −25°C for immunofluorescence evaluation. In cases in which the remaining sclera is thin, scleral graft is used to maintain the integrity of the globe. A template is made from plastic surgical drape to approximate the area of resected sclera. Frozen or glycerine-preserved full-thickness human donor sclera is then cut to size, using this template. The graft is secured with 10-0 nylon sutures to the edges of the resection site and the knots are buried. Conjunctiva is pulled down over the graft whenever enough tissue is present and is sutured with 8-0 Vicryl.

Summary

Histopathologically, most cases of episcleritis and diffuse or nodular scleritis show chronic, nongranulomatous inflammation with lymphocytes and plasma cells, vascular dilitation, and edema. By contrast, most cases of necrotizing scleritis show chronic granulomatous inflammation with epithelioid cells, multinucleated giant cells, lymphocytes, plasma cells, and less often neutrophils. Mast cells and eosinophils can sometimes be seen in the granuloma and around vessels. T lymphocyte subset and surface glycoprotein studies in necrotizing scleritis show a predominance of macrophages and T lymphocytes, with a high T helper/T suppressor ratio, and a marked increase in HLA-DR glycoproteins. These findings suggest an underlying cell-mediated reaction (type IV hypersensitivity reaction) in which the tissue injury is the result of macrophage and lymphocyte immune interaction and enzyme liberation, with subsequent extracellular matrix component degradation.

Comparison of extracellular matrix components between normal and necrotizing scleritis specimens shows a decrease in dermatan sulfate and chondroitin sulfate, without obvious differences in collagen types I, III, V, and VI; these findings suggest that proteoglycans may be the first extracellular matrix components to be degraded in necrotizing scleritis.

The presence of inflammatory microangiopathy in many of the diffuse and nodular recurrent scleritis specimens and most of the necrotizing scleritis specimens suggests and underlying immune complex reaction (type III hypersensitivity reaction), in which the vascular injury is the result of antigen–antibody conjugation within and outside the vessel wall, with subsequent activation of complement.

Demonstration of necrotizing vasculitis with or without granulomas in biopsy material of involved extraocular tissues confirms the diagnosis of systemic vasculitic diseases in patients with compatible multisystem clinical findings. Inflammatory microangiopathy in scleral or conjunctival specimens from patients with scleritis further strengthens the concept of an underlying vasculitic disease. Because noninfectious necrotizing scleritis is highly associated with the presence of inflammatory microangiopathy, scleral and/or conjunctival biopsy is not necessary to prove a vasculitic process. The presence of necrotizing scleritis should be regarded as an ominous sign because it indicates an ocular and probably a systemic vasculitic process that should be treated with a high dosage of corticosteroids or other immunosuppressive drugs. Because noninfectious recurrent diffuse or nodular scleritis is less highly associated with inflammatory microangiopathy, scleral biopsy may be helpful in detecting a local and systemic vasculitic process that should be treated with a high dosage of corticosteroids or other immunosuppressive drugs.

Pathological detection of granulomas with or without inflammatory microangiopathy in scleral and/or conjunctival specimens confirms the diagnosis of Wegener's granulomatosis in a patient with necrotizing, diffuse, or nodular scleritis with complete and, especially, limited clinical features, particularly if ANCA testing is borderline or low positive. Pathological detection of granulomas with or without inflammatory microangiopathy in sclera and/or conjunctival specimens confirms the diagnosis of the highly limited form of Wegener's granulomatosis in a patient with necrotizing, diffuse, or nodular scleritis and positive ANCA testing. In the absence of granulomas in sclera and/or conjunctival specimens, a positive ANCA test in a patient with necrotizing, diffuse, or nodular scleritis is suggestive of highly limited Wegener's granulomatosis, although not diagnostic. In the absence of positive ANCA testing, the presence of granulomas without systemic clinical features does not support the diagnosis of Wegener's granulomatosis.

In infectious scleritis, stainings and cultures of scleral scrapings may demonstrate the microorganism implicated. However, when scrapings are negative, analysis of conjunctival and scleral specimens by histopathological (stainings and cultures), tissue homogenization (culture or cell culture lines), and indirect immunofluorescence (anti-microbe antibodies) techniques may be important for microbe isolation.

References

1. Nathan CF: Secretory products of macrophages. J Clin Invest 79:319, 1987.
2. Adams DO, Hamilton TA: Phagocytic cells: cytotoxic activities of macrophages. In Gallin JI, Goldstein IM, Snyderman R (Eds): *Inflammation: Basic Principles and Clinical Correlates*. Raven, New York, 1988, pp 471–492.
3. Tse HY, Rosenthal AS: Lymphocytes: interaction with macrophages. In Gallin JI, Goldstein IM, Snyderman R (Eds): *Inflammation: Basic Principles and Clinical Correlates*. Raven, New York, 1988, pp 631–649.
4. Adams DO, Hamilton TA: Molecular bases of signal transduction in macrophage activation induced by IFN gamma and by second signals. Immunol Rev 97:1, 1987.
5. Adams DO: The biology of the granuloma. In Ioachim HL (Ed): *Pathology of Granulomas*. Raven, New York, 1983, pp 1–20.
6. Adams DO: The granulomatous inflammatory response: a review. Am J Pathol 84:164, 1976.
7. Postlethwaite AE, Jackson BK, Beachey EH, Kang AH: Formation of multinucleated giant cells from human monocyte precursors. J Exp Med 155:168, 1982.
8. Unanue ER, Benacerraf B: Immunological events in experimentally induced granulomas. Am J Pathol 71:349, 1973.
9. Weinberg JB, Hobbs MM, Misunokis MA: Recombinant human gamma interferon induces human monocyte polykaryon formation. Proc Natl Acad Sci USA 81:4554, 1984.
10. McInnes A, Rennick DM: Interleukin-4 induces cultured monocytes/macrophages to form giant multinucleated cells. J Exp Med 167:598, 1988.
11. Neumann E: Die Picrocarminforbung und ihre Anwendung auf die Entzundungslehre. Archiv für mikroscopische Anatomie, und Entwicklungsmechanik 18:130, 1880.
12. Gitlin D, Craig JM, Janeway CA: Studies on the nature of fibrinoid and the collagen diseases. Am J Pathol 33:55, 1957.
13. Warren BA, Vales O: The release of vesicles from platelets following adhesion to vessel walls *in vitro*. Br J Exp Pathol 53:206, 1972.
14. Johnsen ULH, Lyberg T, Galdal KS, Prydz H: Platelets stimulate thromboplastin synthesis in human endothelial cells. Thromb Haemost 49:69, 1983.
15. Annamalai AE, Stewart GJ, Hansel B, Memoli M, Chiu HC, Manuel DW, Doshi K, colman RW: Expression of factor V on human umbilical vein endothelial cells is modulated by cell injury. Arteriosclerosis 6:196, 1986.
16. Groenewegen G, Buurman WA: Vascular endothelium cells present alloantigens to unprimed lymphocytes. Scand J Immunol 19:269, 1984.

2Tshell do it.

17. Hirschberg H, Bergh OJ, Thorsby E: Antigen-presenting properties of human vascular endothelial cells. J Exp Med 152:249, 1980.
18. Wagner CR, Vetto RM, Burger DR: The mechanism of antigen presentation by endothelial cells. Immunobiology 168:453, 1984.
19. Masuyama J, Minato N, Kano S: Mechanisms of lymphocyte adhesion to human vascular endothelial cells in culture. T lymphocyte adhesion to endothelial cells through endothelial HLA-DR antigens induced by gamma interferon. J Clin Invest 77:1596, 1986.
20. Folkman J: Angiogenesis: initiation and control. Ann NY Acad Sci 401:212, 1983.
21. Watson PG: Diseases of the sclera and episclera. In Tasman W, Jaeger EA (Eds): Duane's Clinical Ophthalmology, rev ed. Lippincott, Philadelphia, 1989, pp 13–17.
22. McCarthy JL: Episcleral nodules and erythema nodosum. Am J Ophthalmol 51:60, 1961.
23. Edström G, Osterlind G: Case of nodular rheumatic episcleritis. Acta Ophthalmol 26:1, 1948.
24. Mundy WL, Howard RM, Stillman PM, Bevans M: Cortisone therapy in the case of rheumatoid nodules of the eye in rheumatoid arthritis. Arch Ophthalmol 45:531, 1951.
25. Fienberg R, Colpoys FL: Involution of rheumatoid nodules treated with cortisone and of non-treated rheumatoid nodules. Am J Pathol 27:925, 1951.
26. Ferry AP: Histopathology of rheumatoid episcleral nodules, an extra-articular manifestation of rheumatoid arthritis. Arch Ophthalmol 82:77, 1969.
27. Young RD, Watson PG: Microscopical studies of necrotising scleritis. I. Cellular aspects. Br J Ophthalmol 68:770, 1984.
28. Fong LP, Sainz de la Maza M, Rice BA, Foster CS: Immunopathology of scleritis. Ophthalmology 98:472, 1991.
29. Sevel D: Necrogranulomatous scleritis. Am J Ophthalmol 64:1125, 1967.
30. Rao NA, Marak GE, Hydayat AA: Necrotizing scleritis. A clinicopathologic study of 41 cases. Ophthalmology 92:1542, 1985.
31. Hatsuda T, Tanaka J: Bilateral necrotizing scleritis. Am J Ophthalmol 86:710, 1978.
32. Hogan MJ, Zimmerman LE: Ophthalmic Pathology. W.B. Saunders, Philadelphia, 1962, pp 337–339.
33. Sainz de la Maza M, Tauber J, Foster CS: Scleral grafting for necrotizing scleritis. Ophthalmology 96:306, 1989.
34. Sellers A, Murphy G: Collagenolytic enzymes and their naturally occurring inhibitors. In Hall DA, Jackson DS (Eds): International Review of Connective Tissue Research, Vol 9. Academic Press, New York, 1981, p 151.
35. Young RD, Watson PG: Microscopical studies of necrotising scleritis. II. Collagen degradation in the scleral stroma. Br J Ophthalmol 68:781, 1984.
36. Watson PG, Young RD: Changes at the periphery of a lesion in necrotising scleritis: anterior segment fluorescein angiography correlated with electron microscopy. Br J Ophthalmol 69:656, 1985.
37. Young RD, Powell J, Watson PG: Ultrastructural changes in scleral proteoglycans precede destruction of the collagen fibril matrix in necrotizing scleritis. Histopathology 12:75, 1988.
38. Montes GS, Bezerra MSF, Junqueira LCU: Collagen distribution in tissues. In Ruggeri A, Motta PM (Eds): Ultrastructure of the Connective Tissue Matrix. Martinius Nijhoff, Boston, 1984, Chap 3.
39. Watson PG: Doyne Memorial Lecture, 1982. The nature and the treatment of scleral inflammation. Trans Ophthalmol Soc UK 102:257, 1982.
40. Sainz de la Maza M, Foster CS: Necrotizing scleritis after ocular surgery. A clinicopathologic study. Ophthalmology 98:1720, 1991.
41. Bloomfield SE, Becker CG, Christian CL, Nauheim JS: Bilateral necrotizing scleritis with marginal corneal ulceration after cataract surgery in a patient with vasculitis. Br J Ophthalmol 64:170, 1980.
42. Calthorpe CM, Watson PG, McCartney ACE: Posterior scleritis: a clinical and histopathological survey. Eye 2:267, 1988.
43. Wilhelmus KR, Watson PG, Vasavada AR: Uveitis associated with scleritis. Trans Ophthalmol Soc UK 101:351, 1981.
44. Frayer WC: The histopathology of perilimbal ulceration in Wegener's granulomatosis. Arch Ophthalmol 64:58, 1960.
45. Wilhelmus KR, Grierson I, Watson PG: Histopathologic and clinical associations of scleritis and glaucoma. Am J Ophthalmol 91:697, 1981.
46. Bertelsen TI: Acute sclerotenonitis and ocular myositis complicated by papillitis, retinal detachment and glaucoma. Acta Ophthalmol 38:136, 1960.
47. Fraunfelder FT, Watson PG: Evaluation of eyes enucleated for scleritis. Br J Ophthalmol 60:227, 1976.
48. Fauci AS, Haynes BF, Katz P: The spectrum of vasculitis: clinical, pathologic, immunologic,

5. Pathology in Scleritis: The Massachusetts Eye and Ear Infirmary Experience

and therapeutic considerations. Ann Intern Med 89:660, 1978.

49. McCluskey RT, Fienberg R: Vasculitis in primary vasculitides, granulomatoses, and connective tissue diseases. Hum Pathol 14:305, 1983.

50. Moskowitz RW, Baggenstonss AH, Slocumb CH: Histopathologic classification of periarteritis nodosa: a study of 56 cases confirmed at necropsy. Proc Staff Meet Mayo Clin 38: 345, 1963.

51. Zeek PM: Periarteritis nodosa and other forms of necrotizing angiitis. N Engl J Med 248:764, 1953.

52. Cohen RD, Conn DL, Ilstrup DM: Clinical features, prognosis, and response to treatment in polyarteritis. Mayo Clin Proc 55:146, 1980.

53. Cogan DG: Corneoscleral lesions in periarteritis nodosa and Wegener's granulomatosis. Trans Am Acad Ophthalmol 53:321, 1955.

54. Patalamo VJ, Sommers SC: Biopsy diagnosis of periarteritis nodosa. Arch Pathol 72:1, 1961.

55. Goar EL, Smith LS: Polyarteritis nodosa of the eye. Am J Ophthalmol 35:1619, 1952.

56. Goldstein I, Wexler D: The ocular pathology of periarteritis nodosa. Arch Ophthalmol 2:288, 1929.

57. Helpern M, Trubeck M: Necrotizing arteritis and subacute glomerulonephritis in gonococcic endocarditis. Arch Pathol 15:35, 1933.

58. Boeck J: Ocular changes in periarteritis nodosa. Am J Ophthalmol 42:567, 1956.

59. Sheehan B, Harriman DG, Bradshaw JP: Polyarteritis nodosa with ophthalmic and neurological complications. Arch Ophthalmol 60: 537, 1958.

60. Diaz-Perez JL, Winkelmann RK: Cutaneous periarteritis nodosa. Arch Dermatol 110:407, 1974.

61. Sack M, Cassidy JT, Bole GG: Prognostic factors in polyarteritis. J Rheumatol 2:411, 1975.

62. Dyck PJ, Conn DL, Okazaki H: Necrotizing angiopathic neuropathy: three-dimensional morphology of fiber degeneration related to sites of occluded vessels. Mayo Clin Proc 47:461, 1972.

63. Churg J, Strauss L: Allergic granulomatosis, allergic angiitis, and periarteritis nodosa. Am J Pathol 27:277, 1951.

64. Dicken CH, Winkelmann RK: The Churg–Strauss granuloma: cutaneous, necrotizing, palisading granuloma in vasculitis syndromes. Arch Pathol Lab Med 102:576, 1978.

65. Strauss L, Churg J, Zak FG: Cutaneous lesions of allergic granulomatosis. A histopathologic study. J Invest Dermatol 17:349, 1951.

66. Crotty CP, Deremee RA, Winkelmann RK: Cutaneous clinicopathologic correlation of allergic granulomatosis. J Am Acad Dermatol 5:571, 1981.

67. Chumbley LC, Harrison EG Jr, Deremee RA: Allergic granulomatosis and angiitis (Churg–Strauss syndrome). Report and analysis of 30 cases. Mayo Clin Proc 52:477, 1977.

68. Lanham JG, Elkon KB, Pusey CD, Huges GR: Systemic vasculitis with asthma and eosinophilia: a clinical approach to the Churg–Strauss syndrome. Medicine (Baltimore) 63:65, 1984.

69. Cury D, Breakey AS, Payne BF: Allergic granulomatous angiitis associated with uveoscleritis and papilledema. Arch Ophthalmol 55:261, 1950.

70. Nissim F, Von der Valde J, Czernobilsky B: A limited form of Churg–Strauss syndrome. Arch Pathol Lab Med 106:305, 1982.

71. Klinger H: Grenzformen der Periarteritis nodosa. Frankfurt Z Pathol 42:455, 1931.

72. Wegener F: Über generalisierte, septische Gefäserkrankungen. Verh Dtsch Ges Pathol 29:202, 1936.

73. Wegener F: Über eine eigenartige rhinogene Granulomatose mit besonderer Beteiligung des Arteriensystems und der Nieren. Beitr Pathol Anat Allg Pathol 102:36, 1939.

74. Godman GC, Churg J: Wegener's granulomatosis: pathology and review of the literature. Arch Pathol 58:533, 1954.

75. Fauci AS, Wolff SM: Wegener's granulomatosis: studies in eighteen patients and a review of the literature. Medicine (Baltimore) 52:535, 1973.

76. Wolff SM, Fauci AS, Horn RG, Dale DC: Wegener's granulomatosis. Ann Intern Med 81:513, 1974.

77. Carrington CB, Leibow AA: Limited forms of angiitis and granulomatosis of Wegener's type. Am J Med 41:497, 1966.

78. Niffenegger JH, Jakobiec FA, Raizman MB, Foster CS: Pathologic diagnosis of very limited (ocular or orbital) Wegener's granulomatosis (in press).

79. Walton EW: Giant cell granuloma of the respiratory tract (Wegener's granulomatosis). Br Med J 2:265, 1958.

80. Fahey J, Leonard E, Churg J, et al.: Wegener's granulomatosis. Am J Med 17:168, 1973.

81. Haynes BF, Fishman ML, Fauci AS, Wolff SM: The ocular manifestations of Wegener's granulomatosis. Fifteen years' experience and review of the literature. Am J Med 63:131, 1977.

82. Fauci AS, Haynes BF, Katz P, Wolff SM: Wegener's granulomatosis: prospective clinical and therapeutic experience with 85 patients over 21 years. Ann Intern Med 98:76, 1983.

83. Spalton DJ, Graham EM, Page NGR, Sanders MD: Ocular changes in limited forms of Wegener's granulomatosis. Br J Ophthalmol 65:553, 1981.

84. Bullen CL, Liesegang TJ, McDonald TJ, DeRemee RA: Ocular complications of Wegener's granulomatosis. Ophthalmology 90:279, 1983.

85. Cutler WM, Blatt IM: The ocular manifestations of lethal midline granuloma (Wegener's granulomatosis). Am J Ophthalmol 42:21, 1956.

86. Straatsma BR: Ocular manifestations of Wegener's granulomatosis. Am J Ophthalmol 44:789, 1957.

87. Coppeto JR, Yamase H, Monteiro MLR: Chronic ophthalmic Wegener's granulomatosis. J Clin Neuro-ophthalmol 5:17, 1985.

88. Brubacker R, Font T, Shepherd E: Granulomatous sclerouveitis. Regression of ocular lesions with cyclophosphamide and prednisone. Arch Ophthalmol 86:517, 1971.

89. Sacks RD, Stock EL, Crawford SE, Greenwald MJ, O'Grady RB: Scleritis and Wegener's granulomatosis in children. Am J Ophthalmol 111:430, 1991.

90. Wegener F: About the so-called Wegener's granulomatosis. Am J Med 19:829, 1955.

91. Boudes P: Purely granulomatous Wegener's granulomatosis: a new concept for an old disease. Semin Arthritis Rheum 19:365, 1990.

92. Hu CH, O'Laughlin S, Winkelmann RK: Cutaneous manifestations of Wegener's granulomatosis. Arch Dermatol 113:175, 1977.

93. Frayer WC: The histopathology of perilimbal ulceration in Wegener's granulomatosis. Arch Ophthalmol 64:58, 1960.

94. Foster CS, Yee M: Corneoscleral manifestations of Graves's disease, the acquired connective tissue disorders, and systemic vasculitis. Int Ophthalmol Clin 23(1):131, 1983.

95. Cohen-Tervaert JW, van der Woude FJ, Fauci AS, Ambrus JL, Velosa J, Keane WF, Meijers, van der Giessen M: Association between active Wegener's granulomatosis and anticytoplasmic antibodies. Arch Intern Med 149:2461, 1989.

96. Nölle B, Specks U, Lüdemann J, Rohrbach MS, DeRemee RA, Gross WL: Anticytoplasmic autoantibodies: their immunodiagnostic value in Wegener's granulomatosis. Ann Intern Med 111:28, 1989.

97. Soukiasian SH, Foster CS, Niles JL, Raizman MB: Diagnostic value of anti-neutrophil cytoplasmic antibodies (ANCA) in scleritis associated with Wegener's granulomatosis. Ophthalmology 99:125, 1992.

98. Kalina PH, Garrity JA, Herman DC, DcReemee RA, Specks U: Role of testing for anticytoplasmic autoantibodies in the differential diagnosis of scleritis and orbital pseudotumor. Mayo Clin Proc 65:1110, 1990.

99. Rodnan GP, Schumacher HR, Zavifler NJ: *Primer on the Rheumatic Diseases*, 8th ed. Arthritis Foundation, Atlanta, GA, 1983, p 38.

100. Sokoloff L: The pathophysiology of peripheral blood vessels in collagen diseases. In Orbison JL, Smith DE (Eds): *The Peripheral Blood Vessels*. Williams & Wilkins, Baltimore, 1963, p 297.

101. Nowoslawski A, Brzosko WJ: Immunopathology of rheumatoid arthritis. II. The rheumatoid nodule (the rheumatoid granuloma). Pathol Eur 2:302, 1967.

102. Harris ED Jr: A collagenolytic system produced by primary cultures of rheumatoid nodule tissue. J Clin Invest 51:2973, 1972.

103. Sevel D: Rheumatoid nodule of the sclera. Trans Ophthalmol Soc UK 85:357, 1965.

104. Abel T, Andrews B, Cunningham P, Brunner CM, Davis JS IV, Horwitz DA: Rheumatoid vasculitis: effect of cyclophosphamide on the clinical course and levels of circulating immune complexes. Ann Rheum Dis 93:407, 1980.

105. Mongan ES, Cass RM, Jacox RF, Vaughan JH: A study of the relation of seronegative and seropositive rheumatoid arthritis to each other and to necrotizing vasculitis. Am J Med 47:23, 1969.

106. Weinstein A, Peters K, Brown D, Bluestone R: Metabolism of the third component of complement (C3) in patients with rheumatoid arthritis. Arthritis Rheum 15:49, 1972.

107. Conn DL, McDuffie FC, Dyck PJ: Immunopathologic study of sural nerves in rheumatoid arthritis. Arthritis Rheum 15:135, 1972.

108. Weisman M, Zvaifler N: Cryoimmunoglobulinemia in rheumatoid arthritis. J Clin Invest 56:725, 1975.

109. Qismorio F, Beardmore T, Kaufman R, Mongan ES: IgG rheumatoid factor and anti-nuclear antibodies in rheumatoid vasculitis. Clin Exp Immunol 52:333, 1983.

110. Rapoport RJ, Kozin F, Mackel SE, Jordon RE: Cutaneous vascular immunofluorescence in rheumatoid arthritis. Correlation with circulating immune complexes and vasculitis. Am J Med 68:325, 1980.

111. Scott DGI, Bacon PA, Tribe CR: Systemic rheumatoid vasculitis: a clinical and laboratory study of 50 cases. Medicine 60:288, 1981.

112. Scott DGI, Bacon PA, Allen C, Elson CJ, Wallington T: IgG rheumatoid factor, complement, and immune complexes in rheumatoid synovitis and vasculitis: comparative and serial studies during cytotoxic therapy. Clin Exp Immunol 43:54, 1981.

113. Sokoloff L, Bunim JJ: Vascular lesions in rheumatoid arthritis. J Chronic Dis 5:668, 1957.

114. Douglas W: The digital artery lesion of rheumatoid arthritis. Ann Rheum Dis 24:40, 1965.

115. Ferguson RH, Slocumb CH: Peripheral neuropathy in rheumatoid arthritis. Bull Rheum Dis 11:251, 1961.

116. Hunder GG, McDuffie FC: Hypocomplementemia in rheumatoid arthritis. Am J Med 54:461, 1973.

117. Collins DH: The subcutaneous nodule of rheumatoid arthritis. J Pathol Bacteriol 45:97, 1937.

118. Bennett GA, Zeller JW, Bauer W: Subcutaneous nodules of rheumatoid arthritis and rheumatic fever: a pathologic study. Arch Pathol 30:70, 1940.

119. Kaye BR, Kaye RL, Bobrove A: Rheumatoid nodules. Review of the spectrum of associated conditions and proposal of a new classification, with a report of four seronegative cases. Am Rheum Dis 23:345, 1964.

120. Swezey RL: Myocardial infarction due to rheumatoid arteritis. JAMA 199:191, 1967.

121. Cobb S, Anderson F, Baurer W: Length of life and cause of death in rheumatoid arthritis. N Engl J Med 249:553, 1953.

122. Jayson MI, Jones DE: Scleritis and rheumatoid arthritis. Ann Rheum Dis 5:668, 1957.

123. Foster CS, Forstot SL, Wilson LA: Mortality rate in rheumatoid arthritis patients developing necrotizing scleritis or peripheral ulcerative keratitis. Ophthalmology 91:1253, 1984.

124. Pavan-Langston D: Varicella-zoster ophthalmicus. Int Ophthalmol Clin 15(4):171, 1975.

125. Ostler HB, Thygeson P: The ocular manifestations of herpes zoster, varicella, infectious mononucleosis, and cytomegalovirus disease. Surv Ophthalmol 21:148, 1976.

126. Hedges TR III, Albert DM: The progression of the ocular abnormalities of herpes zoster; histopathologic observations in nine cases. Ophthalmology 89:165, 1982.

127. Nanda M, Pflugfelder SC, Holland S: *Mycobacterium tuberculosis scleritis*. Am J Ophthalmol 108:736, 1989.

128. Tamesis RR, Foster CS: Ocular syphilis. Ophthalmology 97:1281, 1990.

129. Wilhelmus KR, Yokoyama CM: Syphilitic episcleritis and scleritis: Am J Ophthalmol 104:595, 1987.

130. Reynolds MG, Alfonso E: Infectious scleritis and keratoscleritis: management and outcome. Am J Ophthalmol 112:543, 1991.

131. Raber IM, Laibson PR, Kurz GH, Bernardino VB: *Pseudomonas* corneoscleral ulcers. Am J Ophthalmol 92:353, 1981.

132. Codère F, Brownstein S, Jackson WB: *Pseudomonas aeruginosa* scleritis. Am J Ophthalmol 91:706, 1981.

133. Alfonso E, Kenyon KR, Ormerod LD, Stevens R, Wagoner MD, Albert DM: *Pseudomonas* corneoscleritis. Am J Ophthalmol 103:90, 1987.

134. Farrell PLR, Smith RE: Bacterial corneoscleritis complicating pterygium excision. Am J Ophthalmol 107:515, 1989.

135. Altman AJ, Cohen EJ, Berger ST, Mondino BJ: Scleritis and *Streptococcus pneumoniae*. Cornea 10(4):341, 1991.

136. Friedman AH, Henkind P: Unusual causes of episcleritis. Trans Am Acad Ophthalmol Otolaryngol 78:890, 1974.

137. Stenson S, Brookner A, Rosenthal S: Bilateral endogenous necrotizing scleritis due to *Aspergillus oryzae*. Ann Ophthalmol 14:67, 1982.

138. Lindquist TD, Fritsche TR, Grutzmacher RD: Scleral ectasia secondary to *Acanthamoeba* keratitis. Cornea 9:74, 1990.

139. Margo CE, Hidayat AA, Polack F: Ciliary body granuloma simulating malignant melanoma after herpes zoster ophthalmicus. Cornea 1:147, 1982.

140. Esiri MM, Tomlinson AH: Herpes zoster: demonstration of virus in trigeminal nerve and ganglion by immunofluorescence and electron microscopy. J Neurol Sci 15:35, 1972.

141. Nagashima K, Nakazawa M, Endo H: Pathology of the human spinal ganglia in varicella-

zoster virus infection. Acta Neuropathol 33: 105, 1975.

142. Hasegawa T: Further electron microscopic observations of herpes zoster virus. Arch Dermatol 103:45, 1971.

143. Ruppenthal M: Changes in central nervous system in herpes zoster. Acta Neuropathol 52:59, 1980.

144. Pavan-Langston D, McCulley J: Herpes zoster dendritic keratitis. Arch Ophthalmol 89:25, 1973.

145. McCormick WF, Rodnitzky RL, Schochet SS Jr, McKee AP: Varicella-zoster encephalomyelitis: a morphologic and virologic study. Arch Neurol 21:559, 1969.

146. Hogan EL, Krigman MR: Herpes zoster myelitis: evidence for viral invasion of the spinal cord. Arch Neurol 21:559, 1969.

147. Ghatak NR, Zimmerman HM: Spinal ganglion in herpes zoster. A light and electron microscopic study. Arch Pathol 95:411, 1973.

148. Bastian FO, Rabson AS, Yee CL, Trankla TS: Herpesvirus varicellae. Isolated from human dorsal root ganglia. Arch Pathol 97:331, 1974.

149. Schwartz JN, Cashwell F, Hawkins HK, Klintworth GK: Necrotizing retinopathy with herpes zoster ophthalmicus: a light and electron microscopical study. Arch Pathol Lab Med 100:386, 1976.

150. Witmer R, Iwamoto T: Electron microscope observation of herpes-like particles in the iris. Arch Ophthalmol 79:331, 1968; and Witmer R: Personal communication, 1980.

151. Weller TH, Witton HM, Bell EJ: The etiologic agents of varicella and herpes zoster. Isolation, propagation, and cultural characteristics in vitro. J Exp Med 108:843, 1958.

152. Solomon AR, Rasmussen JE, Weiss JS: A comparison of the Tzanck smear and viral isolation in varicella and herpes zoster. Arch Dermatol 122:282, 1986.

153. Gold E: Serologic and virus-isolation studies of patients with varicella or herpes-zoster infection. N Engl J Med 274:181, 1966.

154. Lam MT, Pazin GJ, JA Armstrong, Ho M: Herpes simplex infection in acute myelogenous leukemia and other hematologic malignancies: a prospective study. Cancer 48:2168, 1981.

155. Leming PD, Martin SE, Zwelling LA: Atypical herpes simplex (HSV) infection in a patient with Hodgkin's disease. Cancer 54:3043, 1984.

156. Orton PW, Huff JC, Tonnesen MG, Weston WL: Detection of a herpes simplex viral antigen in skin lesions of erythema multiforme. Ann Int Med 101:48, 1984.

157. Foster CS, Fong LP, Azar D, Kenyon KR: Episodic conjunctival inflammation after Stevens–Johnson syndrome. Ophthalmology 95:453, 1988.

158. Glassroth J, Robins AG, Snider DE Jr: Tuberculosis in the 1980's. N Engl J Med 302:1441, 1980.

159. Donahue HC: Ophthalmologic experience in a tuberculosis sanatorium. Am J Ophthalmol 64:742, 1967.

160. Shumomura Y, Tader R, Yuam T: Ocular disorders in pulmonary tuberculosis. Folia Ophthalmol Jpn 30:1973, 1979.

161. Phillips S, Williams ML, Maiden SD: Chronic miliary tuberculosis. Am Rev Tuberculosis 62:549, 1950.

162. Bell GH: Report of a case of tuberculosis of the sclera of probable primary origin. Trans Am Ophthalmol Soc 13:787, 1914.

163. Sarda RP, Mehrotra AS, Asnani K: Nodular episcleritis (a proved case of tubercular origin). Indian J Ocular Pathol 3:24, 1969.

164. Swan KC: Some comtemporary concepts of scleral disease. Arch Ophthalmol 45:630, 1951.

165. Finnoff WC: Tuberculosis in etiology of acute iritis. Am J Ophthalmol 14:127, 1931.

166. Brini A, Quéré M, Achard M: Sclerite nodulaire nécrosante (presence de bacille de Koch). Bull Soc d'Ophtalmol France 7:822, 1953.

167. Andreani DG: Tuberculoma of the sclera. Giornale Italiano di Oftalmologia 7:506, 1954.

168. Walker C: Conglomerate tuberculosis of the iris with scleral perforation. Trans Ophthalmol Soc UK 86:169, 1966.

169. Wilner G, Nassar SA, Siket A, Azar HA: Fluorescent staining for mycobacteria in sarcoid and tuberculous granulomas. Am J Clin Pathol 51:584, 1969.

170. Evans JJ: Diffuse gummatous infiltration of scleral and episcleral tissues. Trans Ophthalmol Soc UK 25:188, 1905.

171. Trantas M: Bourrelet périkératique syphilitique. Arch d'Ophtalmol 31:320, 1911.

172. Bhaduri BN, Basu SK: Scleral gumma. Br J Ophthalmol 40:504, 1956.

173. Yobs AR, Brown, L, Hunter EF: Fluorescent antibody technique in early syphilis. Arch Pathol 77:220, 1964.

174. Tourville DR, Byrd LH, Kim DU, Zajd D, Lee I, Reichman LB, Baskin S: Treponemal antigen in immunopathogenesis of syphilitic glomerulonephritis. Am J Pathol 82:479, 1976.

175. Bansal RC, Cohn H, Fani K, Lynfield YL: Nephrotic syndrome and granulomatous hepatitis. Arch Dermatol 114:1228, 1978.

176. Beckett JH, Bigbee JW: Immunoperoxidase localization of *Treponema pallidum*. Arch Pathol 103:135, 1979.

6
Noninfectious Scleritis: The Massachusetts Eye and Ear Infirmary Experience

The intrinsic nature of scleritis poses an ultimate challenge to the skill of the managing ophthalmologist. The chronicity of the disease, its tendency to exacerbate and remit, its relationship with many ocular and systemic diseases, and its variable response to specific treatment combine to complicate management.

Scleritis may occur in association with a variety of noninfectious and infectious local and systemic disorders. Within the noninfectious universe, several types of diseases—immune mediated, dermatological, metabolic, foreign body induced, and chemical substance induced—can cause scleritis (Table 6.1).

Systemic immune-mediated diseases, particularly the vasculitides, are the most severe and destructive conditions that may involve sclera. The presence, the degree, and the nature of scleritis may correlate with the chronicity, severity, and activity of the systemic immune-mediated associated disease. For example, diffuse or nodular scleritis may progress to necrotizing scleritis in association with the development of a vasculitic process in collagen diseases such as rheumatoid arthritis or systemic lupus erythematosus; necrotizing scleritis may appear suddenly in association with primarily vasculitic diseases such as polyarteritis nodosa. Scleritis also correlates with the type of vasculitic involvement of the associated disease. For example, scleritis is frequently seen in association with vasculitic diseases that affect predominantly small- and medium-sized vessels such as rheumatoid arthritis, systemic lupus erythematosus, arthritis

and inflammatory bowel disease, Wegener's granulomatosis, or polyarteritis nodosa; scleritis is less commonly found in association with vasculitic diseases that affect predominantly large-sized arteries such as ankylosing spondylitis, Reiter's syndrome, or giant cell arteritis. In some cases, scleritis may antedate the onset of a potentially lethal systemic immune-mediated disease. Early diagnosis and subsequent therapy of the underlying disease may improve the ocular and life prognoses.

Dermatological and metabolic conditions may secondarily cause scleritis. Foreign bodies embedded in the sclera may excite a granulomatous inflammatory reaction, and scleral acid or alkali chemical injuries may lead to scleritis and subsequent collagen destruction.

The presence of scleritis, therefore, demands a thorough systemic and ocular evaluation to define any associated disease. A detailed past general and ocular history, exhaustive review of systems, standard physical examination, meticulous slit-lamp examination, and appropriate ancillary tests must be included as part of the diagnostic strategy for the patient with scleritis.

Ophthalmologists are not only "eye doctors." They are physicians who must consider the systemic manifestations of the patient and decide whether or not there is any interconnection between systemic and ocular findings. They must be competent enough to promptly diagnose and treat an underlying systemic disease that is associated with ocular inflammation such as scleritis. Ophthalmolo-

TABLE 6.1. Classification of noninfectious diseases associated with scleritis.

Associated with systemic immune-mediated diseases
  Vasculitides
    Primarily small- and medium-sized vessel vasculitic diseases
      Connective tissue diseases in which vasculitis may occur
        Adult rheumatoid arthritis
        Systemic lupus erythematosus
        Relapsing polychondritis
        Juvenile rheumatoid arthritis
        Sjögren's syndrome
        Dermatomyositis
      Inflammatory conditions in which vasculitis may occur
        Arthritis and inflammatory bowel disease
        Psoriatic arthritis
      Primarily vasculitic (and/or granulomatous) diseases
        Polyarteritis nodosa
        Behçet's disease
        Cogan's syndrome
        Allergic granulomatous angiitis (Churg–Strauss syndrome)
        Wegener's granulomatosis
        Schönlein–Henoch purpura
    Primarily large-sized vessel vasculitic diseases
      Inflammatory conditions in which vasculitis may occur
        Ankylosing spondylitis
        Reiter's syndrome
      Primarily vasculitic diseases
        Giant cell arteritis
        Takayasu's arteritis
  Miscellaneous
    Thyroid disorders
    Sarcoidosis
    Vogt-Koyanagi–Harada syndrome
    Sympathetic ophthalmia
    Atopy
Associated with dermatological diseases
  Rosacea
Associated with metabolic diseases
  Gout
Associated with foreign bodies
Associated with chemical injuries
Idiopathic

---

gists, therefore, must remain current with the systemic disorders that are associated with scleritis.

This chapter focuses on the systemic and ocular manifestations of the noninfectious diseases that may be associated with scleritis. Furthermore, it analyzes the presence of other ocular manifestations, occurring before, during, or after the onset of scleritis, that may be helpful in diagnosing the underlying systemic disease.

6.1. Systemic Immune-Mediated Disease-Associated Scleritis: Vasculitides

6.1.1. Adult Rheumatoid Arthritis

Rheumatoid arthritis (RA) is a chronic inflammatory systemic disease of unknown cause. Although the synovial membrane of the joints is the main target of damage, patients often

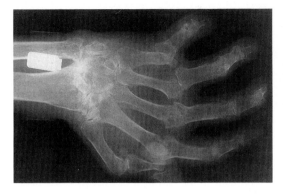

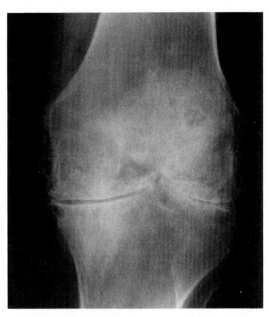

FIGURE 6.1. Hand and wrist X ray of patient with rheumatoid arthritis. Note the arthritic changes in the metacarpal bones, with both bony destruction and new bone formation and fusion of the articulation between the metacarpals. Note also the bony destruction of the distal intraphalangeal joints, the ulnar deviation, and the formation of the Z deformity.

FIGURE 6.2. X Ray of knee joint of a patient with rheumatoid arthritis. Note the hyperostosis and collapse of the joint space.

have involvement of extraarticular tissues such as eyes, skin, lungs, heart, and peripheral nerves.

6.1.1.1. Epidemiology

Definite RA has a worldwide prevalence of about 1% of the population (0.3 to 2.1%). Onset is most frequent in the fourth to fifth decade of life, women are three times more likely to be affected than men, and there is no racial predilection.[1]

6.1.1.2.2. Signs and Symptoms of Joint Involvement

Pain, stiffness, swelling, tenderness, and limitation of motion in the involved joints are the characteristic RA complaints, often associated with constitutional symptoms such as weakness, fatigue, anorexia, and weight loss. Morning stiffness lasting more than 1 h is indicative of joint inflammation; its duration can be used to assess disease activity. Metacarpophalangeal and proximal interphalangeal joints are the joints most commonly involved in RA, often leading to hyperextension of the proximal interphalangeal joints and flexion of the distal interphalangeal joints (swan-neck deformity), and radial deviation of the wrist and ulnar deviation of the fingers (Z deformity) (Fig. 6.1).[4–7] Wrist joint involvement can produce limitation of motion, deformity, and compression of the median nerve (carpal tunnel syndrome). Elbow and knee synovial inflammation and proliferation may lead to loss of full extension (Fig. 6.2). Ankle and foot arthritis may cause deformities (hallux valgus and plantar subluxation of metatarsal heads) and severe pain during ambulation (Fig. 6.3). Cervical spine osteochondral destruction may lead to atlantoaxial subluxation, which may cause paresthesias in the shoulders or arms during neck movement, pain radiating up into the occiput, and, less commonly, slowly progressive spastic quadriparesis, often with painless sensory loss of the hands. Other joints that

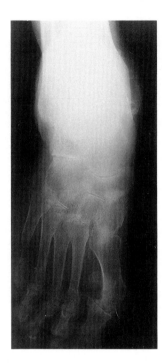

FIGURE 6.3. X Ray of foot and ankle of a patient with rheumatoid arthritis. Note the loss of joint spaces between the metatarsal bones.

TABLE 6.2. Extraarticular clinical features of rheumatoid arthritis.

Rheumatoid nodules
Vasculitis
  Digital arteritis
  Cutaneous ulceration
  Peripheral neuropathy
  Organ infarction
Pulmonary involvement
  Pleural disease
  Rheumatoid nodules
  Diffuse interstitial fibrosis
  Pneumoconiosis
  Infection
  Arteritis
Cardiac involvement
  Pericarditis
  Myocarditis
  Endocarditis
  Coronary arteritis
Neurological involvement
  Compression neuropathy
  Distal sensory neuropathy
  Distal sensorimotor neuropathy
Lymphadenopathy
Laryngeal involvement
  Cricoarytenoid joint involvement
  Vocal cord paralysis
  Vocal cord nodules
Felty's syndrome
Amyloidosis
Miscellaneous
  Gastrointestinal involvement
  Kidney involvement
  Bone involvement
Ocular involvement

may be affected are the temporomandibular, cricoarytenoid, ossicles of the ear, sternoclavicular, and manubriosternal joints. Hip involvement is uncommon. Thoracic and lumbar spine joint disease cannot be ascribed to rheumatoid arthritis.

6.1.1.2.3. Extraarticular Systemic Manifestations

Rheumatoid arthritis is a systemic disease rather than a localized inflammatory disorder of the joints. In general, patients with either high titers of rheumatoid factor or severe joint disease have a higher incidence of extraarticular manifestations than do patients without these findings.[6,7] Extraarticular manifestations in RA are listed in Table 6.2 and are briefly described here.

There is strong evidence to suggest that RA has a genetic basis; a high degree of association exists between *HLA-DR4* (subtypes *Dw4* and *Dw14*) and Caucasian RA patients, predominantly seropositive for rheumatoid factor (70% compared with 28% of control individuals); subtypes *Dw4* and *Dw14* are present in 50 and 35% of the patients, respectively.[2] Thus, *HLA-Dw4* is the major HLA gene accounting for susceptibility to RA.

6.1.1.2. Systemic Manifestations

6.1.1.2.1. Onset

In 55 to 70% of patients, RA begins with the insidious development of malaise, anorexia, fatigue, weakness, weight loss, and diffuse musculoskeletal pain.[3,4] Although asymmetrical involvement of peripheral joints may then appear, it gradually becomes symmetrical. In 8 to 15% of patients, RA begins with an acute onset of symptoms. A rapid development of polyarthritis may appear, accompanied by fever, splenomegaly, and lymphadenopathy. In 15 to 20% of patients, RA begins with an intermediate onset over a period of several weeks.

6.1.1.2.3.1. Tegument. Subcutaneous rheumatoid nodules occur in about 20 to 30% of patients with definite or classic RA. They also may (rarely) appear prior to the onset of the arthritis. They almost always occur in patients with rheumatoid factor, although without correlation with the titer.[8,9] Subcutaneous rheumatoid nodules are usually seen on the extensor surface of the forearms, the olecranon, the Achilles' tendons, the buttock, the fingertip pads, and other areas subjected to mechanical trauma and soft tissue stress. Nodules vary in consistency from a soft, completely mobile mass to a firm rubbery lesion attached to the subjacent periosteum. They also vary in size from a few millimeters up to 3 cm in diameter. Although nodules in patients with RA are almost always of rheumatoid etiology, other possible causes are trauma, tophi (gout),[10] xanthomatosis (type II hyperlipoproteinemia),[11] multiple myeloma (amyloidosis),[12,13] basal cell carcinoma,[14] granuloma annulare,[15] systemic lupus erythematosus,[16,17] rheumatic fever, and reticulohistiocytosis.[18] Nodules are asymptomatic, requiring no treatment, unless they are constantly subject to pressure (feet, hands), in which case erosion and ulceration may occur and may cause local, articular, or systemic infections. Excision of these nodules is at least of temporary benefit, but recurrence is common. Nodules may disappear or new nodule formation may cease in the course of gold salts or penicillamine therapy.

The presence of subcutaneous nodules has been associated with rheumatoid factor seropositivity and more severe erosive articular disease,[8,9,19] and with the extraarticular manifestations of RA, particularly rheumatoid vasculitis.[8,9,19–22] Patients with subcutaneous nodules have a poorer prognosis than do RA patients without rheumatoid nodules.[8,23,24]

6.1.1.2.3.2. Vessels. Rheumatoid vasculitis presents classically as (1) digital arteritis, a noninflammatory obliterative endarteritis ranging from splinter infarcts in the nailbeds to gangrene of the fingertips[25]; (2) cutaneous ulceration, an inflammatory infiltration with fibrinoid necrosis of the cutaneous venule walls on the lower legs, which clinically appears as palpable purpura or urticaria; (3) peripheral neuropathy, a mild distal sensory neuropathy or a severe sensorimotor neuropathy (mononeuritis multiplex), the latter characterized by severe arterial damage on nerve biopsy specimens[26]; or (4) organ infarction, an arteritis with marked inflammatory infiltration, fibrinoid necrosis, and thrombosis of both small- and medium-sized arteries of different organs such as lungs, heart, bowel, spleen, liver, pancreas, lymph nodes, and testis[27,28]; the kidney is rarely involved by vasculitis but often is compromised by amyloidosis or toxicity from therapy. An inflammatory microangiopathy is also the cause of some ocular diseases such as scleritis and peripheral ulcerative keratitis, and rheumatologists are beginning to recognize that the eye is an especially sensitive barometer for potentially lethal but occult rheumatoid vasculitis.[29]

Rheumatoid vasculitis usually occurs in patients whose RA has existed for more than 10 years and who have significant joint destruction and erosion, rheumatoid nodules, high levels of rheumatoid factor, anti-nuclear antibodies, and circulating immune complexes, and depressed complement levels.[30–32] It has been suggested that patients with rheumatoid vasculitis may have a genetic susceptibility, because 88% of them are *HLA-DRw4* positive.[30] The occurrence of vasculitis in a patient with rheumatoid arthritis should be cause for great concern, because it is often a sign of life-threatening lesions. The rapid rate of appearance of new areas of involvement indicates widespread vasculitic disease. Palpable purpura tends to subside most quickly. Digital arteritis is also self-limited, although these necrotic lesions last longer. Motor neuropathy, visceral infarctions, weight loss, renal impairment, and histological evidence of vasculitis on rectal biopsy contribute to a poor prognosis.[33,34] Patients with RA may develop widespread necrotizing lesions involving mediumsized arteries in a variety of sites, producing a condition similar to polyarteritis nodosa. Some of the clinical features of rheumatoid vasculitis are more extensively described as the involved organs are reviewed.

6.1.1.2.3.3. Lung.

Pleuropulmonary manifestations (Fig. 6.4) include (1) pleural disease, (2) rheumatoid nodules, (3) diffuse interstitial fibrosis, (4) pneumoconiosis (Caplan's syndrome), (5) infections, and (6) arteritis.

Pleural involvement is found at autopsy in more than 40% of patients with RA, but clinical disease during life is seen less frequently.[35] Although pleural disease in RA most commonly appears within 5 years after joint involvement (50%), it can, however, occur years prior to (5%) or simultaneously with (20%) the onset of clinical synovitis. The presence of pleural disease with or without effusion does not correlate with the severity of arthritis, but it does correlate with the presence of extraarticular lesions. Pleural effusion may be unilateral or bilateral and may be associated with nodules or fibrosis. Respiratory symptoms include dyspnea, chest pain, cough, and sometimes fever. The fluid is an exudate containing leukocytes, predominantly lymphocytes, elevated lactate dehydrogenase levels, rheumatoid factor titers equal to or greater than those in serum, low complement levels, and low glucose concentrations. The latter, due to impaired transport of glucose into the pleural cavity,[36] helps to differentiate this effusion from other nonpurulent effusions, because the only other condition that usually has low glucose concentrations in pleural fluid is sepsis, particularly tuberculosis. Tuberculosis may be excluded after a needle biopsy. Pleural disease usually improves spontaneously within a few months, although in some patients persistent effusion may lead to pleural thickening or empyema.

Parenchymal pulmonary rheumatoid nodules may occur at any time after the onset of arthritis and occasionally may antedate or appear simultaneously with joint involvement.[37] Patients with intrapulmonary nodules have more subcutaneous nodules and other extraarticular manifestations, particularly cardiac lesions. Whether single or in clusters, they are usually asymptomatic. Differential diagnosis with malignancy, tuberculosis, and fungal infection may require needle biopsy. Nodules may cavitate, leading to a bronchopleural fistula.[38] Effective therapy of rheumatoid arthritis may clear or diminish the nodules.

Diffuse interstitial fibrosis may follow (70%), precede (11%), or occur simultaneously (18%) with the onset of arthritis.[39] Although patients with diffuse interstitial fibrosis have a high incidence of associated subcutaneous nodules, the arthritis does not seem to be more severe. The most common symptoms are dyspnea and cough, but chest pain, fever, and hemoptysis occur occasionally. Ten percent of patients are asymptomatic at the time of diagnosis. The most common signs are basal crepitations,

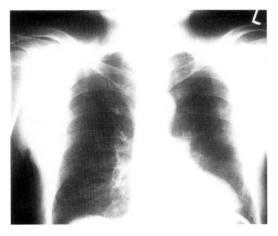

FIGURE 6.4. Chest X ray of patient with rheumatoid arthritis.

finger clubbing, and, in severe cases, cyanosis. Differential diagnosis includes Hamman–Rich syndrome, hypersensitivity pneumonitis, and sarcoidosis. The finding of intrapulmonary nodules or low glucose levels in pleural effusions helps to diagnose this fibrosis as being part of rheumatoid arthritis. Radiographic changes show a bilateral reticular or reticulonodular honeycomb-type pattern[40–42] and respiratory function tests demonstrate a restrictive defect with abnormal diffusing capacity.[43] Although pulmonary insufficiency and even death may occur, diffuse pulmonary fibrosis ascribed to RA is usually slowly progressive and has a better prognosis than idiopathic diffuse pulmonary fibrosis. The treatment of choice is effective control of the rheumatoid synovitis.

Rheumatoid pneumoconiosis was initially described by Caplan[44] as a nodular lung disease among coal miners with RA, but it can also appear in chalk, asbestos, gold, and silica workers.[45,46] Rheumatoid arthritis and pneumoconiosis are synergistic and may produce a violent fibroblastic reaction to the dust, leading to multiple peripheral nodules greater than 1 cm in diameter, often with cavitation. Nodular lung disease appears in a small number of patients with RA and pneumoconiosis, usually after the onset of arthritis; the nodules rarely may antedate the articular disease.[47] The prognosis depends on the severity of the pneumoconiosis. Removal from exposure to inhalants and control of the arthritis are the treatments of choice.

Pulmonary infections, including bronchiectasis, acute bronchitis, chronic bronchitis, and pneumonia are more common in patients with RA.[48] Interestingly, most of the pulmonary infections usually antedate the onset of arthritis by many years.

Pulmonary arteritis, although rare, may cause pulmonary hypertension. It is occasionally associated with digital arteritis.

6.1.1.2.3.4. Heart. Postmortem studies show that 30 to 50% of patients with classic RA have cardiac manifestations.[49–53] Cardiac involvement can be classified as follows: (1) pericarditis, (2) myocarditis, (3) endocarditis (valvular), and (4) coronary arteritis.

Pericarditis is the most common cardiac manifestation of RA. Although necropsy studies show that 40% of patients with RA have evidence of pericarditis, clinical disease is diagnosed only in 10%.[54] However, if echocardiographic studies are performed, the incidence of clinical pericarditis (15 to 40%) closely approximates the incidence of pericarditis in necropsy studies.[55,56] Patients with pericarditis in RA usually show a high incidence of subcutaneous nodules (up to 47%), anemia, and high sedimentation rates.[57,58] The presence of pericarditis does not correlate with the duration of the arthritis; in fact, it can precede the onset of arthritis.[58] Pericardial rheumatoid nodules are rarely found. The majority of patients are asymptomatic but pain and congestive heart failure may occur. Signs consist of pericardial friction or paradoxical pulse. Pericardial fluid is an exudate containing leukocytes, rheumatoid factor titers equal to or greater than those in serum, high lactate dehydrogenase, low complement, low glucose, immune complexes, lymphokines (migration inhibition factor), and cholesterol crystals. Symptomatic patients usually respond to salicylates or nonsteroidal antiinflammatory drugs but if pain is refractory or systemic vasculitis is present, steroids should be used. In case of severe systemic vasculitis, cytotoxic agents are recommended.

Myocarditis in RA can be interstitial or granulomatous. Interstitial myocarditis, occurring in 4 to 30% of RA patients at autopsy, is usually a focal inflammation of the myocardium, although occasionally a diffuse, necrotizing process may occur.[49,50,59–61] It is characterized microscopically by focal or diffuse inflammatory infiltration of plasma cells, lymphocytes, and histiocytes. Focal interstitial myocarditis is clinically silent, but diffuse interstitial myocarditis may show congestive heart failure, conduction abnormalities, and pulmonic and systemic embolizations.

Granulomatous myocarditis, occurring in 5% of RA patients at autopsy, is characterized by the presence of grayish yellow nodules that histologically resemble subcutaneous rheumatoid nodules.[50,62] Patients are usually asymptomatic unless the nodules are located in critical areas such as the conduction system, where they can cause conduction abnormalities.[63]

Endocarditis (valvular) is found in 30 to 40% of RA patients at autopsy.[64–66] The mitral, aortic, tricuspid, and pulmonic valves are affected, in decreasing order of frequency.[67] The entire valve may be involved by a nonspecific inflammation, resulting in either stenosis or insufficiency. In a specific, granulomatous inflammation, inflammatory nodules involve the central core of the leaflet, leaving a small rim of uninvolved tissue in the periphery. The nodules can spread to involve the base of the aorta in severe cases.[68] These nodules, seen in 5 to 15% of cases, are histologically identical to subcutaneous nodules.[69]

Coronary arteritis is found in 15 to 20% of patients with RA at autopsy.[26] It is usually clinically silent, but anginal chest pain or myocardial infarction may occasionally occur, particularly in patients with severe systemic vasculitis or in young patients without atherosclerotic coronary artery disease.[70–72]

6.1.1.2.3.5. Nervous System.

Although both the central and peripheral nervous system can be damaged in RA, peripheral neurological involvement is much more common. The major causes of peripheral neuropathy in RA include (1) compression neuropathy (carpal tunnel syndrome), and (2) angiopathic neuropathy (distal sensory neuropathy and distal sensorimotor neuropathy).

Compression neuropathy, specifically a carpal tunnel syndrome, may be the presenting feature of RA or may occur at any time during the clinical course. The proliferative synovitis compresses the nerve within a bony canal. The diagnosis is suggested by the characteristic symptoms such as paresthesias in the area of the median nerve distribution and nocturnal pain in the arm or hand, and is confirmed by nerve conduction studies. However, electrodiagnostic abnormalities showing compression of the median nerve are relatively common in asymptomatic patients with RA. Ulnar, radial, sciatic, or posterior tibial (tarsal tunnel syndrome) nerve entrapments also may occur in RA. Although entrapment neuropathies usually are related to the severity of arthritis, they do not correlate with the duration of RA, rheumatoid factor, sex, acute-phase reactant levels, or other extraarticular features.

Angiopathic neuropathy is the result of axonal degeneration of nerve fibers, caused by occlusion of vasa nervorum and resultant ischemia of the peripheral nerve. The milder form is distal sensory neuropathy, which may precede the onset of arthritis, although it more often appears many years after the joint disease.[73] The clinical picture is characterized by symmetrical burning, numbness, or tingling of lower limbs with distal loss of vibration sense and proprioception; occasionally, the upper limbs are involved in a stocking-glove distribution.[74,75] There is usually a concomitant motor deficit that can be detected by electromyogram, but this is often not clinically demonstrable, particularly in patients with joint pain or deformity.[76] Muscle wasting, weakness, and loss of tendon reflexes are frequently present. Distal sensory neuropathy is a manifestation seen in vasculitis that may occur alone, without widespread vascular involvement. The prognosis is good with effective treatment of RA, although in a small number of cases the disorder progresses to the more ominous sensorimotor neuropathy.

Less common but more severe is distal sensorimotor neuropathy, which may present as an abrupt painful asymmetric multiple mononeuropathy (mononeuritis multiplex) characterized initially by severe pain and paresthesias of individual peripheral nerves followed hours to days later by a wristdrop, a footdrop, or motor weakness in another involved peripheral nerve. Asymmetric multiple mononeuropathy may progress to symmetric polyneuropathy. Electromyogram abnormalities corroborate the clinical findings, and in questionable cases biopsy of an involved sural nerve will confirm the diagnosis. This type of neuropathy is seen in patients with long-standing rheumatoid arthritis (average duration, 10 years), severe joint deformities, rheumatoid nodules, anemia, anorexia, fever, high titers of rheumatoid factor, and low serum complement levels. Males are afflicted as commonly as females, unlike uncomplicated RA, in which there is a female preponderance. Patients with sensorimotor neuropathy frequently have skin vasculitic lesions such as nailfold infarcts, leg ulcers, and digital gangrene, and widespread underlying vasculitis that may extend to involve mesenteric, coronary, or cerebral arteries. Prognosis is poor, with a 42% mortality rate for patients with a sensorimotor neuropathy involving three or four extremities.[34] Treatment must include systemic immunosuppression.

6.1.1.2.3.6. Lymph Nodes. Asymptomatic enlarged, firm, and mobile lymph nodes are often found in patients with active synovitis.[77–79] The nodes most commonly involved are axillary, epitrochlear, and inguinal, and their presence does not correlate with erythrocyte sedimentation rate, C-reactive protein, anemia, or disease severity. Effective treatment of proliferative synovitis may improve or correct lymphadenopathy. Development of lymphoma occurs with greater frequency in RA patients who also have Sjögren's syndrome,[80] a disorder associated with increased risk for this neoplasm.[81]

6.1.1.2.3.7. Larynx. Laryngeal manifestations in RA include (1) cricoarytenoid joint involvement, (2) vocal cord paralysis, and (3) vocal cord nodules.

Cricoarytenoid joint involvement may be found in nearly 50% of RA cases at autopsy and approximately 25% of living patients with RA. Signs and symptoms may be subtle and include tenderness on palpation, hoarseness, tightness of the throat, difficulty in swallowing, and mild dyspnea. Laryngoscopy may show, in severe cases, edema of the cricoarytenoid joint and the vocal cords.

Vocal cord paralysis in patients with RA is secondary to neuropathy affecting intrinsic laryngeal muscles.

Vocal cord nodules may also appear in patients with RA. Signs and symptoms may resemble those of a tumor.

6.1.1.2.3.8. Felty's Syndrome. Felty's syndrome consists of RA, splenomegaly, and leukopenia.[82] It is most common in the fourth through the sixth decades of life and usually occurs after 10 years of arthritis. Patients with Felty's syndrome have more erosive and deforming articular disease, a more elevated erythrocyte sedimentation rate, higher rheumatoid factor titers, and more extraarticular manifestations than do other patients with RA.[83,84]

Extraarticular manifestations include subcutaneous nodules, leg ulcers, lymphadenopathy, pleuritis, and neuropathy. Patients with Felty's syndrome are more susceptible to infection than are other patients with RA.[85–88] Splenectomy and effective control of RA are the treatments of choice.[89,90]

6.1.1.2.3.9. Amyloidosis. Amyloidosis may be found in 20 to 60% of rheumatoid cases at autopsy but it is not commonly evident in living patients.[91,92] The main indicator is proteinuria due to the deposition of amyloid in the glomerulus. Other possible involved organs are the heart, liver, spleen, intestinal wall, and skin. Diagnosis is confirmed by Congo red staining of involved tissue (skin, rectal, and gingival tissues).[93,94] Effective suppression of RA is the treatment of choice.[95]

6.1.1.2.3.10. Miscellaneous. Specific hepatic lesions are uncommon in the early course of RA, although liver function tests yield mildly elevated results in almost half the patients; serum alkaline phosphatase, 5′-nucleotidase, and γ-glutamyl transpeptidase are the enzymes usually found to be elevated.[96] γ-Glutamyl transpeptidase increases with arthritis activity in a way similar to the C-reactive protein. Nonspecific hepatomegaly is present in 10 to 20% of patients.[97]

Although gastrointestinal involvement is unlikely in uncomplicated RA, infarction, hemorrhage, or perforation of the bowel may occur in rheumatoid vasculitis.[98,99] Vasculitis also may involve pancreatic or peritoneal vessels. Gastric ulcers are common in patients with RA but they are mostly caused by nonsteroidal antiinflammatory drugs used in treating the disease.[100]

Direct kidney involvement is rare in RA but amyloidosis and toxicity from therapy may be indirect causes of renal disease.[99–103] Amyloid deposits may lead to renal failure. Drugs that may cause nephritis are phenacetin, salicylates, D-penicillamine, and gold salts.[104,105]

Bone involvement, such as osteoporosis, correlates with the duration of RA, age and sex of the patient, and use of steroids. Osteomalacia also may occur, but only 10 or more years after the onset of arthritis.[106]

6.1.1.3. Ocular Manifestations

Although keratoconjunctivitis sicca is the most common ocular manifestation in adult RA, scleritis and peripheral keratitis are the most severe. Other ocular manifestations in RA include episcleritis and ocular motility disturbances. Some of peripheral keratitis and ocular motility disturbances are caused by contiguous scleritis. Uveitis, glaucoma, and funduscopic changes are rarely seen in RA except as an extension of scleral inflammation.

6.1.1.3.1 Keratoconjunctivitis Sicca

Keratoconjunctivitis sicca (KCS) or dry eye syndrome appears in 11 to 35% of patients with RA, with women being affected far more often than men (9:1).[107–110] It is bilateral and onset usually occurs in the fourth to fifth decade. Keratoconjunctivitis sicca results from decreased tear secretion by the main and accessory lacrimal glands, leading to reduction of the middle or aqueous layer of the tear film; occasionally, the outermost or oily layer and the innermost or mucoid layer also are abnormal. Characteristic complaints are itching, burning, foreign body sensation, and (less often) photophobia, inability to form tears, or excess tearing due to irritation from dryness; the condition occasionally may be asymptomatic.[111] Characteristic signs are slight redness, papillary conjunctivitis, decreased tear break-up time, mucous debris in the conjunctival sac, mucous debris and desquamated epithelial cells attached to the cornea (filamen-

tary keratitis), and punctate gray corneal opacities (superficial punctate keratitis). Specific diagnostic tests include 1% rose bengal dye, which attaches to abnormal corneal and conjunctival epithelial cells (Fig. 6.5; see color insert) (van Bijsterveld scoring system: staining score of 3 or more on a scale from 0 to 3 in each of three zones of the eye—medial, corneal, and lateral—is considered abnormal), and Shirmer's tear test, which quantitates physiological tear secretion (5 mm or less of filter paper wetting in 5 min indicates low tear secretion). Chronic drying may lead to recurrent blepharitis, conjunctivitis, and corneal ulceration. The severity of KCS symptoms correlates with age and duration of RA, but does not correlate with the severity of the arthritis.[107] When dryness of the mouth (xerostomia) is associated with KCS in patients with a connective tissue disease (usually RA), the resultant triad is a multisystem autoimmune disorder known as Sjögren's syndrome.[112,113] The presence of either xerostomia or KCS with a connective tissue disease is still accepted as sufficient.

Sjögren's syndrome occurs more often in patients with rheumatoid scleritis compared with its incidence in the general rheumatoid population.[114] Keratoconjunctivitis sicca was present in 4 of our 32 patients with rheumatoid scleritis (12.5%); of those, 2 developed sterile corneal ulcers (3 eyes). Interestingly, two of the four patients (one with bilateral corneal ulcers) had non-Hodgkin's lymphomas, a neoplasm that appears to be more frequent in patients with RA and Sjögren's syndrome.[80]

Use of artificial tear substitutes and punctal occlusion, initially with punctal plugs and then permanently with cautery, may be necessary adjunctive measures. Lid scrubs and hot compresses with or without systemic tetracyclines are indicated if there is meibomian gland dysfunction or blepharitis associated. The use of slow-release artificial tear inserts without preservatives may provide continuous lubrication in the presence of some moisture. Occasionally, partial tarsorraphy may be required to decrease evaporation. In addition to its immunosuppressive effects, cyclosporine A (CsA) may activate regulatory prolactin receptors in lacrimal tissue by binding to the cytosolic binding protein cyclophilin (a natural ligand of prolactin).[115,116] Prolactin, which is found in lacrimal acini, may be important in tear regulation.[117] Although additional experimentation is needed, oral CsA (3 to 5 mg/kg per day) alone or in combination with fluorocortolone has been shown to increase tear flow in patients with Sjögren's syndrome.[118,119] Topical CsA also has increased lacrimation in dogs with spontaneous KCS.[120] A prospective, randomized, double-masked, multicenter clinical trial is currently in progress to assess the safety and comparative efficacy of three concentrations of topical CsA ointment versus placebo in patients with KCS refractory to conventional therapy.

6.1.1.3.2. Scleritis

Rheumatoid arthritis is by far the most common systemic condition associated with scleritis. The reported incidence of RA in patients with scleritis ranges from 10 to 33% (Table 6.3).[114,121–125] Conversely, the reported incidence of scleritis in patients with RA ranges from 0.15 to 6.3%.[114] Rheumatoid scleritis is most common in the sixth decade of life, affects women more frequently than men, and

is often bilateral.[114,124,126] Diffuse anterior scleritis is the most frequent type of scleritis in patients with RA[114,124]; however, cases of scleromalacia perforans anterior scleritis in which a systemic diagnosis can be ascribed, are almost exclusively due to RA.[122] Although posterior rheumatoid scleritis is uncommon, it is usually accompanied by diffuse anterior scleritis.[114] In our own series of 172 patients with scleritis, 32 patients had RA (18.6%) (Table 6.4). The mean age of our patients was 61 years (range, 31 to 80 years) and the scleritis was more common in women than in men (18 females and 14 males). The predominance of women with rheumatoid scleritis (1.3:1) was lower than the predominance of women with scleritis without RA (1.6:1), and lower than the predominance of women with RA without scleritis (3:1). Seventeen patients (53%) had bilateral scleritis. Diffuse anterior scleritis (34%) and necrotizing anterior scleritis (34%) were the types most frequently encountered. The percentage of necrotizing scleritis in our RA population was higher than that reported by other authors,[114,122] probably because of the highly selected referral patient characteristics of our Immunology Service, thus biasing the results. All four patients in our study who had scleromalacia perforans with associated systemic disease had RA. The only case of

TABLE 6.3. Incidence of rheumatoid arthritis in episcleritis and scleritis.

Authors	Date of study	No. of episcleritis patients	No. of rheumatoid arthritis patients	Percentage
Lyne and Pitkeathley[121]	1968	55	3	5.5
McGavin et al.[114]	1976	35	2	5.7
Watson and Hayreh[122]	1976	159	7	4.4
Present study	1992	94	3	3.2
		No. of scleritis patients		
Lyne and Pitkeathley[121]	1968	31	9	29.0
McGavin et al.[114]	1976	27	9	33.3
Watson and Hayreh[122]	1976	207	21	10.1
Tuft and Watson[123]	1991	290	30	10.3
Present study	1992	172	32	18.6

TABLE 6.4. Incidence of rheumatoid arthritis in episcleritis and scleritis subtypes.

Diagnosis[a]	Incidence of rheumatoid arthritis		Diagnosis (subtype)	Incidence of rheumatoid arthritis by subtype	
	No. (%) of patients	No. of eyes		No. (%) of patients	No. of eyes
Episcleritis (n = 94)	3 (3.19)	3	Simple	1 (33.33)	1
			Nodular	2 (66.67)	2
Scleritis (n = 172)	32 (18.60)	49	Diffuse	11 (34.37)	15
Total:	35 (13.16)	52	Nodular	5 (15.62)	6
			Necrotizing	11 (34.37)	18
			Scleromalacia	4 (12.51)	8
			Posterior	1 (3.13)	2

[a] Total number of patients.

rheumatoid posterior scleritis had concomitant diffuse anterior scleral involvement.

Although scleritis may be the initial sign of rheumatoid disease,[125,126] it usually presents in patients with long-standing RA, usually 13 or 14 years after the onset of arthritis.[114,127] Patients with rheumatoid scleritis have more advanced joint disease and more extraarticular manifestations than do rheumatoid patients without scleritis.[114,121,125,127,128] Many of the extraarticular manifestations reflect an underlying rheumatoid vasculitis.[129] Although subcutaneous nodules appear in 20 to 30% of patients with classic RA, their presence increases to 50% in patients with rheumatoid scleritis.[114] Pulmonary disorders such as pleural effusion, rheumatoid nodules of lung, and pneumonia are more commonly present in patients with rheumatoid scleritis than in rheumatoid patients without scleritis.[114] Cardiac manifestations such as pericarditis,[114,129,130] valvular disease,[114,125,126] conduction abnormalities,[114] and myocardial infarction[114,129] have been described in association with rheumatoid scleritis. Myocardial ischemia is also more frequent in rheumatoid patients with scleritis.[114] Peripheral neuropathies, skin ulcers, and amyloidosis also have been described in rheumatoid patients with scleritis.[114,129]

Exacerbation of scleritis often occurs at times of increased activity of RA,[121,125,127,131,132] and a progression from diffuse or nodular scleritis

to necrotizing scleritis may indicate the onset of rheumatoid vasculitis elsewhere in the body.[122] Necrotizing scleritis also may appear after surgical trauma to the sclera. The mean time of presentation of scleritis in our series of 32 patients with rheumatoid scleritis was 16 years after the onset of arthritis. In two cases, scleritis was the initial manifestation whose study led to the diagnosis of rheumatoid arthritis. Most patients with rheumatoid scleritis, especially those with necrotizing scleritis, had deforming joint disease and extraarticular RA manifestations. The most frequent extraarticular manifestations were subcutaneous nodules and skin vasculitic lesions. Other extraarticular manifestations included (1) pulmonary disorders such as pleural effusion, pneumonia, and rheumatoid nodules of the lung, (2) cardiac abnormalities such as conduction defects, mitral valvular disease, myocardial infarction, and pericarditis, (3) neurological involvement such as carpal tunnel syndrome, sensory neuropathy, and sensorimotor neuropathy, (4) lymphadenopathy and non-Hodgkin's lymphoma, (5) amyloidosis, (6) mild elevation of liver function tests, (7) gastrointestinal disorders such as gastroduodenal ulcers in patients who had received long-term steroidal or nonsteroidal therapy, (8) kidney involvement secondary to gold treatment, and (9) bone abnormalities such as osteoporosis in patients who had received long-term steroidal therapy. Necrotizing scleritis appeared an average of 16 weeks after ocular surgery in four patients with RA.

The prognosis for life is poorer in patients with RA complicated by scleritis when compared with RA patients without scleritis.[114,122,125,127–129] Thirty-six to 45% of patients with rheumatoid scleritis will be dead within 3 years of the onset of scleritis. This compares to an 18% three-year mortality in patients with RA without scleritis.[114,127] Most causes of death are due to extraarticular RA vasculitic manifestations.[122,129] Necrotizing scleritis is the type of scleritis most predictive of these deaths.[122,129]

Because the presence of necrotizing scleritis in RA may indicate an underlying potentially lethal systemic vasculitis, it is essential to detect both the ocular and systemic conditions as early as possible, so that vigorous treatment can favorably alter not only the ocular but also the life prognosis in these patients.

Scleral inflammation in RA may extend to the adjacent structures and may cause keratitis; anterior uveitis; glaucoma; cataract, retinal, choroidal, and optic nerve changes; and motility disturbances. Some of these complications may affect visual acuity. In our series of 32 (49 eyes) patients with rheumatoid scleritis, a decrease in visual acuity (loss of vision equal or greater to two Snellen lines at the end of the follow-up period, or vision equal to or worse than 20/80 at the first examination) occurred in 19 patients (59%).

6.1.1.3.2.1. Keratitis. Corneal involvement associated with scleritis in patients with RA can be classified depending on whether or not thinning, infiltration, or ulceration of the cornea occurs. Peripheral corneal thinning, acute or sclerosing stromal keratitis, and peripheral ulcerative keratitis (PUK) are the most common corneal abnormalities associated with rheumatoid scleritis.

The reported incidence of keratitis associated with rheumatoid scleritis ranges from 36 to 43.5%.[114,127] In our series of 32 patients with rheumatoid scleritis, 16 patients (27 eyes) had keratitis (50%) (Table 6.5); of those, 2 patients had corneal thinning, 1 patient had acute stromal keratitis, 3 patients had sclerosing stromal keratitis, and 10 patients had PUK. Corneal involvement in rheumatoid scleritis, particularly PUK, was most frequently associated with the necrotizing variety of scleritis (Fig. 6.6). The percentage of PUK in our patients with rheumatoid scleritis was higher than that reported by other authors,[114] probably reflecting the high selection of patients who come to our Immunology Service following referral from other ophthalmology departments.

Keratitis in RA also may occur in the absence of adjacent scleritis.[122,133–139]

6.1.1.3.2.2. Anterior Uveitis. Anterior uveitis in RA is almost always caused by extension of scleral inflammation, but anterior uveitis in the absence of scleritis has no higher incidence in

TABLE 6.5. Incidence of peripheral keratitis in rheumatoid scleritis patients.

Keratitis	Scleritis subtype[a]					No. (%) of patients
	D	N	NE	SC	P	
Corneal thinning	0	0	2	0	0	2
Acute stromal keratitis	0	0	1	0	0	1
Sclerosing stromal keratitis	1	1	0	1	0	3
Perpheral ulcerative keratitis	4	0	6	0	0	10
Total:	5	1	9	1	0	16 (50)

[a] D, Diffuse; N, nodular; NE, necrotizing; SC, scleromalacia perforans; P, posterior.

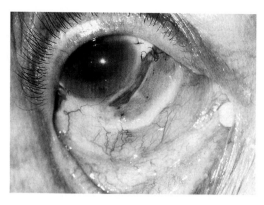

FIGURE 6.6. Necrotizing scleritis and peripheral ulcerative keratitis in a patient with rheumatoid arthritis. Surgical correction of the problem has been attempted, with the predictable result of destruction of the inlay "tectonic" scleral graft that the surgeon has used.

adult RA than in the general population.[140] In our series of 32 patients with rheumatoid scleritis, 14 (44%) had at least one episode of anterior uveitis; of those, 7 patients (50%) had necrotizing anterior scleritis, 5 patients had diffuse anterior scleritis, and 2 patients had nodular anterior scleritis. One of the patients with anterior uveitis and nodular anterior scleritis also had posterior uveitis and posterior scleritis. The incidence of anterior uveitis in our series of 140 patients with nonrheumatoid scleritis was similar (42%), indicating that there is no correlation between anterior uveitis and RA per se.

6.1.1.3.2.3. Glaucoma. Increased intraocular pressure may be caused by the adjacent rheumatoid scleral inflammation with or without uveitis. The reported incidence of glaucoma in patients with rheumatoid scleritis is approximately 19%,[114] although a histological study of enucleated eyes increases the percentage to 45%.[127] The mechanisms implicated in the development of glaucoma in patients with rheumatoid scleritis are the same as the ones implicated in patients with nonrheumatoid scleritis (see Section 4.2.6.3).

6.1.1.3.2.4. Cataract. Long-term systemic steroid treatment in patients with RA without scleritis may lead to the development of pos-terior subcapsular cataract. The combination of long-term systemic steroid treatment with long-standing rheumatoid scleritis with or without uveitis increases the risk of development of posterior subcapsular cataract by threefold.[114]

6.1.1.3.2.5. Retinal, Choroidal, and Optic Nerve Changes. Funduscopic changes in patients with RA can be seen in association with posterior scleritis, including choroidal folds, retinal striae, subretinal mass, annular ciliochoroidal detachment, serous retinal detachment, disk edema, and macular edema.[131] In our series of 32 patients with rheumatoid scleritis, the only patient with posterior scleritis had a choroidal detachment and a serous retinal detachment.

Funduscopic changes in patients with RA, although uncommon, also can be seen in the absence of scleritis. Cotton-wool spots have been correlated with exacerbation and improvement of RA.[141,142] Ischemic optic neuropathy and posterior ciliary arteritis have been reported in a patient with rheumatoid vasculitis.[143] One of our 32 patients with rheumatoid scleritis developed bilateral ischemic optic neuropathy concomitantly with the onset of bilateral necrotizing scleritis and bilateral peripheral ulcerative keratitis.

6.1.1.3.2.6. Motility Disturbances. Motility disturbances have been found to occur in 12.9% of patients with rheumatoid scleritis, although this incidence is not significantly different when compared with patients with nonrheumatoid scleritis.[125]

Some ocular motility disturbances in rheumatoid scleritis may be the result of the extension of scleral inflammation, particularly posterior scleritis, to the extraocular muscles.[114] Symptoms and signs of orbital myositis in posterior scleritis are pain, diplopia, visual loss, chemosis, lid edema, and limitation of ocular movements. In our series of patients with rheumatoid scleritis, the only patient who had posterior scleritis also had restriction of the medial rectus muscle.

Whether or not associated with rheumatoid scleritis, formation of rheumatoid nodules on the posterior tendon of the superior oblique muscle may account for the occurrence of Brown's syndrome, which consists of inability to raise the adducted eye above the mid-horizontal plane, with a smaller elevation deficiency when the eye is in abduction.[144,145] Slight downshoot of the adducting involved eye is often present. Diplopia, particularly noted in upgaze, and a clicking feeling as the tendon of the superior oblique passes through the trochlea, may be the presenting symptoms. One of our patients with rheumatoid scleritis had Brown's syndrome. The patient was a 58-year-old female with seropositive RA for 41 years and bilateral necrotizing scleritis for 3 years. She had severe, often incapacitating, articular lesions, and had extraarticular manifestations such as rheumatoid nodules, mitral valvulopathy, pleural disease, frequent respiratory infections, and osteoporosis. She developed vertical diplopia on upward–inward gaze associated with an exacerbation of RA. She was diagnosed with left Brown's syndrome. Diplopia disappeared simultaneously with clinical improvement of the RA.

Rheumatoid vasculitis with or without rheumatoid scleritis may involve the nervous system, leading to pupillary abnormalities and oculomotor palsies.[146–148]

6.1.1.3.3. Episcleritis.

There is no evidence of any significant relationship between episcleritis and RA.[107] The reported incidence of RA in patients with episcleritis ranges from 4.4 to 5.7% (Table 6.3).[114,121,122] Conversely, the incidence of episcleritis in patients with RA, as reported in one study,[114] is 0.17% (7 of 4210 RA patients). Rheumatoid episcleritis affects women more frequently than men, is most common in the sixth decade of life, and is unilateral as often as it is bilateral.[114] Episcleritis in RA may be simple or nodular.[114,122] In our own series of 94 patients with episcleritis, 3 patients had RA (3.2%) (Table 6.4), 2 females and 1 male. The mean age of patients with rheumatoid episcleritis was 62 years (range, 52 to 69 years); the two cases with nodular episcleritis were unilateral and the case with simple episcleritis was bilateral.

Although only 10% of patients with episcleritis have an underlying connective tissue or vasculitic disease, RA is the most common diagnosis.[121,122] In our series of 94 patients with episcleritis, 13% had an underlying connective tissue disease or vasculitic disease; RA and arthritis associated with inflammatory bowel disease were the most common diagnoses.

Bilateral episcleral nodules may occur in patients with concomitant active joint manifestations of RA (rheumatoid nodules)[149–152]; however, they also may appear in patients with inactive RA (rheumatoid nodulosis),[153] or in patients without any underlying disease (pseudorheumatoid nodules).[154–156]

Although keratitis such as peripheral thinning, acute stromal keratitis, and sclerosing keratitis may occur more frequently in rheumatoid episcleritis than in nonrheumatoid episcleritis, it is never severe.[114] Mild anterior uveitis occurs in a small minority of patients with rheumatoid episcleritis.[114] None of our three patients had either keratitis or anterior uveitis, and none had changes in visual acuity.

6.1.1.4. Laboratory Findings

Although no laboratory tests are specific for diagnosing RA, some of them are valuable in prognosis and management.

6.1.1.4.1. Rheumatoid Factor

The association of positive serum rheumatoid factor (RF) with RA, initially described by Waaler, Rose, and others, is well known.[157,158] Rheumatoid factor is generally defined as an autoantibody (generally IgM, but also IgG and IgA) that reacts with certain epitopes in the Fc fragment of the IgG molecule. Approximately 70 to 90% of patients with definite or classic RA have positive serum RF ("seropositive RA"). Rheumatoid factor is also positive in the sera of a lesser proportion of patients with other rheumatic diseases (systemic lupus erythematosus, scleroderma, and Sjögren's syndrome), viral, bacterial, and parasitic infections, chronic inflammatory diseases, and neoplasms after chemotherapy or radiotherapy (see Chapter 3, Table 3.8). Positive RF is also observed in healthy individuals during the course of secondary immune responses,[159] and in 10 to 20% of nonrheumatic individuals over 65 years old who will not develop RA. Nonetheless, persistent positivity of RF frequently precedes the onset of RA,[160,161] with the risk of developing RA strongly correlated with the titer of serum RF.[162]

Despite some overlap, clinical differences between seropositive and seronegative patients clearly exist. The presence of RF in RA, particularly if present in high titer, is associated with more severe articular disease, both radiographically and functionally, and with a higher frequency of extraarticular manifestations than is observed in seronegative RA, including subcutaneous nodules, vasculitis, and neuropathy.[9,20,163–166]

Patients with rheumatoid scleritis usually have positive RF; RF titers are high in some of them.[114] In our series of 32 patients with rheumatoid scleritis, RF was positive in all but 2 (94%), with a mean titer of 2805 (normal, <60). Within the subset of 11 patients with necrotizing scleritis and RA, RF was positive in all of them and the mean titer was 3577.

6.1.1.4.2. Complete Blood Count

Patients with RA often have anemia, thrombocytosis, and eosinophilia. Suppression of proliferative synovitis may reduce or eliminate hematological abnormalities.

Rheumatoid arthritis patients usually have normocytic hypochromic anemia that tends to follow the erythrocyte sedimentation rate, the C-reactive protein levels, and the activity of synovitis.[167,168] The pathogenesis of the anemia seems to be related to ineffective erythropoiesis.[168]

Mild thrombocytosis is often associated with RA. It also correlates with the erythrocyte sedimentation rate, the C-reactive protein levels, the activity of synovitis, and the presence of extraarticular manifestations.[169] The mechanism of thrombocytosis is unknown.

Eosinophilia (5% of total white blood cell count or greater) appears frequently in RA patients with severe deforming articular disease,[170] pleuritic nodules, low complement levels, and high prevalence of vasculitis.[171]

6.1.1.4.3. Acute-Phase Reactants

The erythrocyte sedimentation rate (ESR) and the C-reactive protein (CRP) level are elevated in almost all patients with RA, and generally these elevations correlate with disease activity.[172–174] Improvement in ESR and CRP on treatment indicates that a remission has been induced and that progressive joint destruction will be retarded or prevented. The ESR is the most important laboratory criterion of the American Rheumatism Association criteria for determining remission.[175]

Patients with rheumatoid scleritis have higher ESR values than do RA patients without scleritis.[114]

6.1.1.4.4. Synovial Fluid Analysis

The synovial fluid in RA is usually turbid, with reduced viscosity, poor mucin clot formation, slightly decreased glucose concentration, and increased protein content. White cell count varies between 2000 and 75,000; 50% or more of the cells are neutrophils. Total hemolytic complement (C3 and C4) in synovial fluid is less than 30% of the usually normal serum complement, reflecting activation of the classic complement pathway by locally produced immune complexes.[176] Synovial histopathology may also be helpful in RA diagnosis.

6.1.1.4.5. Circulating Immune Complexes

Although the presence of circulating immune complexes (CICs) is not specific to any particular disease, their detection may have some diagnostic and prognostic significance in RA. In early arthritis, CICs may be detected several months prior to the definite diagnosis of RA.[177] The presence of CICs may help to distinguish seronegative RA from other arthropathies, because CICs are found in 70% of patients with seronegative RA.[178] Circulating immune complex levels may correlate with disease activity, although not as well as the ESR, CRP, or IgG RF.[179] Patients with rheumatoid vasculitis have high levels of CICs.[30] In our series of patients with rheumatoid scleritis, CICs were detected in all but 2 patients in which the test was done (16 patients). The mean titer of CICs by Raji cell assay was 236 units/ml (normal, 0–50).

6.1.1.4.6. Anti-Nuclear Antibodies

The frequency of anti-nuclear antibodies (ANAs) in rheumatoid sera is about 40%, when measured by indirect immunofluorescence. The most common pattern of ANA staining is the homogeneous pattern, which correlates with the presence of anti-DNA–histone antibodies. The second most common pattern of ANA staining is the speckled pattern, which correlates with the presence of a variety of antibodies directed against nonhistone nuclear proteins; these antibodies include Sm, nRNP, anti-La, Scl_{70}, and other unidentified antigens. Rheumatoid vasculitis may occur in patients with high levels of anti-nuclear antibodies.[30]

6.1.1.4.7. Complement

Reduced serum complement occurs in seropositive RA in which circulating immune complexes are present.[1] Rheumatoid vasculitis may occur in patients with depressed complement levels.[30–32]

6.1.1.4.8. Cryoglobulins

Serum cryoglobulins in patients with RA contain immune complex materials. Elevated cryoglobulin levels occur most frequently in seropositive RA patients with rheumatoid vasculitis and with Felty's syndrome.[1] Serum cryoglobulin levels correlate inversely with serum complement levels.

6.1.1.4.9. Radiographic Evaluation

Radiological findings range from periarticular tissue swelling early in the disease to juxtaarticular osteopenia, loss of articular cartilage, bone erosions, and joint deformities in advanced disease.

6.1.1.5. Diagnosis

The diagnosis of RA is essentially clinical, although the presence of RF, inflammatory synovial fluid, characteristic histological changes in synovial membrane or nodules, and radiographic findings of periarticular osteoporosis and erosions of the affected joints support the diagnosis. The American Rheumatism Association has developed a set of diagnostic criteria for the diagnosis of RA (Table 6.6). A diagnosis of classic RA may be made in the presence of seven of these criteria, whereas definite RA is diagnosed in the presence of five, and probable RA in the presence of three. Exclusions are based on the presence of criteria for other diseases. These include heel pain, conjunctivitis, and urethritis in Reiter's syn-

TABLE 6.6. American Rheumatism Association criteria for the diagnosis of rheumatoid arthritis.[a,b]

1. Morning stiffness
2. Pain on motion or tenderness in at least one joint[a]
3. Swelling of one joint (soft tissue or fluid, not bony overgrowth alone)[a]
4. Swelling of at least one other joint[a] with an interval free of symptoms no longer than 3 months
5. Symmetrical joint swelling[a] with simultaneous involvement of the same joint, right and left. Terminal phalangeal joint involvement is rare in RA and therefore does not satisfy this criterion.
6. Subcutaneous nodules[a] over bony prominences, extensor surfaces, or in juxtaarticular regions
7. Typical roentgenographic changes that must include at least bony decalcification localized to or greatest around the involved joints; degenerative changes do not exclude diagnosis of RA
8. Positive test for rheumatoid factor in serum (1:64 or greater)
9. Synovial fluid; a poor mucin precipitate on adding synovial fluid to dilute acetic acid
10. Synovial histopathology consistent with RA (marked villous hypertrophy, proliferation of synovial cells, lymphocyte/plasma cell infiltration in subsynovium, fibrin deposition within or on microvilli, foci of cell necrosis)
11. Characteristic histopathology of rheumatoid nodules biopsied from any site (granulomatous foci with central zones of cell necrosis, surrounded by proliferated fixed cells, and peripheral fibrosis and chronic inflammatory cell infiltration, predominantly perivascular)

[a] Observed by a physician.
[b] Classic RA, seven criteria needed; definite RA, five criteria needed; probable RA, three criteria needed; possible RA, two criteria (1, 2, 3, or 6), elevated erythrocyte sedimentation rate (ESR) or C-reactive protein, or iritis. To meet criteria 1 to 5, symptoms or signs must be present for at least 6 weeks.

drome, spondylitis in ankylosing spondylitis, tophi in gout, butterfly rash in systemic lupus erythematosus, and so on.

6.1.2. Systemic Lupus Erythematosus

Systemic lupus erythematosus (SLE) is a chronic multisystem disease of unknown etiology. The clinical course of SLE may be mild or severe and recurrent or continuous with a wide range of inflammatory manifestations in almost any organ of the body.

6.1.2.1. Epidemiology

The prevalence of SLE in urban areas of the United States ranges from 15.5 to 50.0 cases per 100,000. Onset of symptoms is more frequent between ages 15 and 45 years, women are nine times more likely to be affected than men, and it is more common among blacks than among whites.[180,181] The prevalence of SLE among black women in the United States between ages 15 and 64 years is 1 case per 245, whereas that for all women of the same ages is 1 per 700.[180] Systemic lupus erythematosus occurs in relatives of patients with the disease with a frequency between 0.4 and 5%, representing a several hundredfold increase over that of the general population.[182] Analysis of SLE families suggests that both genetic predisposition and environmental stimuli are important in the development of the disease; multiple interacting genes, within and outside of the major histocompatibility complex (MHC),[183] and environmental stimuli such as viral infection, ultraviolet irradiation, or contact with certain drugs (hydralazine, procainamide, penicillin, sulfonamides, gold, phenytoin, isoniazide, and methyldopa),[184] may induce immunological alterations resulting in formation of autoantibodies, including anti-nuclear antibody.

6.1.2.2. Systemic Manifestations

Because constitutional symptoms are usually present at the time of diagnosis, any patient with fatigue, loss of weight, fever, malaise, and anorexia who is found to have anti-nuclear antibodies in serum should be carefully studied

TABLE 6.7. Common systemic manifestations of systemic lupus erythematosus.

Articular: Arthralgias, arthritis
Cutaneous: Rash, alopecia, ulcers, photosensitivity
Renal: Glomerulonephritis
Cardiovascular: Pericarditis, Raynaud's phenomenon, thrombophlebitis
Gastrointestinal: Nausea, vomiting, abdominal pain
Neurological: Behavioral disturbance, seizures, mononeuritis
Pulmonary: Pleural effusions, pleurisy, pneumonitis
Miscellaneous: Splenomegaly, lymphadenopathy, parotid swelling
Ocular: Keratitis, episcleritis, scleritis, retinopathy

for possible SLE. Although almost any organ in the body can be affected, the most common systemic manifestations are shown in Table 6.7 and are described here.

6.1.2.2.1. Musculoskeletal

Joint disease is the most common involvement of SLE (95%) and occurs as the initial manifestation of the disease in many cases (55%).[185,186] In some SLE patients joint pain or swelling may precede the onset of multisystem disease by 6 months to 5 years. The joint involvement is symmetrical and most commonly affects the proximal interphalangeal, knee, wrist, and metacarpophalangeal joints. Some SLE patients (about 15%) develop deforming arthritis changes such as swan-neck deformities and ulnar deviation of the fingers, similar to those seen in RA patients. Erosive arthritis is rare in SLE.[187] Myalgia, proximal muscle weakness, or muscle tenderness is common in patients with active disease.[188] Rheumatoid nodules occur in 5 to 7% of patients with SLE.[16,17]

6.1.2.2.2. Tegument

Cutaneous abnormalities occur in 80% of SLE patients and may be the first manifestation of the disease in many cases (about 20%).[189] The typical lesion, the butterfly facial rash, is slightly edematous and is located on both cheeks and across the bridge of the nose (Fig. 6.7). Although the rash is present in about half the patients at the moment of diagnosis, it may

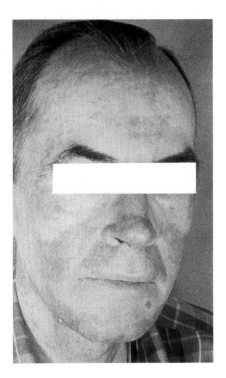

FIGURE 6.7. Typical butterfly rash in a patient with systemic lupus erythematosus.

be the first manifestation of the disease, preceding the multisystem involvement by weeks or months. The rash may be continuous or intermittent and is exacerbated by ultraviolet exposure, by alcohol ingestion, or by nervousness. The second most common rash is a maculopapular eruption, frequently pruritic, and located any place on the body.

Alopecia occurs in 25 to 40% of the patients with SLE. Because in many patients recurrent diffuse alopecia may be the first manifestation of an impending SLE flare-up, its presence should be viewed as evidence of disease activity. Periungual erythema, atrophic blanche lesions, hives or angioneurotic edema, urticaria, bullous lesions, and nail deformities have also been described.

6.1.2.2.3. Vessels

Aside from RA, the connective tissue disease in which vasculitis occurs most frequently is SLE. Skin vasculitic lesions, noted in about 20% of patients with SLE, are most commonly located on the extensor surface of the forearm and on the fingertips, but they also may be on the palms, on the soles of the feet, and on the lower legs near the malleoli. These lesions may ulcerate, particularly during periods of disease exacerbation. Livedo reticularis, purpura, and splinter hemorrhages may also be noted in severe active disease. Mucosal vasculitic lesions such as mucous membrane ulcers (nasal septum, palate, larynx, pharynx, and vagina) may be the first manifestation of an impending SLE flare-up.

Raynaud's phenomenon may occur in about 20% of SLE patients (Fig. 6.8; see color insert). It is usually present with other manifestations at the time of diagnosis but occasionally may precede the onset of multisystem disease.[190] Raynaud's phenomenon may gradually disappear as the disease goes into remission, although in active SLE may result in digital gangrene with amputation of the fingertips. Deep vein thrombosis also may occur and may be migratory and recurrent.[190]

Peripheral neuropathy and cranial nerve involvement are characterized by arterial damage in nerve biopsy specimens. Psychosis, seizures, hemiparesis, and chorea may be the result of vasculitic cerebral involvement.[190,191]

Organ infarction such as cerebral thrombosis and hemorrhages, myocardial infarction, diffuse proliferative lupus nephritis, or bowel perforation may be caused by an arteritis of both small- and medium-sized arteries. Widespread necrotizing arteritis mimicking polyarteritis nodosa has been described in a few patients with SLE.

6.1.2.2.4. Kidney

Although only 40 to 50% of patients have clinical evidence of renal disease (proteinuria or hematuria, nephrotic syndrome, or renal failure), nearly all show changes on renal biopsy. The spectrum of kidney involvement includes (1) focal proliferative lupus nephritis (mild), (2) diffuse proliferative lupus nephritis (severe), (3) membranous lupus nephritis (moderate), and (4) mesangial lupus nephritis (minimal).[192] Hypertension is commonly associated. The extent and severity of the renal lesions correlate with the severity of the disease, and end-stage renal disease is the most common cause of death in patients with SLE.

6.1.2.2.5. Heart

The most frequent cardiac manifestation in SLE is pericarditis, which occurs in about 25% of patients, often during acute exacerbations. Although a pericardial rub is easily detected, echocardiography is most helpful in detecting pericardial thickening.[193] Myocardial involvement may present as tachycardia, cardiac enlargement, congestive heart disease, arrhythmias, conduction defects, or even cardiac failure. Deaths caused by myocardial infarction from coronary arteritis have been reported early in the course of the disease in young patients.[190,194,195] Atypical verrucous endocarditis, termed Libman–Sacks endocarditis, is usually of little clinical significance and is not easily diagnosed in life. The pathological findings at necropsy reveal ovoid vegetations, from 1 to 4 mm of diameter, made up of degenerating valve tissue with fibrin and platelet thrombi. Although the original descriptions by Libman and Sacks[196] were observed on the tricuspid valve, more recent series show a higher incidence of lesions on the mitral valve.[197] Subacute bacterial endocarditis may occur when microorganisms become implanted on the leaflets previously deformed by Libman–Sacks endocarditis.

6.1.2.2.6. Nervous System

Central nervous system involvement is the second most frequent SLE-related cause of death (after renal involvement).[198] The most common neurological manifestation is psychiatric illness (organic brain syndrome) characterized by impairment of orientation, perception, memory, and intellectual function.[199] The second most common is seizures, especially grand mal seizure; petit mal, psychomotor epilepsy, temporal lobe epilepsy, and Jacksonian seizures may also appear. Seizures may be present at the time of diagnosis or later in the course of the disease, but in most cases they occur along with clinical and laboratory evidence of severe systemic disease. Systemic lupus erythematosus patients with central nervous system disease (organic brain syndrome or seizures) are more likely to have evidence of vasculitis of other systems than are those without central nervous system findings.[198] Chorea, recurrent headaches, hemiparesis, and cerebellar signs may occur along with other manifestations of the disease during an exacerbation. Cranial nerves such as the ophthalmic, trochlear, abducens, and less commonly the trigeminal and facial, may be involved in episodes of active systemic disease when evidence of vasculitis is present in other systems.[199] Peripheral neuropathy occurs in about 14% of patients. The most common abnormality is sensory, although occasionally a sensorimotor disturbance may be seen.[198] Psychological abnormalities such as depression and less often anxiety, are reactions to the disease and to the disfigurement caused by both the disease and the corticosteroid therapy.[199]

6.1.2.2.7. Lung

Pleuropulmonary manifestations, which occur in 50 to 75% of SLE patients, include pleurisy with or without effusion, acute pneumonitis, and diffuse interstitial pneumonitis.[200,201] Pleural effusions in SLE are exudates with more than 3.0 g of protein per 100 ml, more than 55 mg per 100 ml of glucose, and occasional lupus erythematosus (LE) cells; pleuritic pain is the usual complaint. Acute pneumonitis may present with dyspnea and, less often, cough or hemoptysis as symptoms, and diffuse acinar infiltrates, especially in the lung bases, as chest X-ray findings; lung function studies may reveal hypoxemia. Diffuse interstitial pneumonitis diagnosis is based on the symptom of dyspnea on exertion, on the physical findings of poor diaphragmatic movement and decreased resonance to percussion over the bases, and on the radiographic evidence of persistent, diffuse interstitial infiltrates; lung function studies reveal a restrictive pattern. Pulmonary involvement may occur in SLE patients with no dyspnea and no radiographic abnormalities; the only disturbance in these patients is an impairment in the diffusion capacity.

6.1.2.2.8. Miscellaneous

Gastrointestinal symptoms such as anorexia, nausea, vomiting, dysphagia, or abdominal pain may occur in SLE and may mimic an acute surgical abdomen. Acute pancreatitis may result from active SLE or from glucocorticoid therapy. Elevated serum levels of liver enzymes are common in active SLE but they return to normal with response of the disease to therapy.[202] Slight to moderate splenomegaly may occur in 20% of SLE patients; lack of splenic activity is uncommon.[203] Lymph nodes are enlarged in 50% of SLE patients at the time of clinical disease activity. The parotid gland may also be enlarged during periods of active SLE.[190]

6.1.2.3. Ocular Involvement

The ocular manifestations in SLE are important because they may be the initial manifestation of the disease or may serve as a barometer of the severity and prognosis of the systemic involvement. Unlike other collagen diseases, which have a frank predilection for either anterior or posterior segment involvement, SLE may affect every structure of the eye. Any patient who develops retinal vasculitis and scleritis must be carefully studied for SLE.

6.1.2.3.1. Scleritis

The reported incidence of SLE in patients with scleritis is about 1%.[122,123] The presence of scleritis is a reasonably accurate guide to the systemic activity in a patient with SLE; the scleritis attacks become more severe and recurrent as the systemic disease deteriorates. Occasionally, scleritis may be the initial manifestation of SLE.[204] Systemic lupus erythematosus scleritis generally takes the form of diffuse anterior scleritis or nodular anterior scleritis but necrotizing anterior scleritis may also occur, especially when systemic vasculitic lesions become significant.[123,204,205] Posterior scleritis, although uncommon, may also be an SLE manifestation.[206] Any patient who presents with any type of scleritis should be screened for SLE; scleritis will resolve with adequate control of systemic disease. Scleral inflammation in SLE may extend to the adjacent structures and may cause keratitis and anterior uveitis. Although anterior uveitis is an unusual isolated finding in SLE (reported incidence of uveitis in patients with SLE ranges from 0.5 to 1.6%),[207] its incidence increases with the presence of SLE scleritis.

In our own series of 172 patients with scleritis, 7 patients had SLE (4%); of those, 2 patients (28%) had bilateral scleritis. All patients were women with a mean age of 39 years (range, 22 to 57 years). Four patients had diffuse anterior scleritis, two patients had nodular anterior scleritis, and one patient had posterior scleritis. The mean time of presentation of scleritis was 6 months after the SLE diagnosis. In most cases scleritis appeared at the time of exacerbation of the systemic disease. In one case, scleritis (nodular) was the initial manifestation whose study led to the diagnosis of SLE. Four of seven patients (57%) with SLE scleritis had had at least one episode of anterior uveitis; of those, two patients had diffuse anterior scleritis, one patient had nodular anterior scleritis, and one patient had posterior scleritis. The patient with posterior scleritis and anterior uveitis also had posterior uveitis. A decrease in visual acuity (equal to or greater than two Snellen lines at the end of the follow-up period or vision equal to or worse than 20/80 at the first examination) occurred in 22% of the eyes.

6.1.2.3.2. Episcleritis

Although episcleritis may occur in patients with SLE, the incidence is low. In the Watson and Hayreh[122] series of 159 patients with episcleritis, there were no patients with SLE. Conversely, two studies reported the incidence of episcleritis in patients with SLE as 0.5 and 1.9% (1 of 200 SLE patients and 2 of 105 SLE patients, respectively).[208,209] Occasionally, episcleritis may be the first manifestation of SLE.[210] In our own series of 94 patients with episcleritis, one patient had SLE (1%); the patient was a 28-year-old female with recurrent unilateral simple episcleritis without keratitis or anterior uveitis and without decrease of visual acuity.

6.1.2.3.3. Other Ocular Findings

Aside from scleritis and episcleritis, anterior segment involvement in SLE may include conjunctivitis, keratitis, and anterior uveitis. Conjunctivitis may affect bulbar, fornix, and tarsal regions and may eventually leave subepithelial fibrosis with shrinkage of the conjunctiva. Although superficial punctate keratitis is the most common corneal problem, stromal infiltration, peripheral ulceration, and vascularization may also occur.[211–214] Keratoconjunctivitis sicca may be associated with SLE (Sjögren's syndrome) but its incidence is low.[215–218] Anterior uveitis may rarely occur in the absence of other ocular lesions.[205,207] Although anterior uveitis may cause secondary glaucoma, it is never severe and responds well to adequate therapy. Posterior segment involvement is more common and serves as a better barometer of the severity of the disease than do anterior segment manifestations. The most frequent posterior segment manifestations include cotton-wool spots, retinal hemorrhages, retinal edema, and optic disk edema; other reported fundus changes include retinal hard exudates, retinal vasculitis, central retinal vein occlusion, arteriolar narrowing, arteriovenous crossing changes, macular pigmentary mottling, and retinal scarring.[207] Although some of these manifestations may be a reflection of a hypertensive retinopathy, they may appear as independent signs as well; in cases of associated hypertension, the decision as to whether the retinal lesions are secondary to high blood pressure or to SLE immunological abnormalities may be difficult; the presence of anterior segment manifestations such as scleritis or episcleritis may be helpful in this regard, because they are reflections of the disease process. Several authors have emphasized that the presence of retinal lesions correlates with the systemic course of the disease[219–222]; Rothfield[222] found an association between the presence of hard exudates and central nervous system disease activity (seizures and organic brain disease). Regan and Foster,[223] however, think that localized manifestations of the disease (eye, skin, and kidney) may sometimes occur, and therefore that retinal vasculitis also may appear without exacerbation of SLE.[223] Whichever the case is, if a patient with SLE develops retinopathy, a thorough search for systemic evidence of disease activity must be performed promptly and, if positive, aggressive therapy must be instituted to control both systemic and ocular abnormalities. Central nervous system SLE vasculitis may produce ocular abnormalities such as internuclear ophthalmoplegia, nystagmus, cranial nerve palsies (second, third, fifth, sixth, or seventh nerve palsies), homonymous hemianopia, and papilledema.[199,224]

6.1.2.4. Laboratory Findings

The LE phenomenon (LE cells) consists of the phagocytosis of antibodies against nucleoproteins (DNA–histone) by neutrophils. Lupus erythematosus cells occur in 70 to 80% of SLE patients but this test has been replaced by the anti-nuclear antibody (ANA) test, which is more sensitive and specific. The presence of ANAs is helpful in supporting the diagnosis of SLE. Antinuclear antibodies are found in 98% of active SLE patients and in 90% of SLE patients in remission, and ANA titers generally correlate with the level of disease activity.[225] Antinuclear antibodies are not, however, specific for the disease; other autoimmune diseases, acute viral infections, and chronic inflammatory processes may cause ANA positivity (see Section 3.2.1.2). Various anti-nuclear antibodies (antibodies to DNA–histone, double-stranded DNA [dsDNA] and single-stranded DNA [ssDNA], RNA, histone, nuclear ribonucleoprotein [nRNP], Sm, and phospholipids) may develop in SLE. Anti-dsDNA and anti-Sm antibodies are highly specific for SLE (Table 3.9), but they are found in only about 70 and 30% of SLE patients, respectively. Antibodies to Ro/SSA and La/SSB/Ha occur in SLE and in Sjögren's syndrome. Antibodies to nRNP also can be detected in patients with mixed connective tissue disease, an entity with overlapping features of SLE, scleroderma, and polymyositis. Antibodies to phospholipids (anti-cardiolipin) are responsible for the false-positive syphilis tests in some SLE patients. Patients with anti-cardiolipin antibodies are at increased risk for venous or arterial thrombosis and for repeated spontaneous abortions. Antibodies to coagulation factors VIII, IX, XI, or XII, to platelets, or to immunoglobulins (rheumatoid factor) also may occur in SLE patients; these abnormalities also may be seen in other diseases.

The presence of low serum complement (C3 and C4, as determined by CH50 [total hemolytic complement]) levels coupled with the presence of anti-DNA antibodies is highly specific for SLE.[226] Low serum complement levels, serum cryoglobulins, or serum immune complexes may correlate with exacerbation of the disease.

Urinalysis in active nephritis may show proteinuria, microscopic hematuria, and cellular casts; this test and the serum creatinine test should be done periodically in patients with SLE.

Normochromic and normocytic anemia (due to retarded erythropoiesis), neutropenia, lymphocytopenia, and thrombocytopenia are frequent findings. A hemolytic anemia with reticulocytosis and low hematocrit, with or without positive Coombs' test, may antedate the other manifestations of the disease by many years. Elevation of the erythrocyte sedimentation rate is common in active SLE.[190]

6.1.2.5. Diagnosis

There is no clinical or laboratory abnormality that is pathognomonic for SLE. Because SLE patients show marked variability in their clinical manifestations and laboratory findings, a group of several criteria has been developed in an attempt to include SLE patients and to exclude patients with other disorders and thereby establish a diagnosis of SLE. The American Rheumatism Association developed in 1971 and revised in 1982 a set of 11 diagnostic criteria for the diagnosis of SLE (Table 6.8). A diagnosis of SLE may be made in the presence of four or more of these criteria, serially or simultaneously, during any interval of observation. Our experience, extending over the past 20 years, with a large number of patients with scleritis, episcleritis, anterior uveitis, and retinal vasculitis, shows unequivocally that patients who eventually fulfil the criteria for the diagnosis of SLE may fall short of satisfying the criteria for many years while experiencing their recurrent ocular inflammatory problem. Two or three of the established SLE diagnostic criteria may be present (most often ANA positivity, episodic mouth sores, photosensitivity, anemia, or arthritis) coincident with or prior to the onset of the ocular inflammation. Over the ensuing years, other SLE manifestations such as typical rash, glomerulonephritis, or CNS vasculitis appear, allowing definitive establishment of the diagnosis. We believe that ocular inflammation (scleritis, episcleritis, anterior uveitis, or retinal vasculitis) should be added to the SLE diagnostic criteria list. We do not know whether or not earlier definitive diagnosis establishment with earlier systemic therapy would favorably alter the prognosis for SLE patients; that possibility can be answered only by a large, prospective controlled clinical trial.

6.1.3. Ankylosing Spondylitis

Ankylosing spondylitis (AS) (Bekhterev's disease, Marie–Strümpell disease, rheumatoid spondylitis) is a chronic inflammatory systemic disease of unknown cause that primarily involves the joints of the spine, sacroiliac joints, and periarticular soft tissues. The disease is the prototype of a group of disorders referred to as spondyloarthropathies, and characterized by common features that differentiate them from rheumatoid arthritis. These features include (1) radiographic sacroiliitis with or without accompanying spondylitis, with a marked tendency toward calcification and ossification of ligaments (ankylosis), (2) inflammatory peripheral arthritis, often asymmetric, with lack of rheumatoid nodules, (3) no association with rheumatoid factor or anti-nuclear antibody, (4) strong association with HLA-B27, (5) tendency for ocular inflammation (especially anterior uveitis and conjunctivitis), (6) variable mucocutaneous lesions, and (7) occasional cardiac abnormalities. The spondyloarthropathies include ankylosing spondylitis, Reiter's syndrome, psoriatic arthritis, and enteropathic (inflammatory bowel disease) arthritis (Table 6.9).[227]

TABLE 6.8. American Rheumatism Association revised criteria for the diagnosis of systemic lupus erythenatosus (1982).

Four or more of the following:

1. Malar rash: Fixed erythema, flat or raised, over the malar eminences, tending to spare the nasolabial folds
2. Discoid rash: Erythematous raised patches with adherent keratotic scaling and follicular plugging; atrophic scarring may occur in older lesions
3. Photosensitivity: Skin rash as a result of unusual reaction to sunlight, by patient history or physician observation
4. Oral or nasopharyngeal ulceration, usually painless, observed by a physician
5. Arthritis: Nonerosive arthritis involving two or more peripheral joints, characterized by tenderness, swelling, or effusion
6. Serositis
   a. Pleuritis: Convincing history of pleuritic pain or rub heard by a physician or evidence of pleural effusion, OR
   b. Pericarditis: Documented by ECG or rub or evidence of pericardial effusion
7. Renal disorder
   a. Persistent proteinuria greater than 0.5 g/day or   greater than 3+ if quantitation not performed OR
   b. Cellular casts: May be red, hemoglobulin, granular, tubular, or mixed
8. Neurological disorder
   a. Seizures: In the absence of offending drugs or known metabolic derangements, e.g., uremia, ketoacidosis, or electrolyte imbalance OR
   b. Psychosis: In the absence of offending drugs or known metabolic derangements, e.g., uremia, ketoacidosis, or electrolye imbalance
9. Hematological disorder
   a. Hemolytic anemia: With reticulocytosis OR
   b. Leukopenia: Less than 4000/mm total on two or more occasions
   c. Lymphopenia: Less than 1500/mm on two or more occasions OR
   d. Thrombocytopenia: Less than 100,000/mm in the absence of offending drugs
10. Immunological disorder
    a. Positive LE cell preparation
    b. Anti-DNA antibody to native DNA in abnormal titer
    c. Anti-Sm: Presence of antibody to Sm nuclear antigen OR
    d. False-positive serological test for syphilis known to be positive for at least 6 months and confirmed by *Treponema pallidum* immobilization or fluorescent treponemal antibody absorption test
11. Anti-nuclear antibody: An abnormal titer of anti-nuclear antibody by immunofluorescence or an equivalent assay at any point in time and in the absence of drugs known to be associated with "drug-induced lupus syndrome"

6.1.3.1. Epidemiology

Ankylosing spondylitis has a prevalence of about 1% in the general population. It is seen mainly in Caucasians and is exceptionally rare in Japanese and black Africans. Onset is more frequent between 15 and 40 years of age, and clinical evidence of AS is three to four times more frequent in men than in women. However, if radioisotope studies that detect subclinical sacroiliitis are taken into account, AS occurs almost as frequently in females as in males (although with milder and more peripheral disease).[228] There is a definitive correlation between the prevalence of the disease and the presence of the histocompatibility antigen HLA-B27.[229] More than 90% of AS Caucasian patients and 52% of their first-degree relatives are HLA-B27 positive, compared with only 6% of a control population.[230] Between 1 and 10% of the HLA-B27-positive adults in the general population and 20 to 30% of the HLA-B27-positive first-degree relatives of spondylitis patients are likely to suffer from AS.[231]

TABLE 6.9. Clinical manifestations in spondyloarthropathies.[a]

Parameter	AS	RS with spondylitis	Psoriatic spondylitis	IBD with spondylitis
Age predilection	15–40	18–40	Variable	Variable
Sex predilection	M > F	M > F	M > F	M = F
HLA-B27	>90%	75–90%	50%	50–70%
Prostatitis	+	+	−	+/−
Urethritis	−	+	−	−
Conjunctivitis	+/−	+	+	+/−
Anterior uveitis	+	+	+	+
Scleritis	+/−	+/−	+/−	+
Episcleritis	−	+/−	+/−	+
Mucosal involvement	−	+	−	+/−
Spinal involvement	+	+/−	+	+

[a] AS, Ankylosing spondylitis; RS, Reiter's syndrome; IBD, inflammatory bowel disease.

6.1.3.2. Systemic Manifestations

6.1.3.2.1. Articular Involvement

The most characteristic early manifestation of AS is low back pain, which is of insidious onset, dull in character, unilateral and intermittent at first, and initially felt deep in the gluteal region. Because symptoms often are ascribed to lumbar disk disease, diagnosis is usually delayed. The pain becomes bilateral, persistent, and localized in the lumbar spine, with occasional irradiation to the iliac crest or to the dorsal thigh within a few months of onset of symptoms. Morning stiffness, which usually lasts longer than is seen in mechanical spinal problems, is typical. Both the pain and the stiffness improve with exercise and worsen with rest. The lumbar spine progressively loses its normal lordosis, leading to limitation of movement (Fig. 6.9). If the thoracic spine is affected, costovertebral and sternomanubrial joint and tendon involvement may cause kyphosis and chest pain, especially on inspiration, sneezing, or coughing. Cervical spine spondylitis may result in cervical arthralgias, limitation of motion, or cord compression. A sudden exacerbation of back pain, especially in the cervical region, may follow a fracture after minimal or even unrecognized injury.[232] Only a few patients progress to the end stage of "bamboo spine" now, because of the earlier recognition and better treatment of AS today

compared to 30 years ago (Fig. 6.10). Bamboo spine is caused by the fusion of the calcified annulus fibrosus with the vertebral bodies through the characteristic syndesmophytes.

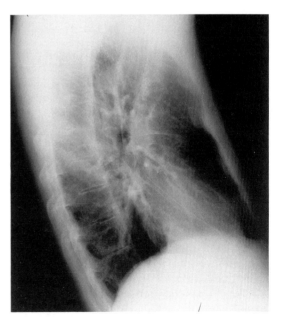

FIGURE 6.9. Lateral chest X ray of patient with ankylosing spondylitis. Note the kyphosis, the soft tissue calcifications in the fibers of the annulus of the disk, and the anterior and lateral vertebral ligaments, creating the so-called "bamboo spine." New bone formation (syndesmophyte) bridges the disk space and fuses the spine.

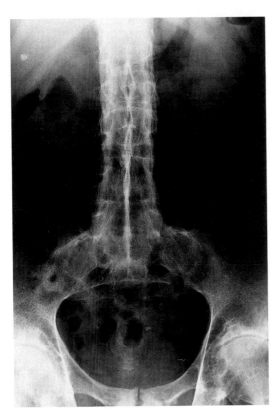

FIGURE 6.10. Abdominal flat plate X ray of patient with ankylosing spondylitis. Note the calcification in the anterior and lateral vertebral ligaments, the "bamboo spine," and the syndesmophytes. Note also the complete obliteration of the sacroiliac joints, erosion and reactive sclerosis in the pubic symphysis and adjacent bone, and the narrowing of the hip joints, with juxtaarticular sclerosis and cyst-like erosions in the acetabular and femoral heads.

Peripheral arthritis is present at some stage of the disease in 35% of AS patients. Although any joint may be involved, the hips, shoulders, and knees are most frequently affected. Pain, swelling, and effusion may be transient, but crippling changes similar to those found in RA may occur after a disease duration of 10 or more years. Peripheral arthritis may be the initial manifestation in 20% of patients with AS.

Insertional tendonitis such as plantar fasciitis, dactylitis, or Achilles tendinitis may be painful and recurrent but they do not leave serious sequelae apart from occasional new bone formation (plantar spur).

Although physical signs may be minimal in the early stages of AS, tenderness and spasm of the paraverterbral muscles, and limitation of motion of the lumbar spine, may occur. Direct pressure over involved joints and tendons may elicit pain.

6.1.3.2.2. Extraarticular Systemic Manifestations

Although extraarticular systemic manifestations are uncommon in patients with AS, many body systems may become affected, especially after years of active disease. Constitutional symptoms include fever, malaise, anorexia, and weight loss.

Cardiovascular involvement is more frequent in patients with severe spondylitis, marked peripheral arthritis, and prominent systemic manifestations.[233] Aortic incompetence, conduction abnormalities (including complete heart block, causing Adams–Stokes disease), cardiomegaly, ascending aortitis, and pericarditis are the primary abnormalities that may occur in AS patients.[234,235] Vasculitis in AS is predominantly a large-artery arteritis.

Ankylosing spondylitis pulmonary disease is characterized by progressive fibrotic changes of the upper lobes of the lungs, with eventual cyst formation and parenchymal destruction. These lesions may become invaded with *Aspergillus* and form a mycetoma.[233] Death may follow massive hemoptysis.

Neurological manifestations in AS patients are most often related to subluxations, fracture dislocations, or cauda equina syndrome.[233] Atlantoaxial subluxation and cervical spine fracture dislocation are the most frequent problems. Cauda equina syndrome, occurring in the later stages of the disease, is due to lumbar central midline disk herniation causing paralysis of the sacral roots; its diagnosis requires emergency neurosurgery (laminectomy). It presents with leg or buttock pain with sensory and motor impairment, and with bowel and bladder dysfunction. Multiple sclerosis may be associated with AS more often than would be expected by chance alone.[236]

Genitourinary disease in AS patients can include chronic prostatitis, which appears to be more frequent in patients with AS than in normal patients or patients with rheumatoid arthritis.[237]

Renal involvement with clinical manifestations is a rare complication of AS in spite of recognized pathological changes detected in electron microscopy and immunofluorescence studies.[238,239] Renal damage may occasionally be caused by amyloidosis after many years of disease,[240] or by IgA nephropathy.[241]

6.1.3.3. Ocular Manifestations

Although anterior uveitis is the most common ocular manifestation in AS, scleritis may occasionally occur. Other ocular problems include conjunctivitis and the complications of uveitis and/or scleritis such as cataract, seclusion of the pupil, iris bombe, secondary glaucoma, or macular edema. Episcleritis does not occur in patients with AS more commonly than in normal control populations.

6.1.3.3.1. Anterior Uveitis

Anterior uveitis, the most common extraarticular manifestation of AS, occurs in approximately 25% of patients either before the onset of the disease or at some point thereafter.[233,242] Conversely, AS is the most common systemic condition associated with anterior uveitis in men: 17 to 31% of men with anterior uveitis have AS.[230] The clinical association between anterior uveitis and AS becomes strengthened by the finding that 50% of patients with anterior uveitis, and 90% of patients with anterior uveitis and a rheumatic disease, are *HLA-B27* positive.[230] The presence of anterior uveitis does not correlate with the severity of the spondylitis but may be more frequent in patients with peripheral involvement. It is typically unilateral but may become bilateral. The characteristic symptoms of anterior uveitis in AS are acute onset of pain, photophobia, redness, and blurred vision, although it may be mild or even asymptomatic. The characteristic signs are prominent ciliary injection, fine whitish-gray keratic precipitates, and fibrinous exudation in the anterior chamber that contributes to the formation of posterior synechiae. An underrecognized fact, which is clear from our experience with a large number of patients with uveitis, is that AS *HLA-B27* patients may develop a violent, explosive onset of anterior uveitis with hypopyon. The posterior segment is usually spared, although cystoid macular edema and, in our experience, retinal vasculitis, may occasionally occur. Individual attacks of uveitis usually subside without residual visual impairment in 4 to 8 weeks, but they may recur over a period of years and become bilateral. Immediate ocular application of topical steroids and mydriatics by the patient as soon as the first symptoms appear may abort the attack, provided he is soon seen by an ophthalmologist who can manage the attack and detect the ocular complications either of the treatment or of the disease (e.g., glaucoma, cataract, and macular edema). Ankylosing spondylitis must always be considered in the differential diagnosis of anterior uveitis.

6.1.3.3.2. Scleritis

Scleritis may occur in AS with or without anterior uveitis. The reported incidence of AS in patients with scleritis ranges from 0.34 to 0.48%.[122,123] Occasionally, scleritis may be the initial manifestation of AS, preceding the disease by many years.[197] Ankylosing spondylitis scleritis generally takes the form of mild to moderate diffuse anterior scleritis that, in spite of recurrences, never progresses to necrotizing anterior scleritis.[122,197,243] Anterior uveitis may appear following the onset of scleritis, in which case it is impossible to know if the uveitis is a reflection of the associated scleritis, or represents an independent effect of the disease, or both.

In our own series of 172 patients with scleritis, 1 patient had AS (0.93%). The patient was a 66-year-old male diagnosed with AS 14 years previously. He had recurrent anterior uveitis in the left eye; onset of moderate diffuse anterior scleritis in both eyes occurred 1 year after the onset of anterior uveitis in the left eye. The scleritis recurred in both eyes during the 3-year follow-up; some of the recurrences were associated with anterior uveitis in the left eye.

There were no corneal lesions, glaucoma, cataract, or macular edema, and final visual acuity was not affected. The patient had marked spondylitis, prominent peripheral arthritis, and a cardiac conduction defect. Although scleritis may precede the articular involvement of AS, it usually occurs after years of active AS disease, especially in patients with marked articular and extraarticular manifestations. Any patient who develops diffuse anterior scleritis after recurrent anterior uveitis should be examined for AS.

6.1.3.4. Laboratory Findings and Radiological Evaluation

Serum alkaline phosphatase, serum creatinine phosphokinase, and erythrocyte sedimentation rate are frequently elevated in patients with AS. There appears to be little or no correlation between erythrocyte sedimentation rate and disease severity or prognosis. Circulating immune complexes may be found,[244] but tests for rheumatoid factor and anti-nuclear antibodies are negative.[233]

Radiographic evaluation confirms the diagnosis by showing blurring of the subchondral bone plate, sclerosis, erosions, joint space narrowing, or ankylosis of sacroiliac joints (Fig. 6.11), characteristics of sacroiliitis, or erosions, vertebral squaring, syndesmophyte formation, ossification, or ankylosis of vertebral joints, characteristic of spondylitis. Bony erosions and osteitis may be seen at sites of osseous attachments of tendons and ligaments.[233]

Radionucleotide and computerized tomography scanning studies can disclose early AS lesions not detectable by conventional X ray.

6.1.3.5. Diagnosis

The diagnosis of AS depends on suspicion, history, clinical evaluation, and radiological confirmation. *HLA-B27* typing cannot be used as a screening test because a majority of *HLA-B27* individuals in the general population remains unaffected, and AS may occasionally occur in *HLA-B27*-negative individuals. Furthermore, most patients with AS can be readily diagnosed on the basis of clinical and radiological findings, and therefore do not need the *HLA-B27* test. In cases of clinical suspicion of AS but with radiologic findings of sacroiliitis difficult to recognize with certainty, the finding of *HLA-B27* positivity increases the probability that the presumptive diagnosis is correct; however, it does not establish the diagnosis.

6.1.4. Reiter's Syndrome

Reiter's syndrome (RS) is a "reactive arthritis" that follows certain enteric or genitourinary infections in genetically susceptible individuals. Reactive arthritis may follow either *Shigella*,

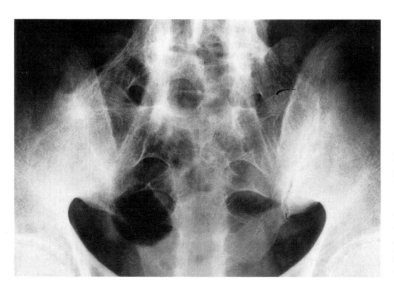

FIGURE 6.11. Lumbosacral spine film of patient with Reiter's syndrome, including ankylosing spondylitis. Note the complete obliteration of the right sacroiliac joint, with pronounced reactive sclerosis of the left sacroiliac joint due to bony ankylosis.

Salmonella, *Yersinia*, or *Campylobacter* enteric infections (postdysenteric), or *Chlamydia trachomatis* or *Mycoplasma* genitourinary infections (postvenereal).[245,246] Although in the United States most patients have the postvenereal form of the disease, in Europe and in the rest of the world the postdysenteric form is most frequent. Reiter's syndrome was initially described by H. Reiter[247] as a nonspecific (nongonococcal) urethritis, acute polyarthritis, and conjunctivitis, but only a minority of cases shows this classic triad. The major manifestations are arthritis (seronegative asymmetric arthropathy, predominantly in the lower extremity), nonspecific urethritis/cervicitis, inflammatory eye disease (conjunctivitis or uveitis), and mucocutaneous lesions (balanitis, oral ulceration, or keratodermia).[248]

The cooccurrence of severe RS, psoriasis, or psoriatic arthritis with the acquired immunodeficiency syndrome (AIDS) emphasizes the connection between immunological factors relevant to these diseases.[249–251]

6.1.4.1. Epidemiology

The prevalence of RS is difficult to assess because of the lack of a definite diagnostic test, forgotten venereal or enteric history, silent mucocutaneous lesions, overlooked eye or skin lesions, asymptomatic urethritis or cervicitis disease, ankylosing spondylitis or seronegative rheumatoid arthritis misdiagnosis, or fragmented care by subspecialty physicians. However, some studies have shown that RS is a relatively common rheumatic disease: RS develops in about 1% of men seen at hospital clinics for nonspecific urethritis, 2 to 3% of patients with *Salmonella* and *Campylobacter* enteritis, and in a higher proportion of those with *Yersinia* infection.[245,248] The onset of symptoms is most frequent between the ages of 18 and 40 years. The sex distribution shows a definite male predilection, but the extent of this is unclear because the diagnosis in females is more difficult to establish. As discussed earlier, ankylosing spondylitis occurs now more frequently in females than was previously believed, and it is likely that RS in females will be more easily detected in the future. *HLA-B27* is present in about 75 to 90% of patients with RS and in only 6% of normal control western Caucasian populations.[245,248]

6.1.4.2. Systemic Manifestations

6.1.4.2.1. Articular Involvement

Arthritis is usually of acute onset, oligoarticular, asymmetric, seronegative, and often persisting or recurring.[245] It occurs within a month of onset of the enteric or genitourinary infection. Lower extremity joints, particularly the knees and the ankles, are the joints most often affected. Low back pain may occur as a result of sacroiliitis or spondylitis (Fig. 6.11). Other rheumatological manifestations involve ligaments, tendons, and fascias; they include dactylitis ("sausage digits"), Achilles tendinitis, plantar fasciitis or calcaneal periostitis ("painful heel syndrome"), and chest wall pain.[245] Reiter's syndrome rheumatological attacks have a mean duration of 3 months, ranging from 2 weeks to more than a year; 50% of patients will have one or more recurrences. Although complete recovery eventually occurs in most patients, those who have had persisting or recurrent attacks may develop permanent joint deformities.

6.1.4.2.2. Extraarticular Systemic Manifestations

Reiter's syndrome patients with severe disease may have constitutional symptoms such as fever, malaise, anorexia, and weight loss.

Genitourinary involvement occurs in RS regardless of whether the disease follows an enteric or a genitourinary infection. The most common problem, occurring in 90% of patients, is urethritis; prostatitis, seminal vesiculitis, epididymitis, cystitis, orchitis, and urethral strictures may also occur. Urethritis is characterized by mild, serous, and transient urethral discharge, often asymptomatic; the discharge sometimes may be mucopurulent and may be accompanied by dysuria. Females may have cervicitis, nonspecific vaginitis, or urethritis, all of which are usually asymptomatic.[245]

Mucocutaneous lesions occur in over 50% of RS patients. The most frequent skin lesion

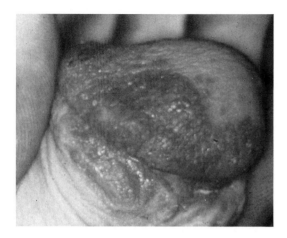

FIGURE 6.12. Circinate balanitis. Note the well-demarcated borders of the superficial erosions on the glans penis, extending over the corona onto the prepuce.

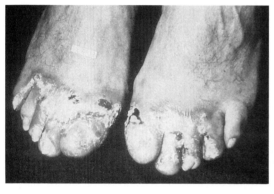

FIGURE 6.13. Keratoderma blennorrhagicum in a patient with Reiter's syndrome. Note the pronounced pustular and hyperkeratotic form of this dermatitis, which began approximately 3 months prior to the taking of this photograph.

is circinate balanitis, which begins as painless small vesicles on the glans penis (Fig. 6.12). These lesions rupture to form superficial erosions, which may coalesce to form well-demarcated borders (circinate). In circumcised patients the lesions become dry and scaly; in uncircumcised patients the lesions remain moist and sometimes become secondarily infected. A less frequent although characteristic

skin lesion in RS is keratoderma blennorrhagicum (Fig. 6.13), which affects primarily soles, palms, and glans penis, and less often limbs, trunk, scrotum, and scalp.[245] It begins as small macules that evolve into papules, vesicles, or pustules that coalesce to form hyperkeratotic scaly nodules that persist for days, weeks, or months; they usually then heal without scarring but can recur. In severe cases, keratoderma blennorrhagicum may affect the whole body, with generalized exfoliation and even death.[252] Oral mucosal lesions occur in about 10% of patients; these affect the palate, tongue, buccal mucosa, and lips. They begin as small papules that evolve into painless shallow ulcers, often with an irregular border that heals within a few days or weeks.[253] Nail involvement may occur as subungual pustules or as yellow and thickened nail plates caused by accumulation of subungual hyperkeratotic material (Fig. 6.14). Inflammatory areas of the adjacent skin may mimic paronychiae.

Other, less common extraarticular systemic manifestations include cardiac conduction abnormalities, pericarditis, aortitis, amyloidosis, thrombophlebitis, pleuritis, nonspecific diarrhea, neuropathy, and meningoencephalitis.[253]

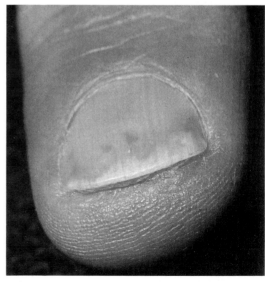

FIGURE 6.14. Subungual hyperkeratosis and nail pitting in a patient with Reiter's syndrome.

As in ankylosing spondylitis, vasculitis in RS is predominantly a large-artery arteritis.

The presence of unusual clinical manifestations such as seborrheic-like dermatitis (malar rash), oral thrush, hairy leukoplakia, persistent lymphadenopathy, prominent constitutional features, or rapid progression of articular manifestations in a patient with RS should alert the physician to the possibility of AIDS.[254] The review of systems in a patient with RS should include information regarding sexual and drug-related behaviors.

6.1.4.3. Ocular Manifestations

Although conjunctivitis and anterior uveitis are the most common ocular manifestation in RS, scleritis and episcleritis may occasionally occur. Other potential ocular problems include keratitis, retinitis, secondary glaucoma, and optic neuritis. Ophthalmic involvement usually follows rheumatological and genitourinary manifestations. In a study performed on 113 patients with RS, ocular manifestations developed within a mean of 2.9 years after the diagnosis of RS.[255]

6.1.4.3.1. Conjunctivitis

Conjunctivitis is the most common ocular problem in RS, occurring in 58% of patients.[255] It usually appears within a few weeks of the onset of arthritis or urethritis, but occasionally may be the first manifestation of the disease.[256] The conjunctivitis is usually mild, bilateral, with mucopurulent discharge, and with a papillary or follicular reaction. It lasts 7 to 10 days without treatment, and cultures are negative. Rarely, a small, nontender, enlarged preauricular lymph node and mild symblepharon formation may occur.

6.1.4.3.2. Anterior Uveitis

Anterior uveitis occurs in about 12% of patients with RS.[255] It is usually unilateral, nongranulomatous, with fine to medium-sized white keratic precipitates, mild cellular reaction, and flare. Posterior iris–lens synechiae and some cells in the vitreous are occasionally seen and there is no hypopyon; in severe cases, however, explosive uveitis with hypopyon may occur. Sec-

ondary glaucoma can develop from posterior iris–lens synechiae (pupillary block), peripheral anterior synechiae, or trabeculitis.[255,256] Anterior uveitis usually appears in recurrent rather than initial attacks of the disease. It is more frequent in patients who are *HLA-B27* positive and/or who have sacroiliitis.[253] Reiter's syndrome must always be considered in the differential diagnosis of anterior uveitis.

6.1.4.3.3. Scleritis

Although rare, scleritis may occur in patients with RS. It usually occurs in the later stages of the disease, and after other ocular manifestations such as conjunctivitis or anterior uveitis have developed. Diffuse anterior scleritis is the most frequent type of scleritis in patients with RS, and although it may be recurrent it never progresses to necrotizing scleritis.

In our own series of 172 patients with scleritis, 3 patients had RS (1.74%), including 2 men and 1 woman with a mean age of 37 years (range, 23 to 52 years). Two patients had diffuse anterior scleritis and one patient had nodular anterior scleritis. In all patients the scleritis was recurrent and unilateral, although in one patient both eyes were involved at different times. The scleritis appeared an average of 6 years after the RS diagnosis in two patients and was the initial manifestation whose study led to the RS diagnosis in the third patient. Scleritis occurred after several episodes of conjunctivitis and/or anterior uveitis and was associated with the presence of moderate anterior uveitis in all patients. Secondary glaucoma developed in one but responded to sclerouveitis antiinflammatory therapy. There were no corneal lesions, cataract, or macular edema, and although the initial visual acuity (during sclerouveitis attack) was worse than 20/80 in one patient, the final visual acuity was not affected. Any patient who develops diffuse or nodular anterior scleritis after recurrent anterior uveitis should be examined for RS or ankylosing spondylitis.

6.1.4.3.4. Episcleritis

Episcleritis is also rare in RS.[253,255,257] It may take the form of simple or nodular episcleritis and usually occurs after years of active RS. In our own series of 94 patients with episcleritis, 1 patient had RS (1.06%). The patient was a 26-year-old male with a seronegative asymmetric polyarthritis, sacroiliitis, circinate balanitis, oral mucosal ulcers, psoriasiform skin eruptions, and recurrent episodes of papillary conjunctivitis. Bilateral simple episcleritis appeared 6 years after the onset of the disease and responded well to oral nonsteroidal antiinflammatory therapy. There were no corneal lesions, cataract, macular edema, or decrease in visual acuity.

6.1.4.3.5. Other Ocular Findings

Keratitis in RS may be isolated but usually occurs associated with conjunctivitis and, less often, with anterior uveitis. It consists of punctate epithelial lesions that may coalesce to form an ulcer. Occasionally, subjacent anterior stroma infiltrates or micropannus occurs. [255,256]

Disk edema and recurrent retinal edema have been occasionally reported in RS but, as in ankylosing spondylitis-associated uveitis, posterior segment manifestations are rare.[258,259]

6.1.4.4. Laboratory and Radiographic Findings

The erythrocyte sedimentation rate is frequently elevated, but there is little or no correlation between the sedimentation rate and disease severity or prognosis. Mild hypo- or normochromic anemia or leukocytosis may be present, and serum proteins may be elevated. Circulating immune complexes may be found.[244] Tests for rheumatoid factor and antinuclear antibodies are negative.[255] Synovial fluid analysis and synovial biopsy are rarely contributory in the differential diagnosis of inflammatory joint disease. The synovial fluid–serum complement ratio is reduced.

Radiographic findings appear with progression of disease: erosions, joint space narrowing, and osteoporosis. New bone reaction and osteitis may be seen at sites of osseous attachments (pelvis, metatarsals, tarsal bones, and phalanges) of tendons and ligaments. Sacroiliitis and spondylitis indistinguishable from that seen in ankylosing spondylitis may occur, or they may be asymmetric.

6.1.4.5. Diagnosis

The diagnosis of RS is essentially clinical (Table 6.10). The major manifestations of RS are arthritis, nonspecific urethritis/cervicitis, inflammatory eye disease, and mucocutaneous lesions. The presence of arthritis and at least two of the other three manifestations establishes the diagnosis of Reiter's syndrome.[248] Many cases of suspected RS are never confirmed because major manifestations are too subtle; minor criteria have therefore been proposed to allow the diagnosis of probable or possible RS.[254] As in ankylosing spondylitis, the finding of *HLA-B27* increases the probability that the presumptive diagnosis is correct but it does not establish the diagnosis.

TABLE 6.10. Criteria for the diagnosis of Reiter's syndrome.[a]

Major criteria	Minor criteria
Polyarthritis	Plantar fasciitis, Achilles tendinitis, lower back pain, sacroiliitis, spondylitis
Conjunctivitis or anterior uveitis	Keratitis
Urethritis/cervicitis	Cystitis, prostatitis
Balanitis circinata, oral ulceration, or keratoderma blennorrhagicum	Psoriasiform eruptions, nail changes
	Diarrhea

[a] Reiter's syndrome (RS) diagnosis (modified from Ref. 243): definite RS, arthritis (seronegative asymmetric) and two or more other major criteria; probable RS, two major and two minor (found in different systems) criteria; possible RS, two major and one minor criterion.

6.1.5. Psoriatic Arthritis

Psoriatic arthritis (PA) is defined as the triad of psoriasis (skin and/or nail), idiopathic inflammatory arthritis (peripheral and/or spinal), and a negative test for rheumatoid factor.[227,251,260]

6.1.5.1. Epidemiology

Psoriasis occurs in 1 to 2% of the white population and affects individuals in the second and third decade of life. Psoriatic arthritis, occurring in about 5 to 7% of patients with psoriasis, has a estimated prevalence in the population of 0.10%. Onset is more frequent between 30 and 40 years of age and women are slightly more frequently involved than men (1.04:1). Family history may be obtained in one-third of patients, implying a role for genetic and/or environmental factors. Psoriasis and PA are associated with *HLA-B13, -B17, -B27, -Bw37, -Bw38, -Bw39*, and *-Cw6* genes. The association of *HLA-B27* is with psoriatic sacroiliitis and spondylitis (50%) but not with psoriatic peripheral arthritis or psoriasis.[227,261] The developments of guttate psoriasis following streptococcal infections, and of PA following trauma to the joint, have been recognized for many years.[227,260]

6.1.5.2. Systemic Manifestations

Psoriatic arthritis is characterized by skin and articular involvement. Other systemic findings such as amyloidosis, apical pulmonary fibrosis, and aortic insufficiency are seen only rarely.[227] Pustular skin lesions, due to small-vessel vasculitis, may occasionally appear.

6.1.5.2.1. Skin and Articular Involvement

The skin disease usually precedes the articular involvement by many years,[262,263] but in about 10% of patients with PA arthritis appears at the same time as psoriasis. Rarely, arthritis may precede psoriasis.

   Skin lesions in patients with PA commonly begin on the elbows, followed by appearance on the legs, scalp, *abdomen*, and back (Fig. 6.15). Although arthritis is more common in patients with severe skin involvement than in those with mild involvement,[264,265] a careful

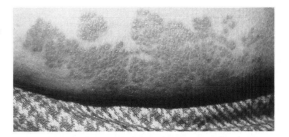

FIGURE 6.15. Psoriasis: typical scaly, erythematous dermatitis of psoriasis on the abdomen, with some areas having characteristic silver borders.

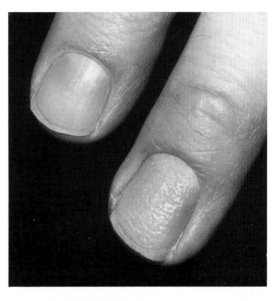

FIGURE 6.16. Nail pitting in a patient with psoriasis; the pattern is nearly pathognomonic for this disease.

search for minimal psoriatic lesions in the axilla, under the breast, in the umbilicus, or on the genitalia needs to be made in cases in which PA is suspected from the pattern of arthritis. Nail changes are more frequent in patients with PA (80%) than in patients with psoriasis without arthritis (30%). They are characterized by onycholysis, pitting, ridging, and nail discoloration or fragmentation (Fig. 6.16).

   There are at least five patterns of joint involvement in PA[262,263]: (1) Asymmetric monoarticular arthritis (5 to 10%) involves the distal interphalangeal joints of the fingers and toes, and is often associated with diffuse swelling of the digits (sausage digits) and with nail lesions; (2) chronic asymmetric oligoarticular arthritis (50 to 70%) affects two or three joints at a time; (3) chronic symmetric polyarthritis (15 to 25%) resembles rheumatoid arthritis but the test for rheumatoid factor is negative; (4) spondyloarthritis (20 to 30%) is characterized by sacroiliitis with or without spondylitis, is more common in males than in females, and has strong association with *HLA-B27*; (5) erosive "arthritis mutilans," the most uncommon subtype, shows a severe destructive and deforming polyarthritis with ankylosing of joints, "telescoping" of digits, and possible ankylosis of the spine. Apart from this deforming group, PA is not a severe disease; the pain and disability are much less than those produced by rheumatoid arthritis.[266]

6.1.5.3. Ocular Manifestations

Eye lesions of psoriasis consist of conjunctivitis and anterior uveitis and occasionally scleritis and episcleritis.[267] Anterior uveitis is usually mild with fine endothelial keratic precipitates. Psoriatic arthritis must always be considered in the differential diagnosis of anterior uveitis.

6.1.5.3.1. Scleritis

The reported incidence of PA in patients with scleritis is 1.44%.[122] Conversely, the reported incidence of scleritis in patients with PA is 1.8%.[267] Scleritis in PA usually appears after many years of active disease and, although diffuse anterior scleritis is often seen,[205] it may take almost any form of scleritis.

In our own series of 172 patients with scleritis, 2 patients had PA (1.16%). Both patients were female with a mean age of 70 years. One patient had unilateral necrotizing scleritis, which appeared 2 months after cataract surgery, and the other patient had bilateral posterior scleritis with choroidal folds, subretinal mass, choroidal detachment, and bilateral diffuse anterior scleritis. Both patients had had PA for many years. The patient with necrotizing scleritis developed sclerosing stromal keratitis. There was no conjunctivitis, anterior uveitis, glaucoma, cataract, or macular edema, and final visual acuity was not decreased Any pa-

tient who develops scleritis should be questioned and examined for skin and nail lesions.

6.1.5.3.2. Episcleritis

Episcleritis is also uncommon in PA and usually occurs after years of active disease. In our own series of 94 patients with episcleritis, 2 patients had PA (2.12%). Both patients were females with a mean age of 47 years, with chronic seronegative asymmetric oligoarthritis and skin psoriatic lesions, especially in legs and scalp. Bilateral simple episcleritis appeared 5 years and 20 years, respectively, after the onset of the psoriasis and recurred many times. There were no other ocular findings or decrease in visual acuity.

6.1.5.4. Laboratory and Radiographic Findings

Tests for rheumatoid factor and anti-nuclear antibodies are usually negative. The erythrocyte sedimentation rate is frequently elevated and mild anemia may appear. Hyperuricemia may be associated in patients with severe skin involvement and gout has been reported on several occasions.[268]

Radiographic findings depend on the type of articular involvement. Distal interphalangeal joints may show erosions with widening of the joint space and expansion of base of terminal phalanx. Dissolution of bones, especially the metatarsal, may be seen in arthritis mutilans, resulting in a "pencil in cup" appearance or "fish tail" deformity. Sacroiliitis and spondylitis indistinguishable from that seen in ankylosing spondylitis may be seen.[262]

6.1.5.5. Diagnosis

Psoriatic arthritis is diagnosed in the presence of skin psoriatic lesions and the presence of one or more swollen joints for at least 3 months (elbows, wrists, knees, ankles, metacarpophalangeal, proximal interphalangeal, and distal interphalangeal joints of the hands and feet, sacroiliacs, lumbar or cervical spine), with radiologic changes compatible with PA, including erosions in peripheral joints or definite spinal changes. As in ankylosing spondylitis or

Reiter's syndrome, the finding of *HLA-B27* positivity increases the probability that the presumptive diagnosis is correct but does not establish the diagnosis.

6.1.6. Inflammatory Bowel Disease-Associated Arthritis

Crohn's disease (CD) and ulcerative colitis (UC) are inflammatory bowel diseases that may have articular manifestations such as peripheral arthritis or spondyloarthropathy. Crohn's disease is a chronic focal granulomatous disease characterized by transmural inflammation of the gastrointestinal tract, predominantly the terminal ileum and cecum. Ulcerative colitis is a chronic inflammatory disease that affects the colonic mucosa and submucosa, predominantly the rectosigmoid area.[269]

6.1.6.1. Epidemiology

Crohn's disease occurs in 2 to 3 of 100,000 individuals and men are affected more often than women. Ulcerative colitis occurs in 2 to 7 of 100,000 individuals and females are more commonly affected than men. Both diseases have a first peak of incidence between the ages of 12 and 30 years, with a secondary peak at age 50 years. In comparison with the general population, Jews have a higher risk of developing the diseases.

Peripheral arthritis appears in 20% of patients with CD and in 10% of patients with UC, usually those with other extraintestinal manifestations. It most commonly begins between the ages of 25 and 45 years, and women and men are equally involved. Sacroiliitis with or without spondylitis appears in 10% of patients with CD or UC and affects men more commonly than women. This form of arthritis is strongly associated with *HLA-B27*, which is present in 50 to 70% of the patients.

6.1.6.2. Systemic Manifestations

Gastrointestinal and articular manifestations are the hallmarks of inflammatory bowel diseases. Other systemic manifestations include anemia, hepatobiliary disorders, thrombophlebitis, ureteral obstruction, nephrolithiasis, prostatitis, oral ulcerations, erythema nodosum, and pyoderma gangrenosum. Some of these manifestations, particularly the skin lesions, are due to small-sized vessel vasculitis.

6.1.6.2.1. Gastrointestinal and Articular Manifestations

Gastrointestinal symptoms in CD include right lower quadrant colicky pain associated with cramps and constipation, diarrhea, nausea, vomiting, fever, anorexia, and weight loss. Fistulae to the skin or other organs are common. Patients with UC present with left lower quadrant cramping pain, relapsing bloody mucoid diarrhea leading to dehydration and electrolyte imbalance, fever, anorexia, and weight loss.

Peripheral arthritis in both diseases usually occurs 6 months to several years after the onset of intestinal manifestations, although occasionally it may appear at the same time, or preceding colitis. It usually has an acute onset, affects one or a few joints, primarily knees and ankles, and usually resolves within a few weeks without sequelae. Other joints that may be involved are the proximal interphalangeal, elbow, shoulder, and wrists. Arthritis is more common in patients with extensive or severe bowel disease and waxes and wanes with the intestinal activity. Joint involvement in UC is more frequent in patients with colon disease than in patients with isolated rectal involvement. In CD, articular manifestations are more common in patients with colon disease than in patients with small bowel involvement. Patients with UC or CD with other manifestations such as skin lesions (erythema nodosum, pyoderma gangrenosum), mouth ulceration, or uveitis are more likely to develop arthritis. Proctocolectomy may lead to remission of arthritis in many patients with UC but in only a small number of patients with CD.[269]

Sacroiliitis with or without spondylitis, indistinguishable from ankylosing spondylitis, usually precedes the intestinal involvement and progresses independently of the bowel disease or proctocolectomy.[269]

6.1.6.3. Ocular Manifestations

The reported incidence of ocular manifestations in patients with inflammatory bowel diseases ranges from 1.9 to 11.8%.[270–273] The most common eye findings in inflammatory bowel disease patients include episcleritis, anterior uveitis, keratitis, and scleritis; conjunctivitis, macular edema, serous retinal detachment, choroidal infiltrates, orbital pseudotumor, extraocular muscle paresis, retrobulbar neuritis, papillitis, orbital cellulitis, and myositis are seen less frequently.[274,275] Ocular involvement in CD or UC patients is more common in those with arthritis[270,271,275]; other extraintestinal manifestations such as anemia, skin lesions, liver disease, and oral ulcers also are frequently associated with ocular disease. Ocular involvement in CD patients is more likely in those with colitis or ileocolitis than in patients with small bowel involvement alone.[275] Although eye lesions may precede the bowel disease, they often occur with exacerbation of colitis.[270,272,272,275,276] After proctocolectomy, the ocular prognosis is variable.[270] Because effective treatment of the bowel disease may improve the ocular and systemic prognoses, patients with ocular manifestations and gastrointestinal symptoms must be studied to define the nature of their gut involvement. The ophthalmologist may be the first to diagnose an inflammatory bowel disease.

6.1.6.3.1. Anterior Uveitis

Anterior uveitis is usually nongranulomatous, recurrent, with fine white keratic precipitates, moderate cells, and flare. It may occur before, during, or after the initial bowel attack, and often is associated with the presence of arthritis, particularly spondylitis.[271,272,275] Inflammatory bowel disease must always be considered in the differential diagnosis of anterior uveitis.

6.1.6.3.2. Scleritis

The reported incidence of scleritis in patients with inflammatory bowel disease ranges from 2.06 to 9.67%.[121,123] It is more common in patients with arthritis, anemia, skin manifestations, oral ulcers, or liver disease than in patients without extraintestinal manifestations.[272,275] Although scleritis may precede bowel disease, it usually occurs some years after the onset of gut symptoms, particularly during active episodes.[273,275,277] Scleritis associated with inflammatory bowel disease is recurrent and may take the form of almost any type of scleritis, including necrotizing anterior scleritis.[205,275,278] Treatment of the bowel manifestations may control the ocular condition. Knox and co-workers[272] reported that the presence of scleritis or episcleritis in a patient with inflammatory bowel disease is useful in differentiating CD and UC because, in their experience, these ocular lesions are not associated with UC.

In our own series of 172 patients with scleritis, 7 patients had inflammatory bowel diseases (4%), 4 with CD and 3 with UC. The patients were five women and two men with a mean age of 47 years (range, 32 to 68 years). All four patients with CD had arthritis; three patients had peripheral arthritis involving knees, proximal interphalangeal joints, and elbows, and one patient had sacroiliitis and spondylitis. Other extraintestinal manifestations included anemia, sclerosing colangitis, and oral ulcers. The mean time between bowel disease diagnosis and onset of arthritis was 4 years (range, 1 to 10 years) in three patients; the patient with spondyloarthropathy had back abnormalities before the onset of gut manifestations. The mean time between bowel disease diagnosis and onset of scleritis was 10 years (range, 6 to 20 years). Two patients had diffuse anterior scleritis (one bilateral and one unilateral) and two patients had unilateral nodular diffuse anterior scleritis. The scleritis was persistent or recurrent, and often related to episodes of active bowel disease. Proctocolectomy and ileostomy performed in one patient did not alter the frequency of scleritis attacks. Bilateral scleritis occurred after 3 years of almost monthly episodes of recurrent bilateral anterior uveitis in the patient with spondyloarthropathy. Any patient who develops scleritis after recurrent anterior uveitis should be examined for CD. There were no corneal lesions, secondary glaucoma, or macular edema, and final visual acuity was not affected. Crohn's disease must always be included in the differential diagnosis of a patient with scleritis.

Two of the three patients with UC developed necrotizing scleritis 3 weeks after cataract surgery and 1 year after scleral buckle followed by multiple infections, respectively. Both patients had UC for an average of 40 years, had not had any bowel disease exacerbation for many years, and did not have arthritis. Both patients had anterior uveitis: one, several years before the development of scleritis; the other, concomitantly with the onset of scleritis. Final visual acuity was not affected in one patient; the other patient maintained the low visual acuity determined at first examination because of retinal problems. Whether necrotizing scleritis after trauma and/or infection was associated with or independent of UC is unknown. The third patient developed nodular scleritis and mild anterior uveitis 5 years after the diagnosis of UC. She was 5 months pregnant and did not have any exacerbation of her bowel disease. Whether nodular scleritis during pregnancy was associated with or independent of UC is unknown.

6.1.6.3.3. Episcleritis

Episcleritis is common in inflammatory bowel disease.[272,275] Knox and co-workers[272] reported that the presence of episcleritis in UC is a good indicator to consider changing the diagnosis to CD because, in their experience, episcleritis is associated only with CD. Although episcleritis may appear prior to the onset of the gut manifestations,[277] it usually occurs after some years of bowel disease, especially during periods of disease exacerbation.[275] Episcleritis is more frequently seen in patients with arthritis and other extraintestinal manifestations.[270,272,275]

In our own series of 94 patients with episcleritis, 3 patients had inflammatory bowel disease (3.19%); all 3 patients had CD. All were female, with a mean age of 36 years, who developed recurrent simple episcleritis an average of 6 years (range, 5 to 7 years) after the diagnosis of CD. Two patients had had previous episodes of anterior uveitis and continued to have such episodes associated with episcleritis. Peripheral arthritis was present in two patients and anemia

and nasal ulcers were present in one. There were no corneal lesions, glaucoma, or decrease in visual acuity.

6.1.6.3.4. Keratitis

Keratitis in inflammatory bowel disease, specifically in CD, consists of either peripheral small round subepithelial gray infiltrates, probably due to acute inflammation, or peripheral nebulous subepithelial infiltrates, probably due to scarring.[279]

6.1.6.4. Laboratory and Joint Radiological Findings

Inflammatory bowel disease may account for anemia, leukocytosis, elevated sedimentation rate, and evidence of malabsorption or protein loss. Rheumatoid factor and anti-nuclear antibody tests are negative. Radiographs of involved joints show only minimal destructive signs such as cystic changes, narrowing of the joint space, and erosions.

6.1.6.5. Diagnosis

Diagnosis of CD is made on the basis of clinical signs and symptoms combined with characteristic X-ray findings, including deep (collar button) ulcerations, long strictured segments (string sign), and skip areas. Colonoscopy may be helpful when there is colonic involvement, and biopsies may show granuloma formation with transmural inflammation.[280]

Diagnosis of UC is based on clinical presentations along with the exclusion of infectious, parasitic, and neoplastic etiologies. Proctoscopy may reveal friability, edema, ulcerations, and mucopurulent exudate. Characteristic X-ray findings include lack of haustral markings, fine serrations, large ulcerations, and pseudopolyps. Biopsies show microabscesses of the crypts of Lieberkühn and macroscopic ulcerations; the inflammatory response is limited to the mucosa.

6.1.7. Relapsing Polychondritis

Relapsing polychondritis (RP) is an uncommon multisystem disease of unknown cause. Cartilage and other tissues with a high concentration of glycosaminoglycans are the main target of damage. These include the pinnae of the ears, nasal cartilage, eustachian tubes, larynx, trachea, bronchi, joints, vessels, and sclera.[281]

6.1.7.1. Epidemiology

Relapsing polychondritis is most frequent in the fourth decade of life, occurs predominantly in whites, and does not have sexual predilection.

6.1.7.2. Systemic Manifestations

Inflammation of auricular pinnae is the most common feature of the disease, occurring in 88.6% of patients.[282] Recurrent pain, swelling, and tenderness of one or both pinnae lead to resorption of cartilage and soft, pliable, drooping ears. Inflammation of the nasal cartilage occurs in over 50% of patients and may result in a saddle nose deformity (Fig. 6.17). Audio-vestibular involvement occurs in about 50% of patients and includes conductive or sensorineural hearing loss with or without vestibular damage. Impaired conductive hearing may be caused by involvement of the eustachian tube, external auditory meatus, or serous otitis media. Impaired sensorineural hearing or vestibular dysfunction may be caused by vasculitis of the cochlear or vestibular branch of the internal auditory artery.[282] Deafness or dizziness, vertigo, tinnitus, ataxia, nausea, and vomiting are the characteristic complaints. Laryngotracheal inflammation may be present in over 50% of patients and produces cough, hoarseness, dyspnea, pain over the anterior tracheal cartilage, and wheezing. Collapse of the upper airway through inflammation of the glottis, larynx, or subglottic tissue may be the cause of death in 10% of patients. Bronchial disease also can occur, leading to pulmonary infections and respiratory failure. A seronegative nondeforming nonerosive oligoarthritis or polyarthritis may appear in 50 to 80% of patients. Costochondral joints are frequently involved. Aortitis due to large-vessel vasculitis is the cardinal cardiovascular manifestation. It may lead to thoracic or abdominal aortic aneurysms that are silent until dissection or rupture occurs. Aortitis also may produce aor-

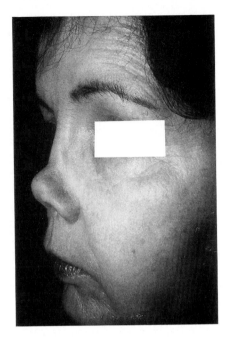

FIGURE 6.17. Relapsing polychondritis: Note the loss of nasal cartilage and the resultant nasal deformity.

tic regurgitation with secondary aortic valve insufficiency, and electrocardiographic abnormalities due to the proximity of the aortic root and the cardiac conduction system.

Manifestations due to small- and medium-sized vessel vasculitis include skin lesions, renal involvement, and neurological abnormalities. Skin lesions include purpura, urticaria, erythema nodosum, livedo reticularis, angioedema, and migratory thrombophlebitis.[283] Renal involvement presenting with proteinuria or microhematuria may be caused by focal proliferative glomerulonephritis with crescent formation.[284] Neurological abnormalities include cranial nerve involvement (second, sixth, seventh, and eighth), seizures, hemiplegia, ataxia, and sensorimotor neuropathy.[283,285]

6.1.7.3. Ocular Manifestations

Ocular manifestations may be the presenting symptom of RP in 20% of patients and will eventually occur in about 60% of patients.[283] Scleritis and episcleritis are the most common findings, but anterior uveitis, retinitis, extraocular muscle palsies, optic neuritis, conjunctivitis, keratitis, and exophthalmos also may occur.[243,283,285–288]

6.1.7.3.1. Scleritis

The reported incidence of RP in patients with scleritis ranges from 0.96 to 2.06%.[122,123] Conversely, about 14% of patients with RP have scleritis.[283] Scleritis may be diffuse anterior, nodular anterior, necrotizing anterior, or posterior,[122,289] and tends to occur with other manifestations of disease activity, such as auricular and nasal chondritis, and arthritis. Scleritis is usually recurrent and is frequently associated with anterior uveitis or peripheral keratitis.[283,290]

In our series of 172 patients with scleritis, 11 patients had RP (6.39%), including nine women and two men, with a mean age of 52 years (range, 26 to 74 years).[291] Systemic manifestations included auricular chondritis (nine patients), nasal chondritis (seven patients), nonerosive arthritis (six patients), cochleovestibular damage (four patients), and respiratory tract chondritis (two patients). Skin and renal lesions (one patient), and central neurological abnormalities and aortic aneurism (one patient) also were present. In 6 of 11 RP patients, scleritis was the presenting manifestation whose study led to the diagnosis of the systemic disease.

Three patients had necrotizing anterior scleritis, two had nodular anterior scleritis, and the scleritis was diffuse anterior in six patients. Scleritis was bilateral in four patients. Peripheral keratitis (seven patients), including corneal thinning (one patient), acute stromal keratitis (two patients), sclerosing keratitis (two patients), and peripheral ulcerative keratitis (two patients), was the most common ocular manifestation associated with RP scleritis. The second most common associated ocular abnormality was mild nongranulomatous anterior uveitis, which was present in six patients with RP scleritis. Other accompanying ocular manifestations were retinitis (two patients), extraocular muscle palsies (two patients), and optic disk edema (one patient). There was no decrease in final visual acuity. Any patient who develops scleritis should be asked and examined for auricular and nasal cartilage lesions.

6.1.7.3.2. Episcleritis

Episcleritis is a common finding in RP, accounting for 39% of RP patients in one series.[283] It may be simple or diffuse, unilateral or bilateral, and recurrent. As in the Watson and Hayreh series,[122] we do not have patients with RP episcleritis without scleritis, probably reflecting the high selection of cases who come to our Immunology Service following referral from other ophthalmology departments.

6.1.7.4. Laboratory Findings

Normochromic or hypochromic anemia, leukocytosis, eosinophilia, elevated erythrocyte sedimentation rate, and albuminuria are nonspecific abnormalities seen in RP.

6.1.7.5. Diagnosis

Relapsing polychondritis is characterized by recurrent chondritis of both auricles, chondritis of nasal cartilages, nonerosive inflammatory polyarthritis, inflammation of ocular structures, chondritis of the respiratory tract, and cochlear and/or vestibular damage. A diagnosis of RP[292,293] may be made in the presence of (1) three or more of these signs; or (2) at least one of these signs and a positive biopsy for vasculitis; or (3) chondritis in two or more separate anatomical locations with response to corticosteroids or dapsone.

6.1.8. Polyarteritis Nodosa

Polyarteritis nodosa (PAN) is a multisystem disease characterized, as it was originally described,[294] and later categorized,[295] by necrotizing vasculitis of small- and medium-sized arteries. The lesions tend to be segmental, with a predilection for bifurcations and branchings of vessels, with some distal involvement of arterioles and adjacent veins. Polyarteritis nodosa may be primary (idiopathic), or secondary to drugs or viral infections (e.g., hepatitis B). Polyarteritis nodosa may involve any organ, but skin, joints, peripheral nerves, gut, and kidney are most frequently involved. Without therapy, the prognosis of PAN is extremely poor, with a 12% 5-year survival in untreated patients. Patients treated with a combination of systemic corticosteroids and immunosuppressive agents have an 80% 5-year survival.[296]

6.1.8.1. Epidemiology

Polyarteritis nodosa is an uncommon disease with an incidence of about 1.8 per 100,000 population.[297] Onset is most frequent in the fourth or fifth decade, men are twice as likely to be affected than women, and there is no racial or familial predisposition.

6.1.8.2. Systemic Manifestations

Systemic manifestations of PAN are protean and may range from mild to fulminating. Constitutional symptoms such as fever, malaise, weight loss, and anorexia may appear along with skin, joint, or neurological manifestations. Visceral involvement such as gut or kidney may present concomitantly with, or after, these features.[298,299] Skin lesions include tender purple nodules (Osler's nodes), palpable purpura, ulcerations, livedo reticularis, or gangrenous plaques. Joint involvement consists of an asymmetric, nondeforming polyarthritis involving predominantly the large joints of the lower extremity. Neurological abnormalities include peripheral nervous system (sensory or sensorimotor neuropathy) and, less commonly, central nervous system (seizures, hemiparesis) manifestations. The presence of sensorimotor neuropathy (mononeuritis multiplex) during the course of PAN does not appear to have as bad a prognosis as does sensorimotor neuropathy complicating rheumatoid arthritis. Gastrointestinal involvement may manifest with abdominal pain, nausea, vomiting, diarrhea, hepatomegaly, ileus, bleeding, infarction, and perforation of visceral organs. Renal disease, occurring in almost 80% of patients, may present as focal or diffuse glomerulonephritis, renal ischemia, or hemorrhagic cystitis. Hypertension is a frequent complication of renal polyarteritis and may lead to uremia, congestive heart failure, and death. Ovarian, testicular, or epididymal involvement is often asymptomatic but infarction with pain may occur, and in some cases may be the presenting manifestation of PAN.

Other less common clinical findings, although frequent pathologically, are cardiac manifestations such as pericarditis, myocarditis, endocarditis, and myocardial infarction. Pulmonary abnormalities such as pleuritis and lung infiltration also may occur; however, they are more common in patients with granulomatous vasculitis (Wegener's granulomatosis, or allergic granulomatous angiitis [Churg–Strauss syndrome]).

6.1.8.3. Ocular Manifestations

Ocular manifestations appear in 10 to 20% of PAN patients. Polyarteritis nodosa may involve every tissue of the eye, depending on which vessels are affected by the vasculitic process. Choroidal vasculitis is the most frequent histological abnormality,[243,300–306] but the presence of yellow subretinal patches is less often appreciated clinically. Retinal vasculitis may lead to retinal hemorrhages, retinal edema, cotton-wool spots, irregular caliber of retinal vessels, and retinal vascular occlusion.[301,305,306] Sometimes the retinopathy may be secondary to concomitant hypertension. Papilledema or papillitis due to optic nerve vasculitis may occur and inflammation of orbital vessels may lead to exophthalmos.[301,302,307–309] Vasculitic involvement of the central and peripheral nervous system may produce third, fifth, sixth, and seventh nerve palsies, homonymous hemianopia, nystagmus, amaurosis fugax, and Horner's syndrome.[307] Anterior uveal vascular inflammation is occasionally seen as anterior uveitis with leakage of protein into the anterior chamber.[305,310] Conjunctival infarction may produce pale yellow, raised and friable conjunctival lesions, chemosis, and subconjunctival hemorrhages.[310] Vascular inflammation of episcleral, scleral, and limbal vessels may lead to episcleritis, scleritis, and sclerokeratitis.[304,305,311–313] Ocular involvement may be the first manifestation of PAN.[204,312,314]

6.1.8.3.1. Scleritis

The reported incidence of PAN in patients with scleritis ranges from 0.68 to 6.45%.[121–123]

Necrotizing anterior scleritis, often associated with peripheral ulcerative keratitis, is the most frequent type of scleritis in patients with PAN.[311–313] Scleritis becomes extremely painful and is highly destructive unless correct diagnosis and control of the underlying systemic disease are achieved. Corneal ulceration is progressive, both circumferentially and centrally, with undermining of the central edge of the ulcer, resulting in overhanging lip of the cornea. Scleral involvement helps to distinguish classic Mooren's ulcer from sclerokeratitis associated with vasculitic diseases such as rheumatoid arthritis, Wegener's granulomatosis, or PAN. In most cases, sclerokeratitis will present after PAN diagnosis, but occasionally may be the presenting manifestation of the disease.[204,312,314]

In our series of 172 patients with scleritis, PAN was diagnosed in 2 patients (1.16%): 1 man and 1 woman, with a mean age of 58 years. One patient had unilateral diffuse scleritis and the other patient had unilateral necrotizing scleritis with peripheral ulcerative keratitis. Polyarteritis nodosa had already been diagnosed 1 year before the onset of nodular scleritis in the first patient. Necrotizing scleritis with peripheral ulcerative keratitis was the first manifestation whose study led to the diagnosis of PAN in the second patient; biopsy of an elbow nodule compatible with PAN and saccular aneurysms in the superior mesenteric artery in the setting of systemic clinical findings such as constitutional symptoms, dizziness, profound quadriceps muscle weakness, tinnitus, skin lesions, and grand mal seizure confirmed the diagnosis of PAN. Prompt and aggressive therapy improved the ocular and systemic prognoses. The ophthalmologist may play an important role in the diagnosis and management of a patient with this potentially lethal vasculitic disease.

6.1.8.3.2. Episcleritis

Although histological involvement of episcleral vessels is frequently seen, episcleritis is less often detected clinically.[299,304] It may be simple or diffuse, and recurrent.[205] Episcleritis in patients with PAN is less common than scleritis.[122]

There are no patients with PAN in our series of patients with episcleritis.

6.1.8.4. Laboratory and Angiographic Findings

There are no laboratory tests that can confirm the diagnosis of PAN. Leukocytosis, eosinophilia, and an elevated erythrocyte sedimentation rate may be seen. In cases with urinary sediment red cells, red cell casts, or proteinuria, renal disease must be suspected. The angiographic finding of small, aneurysmal dilatations in renal, hepatic, and gastrointestinal vessels may be helpful in establishing the diagnosis although they may also be found in systemic lupus erythematosus[315] and fibromuscular dysplasia.[316]

6.1.8.5. Diagnosis

The diagnosis of PAN is based on the histological finding of necrotizing vasculitis of small- and medium-sized muscular arteries in patients with compatible multisystem clinical findings. Biopsy of symptomatic areas such as skin, testes, epididymus, skeletal muscle, or peripheral nerves provides the highest diagnostic yield.[317–319] Blind biopsy of asymptomatic organs rarely establish the diagnosis.

6.1.9. Allergic Granulomatous Angiitis (Churg–Strauss Syndrome)

Allergic granulomatous angiitis (Churg–Strauss syndrome) is a vasculitic disease similar to classic polyarteritis nodosa in that it may affect any organ of the body; however, unlike classic polyarteritis nodosa, pulmonary involvement is a sine qua non of this syndrome. Churg–Strauss syndrome is characterized, as it was originally described,[320] by asthma, eosinophilia, pulmonary infiltrations, vasculitis, and extravascular granulomas.

6.1.9.1. Epidemiology

Although there are no epidemiological studies, Churg–Strauss syndrome is an uncommon disease. Age at onset ranges from 15 to 70 years and men are twice as likely to be affected as women.

6.1.9.2. Systemic Manifestations

Lung involvement is predominant and usually the first manifestation of the disease. There is often a history of asthma, or atopy, or both, sometimes with bronchitis and pneumonitis. After a mean duration of asthma of 8 years,[321] constitutional symptoms such as fever, malaise, and weight loss may appear, heralding the onset of systemic manifestations in skin, peripheral nerves, heart, gastrointestinal tract, and kidney.[321,322] At this time, chest X rays may show evanescent pulmonary infiltrates (Löffler's syndrome), massive nodular infiltrates without cavitation, or diffuse interstitial lung disease. Systemic findings include (1) skin lesions such as subcutaneous nodules, purpura, or ulcerations, (2) peripheral neuropathy such as mononeuritis multiplex, (3) heart abnormalities such as congestive heart failure, (4) gastrointestinal involvement such as infarction, ulceration, or perforation of the stomach, small bowel, or large bowel, and (5) renal disease with eosinophilic granulomatous involvement of the prostate and lower urinary tract.

Polyarthralgias and arthritis are uncommon in Churg–Strauss syndrome. Central nervous system abnormalities such as seizures are unusual.

6.1.9.3. Ocular Manifestations

Ocular manifestations in Churg–Strauss syndrome are rare. A necrotizing eosinophilic granulomatous process may involve conjunctiva,[323] cornea, uveal tract, retina, and optic nerve.[324] Episcleritis and scleritis may occur as part of the ocular involvement.[324] Because ocular abnormalities may be the initial manifestation of the disease,[323] their recognition may lead to early Churg–Strauss syndrome diagnosis and prompt initiation of therapy. There are no cases of Churg–Strauss syndrome in our series of scleritis or episcleritis.

6.1.9.4. Laboratory Findings

The characteristic laboratory finding is eosinophilia. In the original description by Churg and Strauss,[320] eosinophil counts ranged from 5000 to 20,000 eosinophils per mm^3. With patient improvement, eosinophilia decreases. Elevated serum IgE, anemia, and an elevated erythrocyte sedimentation rate also may be found.[321]

6.1.9.5. Diagnosis

Diagnosis of Churg–Strauss syndrome is based on both pathological and clinical findings. Demonstration of necrotizing small-vessel vasculitis and eosinophilic necrotizing intra- and extravascular granulomas on biopsy material confirms the diagnosis of Churg–Strauss syndrome in a patient with compatible multisystem clinical findings and laboratory tests.[319,320,323–328] Involved tissues more commonly biopsied for diagnosis are lung, skin, and peripheral nerves.

6.1.10. Wegener's Granulomatosis

Wegener's granulomatosis (WG) is a systemic disease of unknown etiology characterized, as it was originally described, by granulomatous inflammation of the upper and lower respiratory tract, necrotizing vasculitis, and nephritis.[328–330] A description of classic pathological findings is shown in Table 6.11. Aside from this fulminant, active, generalized, or disseminated form of the disease, an indolent form called limited, initial, or locoregional WG also may occur.[331–335] In the limited form of WG, the respiratory tract is involved and the kidneys are spared; chronic hemorrhagic rhinitis, sinusitis, otitis, ulcerations in the oral cavity, nasolacrimal duct obstruction, orbitopathy, conjunctivitis, keratitis, scleritis, or uveitis also may occur.[332–338] Pathologically, involved tissues reveal necrotizing granulomatous inflammation and vasculitis. A highly limited form of WG has been described by our group[339] in patients with only ocular or orbital disease on the basis of a constellation of histopathological findings and a positive laboratory test (anti-neutrophil cytoplasmic antibodies [ANCAs]).

Untreated WG is rapidly fatal, particularly once there is functional renal impairment;

TABLE 6.11. Classic diagnostic triad for Wegener's granulomatosis.[a]

1. Necrotizing granuloma of the upper and/or lower respiratory tract: There is typically mucosal inflammation and ulceration in the respiratory tract. Mucosal inflammation is characterized by foci of epithelioid cells, multinucleated giant cells, and fibrillar organization with secondary necrosis of fibrillar tissue. Tissue eosinophilia is common.

2. Vasculitis: The vasculitis involves both arteries and veins and is of a focal, necrotizing variety. The vasculitis is granulomatous in nature, featuring multinucleated giant cells. This vasculitis is typically seen in lung tissue, and is variably present elsewhere.

3. Nephritis: The nephritis is a focal, necrotizing glomerulitis with fibrinoid necrosis and thrombosis of capillary loops, sometimes extending beyond Bowman's capsule. Neutrophils are usually present; granulomatous inflammation with giant cells is only occasionally seen.

[a] Based on the pathological findings described by Godman and Churg.[330]

onset of renal disease is associated with a mean survival of 5 months, with a 1-year mortality rate of 82% of patients and a 2-year mortality rate of 90%.[331] Therapy with systemic corticosteroids and immunosuppressive agents may induce remission in 93% of patients.[338] It is imperative, therefore, to establish the diagnosis and initiate appropriate treatment as early as possible in the course of the disease.

6.1.10.1. Epidemiology

Wegener's granulomatosis is a rare disease that typically occurs in patients between 40 and 60 years of age, although presentation at ages ranging from 7 to 75 years has been reported.[338,340] The disease occurs slightly more frequently in men than in women, with a ratio up to 1.5:1.[331,338,341] Wegener's granulomatosis may affect blacks and Hispanics, but is most commonly seen in whites.[338]

6.1.10.2. Clinical Manifestations

Pulmonary infiltrates and sinusitis are the two most common presenting signs of WG.[338] Arthralgias or arthritis, fever, otitis (usually related to eustachian tube obstruction), cough, and (less frequently) functional renal impairment also may be presenting manifestations. Malaise, fatigue, fever, and weight loss are characteristic of the onset of active or generalized WG.

Over the course of WG, lower respiratory tract or upper airway abnormalities (sinusitis, hemorrhagic rhinitis, nasal mucosal ulcerations, and otitis media) are the most common manifestations. Characteristic lower respiratory tract symptoms are cough, hemoptysis, dyspnea, and (less often) pleuritic pain. Chest X-ray findings show multiple, bilateral nodal infiltrates with a tendency toward cavitation, as well as evanescent areas of atelectasis. Pleural effusions and subglottal stenosis of the airway also may occur, but hilar adenopathy is rare.[338] Nasal septal perforation and loss of supporting nasal structures may lead to the characteristic saddle nose deformity. Secondary infections, almost invariably caused by *Staphylococcus aureus*, often complicate upper airway abnormalities.

Renal disease, the second most common manifestation, usually occurs after upper and lower airway manifestations. It may range from mild, focal and segmental glomerulonephritis, with minimal urinary sediment finding or functional impairment, to fulminant, diffuse, necrotizing glomerulonephritis, with proliferative and crescentic changes. Renal disease, once present, may progress rapidly and is associated with a poor prognosis.[342]

Other manifestations include arthralgias and nondeforming arthritis, skin lesions such as papules, vesicles, palpable purpura, ulcers, and subcutaneous nodules, neurological abnormalities such as peripheral neuropathy (mononeuritis multiplex) or cranial nerve palsies, and cardiac involvement such as acute pericarditis and dilated congestive cardiomyopathy.[338]

6.1.10.3. Ocular Manifestations

Ocular manifestations occur in 29 to 58% of WG patients.[338,343–345] They can be divided into two categories: contiguous and focal.[345] Contiguous ocular manifestations such as severe orbital pseudotumor, orbital abscess or cellulitis, or nasolacrimal duct obstruction, occur as a result of the extension of contiguous granulomatous sinusitis of long duration. Orbital inflammation with proptosis is the most common ocular manifestation in WG.[343-345] Focal ocular disease in WG is unrelated to any upper airway disease; it is characterized by a focal vasculitis of the anterior and/or posterior segments of the eye and possibly the orbit. Of the focal ocular manifestations of WG, conjunctivitis, scleritis, episcleritis, and keratitis are most common.[343-345] Ischemic optic neuropathy and retinal artery occlusion are other types of focal eye involvement that can occur in WG. Uveitis,[343-345] chorioretinal ischemia and infarction,[346] and keratoconjunctivitis sicca[347] may occasionally occur. Although most patients with complete or limited WG present with upper and lower airway symptoms, ocular involvement also may be the first sign prompting patients to seek medical attention.[204,338,343,344,348] In the highly limited form of WG, ocular or orbital involvement is the only objective finding of the condition.[339] The ophthalmologist may be the first to diagnose WG.

6.1.10.3.1. Scleritis

The reported incidence of WG in patients with scleritis is about 3.79%.[123] Conversely, the reported incidence of scleritis in patients with WG ranges from 7 to 11%.[342-344] The scleritis may be diffuse, nodular, or necrotizing. Necrotizing scleritis and peripheral ulcerative keratitis are the most malignant ocular manifestations of WG; they can result in ocular perforation, leading to blindness, and possibly loss of the eye.[243] Corneal ulceration, exactly like that seen in rheumatoid arthritis or polyarteritis nodosa, develops after breakdown of the peripheral corneal epithelium and progresses centrally and circumferentially, producing an overhanging lip of the cornea; the biomicroscopic appearance is similar to that of Mooren's ulcer, except that sclera is never involved in the latter. Patients with complete, limited, or highly limited forms of WG may have scleritis at the time of the initial medical

examination.[204,335,339,344,349-351] Scleritis often parallels systemic symptoms and may be the initial manifestation of a systemic disease exacerbation.[343,352] Necrotizing scleritis may appear after surgical trauma of the sclera.

In our series of 172 patients with scleritis, 14 patients had WG (8%). Two patients had complete WG, 10 patients had limited WG, and 2 patients had highly limited WG. The mean age of our patients was 60 years (range, 15 to 81 years) and the scleritis was more common in males than in females (10 males and 4 females). In all patients but one, the presence of scleritis was the first manifestation whose study led to the diagnosis of WG; the mean time between onset of scleritis and diagnosis of WG was 8.5 months. Review of systems in patients with scleritis disclosed upper or lower airway abnormalities in 9 of 14 patients. The scleritis attacks were persistent or recurrent, and often related to episodes of active disease. Necrotizing anterior scleritis was present in 11 patients; in 4 of those, necrotizing anterior scleritis appeared after surgical trauma of the sclera. Two patients had diffuse anterior scleritis and one patient had nodular anterior scleritis. Peripheral ulcerative keratitis was present in 7 of 14 patients (50%) with scleritis; 6 patients had necrotizing anterior scleritis and 1 patient had diffuse anterior scleritis. Anterior uveitis was present in 6 of 14 patients (43%) with scleritis. The incidence of anterior uveitis in our series of 158 patients with scleritis without WG was similar (42%), indicating that there is no correlation between anterior uveitis and WG per se.

Keratitis, uveitis, glaucoma, cataract, and disk edema caused by scleral inflammation may affect visual acuity. A decrease in visual acuity (equal to or greater than two Snellen lines at the end of the follow-up period or vision equal to or worse than 20/80 at the first examination) occurred in 50% of the eyes.

6.1.10.3.2. Episcleritis

Episcleritis may occur in WG but is less frequent than scleritis.[343,345] It may be simple or nodular and often is recurrent. Episcleritis in WG may be the first manifestation that prompts the patient to seek medical advice.[343]

In our series of patients with episcleritis there were no patients with WG.

6.1.10.4. Laboratory Findings

Until recently, there was no specific laboratory diagnostic test for WG. Normochromic normocytic anemia, leukocytosis, thrombocytosis, an elevated sedimentation rate, positive rheumatoid factor, elevated C-reactive protein, and circulating immune complexes are common nonspecific abnormalities found in patients with WG.

It was in 1985 that the presence of ANCA in serum was found to be specific for WG and to correlate with disease activity.[353] Subsequent studies confirmed that ANCA is indeed specific for WG,[341,354,355] with specificity as high as 99% by indirect immunofluorescence techniques and 98% by enzyme-linked immunosorbent assay (ELISA) detection.[341] The sensitivity of ANCA depends on disease activity and extent: sensitivity is 32% for WG patients in full remission after limited disease, 67% for WG patients with active limited disease, and 96% for WG patients with active generalized disease. These findings indicate that a negative ANCA test does not rule out a diagnosis of WG. "False-positive" ANCA titers have been found in only 0.6% of patients, all of whom have glomerulonephritis, pulmonary–renal syndrome, or vasculitis.[341] Although still pending confirmation, relapses of WG seem to be preceded by elevation of ANCA titers.

At least two types of ANCA staining of neutrophils may occur. The classic granular cytoplasmic staining pattern (C-ANCA) is specific for myeloblastin, a neutrophil serine protease referred to as proteinase 3 (PR-3).[356,357] Although C-ANCA is highly specific for WG,[339,340] not all patients positive for C-ANCA fullfil the classic criteria for WG.[358] A perinuclear staining pattern (P-ANCA) is specific for various lysosomal enzymes such as myeloperoxidase, cathepsin G, human leukocyte elastase, or lactoferrin. P-ANCA is a specific marker of idiopathic necrotizing and crescentic glomerulonephritis, a disease frequently associated with microscopic polyarteritis, and occasionally with WG.[356] The absence of granulomata helps to distinguish microscopic polyarteritis from WG, athough the clinical picture is similar. It would seem that WG, microscopic polyarteritis, and idiopathic necrotizing and crescentic glomerulonephritis are part of the spectrum of one disease process. Although C-ANCA is typically the ANCA associated with WG,[358,359] there are cases that fulfill the classic criteria for WG and show the P-ANCA pattern of staining.[360]

The ANCA test must be included in the diagnostic evaluation of patients with ophthalmic manifestations suggestive of systemic vasculitis.[352,361] In a study performed by us on the diagnostic value of ANCA testing in patients with scleritis associated with WG, ANCA titers were highly specific and sensitive for WG in patients with scleritis[362]: of 23 patients with scleritis in which ANCA titers were obtained, all 7 patients with positive titers had limited or generalized WG and none of the 16 patients with negative ANCA titers had WG.

Positive ANCA testing confirms the diagnosis of the highly limited forms of Wegener's granulomatosis in a patient with scleritis and pathological detection of necrotizing granulomas with or without inflammatory microangiopathy.[339]

Either type of ANCA (C-ANCA or P-ANCA) can be found in patients with generalized, limited, or highly limited forms of WG with ophthalmic involvement.[339,361,362]

The discovery of ANCA as a specific and sensitive index of generalized disease in WG is likely to improve the prognosis for patients with this disease by facilitating earlier diagnosis and detection of relapse. However, a single positive ANCA test should be interpreted with caution.

6.1.10.5. Diagnosis

The diagnosis of WG is generally made on the basis of the clinicopathological findings of necrotizing granulomatous lesions of the upper and lower respiratory tract, glomerulonephritis, and frequently vasculitis involving other organ systems. The American College of Rheumatology established criteria for the diagnosis of WG.[363] The presence of two or more of the following four criteria was associated with a sensitivity of 88.2% and a specificity of 92% for WG: (1) abnormal urinary sediment (red cell casts or five blood cells per high power field), (2) abnormal findings on chest radiograph (nodules, cavities, or fixed infiltrates), (3) oral ulcers or nasal discharge, (4) granulomatous inflammation (in the vessel wall, perivascular, or extravascular).

Cultures and special stains must be done to rule out infectious causes of granulomatous inflammation, such as acid-fast bacilli and fungi.

ANCA testing is an important adjunct in the diagnosis of WG because it has been found to be 99% specific and 96% sensitive for the active generalized condition.[341] Because of its high specificity, a positive test is suggestive of WG, even in patients without compatible clinical and histopathological findings. However, because ANCA is positive only in 67% of patients with active limited disease and in 32% of patients in full remission after limited disease,[341] a negative ANCA test does not exclude the diagnosis, especially in patients with limited clinical features and characteristic histological findings.

Pathological detection of necrotizing granulomas with or without vasculitis in involved extraocular tissues (nasal mucosal, sinus tissue, skin, and lung) confirms the diagnosis of WG in a patient with compatible systemic clinical findings with or without positive ANCA testing. Pathological detection of necrotizing granulomas with or without inflammatory microangiopathy in conjunctiva and/or scleral specimens in association with complete and, especially, limited clinical features confirms the diagnosis of WG even if the ANCA test is negative.

In the absence of characteristic ocular histological findings, a positive ANCA test is suggestive of highly limited WG, although not diagnostic. In the absence of positive ANCA test, the presence of characteristic ocular histological findings without systemic clinical features does not support the diagnosis of WG.

6.1.11. Behçet's Disease

Behçet's disease (BD) is a chronic relapsing systemic vasculitis of unknown etiology characterized by oral ulceration, genital ulceration, and ocular inflammation. Although Hippocrates had already noted the association between ocular inflammation and oral and genital ulcers,[364] it was Hulusi Behçet,[365] a Turkish professor of dermatology, who first recognized the disease as a distinct entity in 1937.

6.1.11.1. Epidemiology

The prevalence of BD has a peculiar distribution as most cases have been reported from Japan and the eastern Mediterranean countries, especially along ancient silk trade routes. The highest reported prevalence is in Japan, with 7 to 8.5 cases per 100,000 population.[366] However, the disease may occur worldwide. Our series of cases with ocular BD have been reported from the United States with a higher than expected proportion of Hispanic patients.[367]

Although the number of male patients exceeds females in Turkish,[368] Israeli,[369] and Japanese clinic populations,[370] reports from U.S. clinic populations have equal numbers of male and female patients.[367,371] Male sex and early age of onset of BD are associated with greater severity.[370,372]

There is no association between HLA antigens and BD in Northern European and American populations.[373,374] By contrast, in Japanese and Mediterranean populations, BD is associated with the histocompatibility B5 antigen, and particularly the Bw51 subgroup.[375,376]

6.1.11.2. Systemic Manifestations

Systemic manifestations of BD include oral and genital mucosal ulcers. In addition to that, there may be involvement of the skin, joints, major vessels, gastrointestinal tract, and central nervous system.

Mucosal oral ulcers, ranging from 2 to 10 mm in diameter, are typically round or oval, with a central yellow base, and surrounded by a red halo. They are exceedingly painful and can appear on the buccal mucosa, lips, tongue, and pharynx. These ulcers heal in 3 to 30 days, usually without scarring, and typically are recurrent. Mucosal ulcers of the vulva and vagina in females and of the scrotum and penis in males are similar to the oral ulcers, but tend to be deeper and often scar. Genital ulcerations recur less frequently than oral ulcerations. Nonmucosal genital ulcers are nodular with central ulceration.

The skin lesions typical of BD include erythema nodosum, pustules, and papules, all considered to be manifestations of cutaneous vasculitis. However, because cutaneous vasculitis is common in other systemic diseases, skin lesions are nonspecific. Erythema nodosum is an eruption of tender, raised, red nodules, usually confined to the lower extremities, that usually resolves without ulceration in a matter of weeks. Pustular vasculitis or papulopustular eruption also may occur in BD. A nonspecific skin sensitivity to simple trauma or pathergy test has been reported in patients with BD; the presence of marked redness, swelling, and/or a pustular lesion 24 to 48 h after a sterile skin prick, or after intradermal injection of air or saline, is interpreted as a positive result. However, because this test has a lower positivity rate in British and North American patients with BD, it is not helpful for diagnosis in these clinical populations.[377]

Nonmigrating recurrent seronegative nondeforming arthritis, affecting knees, ankles, and wrist, may occur in up to 60% of patients with BD.[378] Cardiovascular involvement includes venous and arterial occlusion and aneurysms, with venous involvement being twice as common as arterial involvement. Venous involvement includes deep vein occlusion (superior vena cava, inferior vena cava, femoral and subclavian veins, or common iliac and hepatic vein) and superficial thrombophlebitis. Arterial involvement includes stenosis or occlusion of subclavian, renal, carotid, or femoral arteries. Cardiovascular involvement in BD carries a poor prognosis.[378] Gastrointestinal ulcerations may occur, particularly in the lower ileum and right side of the colon; they may perforate and require hemicolectomy and distal ileal resection. Central nervous system manifestations of BD can cause sensory, motor, or neuropsychiatric symptoms. Meningoencephalitis can cause headache, fever, stiff neck, cerebrospinal pleocytosis, and focal neurological deficits.

6.1.11.3. Ocular Manifestations

Ocular involvement may be the presenting manifestation of BD. It also may correlate with systemic exacerbations of the disease, particularly with central nervous system complications.[367] Ocular disease usually begins in one eye but eventually involves both; inflammation is more severe in one eye when it is bilateral. Sterile hypopyon, occurring in one-third of cases, is the classic ocular finding described by Behçet. It may be a late sign and tends to disappear quickly. Sterile hypopyon in BD can be distinguished from an infectious hypopyon in that it does not coagulate; it moves with gravity, changing with position. Anterior uveitis and vasculitic involvement of the retina and optic nerve are much more common than hypopyon in BD. Anterior uveitis may lead to cataract as well as to synechia formation and subsequent glaucoma. Retinal vasculitis can involve small vessels of both the arterial and venous systems and can produce vascular "sheathing" with intraretinal hemorrhages, edema, and exudates, branch and central retinal vein occlusion, arteriolar attenuation, and venous dilatation and tortuosity. Serous retinal detachment is sometimes seen. Optic nerve vasculitis leads to disk hyperemia or edema and eventual optic atrophy.[370] Retinal or optic nerve vasculitis may lead to blindness.

Although much less common, involvement of the anterior segment of the eye may lead to conjunctivitis, keratitis, scleritis, and episcleritis.

6.1.11.3.1. Scleritis

Scleritis is rare in BD.[367] Behçet's disease is also rare in patients with scleritis; the reported incidence of BD in patients with scleritis is about 0.68%.[123] Occasionally, however, it may be the presenting symptom that prompts the patient to seek medical advice and whose study leads to the BD diagnosis. Scleritis may appear as an isolated ocular finding, or may be part of a complex ocular involvement with retinal vasculitis and papillitis. Behçet's disease must be strongly considered in a young patient with recurrent, bilateral retinal vasculitis associated with scleritis. A careful review of systems and dermatological examination are essential in establishing the diagnosis. Scleritis may correlate with systemic disease activity.

Only 1 patient of our 172 patients with scleritis had BD (0.58%). The patient was a 35-year-old white female who presented to us with a third episode of "red and painful left eye"; slit-lamp examination revealed a moderate nodular scleritis with mild anterior uveitis in the left eye. There were no posterior pole abnormalities and visual acuity was not decreased. Review of systems disclosed oral ulcers, genital ulcers, erythema nodosum, and arthritis.

6.1.11.3.2. Episcleritis

Episcleritis is also rare in BD and often appears after other ocular manifestations such as retinal vasculitis or disk edema. Behçet's disease must be strongly considered in a young patient with recurrent, bilateral retinal vasculitis associated with episcleritis. Mucosal and skin examination may be helpful in determining the diagnosis of BD. Like other ocular abnormalities in BD, episcleritis may appear during episodes of active disease. Only 1 patient of our 94 patients with episcleritis had BD (1.06%). The patient was a 42-year-old white female who had simple episcleritis as well as retinal vasculitis and disk edema in the left eye. Vision in the left eye was reduced to the level of counting fingers. The patient had already been diagnosed with BD because of oral ulcers, genital ulcers, papulopustular eruptions in skin, arthritis, gastrointestinal complaints, retinal vasculitis, and optic neuritis. Exacerbation of the systemic disease, in spite of immunosuppressive therapy, was concomitant with the onset of episcleritis and the relapse of retinal vasculitis and optic neuritis.

6.1.11.4. Laboratory Findings

Numerous immunological abnormalities in patients with BD have been detected but none is diagnostic. These abnormalities include elevated circulating immune complexes and decreased complement components, leukocytosis, cryoglobulins, elevated interferon γ, increased chemotactic activity of neutrophils, and elevation of serum immunoglobulins A, G, and M. Furthermore, T cell subsets CD4$^+$ (helper) and CD8$^+$ (suppressor), which are normally in serum in a 2:1 ratio, change to a 1:1 ratio in BD.

6.1.11.5. Diagnosis

The diagnosis of BD is based on a constellation of clinical findings that may occur simultaneously or sequentially.[366,379] The International Study Group (ISG) for BD[380] established in 1990 new, internationally agreed-on diagnostic criteria for BD. These criteria include recurrent oral ulceration plus two of the following: (1) genital ulceration, (2) typical defined eye lesions, (3) typical defined skin lesions, and (4) a positive pathergy test.

The diagnosis of BD should be considered in any young patient with bilateral and recurrent retinal vasculitis or vascular occlusion that may be associated with anterior uveitis, with scleritis, or with episcleritis. Fluorescein angiography may be useful in determining the extent of retinal and disk involvement. Meticulous review of systems and mucosal and skin examination are essential in establishing the diagnosis.

6.1.12. Giant Cell Arteritis

Giant cell arteritis (GCA), also called temporal arteritis, cranial arteritis, or granulomatous arteritis, is a systemic vasculitis of unknown etiology that involves the medium-sized extracranial arteries of the carotid circulation (superficial temporal, vertebral, and ophthalmic), and sometimes the aorta and its primary branches.[381,382] Complications of this vasculitis can lead to blindness, stroke, and death. Certain clinical features, laboratory tests, and histopathological findings are helpful in distinguishing GCA from other vasculitides: the age at onset, temporal headache or tenderness, reduced temporal artery pulsation, transient or irreversible visual loss, polymyalgia rheumatica, an elevated erythrocyte sedimentation rate, and mononuclear or multinucleated giant cells in the internal elasticum of the artery wall.[383]

6.1.12.1. Epidemiology

Giant cell arteritis appears to be relatively common in Europe and in the United States, although the incidence varies with the location of the population studied. It ranges from 17 cases per 100,000 population (age 50 years or older) in Scandinavia to 0.49 cases per 100,000 in Israel.[384,385] Giant cell arteritis occurs in patients over 60 years of age, women are affected about three times as often as men, and is most commonly seen in Caucasians.[386]

The HLA antigens HLA-B8[387] and HLA-DR4[388] may be associated with GCA more commonly than expected by chance alone; however, these associations have not been definitively established.[389,390]

6.1.12.2. Systemic Manifestations

Headache, occurring in more than two-thirds of patients, is the most common systemic manifestation of GCA.[391] Bilateral or unilateral, it usually begins early in the course and is often the initial symptom. The pain is throbbing or shooting in quality, sometimes severe enough to prevent sleep.[392] It is commonly localized to the temporal or occipital areas. Other cranial symptoms such as temporal artery or scalp tenderness, and jaw claudication, are present in the majority of patients. Constitutional symptoms, including fatigue, fever, anorexia, and weight loss, may be present in about half of patients, and may be an initial finding of the disease.[393] Because headache, fever, fatigue, and anorexia are nonspecific manifestations, many patients do not seek medical attention until more specific symptoms such as scalp tenderness or jaw claudication appear, or catastrophic vision loss occurs.

Although medium-sized extracranial arteries of the carotid circulation are the arteries most commonly affected in GCA, the aorta and its branches to the upper extremities and neck also can be involved, leading to cardiovascular and cerebrovascular disease.[387,390] Upper extremity claudication, bruits over the carotid, subclavian, and axillary arteries, and decreased or absent pulses in the neck or arms are some of the findings. Angina pectoris, congestive heart failure, and myocardial infarction secondary to coronary arteritis may occasionally occur. Neurological manifestations such as peripheral neuropathy, hemiparesis, acute hearing loss, confusion, depression, psychosis, and brainstem strokes are not uncommon, occuring in one-third of cases of biopsy-proven temporal arteritis.[394,395]

Forty to 60% of patients with GCA have polymyalgia rheumatica (PMR), a disorder characterized by pain and stiffness involving the neck, and the shoulder and hip girdles[396,397]; In the majority of patients, the shoulder girdle is the first to become symptomatic; in the remainder, hips and neck are involved at onset. Morning stiffness and "gelling" after inactivity are common. Polymyalgia rheumatica may be the initial symptom of GCA in 20 to 40% of patients. Conversely, 15% of patients with PMR may have GCA.[398] Polymalgia rheumatica is not associated with blindness, stroke, and death per se,[396] but may be indirectly associated because of its relationship with GCA.[399] If patients with PMR, even those who are "adequately treated,"[397] develop complaints suggestive of vasculitic involvement, an erythrocyte sedimentation rate should be obtained as soon as possible and, if elevated, treatment with high-dose oral steroids should be started immediately.

6.1.12.3 Ocular Manifestations

Ocular involvement usually occurs several weeks after the onset of systemic manifestations. The most frequent ocular symptom is vision loss. Rates of vision loss as high as 35 to 50% have been reported in early reports,[400–402] but more recent series present a lower rate of vision loss, (7 to 8%) probably reflecting earlier recognition and treatment.[384,394] Vision loss in GCA occurs as a result of arteritic anterior ischemic optic neuropathy (AION), or central or branch retinal artery occlusion. Arteritic AION in GCA is due to occlusion of the two main posterior ciliary arteries that supply the optic nerve and choroid. Arteritic AION in GCA is characterized by transient monocular visual loss or amaurosis fugax, sometimes alternating between the two eyes, persisting for 2 to 3 min, and rarely lasting more than 5 to 30 min. Amaurosis fugax is one of the most important warning symptoms of impending blindness. If the diagnosis and treatment of GCA is missed, sudden, profound vision loss, usually to less than 20/200, may occur in 40 to 50% of patients. It is often bilateral, either simultaneously or sequentially. Other manifestations are color vision deficit, relative afferent pupillary defect (Marcus Gunn pupil), and severe disk edema. Fundus examination may help to distinguish arteritic AION from nonarteritic AION by revealing the chalky appearance of an edematous disk, a cilioretinal artery occlusion, or cotton-wool spots.[403]

Diplopia is also a common complaint in GCA[392] and may be the presenting symptom of GCA. Diplopia is due to sixth nerve palsy in half of the patients; third nerve palsy accounts for the other half. However, ocular motility disturbances in GCA may be the result of muscle ischemia rather than nerve ischemia.

Typically there is no conjunctival, corneal, scleral, episcleral, uveal, or retinal vasculitis in GCA because the arteritic process usually involves only the medium- and large-sized arteries, sparing the ocular tissues. Occasionally, however, small vessels such as the anterior ciliary and long posterior ciliary vessels may be involved, leading to ocular manifestations such as scleritis.[404]

6.1.12.3.1. Scleritis

Scleritis is rare in GCA with or without PMR.[132] However, the diagnosis of GCA must be considered in an elderly patient with a high erythrocyte sedimentation rate, particularly in cases of diplopia or vision loss as symptoms, and AION, central retinal artery occlusion, or branch retinal artery occlusion as signs. The reported incidence of PMR in patients with scleritis is 0.68%.[123] Scleritis may correlate with the activity of the systemic disease.[205] In our series of 172 patients with scleritis, 1 patient had GCA associated with PMR (0.58%). The patient was a 67-year-old male diagnosed with GCA and PMR, and treated with 10 mg of prednisone for 4 years. He developed moderate vision loss with choroidal

folds and retinal deposits in both eyes. There were no signs of disk edema. The erythrocyte sedimentation rate was 88 mm/h. Ultrasonography confirmed the presence of bilateral posterior scleritis. Increased doses of steroids controled the scleral inflammatory process as well as the erythrocyte sedimentation rate.

6.1.12.4. Laboratory Findings

An elevated erythrocyte sedimentation rate is characteristic of most patients with GCA, although 5 to 10% of patients have a normal sedimentation rate.[392,405] Because a normal sedimentation rate does not exclude the diagnosis, elevations of other acute-phase reactants such as C-reactive protein, fibrinogen, and haptoglobin may be helpful in making the diagnosis.[406,407] Leukocytosis and anemia are variably present. Increased serum alkaline phosphatase, glutamic-oxaloacetic transaminase, and γ-glutamyl transferase may also be found in GCA,[391,408] as well as prolonged prothrombin time, and decreased peripheral blood CD8$^+$ (suppressor/cytotoxic) lymphocytes.[409]

6.1.12.5. Diagnosis

The diagnosis of GCA should be considered in any patient over the age of 60 years who has a new onset of headache, transient or irreversible visual loss, polymyalgia rheumatica, unexplained prolonged fever or anemia, and elevated erythrocyte sedimentation rate. Temporal artery biopsy, or less commonly facial or occipital artery biopsy, is necessary to confirm the diagnosis.[410] Because the arterial involvement may be focal, a symptomatic or clinically suspicious arterial segment several centimeters long (1 to 5 cm) should be biopsied and carefully sectioned serially for histopathological examination at several points along its length. The pathological diagnosis is based on the presence of nongranulomatous inflammation with mononuclear cells, or granulomatous inflammation with epithelioid cells with or without Langhans' (foreign body-type) multinucleated giant cells in the arterial wall. Although characteristic of GCA, giant cells need not be present to make the diagnosis pathologically. Because skip areas have been described along the length of affected arteries,[411] patients with GCA and elevated sedimentation rates may have a negative temporal artery biopsy. However, a patient with clinical features suggestive of GCA and an elevated sedimentation rate should have a temporal artery biopsy. The opposite temporal artery may be biopsied if the first biopsy is negative and clinical suspicion of the diagnosis is high.

High-dose oral steroid therapy should be started immediately in a patient with ocular or systemic symptomatology suggestive of GCA and an elevated sedimentation rate, even before performing the biopsy. However, the biopsy should be done within 1 week of initiation of steroid therapy, because the rate of positive biopsy falls from 82% in patients who had received no steroid to 60% in patients who had received up to 1 week of steroid therapy.[412] The false-negative rate has been reported as 5%[413] and 9%[414]; these data may be explained, at least in part, by the inclination of some clinicians to biopsy with minimal evidence of the disease.

6.1.13. Cogan's Syndrome

Cogan's syndrome is a systemic disease of unknown etiology that is typically manifested as nonsyphilitic interstitial keratitis associated with vertigo, tinnitus, and profound deafness. Young adults are most likely to be affected. Atypical forms with ocular manifestations other than keratitis may occur. It is probable that most cases of this syndrome are caused by a small-sized vessel vasculitis of the inner ear and eye.

6.1.13.1. Clinical Manifestations

There are typical and atypical forms of Cogan's syndrome. The typical form, as it was first described by Cogan in 1945,[415] is characterized by an abrupt onset of pain and redness in the eyes, reduced vision, vertigo, nausea, vomiting, noises in the ears, and progressive hearing loss.[415,416] The ocular signs consist of patchy midstromal corneal infiltrates that tend to fluc-

tuate in intensity and distribution, are usually located in the periphery, and are associated with deep corneal vascularization in the later stages of the disease.[415] As the inflammation subsides, deep stromal infiltrates remain; they are interrupted by clear intervals around the now empty old vessels. It has been suggested that nummular anterior stromal keratitis may be an early manifestation of interstitial keratitis; progression to interstitial keratitis may be halted by suppression of nummular anterior stromal keratitis with topical steroid treatment.[417] Either the ocular or the vestibuloauditory symptoms may be affected first, but the time between both types of manifestations never exceeds a few months.[418] A small population of patients (10%) develops a systemic necrotizing vasculitis affecting large arteries, which is manifested by proximal aortitis, aortic insufficiency, and infarction of other organ systems.[419-425] Other abnormalities include myalgias, arthralgias, and arthritis. Whereas severe hearing loss occurs in 60% of patients without treatment, prednisone therapy preserves hearing in 80% of patients.[426] Cogan's syndrome has been described in patients diagnosed with other systemic diseases, such as rheumatoid arthritis or polyarteritis nodosa.[423,424,427]

An atypical form of Cogan's syndrome, accounting for about 30% of the cases, consists of vestibuloauditory dysfunction associated with ocular manifestations other than keratitis (scleritis, episcleritis, anterior uveitis, posterior uveitis, optic neuritis, and orbital pseudotumor).[427-432] Atypical forms of Cogan's syndrome often overlap with other systemic diseases such as Wegener's granulomatosis, polyarteritis nodosa, rheumatoid vasculitis, sarcoidosis, or Vogt-Koyanagi–Harada syndrome. Patients with the atypical form of Cogan's syndrome are more likely to develop a systemic necrotizing vasculitis (21%).[422]

6.1.13.1.1 Scleritis

The atypical form of Cogan's syndrome may become manifest with vestibuloauditory dysfunction and scleritis.[427-429,432] Keratitis may or may not be present. Vestibuloauditory symptoms may be present before or after the scleritis but usually both events are not separated by more than a few months. Although nodular anterior scleritis is a frequent type of scleritis in Cogan's disease, other varieties such as diffuse anterior scleritis and necrotizing anterior scleritis may occur.[205,429]

In our series of 172 patients with scleritis, 1 patient had Cogan's syndrome (0.58%). The patient was a male who had diffuse anterior scleritis in his right eye 1 month before developing bilateral progressive hearing loss. There were no corneal abnormalities. Review of systems revealed arthritis, and laboratory tests disclosed an elevated sedimentation rate and positive circulating immune complexes detected by Raji cell assay. Tests for rheumatoid factor, antinuclear antibodies, and ANCAs were negative. Prednisone therapy seemed to halt both recurrent scleritis and hearing loss.

6.1.13.1.2. Episcleritis

Episcleritis with or without keratitis may also occur in association with vestibuloauditory symptoms as part of atypical Cogan's syndrome.[427,430] In our series of 94 patients with episcleritis, 1 patient had Cogan's syndrome (1.06%). The patient was a 39-year-old woman who developed recurrent simple episcleritis in her left eye 1 month after the onset of progressive sensorineural hearing loss. Systemic evaluation did not show evidence of aortic involvement or systemic vasculitis. Tests for anti-nuclear antibodies, rheumatoid factor, ANCAs, and cryoglobulins were negative; erythrocyte sedimentation rate and circulating immune complexes were elevated and complement levels were decreased. Prednisone controlled recurrences of episcleritis and progression of hearing loss.

6.1.13.2. Laboratory Findings

There are no specific diagnostic tests for Cogan's syndrome. Erythrocyte sedimentation rate and circulating immune complexes are typically elevated. Leukocytosis and, occasionally, eosinophilia may occur. No evidence of syphilis infection is found.

6.1.14. Systemic Immune-Mediated Diseases Associated with Scleritis: Atopy

Atopy (*a* means "without", *topos* means "place") is a term coined by Coca and Cooke[433] in 1923, which refers to "strange reactivity" or "hypersensitivity" to environmental antigens in patients with hereditary backgrounds of allergic disease. The major atopies are seasonal rhinitis (hay fever), perennial rhinitis, bronchial asthma, and atopic dermatitis (eczema). The minor atopies include food allergy, urticaria, and nonhereditary angioedema.

Although conjunctivitis and keratoconjunctivitis (allergic, giant papillary, vernal, and atopic) are the most characteristic ocular manifestations in atopy, scleritis, and particularly episcleritis, also may occur. Exposure to airborne allergens, either occasional (e.g., vapor of printing inks), seasonal (e.g., pollen), or perennial (e.g., house dust mite), may trigger recurrent attacks of episcleritis.[114,122,205,434] Skin testing was investigated by McGavin et al.[114] in 23 patients (17 patients with episcleritis and 6 patients with scleritis). Of the eight patients with episcleritis and one patient with scleritis who had a positive reaction to some allergen, only three gave a clear history of either hay fever or asthma. In the Watson and Hayreh series,[122] 12% of patients with episcleritis and 0.96% of patients with scleritis had a history of asthma or hay fever. Although several of our patients with episcleritis and scleritis had positive skin test results to multiple allergens, only seven patients with episcleritis (7.44%) and one patient with scleritis (0.58%) had a clear history of major atopies with bronchial asthma (four patients), hay fever (four patients), eczema (two patients), and perennial rhinitis (two patients). In two patients, episcleritis was associated with a past history of perennial keratoconjunctivitis and giant papillary conjunctivitis, respectively. Episcleritis was recurrent, almost always bilateral, and simple or nodular. Scleritis was recurrent, bilateral, and diffuse. There were no corneal lesions, cataract, or glaucoma, and the visual acuity was not affected.

The incidence of atopy in patients with episcleritis or scleritis in these studies is not higher than that expected in patients without episcleritis or scleritis (10 to 20% of the general population),[435,436] indicating that there is no significant relationship between atopy and episcleritis or scleritis.

6.1.15. Other Systemic Immune-Mediated Diseases That Rarely May Be Associated with Scleritis and Episcleritis

Juvenile rheumatoid arthritis (JRA) is diagnosed in patients under 16 years of age who have had arthritis for 3 months or more. Juvenile rheumatoid arthritis may be classified in three groups, depending on the number of involved joints at onset: systemic onset group, polyarticular onset group, and pauciarticular onset group.[437] Patients with polyarticular onset of JRA follow a clinical course similar to that of adults with rheumatoid arthritis. Ocular involvement in JRA occurs most commonly in the pauciarticular onset group of JRA; it is characterized by anterior uveitis, which may lead to band keratopathy, cataracts, or secondary glaucoma.[438] However, ocular involvement also may occur in the polyarticular onset group of JRA[439]; it is characterized by scleritis, usually of the diffuse or nodular variety, and episcleritis.[121,205] Juvenile rheumatoid arthritis patients with episcleritis or scleritis are usually girls who are seropositive for rheumatoid factor. Patients with the systemic onset of JRA (Still's disease) do not develop ocular manifestations. Patients with the pauciarticular onset of JRA do not develop scleritis or episcleritis.[243]

Occasionally, scleritis has been associated with dermatomyositis,[440] Sjögren's syndrome,[440] Takayasu's arteritis,[121] and thyroid diseases, including Hashimoto's thyroiditis or thyrotoxicosis.[205] Simple episcleritis may, although rarely, accompany the onset of Schönlein–Henoch purpura, a small-sized vessel vasculitis, which commonly affects young children, especially boys.[205]

Ocular manifestations of sarcoidosis include conjunctival granulomas, infiltration of the lacrimal gland, keratoconjunctivitis sicca, anterior, intermediate, or posterior uveitis, retinal vasculitis, and optic nerve involvement. Scleral and episcleral nodules occur rarely; these may recur when the systemic condition exacerbates.[123,132,441–445] Anterior staphyloma has occasionally been found to be the first ocular manifestation of sarcoidosis.[446]

Because Vogt-Koyanagi–Harada syndrome is caused by an autoimmune attack directed against organs containing melanocytes, ocular involvement is usually characterized by bilateral progressive panuveitis affecting the choroid, ciliary body, and iris. The sclera may contain some melanocytes, especially at the site of emergence of long ciliary nerves anterior to the insertion of the recti muscles. Although uncommon, focal necrotizing scleritis in Vogt-Koyanagi–Harada syndrome may occur and may lead to uveal show and anterior staphyloma.[447] Scleritis also may be caused by an extension of an orbital granulomatous process, or of a uveal granulomatous process such as sympathetic ophthalmia.[440]

6.1.16. Systemic Immune-Mediated Disease-Associated Scleritis after Ocular Surgery

Scleritis, particularly necrotizing anterior scleritis, may appear following surgical trauma of the sclera in patients with autoimmune vasculitic diseases such as rheumatoid arthritis, Wegener's granulomatosis, or inflammatory bowel disease.[448–451] Surgical trauma may favor circulating immune complexes becoming entrapped in episcleral vessels and perforating scleral vessels. Inflammatory microangiopathy may lead to scleral destruction.[452,453] Subcutaneous nodules in rheumatoid arthritis usually appear in areas subjected to mechanical trauma such as the olecranon, the buttock, or the fingertip pads. Pathological studies show vasculitis and fibroblast proliferation; vessel thrombosis and collagenase production result in tissue destruction.[454–456] Cutaneous vascular lesions such as purpura, pustules, vesicles, and ulcers most often appear in areas of repeated low-grade trauma. Pathological studies show cutaneous necrotizing venulitis.[457,458]

Ten of our 11 patients (90.9%) who developed necrotizing scleritis up to 6 months after ocular surgery (interval range, 2 to 4 weeks) had an underlying systemic autoimmune vasculitic disease; these diseases included rheumatoid arthritis, Wegener's granulomatosis, and inflammatory bowel disease (Table 4.21). Appropriate studies led to the discovery and subsequent treatment of the systemic diseases in five patients; the other five had been previously diagnosed. These results emphasize the need for meticulous diagnostic pursuit of systemic autoimmune vasculitic diseases in patients with necrotizing scleritis following intraocular surgery.

Sclerokeratitis may appear following keratoplasty in patients with severe atopy. Lyons et al.[459] reported a series of five severe atopic patients in whom sclerokeratitis developed 1 to 4 weeks after keratoplasty. Serum IgE levels were elevated in all these patients. The scleritis was of the diffuse type and the keratitis was characterized by host stromal inflammation, which, through loosening of the graft sutures, caused protrusion of the graft or incompetence of the graft–host interface. The authors proposed that IgE binding on the surface of mast cells in the conjunctiva with subsequent degranulation could be involved in the pathogenesis of the sclerokeratitis. These results emphasize that severe atopic patients undergoing keratoplasty require prophylactic measures for stabilization of the atopic ocular disease (seasonal timing of the operation, cromolyn sodium and, if necessary, topical steroids), use of interrupted sutures, and frequent postoperative follow-up for detection of sclerokeratitis. High-dose oral steroids at the onset of the condition may adequately suppress the ocular inflammation.

Suture-related episcleritis may occur after transscleral fixation of a posterior chamber intraocular lens in a patient with absence of capsular and zonular support.[460]

6.2 Dermatological Disease-Associated Scleritis

6.2.1. Rosacea

Acne rosacea is a chronic disease characterized by skin manifestations, which include persistent erythema, telangiectasias, papules, and pustules in the flush areas of the face and neck. The classic rhinophyma, caused by sebaceous gland hypertrophy, also is a typical feature of the advanced stage of the disease. Ocular rosacea occurs in 3 to 58% of the cases with acne rosacea, depending on the series, and consists primarily of meibomian gland (modified sebaceous gland) dysfunction associated with the cutaneous disease.[461] Abnormalities in meibomian gland secretions (alteration in melting points of waxes and cholesterol esters, excessive free fatty acids, or biochemical abnormalities)[462] may secondarily inflame the external surface of the eye, causing conjunctivitis, keratitis, and (less frequently) episcleritis and scleritis.[461,463–465] A type IV hypersensitivity reaction may play a significant role in the pathogenesis of the disease.[465] Burning, tearing, eyelid swelling, irritation, photophobia, blurred vision, dryness, and mild itching are the usual symptoms.

The reported incidence of rosacea in patients with episcleritis is 1.88%.[122] In our series of 94 patients with episcleritis, 7 patients had rosacea (7.44%). Rosacea episcleritis may be simple or nodular, and is usually bilateral. The reported incidence of rosacea in patients with scleritis ranges from 0.34 to 0.96%.[122,123] In our series of 172 patients with scleritis, 1 patient had rosacea (0.58%). Rosacea scleritis is usually diffuse or nodular, but scleral perforation occasionally may occur.[132,464] Rosacea episcleritis and scleritis are accompanied by meibomianitis (solidified plugs, dilated glands, pouting orifices, distorted orifices, hordeolum, and chalazion), blepharitis (crusting, decreased cilia, margin thickening or irregularity, and scaling), telangiectasia of lid margins, conjunctivitis (bulbar injection, tarsal papillary hypertrophy, symblepharon), or keratitis (superficial punctate keratopathy, corneal vascularization, peripheral ulcerative keratitis, and corneal perforation). Mechanical and hygienic maneuvers with or without doxycycline is the treatment of choice for rosacea episcleritis and scleritis.

The diagnosis of ocular rosacea is made on the basis of skin clinical findings, although in 20% of cases the ocular manifestations appear first. Meibomian gland dysfunction is a nonspecific ocular finding but, when seen in combination with characteristic skin manifestations, it allows a firm diagnosis of ocular rosacea. Any patient who develops episcleritis or scleritis and meibomian gland dysfunction should be examined for skin manifestations.

6.3 Metabolic Disease-Associated Scleritis

6.3.1. Gout

Gout is a defect of purine metabolism that is manifested by (1) an increase in the serum urate concentration, (2) recurrent attacks of acute arthritis with deposits of monosodium urate monohydrate (tophi) in and around the joints of the extremities (often the big toe), (3) renal disease, and (4) uric acid urolithiasis.

Deposits of monosodium urate monohydrate may also precipitate in the eye, leading to conjunctivitis, episcleritis, or (less commonly) scleritis.[114,122,466] They also may precipitate in the corneal epithelium or Bowman's membrane, and in the iris. The reported incidence of high serum uric acid values in patients with episcleritis is 11%, and that of clinical gout is 7%.[122] The onset of episcleritis in gout is sudden and may be triggered by cold, heat, or indiscretions of diet. Episcleritis is simple or nodular, recurrent, and is often accompanied by conjunctivitis. Occasionally, fine crystals may be seen in the episclera or conjunctiva close to the vessels.[440] Although these crystals have never been biopsied, their presence suggests that a serum uric acid analysis should be performed. Gouty tophi in conjunctiva or episclera have been reported but are extremely unusual.[467–469] The attacks usually last approximately 10 days, in spite of the medication; if the patient recognizes an episcleritis attack is

imminent and initiates the treatment before episcleral inflammation develops, the attack may be aborted. Episcleritis may be accompanied by keratitis (crystals in epithelium and Bowman's membrane) or anterior uveitis. Corneal scrapings reveal urates that can be demonstrated by colorimetry and spectrophotometry.[470] Only one patient with episcleritis had clinical gout in our series (1.06%). The patient had had attacks of bilateral simple episcleritis for 10 years without diagnosis of associated disease. The great toe began to be sensitive and developed an acute arthritis, and the serum uric acid level was elevated. Therapy for gout controlled the arthritis and the episcleritis attacks. Episcleritis may be the first or the only clinical manifestation of the disease.

Scleritis in gout is less frequent than episcleritis.[114,122] The reported incidence of gout in patients with scleritis ranges from 0.34 to 2.41%.[122,123] Only one patient with scleritis had clinical gout in our series (0.58%). Scleritis is more painful than episcleritis and may be accompanied by keratitis or anterior uveitis. Therapy for gout may control the systemic and ocular manifestations.

6.4. Foreign Body Granuloma-Associated Scleritis

A sterile foreign body in the sclera or episclera may produce a granulomatous inflammatory reaction without scleral or episcleral abscess. A history of accidental or surgical injury can usually be elicited. Because the granuloma is confined to the affected area, scleritis secondary to a foreign body is usually nodular and unresponsive to antiinflammatory therapy. Sometimes the nodular process can progress to necrotizing scleritis; scleral thinning may threaten the integrity of the globe. Vegetable matter such as plant hairs or needles, animal matter such as mite mouth parts[443] and caterpillar hairs,[440] and mineral matter such as pieces of stone, talc, and silk or catgut surgical sutures may cause scleral granulomas. The foreign body may occasionally be seen in the scleral nodule or in the adjacent cornea (caterpillar hairs) after meticulous slit-lamp examination, particularly if the episcleral congestion has been cleared with topical phenylephrine (10%). Removal of the noxious material, sometimes through excision of the scleral nodule with or without scleral homografting, should be performed. Some foreign bodies, especially the vegetal ones, may secondarily complicate with infection, often mycotic, and produce a scleral abscess.

In our series of 172 patients with scleritis, 1 patient had scleritis due to a foreign body granulomatous reaction (0.58%). The patient was a 39-year-old man whose left eye had been irritated for several weeks. Ocular examination disclosed a necrotizing scleritis and keratitis in his left eye; visual acuity was 20/60. Smears and cultures were negative and blood tests and orbit and sinuses plain films were normal. Oral prednisone (60 mg/day) was administered but scleral melting continued. Orbital CT scan showed small foreign bodies in the skin anterior to the superior orbital rim and anterior wall of the globe. Foreign body granuloma-associated scleritis was diagnosed. Necrotic scleral tissue was resected and scleral homografting was performed. Scleral tissue histopathology showed granulomatous reaction and necrosis. Scleral inflammation resolved without further recurrences.

6.5. Chemical Injury-Associated Scleritis

In most cases, alkali or acid chemical injuries to the eye are relatively minor and heal without sequelae. Occasionally, strong alkali or acid chemicals may cause severe ocular damage and, if they come into direct contact with the sclera, may cause scleritis and scleral destruction. Alkaline substances produce scleral damage through changes in pH produced by hydroxyl ion. At high pH, cations bind to scleral collagen and glycosaminoglycans by reacting with carboxyl groups, leaving the collagen more susceptible to enzymatic degradation; collagenolytic enzymes are synthesized by inflammatory cells that are attracted to the region of tissue damage. Acid substances

produce scleral damage through changes in pH produced by hydrogen ion and through coagulation and precipitation of tissue proteins caused by interaction with the ionic portion of the acid. Scleral tissue excision and scleral homografting may be performed in severely damaged scleras to retain sufficient integrity after collagen breakdown; donor sclera may act as a matrix for scar tissue, preventing the phtisis of the eye.[440]

In our series of 94 patients with episcleritis, 1 patient had a chemical injury (1.06%). The right eye of a 58-year-old woman was injured with a weak acid substance. Prolonged irrigation with water was performed and topical antibiotics and cycloplegics were administered. Three months later, the patient still had intermittent episodes of redness; simple episcleritis was diagnosed and topical steroid therapy was instituted with subsequent slow tapering of the frequency of application of this medication. Episcleritis resolved without further recurrences.

Summary

Because scleritis may occur in association with a variety of noninfectious local and systemic disorders (autoimmune, dermatological, metabolic, and foreign body reactions), its presence must be regarded in relation to the larger picture of a patient's general health. Scleritis is frequently seen in association with autoimmune vasculitic diseases that affect predominantly small- and medium-sized vessels, such as rheumatoid arthritis (18.6%), Wegener's granulomatosis (8.13%), relapsing polychondritis (6.39%), arthritis and inflammatory bowel disease (4.06%), systematic lupus erythematosus (4%), polyarteritis nodosa (1.16%), psoriatic arthritis (1.16%), Behçet's disease (0.58%), or Cogan's syndrome (0.58%); scleritis is less commonly found in association with autoimmune vasculitic diseases that affect predominantly large-sized arteries, such as Reiter's syndrome (1.74%), ankylosing spondylitis (0.93%), or giant cell arteritis (0.58%).

Scleritis may also be associated with other systemic immune diseases such as atopy

(0.58%), with systemic dermatological diseases such as rosacea (0.58), with systematic metabolic diseases such as gout (0.58%), and with local foreign body reactions (0.58%).

Because some of these systemic diseases are potentially lethal, early diagnosis and subsequent therapy are extremely important. The presence of scleritis demands a meticulous systemic and ocular evaluation. The ophthalmologist must remain current with the systemic disorders that are associated with scleritis.

References

1. Harris ED: Rheumatoid arthritis: the clinical spectrum. In Kelley WN, Harris ED, Ruddy S, Sledge CB: *Textbook of Rheumatology*, 3rd ed. W.B. Saunders, Philadelphia, 1989, pp 915–949.
2. Nepom GT, Byers P, Seyfried C, Healey LA, Wilske KR, Stage D, Nepom BS: HLA genes associated with rheumatoid arthritis: identification of susceptibility alleles using specific oligonucleotide probes. Arthritis Rheum 32:15, 1989.
3. Jacoby RK, Jayson MIV, Cosh JA: Onset, early stages and prognosis of rheumatoid arthritis: a clinical study of 100 patients with 11 year follow-up. Br Med J 2:96, 1973.
4. Fleming A, Crown JM, Corbett M: Early rheumatoid disease. I. Onset. Ann Rheum Dis 35:357, 1976.
5. Fleming A, Benn RT, Corbett M, Wood PH: Early rheumatoid disease. II. Patterns of joint involvement. Ann Rheum Dis 35:361, 1976.
6. Hurd ER: Extra-articular manifestations of rheumatoid arthritis. Semin Rheum Dis 8:151, 1979.
7. Hart FD: Rheumatoid arthritis. Extra-articular manifestations. Br Med J 3:131, 1969.
8. Sharp JT, Calkins E, Cohen AS, Schubart AF, Calabro JJ: Observations on the clinical, chemical, and serologic manifestations of rheumatoid arthritis based on the course of 154 patients. Medicine 43:41, 1964.
9. Masi AT, Maldonado-Cocco JA, Kaplan SB, Feigenbaum SL, Chandler RW: Prospective study of the early course of rheumatoid arthritis in young adults: comparison of patients with and without rheumatoid factor positivity at entry and identification of variables correlating with outcome. Semin Arthritis Rheum 5:299, 1976.
10. Talbott JH, Altman RD, Yu TF: Gouty arthritis masquerading as rheumatoid arthritis or vice versa. Semin Arthritis Rheum 8:77, 1978.
11. Khachadurian AK: Migratory polyarthritis in familial hypercholesterolemia (type II hyperlipoproteinemia). Arthritis Rheum 2:385, 1968.
12. Wiernik PH: Amyloid joint disease. Medicine (Baltimore) 51:465, 1971.
13. Gordon DA, Pruzanski W, Ogyzlo MA, Little HA: Amyloid arthritis simulating rheumatoid disease in five patients with multiple myeloma. Am J Med 55:142, 1973.
14. Healey LA, Wilske KR, Sagebiel RW: Rheumatoid nodules simulating basal-cell carcinoma. N Engl J Med 277:7, 1967.
15. Wood MG, Beerman H: Necrobiosis lipoidica, granuloma anulare. Report of a case with lesions in the galea aponeurotica of a child. Am J Dis Child 96:720, 1958.
16. Hahn BH, Yardley JH, Stevens MB: "Rheumatoid" nodules in systemic lupus erythematosus. Ann Intern Med 72:49, 1970.
17. Dubois EL, Friou GJ, Chandor S: Rheumatoid nodules and rheumatoid granulomas in systemic lupus erythematosus. JAMA 220:515, 1972.
18. Barrow MV, Holubar K: Multicentric reticulohistiocytosis: a review of 33 patients. Medicine (Baltimore) 48:287, 1969.
19. Cats A, Hazevoet HM: Significance of positive tests for rheumatoid factor in the prognosis of rheumatoid arthritis. Ann Rheum Dis 29:254, 1970.
20. Mongan ES, Cass RM, Jacox RF, Vaughan JH: A study of the relation of seronegative and seropositive rheumatoid arthritis to each other and to necrotizing vasculitis. Am J Med 47:23, 1969.
21. Turner R, Collins R, Nomeir AM: Extra-articular manifestations of rheumatoid arthritis. Bull Rheum Dis 29:986, 1978–1979.
22. Sokoloff L, Bunim JJ: Vascular lesions in rheumatoid arthritis. J Chron Dis 5:668, 1957.
23. Duthie JJR, Brown PE, Truelove LH, Barago E, Lawrie AJ: Course and prognosis in rheumatoid arthritis. A further report. Ann Rheum Dis 23:193, 1964.
24. Ragan C, Farrington E: The clinical features of rheumatoid arthritis. JAMA 181:663, 1962.
25. Scott JT, Hourhane DO, Doyle FH, *et al.*: Digital arteritis in rheumatoid disease. Ann Rheum Dis 20:224, 1961.
26. Schmid FR, Cooper NS, Ziff M, McEweh C: Arteritis in rheumatoid arthritis. Am J Med 30:56, 1961.

27. Bienenstock H, Minick R, Rogoff B: Mesenteric arteritis and intestinal infarction in rheumatoid disease. Arch Intern Med 119:359, 1967.

28. Voyles WF, Searles RP, Bankhurst AD: Myocardial infarction caused by rheumatoid vasculitis. Arthritis Rheum 23(7):860, 1980.

29. Fong LP, Sainz de la Maza M, Rice BA, Foster CS: Immunopathology of scleritis. Ophthalmology 98:472, 1991.

30. Scott DG, Bacon PA, Tribe CR: Systemic rheumatoid vasculitis: a clinical and laboratory study of 50 cases. Medicine (Baltimore) 60(4):288, 1981.

31. Scott DGI, Bacon PA, Allen C, Elson CJ, Wallington T: IgG rheumatoid factor, complement, and immune complexes in rheumatoid synovitis and vasculitis: comparative and serial studies during cytotoxic therapy. Clin Exp Immunol 43:54, 1981.

32. Hunder GG, McDuffie FC: Hypocomplementinemia in rheumatoid arthritis. Am J Med 54:461, 1973.

33. Scott DGI, Bacon PA, Elliott PJ, Tribe CR, Wallington TB: Systemic vasculitis in a district general hospital 1972–80: clinical and laboratory features, classification and prognosis of 80 cases. Q J Med 51:292, 1982.

34. Ferguson RH, Slocumb CH: Peripheral neuropathy in rheumatoid arthritis. Bull Rheum Dis 11:251, 1961.

35. Walker WC, Wright V: Pulmonary lesions and rheumatoid arthritis. Medicine 47:501, 1968.

36. Dodson WH, Hollingsworth JW: Pleural effusion in rheumatoid arthritis: impaired transport of glucose. N Engl J Med 275:1337, 1966.

37. Jones SJ: An account of pleural effusions, pulmonary nodules and cavities in rheumatic disease. Br J Dis Chest 72:39, 1978.

38. Portner MM, Gracie WA: Rheumatoid lung disease with cavitary nodules, pneumothorax and eosinophilia. N Engl J Med 275:697, 1966.

39. Brannan HM, Good CA, Divertie MB, Baggenstoss AH: Pulmonary disease associated with rheumatoid arthritis. J Am Med Assoc 189:914, 1964.

40. Dixon AStJ, Ball J: Honeycomb lung and chronic rheumatoid arthritis: a case report. Ann Rheum Dis 16:241, 1957.

41. Stack BHR, Grant IWB: Rheumatoid interstitial lung disease. Br J Dis Chest 59:202, 1965.

42. Walker WC, Wright V: Diffuse interstitial pulmonary fibrosis and rheumatoid arthritis. Ann Rheum Dis 28:252, 1969.

43. Frank ST, Weg JG, Harkleroad LE, Fitch RF: Pulmonary dysfunction in rheumatoid disease. Chest 63:27, 1973.

44. Caplan A: Certain unusual radiographic appearances in the chest of coal miners suffering from RA. Thorax 8:29, 1953.

45. Caplan A, Cowen EDH, Gough J: Rheumatoid pneumoconiosis in a foundry worker. Thorax 13:181, 1958.

46. Chatgidakis CB, Theron C: Rheumatoid pneumoconiosis (Caplan's syndrome): a discussion of the disease and a report of a case in a European Witwatersrand gold miner. Arch Environ Health 2:397, 1961.

47. Hull S, Mathews JA: Pulmonary necrobiotic nodules as a presenting feature of rheumatoid arthritis. Ann Rheum Dis 41:21, 1982.

48. Walker WC: Pulmonary infections and rheumatoid arthritis. Q J Med 36:239, 1967.

49. Catheart ES, Spodick DH: Rheumatoid heart disease: a study of the incidence and nature of cardiac lesions in rheumatoid arthritis. JAMA 266:959, 1962.

50. Bongiglio T, Atwater EC: Heart disease in patients with seropositive rheumatoid arthritis: a controlled autopsy study and review. Arch Intern Med 124:714, 1969.

51. Cosh JA: Arthritis and the heart. Bristol Med Chir J 84:145, 1969.

52. Comess KA, Fenster PE, Gall EP: Cardiac involvement in rheumatoid arthritis. Cardiovasc Res 3:533, 1982.

53. Lie JT: Rheumatoid arthritis and heart disease. Primary Cardiol 40:137, 1982.

54. Kirk J, Cosh J: The pericarditis of rheumatoid arthritis. Q J Med 38:397, 1969.

55. Bacon PA, Gibson DG: Cardiac involvement in rheumatoid arthritis—an echocardiographic study. Ann Rheum Dis 31:426, 1972.

56. MacDonald WJ, Crawford MH, Klippel JH, Zvaifler NJ, O'Rourke RA: Echocardiographic assessment of cardiac structure and function in patients with rheumatoid arthritis. Am J Med 63:890, 1977.

57. Butman S, Espinoza LR, DelCarpio J, Osterland K: Rheumatoid pericarditis: rapid deterioration with evidence of local vasculitis. JAMA 238:2394, 1977.

58. Franco AE, Levine HO, Hall AP: Rheumatoid pericarditis: report of 17 cases diagnosed clinically. Ann Intern Med 77:837, 1972.

59. Khan AH, Spodick DH: Rheumatoid heart disease. Semin Arthritis Rheum 1:327, 1972.

60. Sokoloff L: The heart in rheumatoid arthritis. Am Heart J 45:635, 1953.

61. Leibowitz WB: The heart in rheumatoid arthritis. Ann Intern Med 58:102, 1963.
62. Harris M: Rheumatoid heart disease with complete heart block. J Clin Pathol 23:623, 1970.
63. Hoffman FG, Leight L: Complete atrioventricular block associated with rheumatoid disease. Am J Cardiol 16:585, 1965.
64. Roberts WC, Kehoe JA, Carpenter DF, Golden A: Cardiac valvular lesions in rheumatoid arthritis. Arch Intern Med 122:141, 1968.
65. Cruickshank B: Heart lesions in rheumatoid disease. J Pathol Bacteriol 76:223, 1958.
66. Goehrs HR, Baggenstoss AH, Slocumb CH: Cardiac lesions in rheumatoid arthritis. Arthritis Rheum 3:298, 1960.
67. Roberts WC, Dangel JC, Buklay BH: Nonrheumatic valvular cardiac disease: a clinicopathologic survey of 27 different conditions causing valvular dysfunction. Cardiovasc Clin 5:333, 1973.
68. Reimer KA, Rodgers RF, Oyasu R: Rheumatoid arthritis with rheumatoid heart disease and granulomatous aortitis. JAMA 235:2510, 1976.
69. Bywaters EGL: The relation between heart and joint disease including "rheumatoid heart disease" and chronic postrheumatic arthritis (type Jaccoud). Br Heart J 12:101, 1950.
70. Karten I: Arteritis, myocardial infarction and rheumatoid arthritis. JAMA 210:1717, 1969.
71. Parrillo JE, Fauci AS: Necrotizing vasculitis, coronary angiitis and the cardiologist. Am Heart J 99:547, 1980.
72. Sweezy RL: Myocardial infarction due to rheumatoid arteritis. JAMA 199:855, 1967.
73. Chamberlain MA, Bruckner FE: Rheumatoid neuropathy: clinical and electrophysiological features. Ann Rheum Dis 29:609, 1970.
74. Weller RO, Bruckner FE, Chamberlain MA: Rheumatoid neuropathy: a histological and electrophysiological study. J Neurol Neurosurg Psychiatry 33:592, 1970.
75. Irby R, Adams RA, Toone EC: Peripheral neuritis associated with rheumatoid arthritis. Arthritis Rheum 1:44, 1958.
76. Pallis CA, Scott JT: Peripheral neuropathy in rheumatoid arthritis. Br Med J 1:1141, 1965.
77. Motulsky AG, Weinberg S, Saphir O, Rosenberg E: Lymph nodes in rheumatoid arthritis. Arch Intern Med 90:660, 1952.
78. Nosanshuk JS, Schnitzer B: Follicular hyperplasia in lymph nodes from patients with rheumatoid arthritis. Cancer 24:343, 1969.
79. Robertson MDJ, Hart FD, White WF, Nuki G, Boardman PL: Rheumatoid lymphadenopathy. Ann Rheum Dis 27:153, 1968.
80. Kassan SS, Hoover R, Kimberly RP: Increased incidence of malignancy in Sjögren's syndrome. Arthritis Rheum 20:123, 1977.
81. Whaley K, Webb J, McAvoy BA, Hughes GRC, Lee P, MacSween RNM, Buchanan WW: Sjögren's syndrome. 2. Clinical associations and immunological phenomena. Q J Med 42:513, 1973.
82. Felty AR: Chronic arthritis in the adult, associated with splenomegaly and leucopenia. Johns Hopkins Hosp Bull 35:16, 1924.
83. Ruderman M, Miller LM, Pinals RS: Clinical and serologic observations on 27 patients with Felty's syndrome. Arthritis Rheum 11:377, 1968.
84. Sienknecht CW, Urowitz MB, Pruzanski W, Stein HB: Felty's syndrome. Clinical and serological analysis of 34 cases. Ann Rheum Dis 36:500, 1977.
85. Hurd ER, Andreis M, Ziff M: Phagocytosis of immune complexes by polymorphonuclear leucocytes in patients with Felty's syndrome. Clin Exp Immunol 28:413, 1977.
86. Joyce RA, Boggs DR, Chervenick PA, Lalezari P: Neutrophil kinetics in Felty's syndrome. Am J Med 69:695, 1980.
87. Howe GB, Fordham JN, Brown KA, Currey HLF: Polymorphonuclear cell function in rheumatoid arthritis and in Felty's syndrome. Ann Rheum Dis 40:370, 1981.
88. Gupta RC, Laforce FM, Mills DM: Polymorphonuclear leukocyte inclusions and impaired bacterial killing in patients with Felty's syndrome. J Lab Clin Med 88:183, 1976.
89. Laszlo J, Jones R, Silberman HR, Banks PM: Splenectomy for Felty's syndrome: clinicopathological study of 27 patients. Arch Intern Med 138:597, 1978.
90. Goldberg J, Pinals RS: Felty's syndrome. Semin Arthritis Rheum 10:52, 1980.
91. Cohen AS: Amyloidosis associated with rheumatoid arthritis. Med Clin North Am 52:643, 1968.
92. Husby G: Amyloidosis in rheumatoid arthritis. Ann Clin Res 7:154, 1975.
93. Arapakis G, Tribe CR: Amyloidosis in rheumatoid arthritis investigated by means of rectal biopsy. Ann Rheum Dis 22:256, 1963.
94. Trieger N, Cohen AS, Calkins E: Gingival biopsy as a diagnostic aid in amyloid disease. Arch Oral Biol 1:187, 1959.
95. Falcek HM, Törnroth, Skrifvars B, Wegelius O: Resolution of renal amyloidosis secondary to rheumatoid arthritis. Acta Med Scand 205:651, 1979.

96. Fernandes L, Sullivan S, McFarlane IG, Wojcicka BM, Warnes TW, Eddleston AL, Hamilton EB, Williams R: Studies on the frequency and pathogenesis of liver involvement in rheumatoid arthritis. Ann Rheum Dis 38:501, 1979.

97. Weinblatt ME, Tesser JRP, Gilliam JH: The liver in rheumatic diseases. Semin Arthritis Rheum 11:399, 1981.

98. Mogadam M, Schuman B, Duncan H, Patton RB: Necrotizing colitis associated with rheumatoid arthritis. Gastroenterology 57:168, 1969.

99. Pettersson T, Wegelius D, Skrifvars B: Gastrointestinal disturbances in patients with severe rheumatoid arthritis. Acta Med Scand 188:139, 1970.

100. Atwater EC, Morgan ES, Wieche DR, Jacox RF, Rochester NY: Peptic ulcer and rheumatoid arthritis: a prospective study. Arch Intern Med 115:184, 1965.

101. Brun C, Olsen TX, Rasshou F, Sorensen AW: Renal biopsy in rheumatoid arthritis. Nephron 2:65, 1965.

102. Healey LA, Bulger RJ: Abnormal renal function in rheumatoid arthritis. Arthritis Rheum 10:283, 1967.

103. Pollack VE, Priani CL, Steck IE, et al.: The kidney in rheumatoid arthritis: studies by renal biopsy. Arthritis Rheum 5:1, 1962.

104. Lawson AAH, MacLean N: Renal disease and drug therapy in rheumatoid arthritis. Ann Rheum Dis 25:441, 1966.

105. Samuels B, Lee JC, Engleman EP, Hooper J Jr: Membranous nephropathy in patients with rheumatoid arthritis: relationship to gold therapy. Medicine 57:319, 1977.

106. O'Driscoll S, O'Driscoll M: Osteomalacia in rheumatoid arthritis. Ann Rheum Dis 39:1, 1980.

107. Williamson J: Incidence of eye disease in cases of connective tissue disease. Trans Ophthalmol Soc UK 94:742, 1974.

108. Thompson M, Eadie S: Keratoconjunctivitis sicca and rheumatoid arthritis. Ann Rheum Dis 5:21, 1956.

109. Lackington MC, Charlin VC, Gormas BA: Keratoconjunctivitis sicca y artritis reumatoidea. Rev Med Chil 79:133, 1951.

110. Lamberts DW: Dry eye and tear deficiency. Int Ophthalmol Clin 23(1):123, 1983.

111. Ichikawa Y, Takaya M, Saitoh H: Characterization of sicca symptoms in patients with Sjögren's syndrome, and report of six cases lacking subjective sicca features ("subclinical syndrome"). Exp Clin Med 6:229, 1981.

112. von Grosz S: Aetiologie und Therapy der Keratoconjunctivitis sicca. Klin Monatsbl Augenheilk 97:472, 1936.

113. Sjögren H: Zur Kenntnis der Keratoconjunctivitis sicca. (Keratitis filiformis bei Hypofunktion der Tränen drusen). Acta Ophthalmol Suppl 2:1, 1933.

114. McGavin DDM, Williamson J, Forrester JV, Foulds WS, Buchanan WW, Dick WC, Lee P, MacSween RN, Whaley K: Episcleritis and scleritis: a study of their clinical manifestations and association with rheumatoid arthritis. Br J Ophthalmol 60:192, 1976.

115. Russell DH, Kibler R, Matrisian L, Larson DF, Poulos B, Magun BE: Prolactin receptors on human T and B lymphocytes: antagonism of prolactin binding by cyclosporine. J Immunol 134:3027, 1985.

116. Koletsky AJ, Harking MW, Handshumacker RE: Cyclophilin: distribution and properties in normal and neoplastic tissues. J Immunol 137:1054, 1986.

117. Sullivan DA: Hormonal modulation of tear volume in the rat. Exp Eye Res 42:131, 1986.

118. Leuenberger PM, Miescher PA: Syndrome de Sjögren: Traitement par la ciclosporine: communication preliminaire. Klin Monatsbl Augenheilk 190:290, 1987.

119. Drosos AA, Skopouli FN, Costopoulos JS, Papadimitriou CS, Moutsopoulos HM: Cyclosporine A in primary Sjögren's syndrome: a double blind study. Ann Rheum Dis 45:732, 1986.

120. Kaswan RL, Salisbury MA, Ward DA: Spontaneous canine keratoconjunctivitis sicca. A useful model for human keratoconjunctivitis sicca: treatment with cyclosporine eye drops. Arch Ophthalmol 107:1210, 1989.

121. Lyne AJ, Pitkeathley DA: Episcleritis and scleritis. Arch Ophthalmol 80:171, 1968.

122. Watson PG, Hayreh SS: Scleritis and episcleritis. Br J Ophthalmol 60:163, 1976.

123. Tuft SJ, Watson PG: Progression of scleral disease. Ophthalmology 98:467, 1991.

124. Sevel D: Necrogranulomatous scleritis: clinical and histologic features. Am J Ophthalmol 64:1125, 1967.

125. Jayson MIV, Jones DEP: Scleritis and rheumatoid arthritis. Ann Rheum Dis 30:343, 1971.

126. Kleiner RC, Raber IM, Passero FC: Scleritis, pericarditis, and aortic insufficiency in a patient with rheumatoid arthritis.

127. Sevel D: Rheumatoid nodule of the sclera (a type of necrogranulomatous scleritis). Trans Ophthalmol Soc UK 85:357, 1965.

128. Jones P, Jayson MIV: Rheumatoid scleritis: a long-term follow up. Proc R Soc Med 66:1161, 1973.

129. Foster CS, Forstot SL, Wilson LA: Mortality rate in rheumatoid arthritis patients developing necrotizing scleritis or peripheral ulcerative keratitis. Ophthalmology 91:1253, 1984.

130. Smoleroff JW: Scleral disease in rheumatoid arthritis; report of three cases, in one of which both eyes were studied post mortem. Arch Ophthalmol 29:98, 1943.

131. Hurd ER, Snyder WB, Ziff M: Choroidal nodules and retinal detachments in rheumatoid arthritis. Am J Med 48:273, 1970.

132. Lachman SM, Hazleman BL, Watson PG: Scleritis and associated disease. Br Med J 1:88, 1978.

133. Brown SI, Grayson M: Marginal furrows: a characteristic corneal lesion of rheumatoid arthritis. Arch Ophthalmol 79:563, 1968.

134. Eiferman RA, Carothers DJ, Yankeelov JA: Peripheral rheumatoid ulceration and evidence for conjunctival collagenase production. Am J Ophthalmol 87:703, 1979.

135. Jayson MIV, Easty DL: Ulceration of the cornea in rheumatoid arthritis. Ann Rheum Dis 36:428, 1977.

136. Scharf Y, Meyer E, Nahir M, Zonis S: Marginal mottling of cornea in rheumatoid arthritis. Ann Ophthalmol 16:924, 1984.

137. Lyne AJ: "Contact lens" cornea in rheumatoid arthritis. Br J Ophthalmol 54:410, 1970.

138. Sainz de la Maza M, Foster CS: The diagnosis and treatment of peripheral ulcerative keratitis. Semin Ophthalmol 6(3):133, 1991.

139. Tauber J, Sainz de la Maza M, Hoang-Xuan T, Foster CS: An analysis of therapeutic decision making regarding immunosuppressive chemotherapy for peripheral ulcerative keratitis. Cornea 9(1):66, 1990.

140. Kimura SJ, Hogan MJ, O'Connor GR, EpsTein WV: Uveitis and joint diseases. Arch Ophthalmol 77:309, 1967.

141. Meyer E, Scharf J, Miller B, Zonis S, Nahis M: Fundus lesions in rheumatoid arthritis. Ann Ophthalmol 10:1583, 1978.

142. Martin M, Scott D, Gilbert C, Dieppe PA, Easty DL: Retinal vasculitis in rheumatoid arthritis. Br J Ophthalmol 282:1745, 1981.

143. Crompton J, Iyer P, Begg M: Vasculitis and ischemic optic neuropathy associated with rheumatoid arthritis. Aust J Ophthalmol 8:219, 1980.

144. Killian PJ, McClain B, Lawless OJ: Brown's syndrome: an unusual manifestation of rheumatoid arthritis. Arthritis Rheum 20:1080, 1977.

145. Sandford-Smith JH: Intermittent superior oblique tendon sheath syndrome. Br J Ophthalmol 53:412, 1969.

146. Watson P, Fekete J, Deck J: Central nervous system vasculitis in rheumatoid arthritis. Can J Neurol Sci 4:269, 1977.

147. Ramos M, Mandybur TI: Cerebral vasculitis in rheumatoid arthritis. Arch Neurol 32:271, 1975.

148. Victor DI, Green WR, Stark WJ, Walsh FB: A non-permanent tonic pupil in rheumatoid arthritis. Can J Neurol Sci 4:209, 1977.

149. Edström G, Österlind G: A case of nodular rheumatic episcleritis. Acta Ophthalmol 26:1, 1948.

150. Mundy WL, Howard RY, Stillman PH, Bevans M: Cortisone therapy in case of rheumatoid nodules of the eye in chronic rheumatoid arthritis. Arch Ophthalmol 45:531, 1951.

151. Fienberg R, Colpoys FL Jr: The involution of rheumatoid nodules treated with cortisone and of non-treated rheumatoid nodules. Am J Pathol 27:925, 1951.

152. Ferry AP: The histopathology of rheumatoid episcleral nodules: an extra-articular manifestation of rheumatoid arthritis. Arch Ophthalmol 82:77, 1969.

153. Leibowitz MA, Jakobiec FA, Donnenfeld ED, Stavr M: Bilateral epibulbar rheumatoid nodulosis. A new ocular entity. Ophthalmology 95:1256, 1988.

154. Mesara BW, Brody GL, Oberman HA: "Pseudorheumatoid" subcutaneous nodules. Am J Clin Pathol 45:684, 1966.

155. Rao NA, Font RL: Pseudorheumatoid nodules of the ocular anexa. Am J Ophthalmol 79:471, 1975.

156. Ross MJ, Cohen KL, Peiffer RL Jr, Grimson BS: Episcleral and orbital pseudorheumatoid nodules. Arch Ophthalmol 101:418, 1983.

157. Rose HM, Ragan C, Pearce E, Lipman MO: Differential agglutination of normal and sensitized sheep erythrocytes by sera of patients with rheumatoid arthritis. Proc Soc Exp Biol Med 68:1, 1948.

158. Waaler E: On the occurrence of a factor in human serum activating the specific agglutination of sheep blood corpuscles. Acta Pathol Microbiol Scand 17:172, 1940.

159. Tarkowski A, Czerkinsky C, Nilsson L-A: Simultaneous induction of rheumatoid factor- and antigen-specific antibody-secreting cells

during the secondary immune response in man. Clin Exp Immunol 61:379, 1985.

160. Aho K, Palosuo T, Raunio V, Puska P, Aromaa A, Salonen JT: When does rheumatoid disease start? Arthritis Rheum 28:485, 1985.

161. Ball J, Lawrence JS: The relationship of rheumatoid serum factor to rheumatoid arthritis. Ann Rheum Dis 22:311, 1963.

162. Del Puente A, Knowler WC, Pettitt DJ, Bennett PH: The incidence of rheumatoid arthritis is predicted by rheumatoid factor titer in a longitudinal population study. Arthritis Rheum 31:1239, 1988.

163. Bland JH, Brown EW: Seronegative and seropositive rheumatoid arthritis: clinical, radiological, and biochemical differences. Ann Intern Med 60:88, 1964.

164. Kellgren JH, O'Brien WM: On the natural history of rheumatoid arthritis in relation to the sheep cell agglutination test (SCAT). Arthritis Rheum 5:115, 1962.

165. Jacoby RK, Jayson MIV, Cosh JA: Onset, early stages and prognosis of rheumatoid arthritis: a clinical study of 100 patients with 11-year follow-up. Br Med J 2:96, 1973.

166. Theofilopoulos AN, Burtonboy G, LoSpalluto JJ, Ziff M: IgM rheumatoid factor and low molecular weight IgM: an association with vasculitis. Arthritis Rheum 17:272, 1974.

167. Engstedt L, Strandberg O: Haematological data and clinical activity of the rheumatoid diseases. Acta Med Scand 180:13, 1966.

168. Samson D, Holliday D, Gumpel JM: Role of ineffective erythropoiesis in the anaemia of rheumatoid arthritis. Ann Rheum Dis 36:181, 1977.

169. Hutchinson RM, Davis P, Jayson MIV: Thrombocytosis in rheumatoid arthritis. Ann Rheum Dis 35:138, 1976.

170. Winchester RJ, Litwin SD, Koffler D, Kunkel HG: Observations on the eosinophilia of certain patients with rheumatoid arthritis. Arthritis Rheum 14:650, 1971.

171. Panush RS, Franco AE, Schur PH: Rheumatoid arthritis associated with eosinophilia. Ann Intern Med 75:199, 1971.

172. Fleming A, Crown JM, Corbett M: Prognostic value of early features in rheumatoid disease. Br Med J 1:1243, 1976.

173. Amos RS, Constable TJ, Crockson RA, Crockson AP, McConkery B: Rheumatoid arthritis: relation of serum C-reactive protein and erythrocyte sedimentation rates to radiographic changes. Br Med J 1:195, 1977.

174. Nusinow S, Arnold WJ: Prognostic value of C-reactive protein (CRP) levels in rheumatoid arthritis. Clin Res 30:474, 1982.

175. Roth SH: Remission: the goal of rheumatic disease therapy. J Rheumatol 9(8):120, 1982.

176. Ruddy S, Austen KF: Activation of the complement system in rheumatoid synovitis. Fed Proc 32:134, 1973.

177. Jones VE, Jacoby RK, Wallington T, Holt P: Immune complexes in early arthritis. I. Detection of immune complexes before rheumatoid arthritis is definite. Clin Exp Immunol 44:512, 1981.

178. Zubler RH, Nydegger UE, Perrin LH, Fehr K, McCormick J, Lambert PH, Miescher PA: Circulating and intraarticular immune complexes in patients with rheumatoid arthritis. J Clin Invest 57:1308, 1976.

179. Lessard J, Nunnery E, Cecere F, McDuffy S, Pope RM: Relationship between the articular manifestations of rheumatoid arthritis and circulating immune complexes detected by three methods and specific classes of rheumatoid factors. J Rheumatol 10:411, 1983.

180. Fessel WJ: SLE in the community: incidence, prevalence, outcome and first symptoms; the high prevalence in black women. Arch Intern Med 134:1027, 1974.

181. Siegel M, Lee SL: The epidemiology of systemic lupus erythematosus. Semin Arthritis Rheum 3:1, 1973.

182. Arnett FC, Shulman LE: Studies in familial systemic lupus erythematosus. Medicine 55:313, 1976.

183. Winchester RJ, Nunez-Roldon A: Some genetic aspects of systemic lupus erythematosus. Arthritis Rheum 25:833, 1982.

184. Hess EV: Introduction to drug related lupus. Kroc Foundation Conference on Drug Induced Lupus. Arthritis Rheum 24:979, 1981.

185. Armas-Cruz R, Harnecker, J, Ducach G, Jalil J, Gonzales F: Clinical diagnosis of systemic lupus erythematosus. Am J Med 25:409, 1958.

186. Davis P, Atkins B, Jesse RG, Highes GRV: Criteria for classification of SLE. Br Med J 3:88, 1973.

187. Labowitz R, Schumacher HR: Articular manifestations of systemic lupus erythematosus. Ann Intern Med 74:911, 1971.

188. Isbender DA, Snaith ML: Muscle disease in systemic lupus erythematosus: a study of its nature, frequency and cause. J Rheumatol 8:917, 1981.

189. Gilliam JN, Sontheimer OO: Skin manifestations of SLE. Clin Rheum Dis 8:207, 1982.

190. Ropes MW: *Systemic Lupus Erythematosus.* Harvard University Press, Cambridge, 1976.

191. Ellis SG, Verity MA: Central nervous system involvement in systemic lupus erythematosus: a review of neuropathologic findings in 57 cases, 1955–1977. Semin Arthritis Rheum 8:212, 1979.

192. Pirani CL, Pollack VE: Systemic lupus erythematosus glomerulonephritis. In Andres GA, McCluskey RT (Eds): *Immunologically Mediated Renal Disease: Criteria for Diagnosis.* Marcel Dekker, New York, 1978.

193. Chia GL, Mah EPK, Feng PH: Cardiovascular abnormalities in systemic lupus erythematosus. J Clin Ultrasound 9:237, 1981.

194. Bonfiglio TA, Botti RE, Hagstrom JWC: Coronary arteritis, occlusion and myocardial infarction due to lupus erythematosus. Am Heart J 83:153, 1972.

195. Homcy CJ, Liberthson RR, Fallon JT, Gross S, Miller LM: Ischemic heart disease in systemic lupus erythematosus: report of six cases. Am J Cardiol 49:478, 1982.

196. Libman E, Sacks B: A hitherto undescribed form of valvular and mural endocarditis. Arch Intern Med 33:701, 1924.

197. Buckley BH, Roberts WC: The heart in systemic lupus erythematosus and the changes induced in it by corticosteroid therapy: a study of 36 necropsy patients. Am J Med 58:243, 1975.

198. Feinglass EJ, Arnett FC, Dorsch CA, Zizic RM, Stevens MC: Neuropsychiatric manifestations of systemic lupus erythematosus: diagnosis, clinical spectrum and relationship to other features of the disease. Medicine 55:323, 1976.

199. Klippel JH, Zwaifler NJ: Neuropsychiatric abnormalities in systemic lupus erythematosus. Clin Rheum Dis 1:621, 1975.

200. Haupt HM, Moore GW, Hutchins GM: The lung in systemic lupus erythematosus: analysis of the pathologic changes in 120 patients. Am J Med 71:791, 1981.

201. Matthay RA, Schwartz MI, Petty TL, Stanford RE, Gupta RC, Sahn SA, Steigerwald JC: Pulmonary manifestations of systemic lupus erythematosus: review of twelve cases of acute lupus pneumonitis. Medicine 54:397, 1974.

202. Runyon BA, LaBrecque DR, Anuras S: The spectrum of liver disease in systemic lupus erythematosus: report of 33 hystologically proved cases and review of the literature. Am J Med 69:187, 1980.

203. Dillon AM, Stein HB, English RA: Splenic atrophy in SLE. Ann Intern Med 96:40, 1982.

204. Foster CS: Immunosuppressive therapy for external ocular inflammatory disease. Ophthalmology 87:140, 1980.

205. Watson PG, Hazleman BL: *The Sclera and Systemic Disorders.* W.B. Saunders, Philadelphia, 1976, pp 206–305.

206. Cappaert WE, Purnell EW, Frank KE: Use of B-sector scan ultrasound in the diagnosis of benign choroidal folds. Am J Ophthalmol 84:375, 1977.

207. Gold DH, Morris DA, Henkind P: Ocular findings in systemic lupus erythematosus. Br J Ophthalmol 56:800, 1972.

208. Larson DL: *Systemic Lupus Erythematosus.* Little Brown, Boston, 1961.

209. Harvey AM, Shulman LE, Tumulty PA, Conley CL, Schoenrich EH: Systemic lupus erythematosus: review of the literature and clinical analysis of 138 cases. Medicine 33:291, 1954.

210. Frith P, Burge SM, Millard PR, Wojnarowska F: External ocular findings in lupus erythematosus: a clinical and immunopathological study. Br J Ophthalmol 74:163, 1990.

211. Reeves JA: Keratopathy associated with systemic lupus erythematosus. Arch Ophthalmol 74:159, 1965.

212. Henkind P, Gold DH: Ocular manifestations of rheumatic disorders: natural and iatrogenic. Rheumatology 4:13, 1973.

213. Halmay O, Ludwig K: Bilateral bandshaped deep keratitis and iridocyclitis in systemic lupus erythematosus. Br J Ophthalmol 48:558, 1964.

214. Spaeth GL: Corneal staining in systemic lupus erythematosus. N Engl J Med 276:1168, 1967.

215. Heaton JM: Sjögren's syndrome and systemic lupus erythematosus. Br Med J 1:466, 1959.

216. Bencze G, Lakatos L: Relationship of systemic lupus erythematosus to rheumatoid arthritis, discoid lupus erythematosus, and Sjögren's syndrome. Ann Rheum Dis 22:273, 1963.

217. Dubois EL: The clinical picture of systemic lupus erythematosus. In Dubois EL (Ed): *Lupus Erythematosus.* McGraw-Hill, New York, 1966, pp 129–276.

218. Steinberg AD, Talal N: The coexistence of Sjögren's syndrome and systemic lupus erythematosus. Ann Intern Med 74:55, 1971.

219. Brihaye-Van Geertruyden M, Danis P, Toussaint C: Fundus lesions with disseminated lupus. Arch Ophthalmol 51:799, 1954.

220. Maumenee AE: Retinal lesions in lupus erythematosus. Am J Ophthalmol 23:971, 1940.

221. Clifton F, Greer CH: Ocular changes in acute systemic lupus erythematosus. Br J Ophthalmol 39:1, 1955.

222. Rothfield N: Clinical features of systemic lupus erythematosus. In Kelley WN, Harris ED, Ruddy S, Sledge CB (Eds): *Textbook of Rheumatology*. W.B. Saunders, Philadelphia, 1985, pp 1070–1097.

223. Regan CDJ, Foster CS: Retinal vascular diseases: clinical presentation and diagnosis. Int Ophthalmol Clin 26:25, 1985.

224. Silberberg DH, Laties AM: Increased intracranial pressure in disseminated lupus erythematosus. Arch Neurol 29:88, 1973.

225. Raptk L, Menard HA: Quantitation and characterization of plasma DNA in normals and patients with systemic lupus erythematosus. J Clin Invest 66:1391, 1980.

226. Weinstein A, Bordwell B, Stone B, Tibbetts C, Rothfield NF: Antibodies to native DNA and serum complement (C3) levels: applications to the diagnosis of systemic lupus erythematosus. Am J Med 74:206, 1983.

227. Arnett FC: Seronegative spondylarthropathies. Bull Rheum Dis 37(1):1, 1987.

228. Marks SH, Barnett M, Calin A: Ankylosing spondylitis in women and men: a case-control study. J Rheumatol 10:624, 1983.

229. Woodrow JC: Genetic aspects of spondylarthropathies. Clin Rheum Dis 11:1, 1985.

230. Brewerton DA, Caffrey M, Hart FD, James DCO, Nicholls A, Sturrock RD: Ankylosing spondylitis and HL-A 27. Lancet 1:904, 1973.

231. Van der Linden S, Valkenburg HA, Cats A: Evaluation of diagnostic criteria for ankylosing spondylitis: a proposal for modification of the New York criteria. Arthritis Rheum 27:361, 1984.

232. Hunter T, Dubo H: Spinal fractures complicating ankylosing spondylitis. Ann Intern Med 88:546, 1978.

233. Khan MA: Ankylosing spondylitis. In Calin A (Ed): *Spondyloarthropathies*. Grune & Stratton, Orlando, FL, 1984, pp 69–117.

234. Bergfeldt L, Moller E: Complete heart block—another HLA-B27 associated disease manifestation. Tissue Antigens 21:385, 1983.

235. Bergfeldt L: HLA-B27 associated rheumatic diseases with severe cardiac bradyarrhythmias: clinical features and prevalence in 223 men with permanent pacemaker. Am J Med 75:210, 1983.

236. Khan MA, Kushner I: Ankylosing spondylitis and multiple sclerosis: a possible association. Arthritis Rheum 22:784, 1979.

237. Mason RM, Murray RS, Oates JK, et al.: Prostatitis and ankylosing spondylitis. Rheum Phys Med 1:78, 1971.

238. Calin A: Renal glomerular function in ankylosing spondylitis. Scand J Rheumatol 4:241, 1975.

239. Pasternack A, Tornroth T, Martio J: Ultrastructural studies of renal arteriolar changes in ankylosing spondylitis. Acta Pathol Microbiol Scand Sect A, 79:591, 1971.

240. Jayson MIV, Salmon PR, Harrison W: Amyloidosis in ankylosing spondylitis. Rheum Phys Med 1:78, 1971.

241. Jennette JC, Ferguson AL, Moore MA, Freeman DG: IgA nephropathy associated with seronegative spondylarthropathies. Arthritis Rheum 25:144, 1982.

242. Bluestone R: Ankylosing spondylitis. In McCarthy DJ (Ed): *Arthritis and Allied Conditions*, 10th ed. Lea & Febiger, Philadelphia, 1985, pp 819–840.

243. Hakin KN, Watson PG: Systemic associations of scleritis. Int Ophthalmol Clin 31(3):111, 1991.

244. Rosenbaum JT, Theofilopoulos A, McDevitt HO, Pereira AB, Carson D, Calin A: Presence of circulating immune complexes in Reiter's syndrome and ankylosing spondylitis. Clin Immun Pathol 18:291, 1981.

245. Keat AC: Reiter's syndrome and reactive arthritis in perspective. N Engl J Med 309:1606, 1983.

246. Moller G: Immunology of reactive arthritis and ankylosing spondylitis. Immunol Rev 86:1, 1985.

247. Reiter H: Ueber eine bisher unerkannte Spirochaeteninfektion (Spirochaetosis arthritica). Dtsch Med Wochenschr 42:1435, 1916.

248. Aho K, Leirisalo-Repo M, Reop H: Reactive arthritis. In Panayi GS (Ed): *Seronegative Spondyloarthropathies*, Vol 11. W.B. Saunders, London, 1985, pp 25–40.

249. Winchester R, Bernstein DH, Fisher HD, Enlow R, Solomon G: The co-occurrence of Reiter's syndrome and acquired immunodeficiency. Ann Intern Med 106:19, 1987.

250. Duvic M, Johnson TM, Rapini RP, Freese T, Brewton G, Rios A: Acquired immunodeficiency syndrome-associated psoriasis and Reiter's syndrome. Arch Dermatol 123:1622, 1987.

251. Lin RY: Reiter's syndrome and human immunodeficiency virus infection. Dermatologica 176:39, 1988.

252. Carr JL, Friedman M: Keratodermia blennorrhagicum, report of a case with autopsy. Am J Pathol 20:709, 1944.

253. Calin A: *Spondyloarthropathies*. Grune & Stratton, Orlando, FL, 1984.

254. Buskila D, Langevitz P, Tenenbaum J, Gladman DD: Malar rash in a patient with Reiter's syndrome—a clue for the diagnosis of human immunodeficiency virus infection. J Rheumatol 17:843, 1990.

255. Lee DA, Barker SM, Su WPD, Allen GL, Liesegang TJ, Ilstrup DM: The clinical diagnosis of Reiter's syndrome. Ophthalmology 93:350, 1986.

256. Ostler HB, Dawson CR, Schachter J, Engleman EP: Reiter's syndrome. Am J Ophthalmol 71:986, 1971.

257. Weinberger HW, Ropes MW, Kulka JP, Bauer W: Reiter's syndrome, clinical and pathological observations: a long-term study of 16 cases. Medicine 41:35, 1962.

258. Zewi M: Morbus Reiteri. Acta Ophthalmol 25:47, 1947.

259. Mattson R: Recurrent retinitis in Reiter's disease. Acta Ophthalmol 33:403, 1955.

260. Gerber LH, Espinoza LR: *Psoriatic Arthritis*. Grune & Stratton, Orlando, FL, 1985.

261. Suarez-Almazor ME, Russell AS: Sacroiliitis in psoriasis: relationship to peripheral arthritis and HLA-B27. J Rheumatol 17:804, 1990.

262. Bennet RM: Psoriatic arthritis. In McCarthy DJ (Ed): *Arthritis and Allied Conditions*, 11th ed. Lea & Febiger, Philadelphia, 1989, pp 954–971.

263. Gladman DD, Stafford-Brady F, Chang C, Lewandowski K, Russell ML: Longitudinal study of clinical and radiological progression in psoriatic arthritis. J Rheumatol 17:809, 1990.

264. Leczinsky CG: The incidence of arthropathy in a ten-year series of psoriasis cases. Acta Derm Venereol 28:483, 1948.

265. Little M, Harvie JN, Lester RS: Psoriatic arthritis in severe psoriasis. Can Med Assoc J 112:317, 1975.

266. Roberts MET, Wright V, Hill AGS, *et al.*: Psoriatic arthritis: a follow-up study. Ann Rheum Dis 35:206, 1976.

267. Lambert JR, Wright V: Eye inflammation in psoriatic arthritis. Ann Rheum Dis 35:354, 1976.

268. Bird HA, Wright V: Psoriatic arthritis. Clin Rheum Dis 9:671, 1983.

269. Palumbo PJ, Ward LE, Sauer WG: Musculoskeletal manifestations of inflammatory bowel disease: ulcerative and granulomatous colitis and ulcerative proctitis. Mayo Clin Proc 48:411, 1973.

270. Hopkins DJ, Horan E, Burton IL, Clamp SE, de Dombal FT, Goligher JC: Ocular disorders in a series of 332 patients with Crohn's disease. Br J Ophthalmol 58:732, 1974.

271. Wright R, Lumsden K, Luntz MH, Sevel D, Truelove SC: Abnormalities of the sacroiliac joints and uveitis in ulcerative colitis. Q J Med 34:229, 1965.

272. Knox DL, Schachat AP, Mustonen E: Primary, secondary and coincidental ocular complications of Crohn's disease. Ophthalmology 91:163, 1984.

273. Billson FA, de Dombal FT, Watkinson G, Goligher JC: Ocular complications of ulcerative colitis. Gut 8:102, 1967.

274. Ernst BB, Lowder CY, Meisler D, Gutman FA: Posterior segment manifestations of inflammatory bowel disease. Ophthalmology 98:1272, 1991.

275. Salmon JF, Wright JP, Murray ADN: Ocular inflammation in Crohn's disease. Ophthalmology 98:480, 1991.

276. Ellis PO, Gentry JH: Ocular complications of ulcerative colitis. Am J Ophthalmol 58:779, 1964.

277. Petrelli EA, McKinley M, Troncale FJ: Ocular manifestations of inflammatory bowel disease. Ann Ophthalmol 14:356, 1982.

278. Jameson Evans P, Eustace P: Scleromalacia perforans associated with Crohn's disease. Br J Ophthalmol 57:330, 1973.

279. Knox DL, Snip RC, Stark WJ: The keratopathy of Crohn's disease. Am J Ophthalmol 90:862, 1980.

280. Clark RL, Muhletaler CA, Margulies SI: Colitic arthritis: clinical and radiographic manifestations. Radiology 101:585, 1971.

281. Jaksch-Wartenhorst R: Polychondropathia. Wien Arch Inn Med 6:93, 1923.

282. White JW: Relapsing polychondritis. South Med J 78:448, 1985.

283. Isaak BL, Liesengang TJ, Michet CJ Jr: Ocular and systemic findings in relapsing polychondritis. Ophthalmology 93:681, 1986.

284. Espinoza LR, Richman A, Bocanegra T, Pina I, Vasey FB, Rifkin SI, Germain BF: Immune complex-mediated renal involvement in relapsing polychondritis. Am J Med 71:181, 1981.

285. Sundaram MBM, Raiput AH: Nervous system complications of relapsing polychondritis. Neurology 33:513, 1983.

286. Margargal LE, Donoso LA, Goldberg RE, Gonder J, Brodsky I: Ocular manifestations of relapsing polychondritis. Retina 1:96, 1981.

287. McKay DAR, Watson PG, Lyne AJ: Relapsing polychondritis and eye disease. Br J Ophthalmol 58:600, 1974.

288. Matoba A, Plager S, Barger J, McCulley JP: Keratitis in relapsing polychondritis. Ann Ophthalmol 16:367, 1984.

289. Anderson B Sr: Ocular lesions in relapsing polychondritis and other rheumatoid syndromes. Trans Am Acad Ophthalmol Otolaryngol 71:227, 1967.

290. Michelson JB: Melting corneas with collapsing nose. Surv Ophthalmol 29:148, 1984.

291. Hoangh-Xuan T, Foster CS, Rice BA: Scleritis in relapsing polychondritis. Response to therapy. Ophthalmology 97:892, 1990.

292. McAdam LP, O'Hanlan MA, Bluestone R, Pearson CM: Relapsing polychondritis: prospective study of 23 patients and a review of the literature. Medicine 55:193, 1976.

293. Damiani JM, Levine HL: Relapsing polychondritis—report of ten cases. Laryngoscope 89:929, 1979.

294. Kussmaul A, Maier K: Über eine bischer nicht beschreibene eigenthümliche Arterienerkrankung (Periarteritis nodosa), die mit Morbus Brightii und rapid fortschreitender allgemeiner Müskellähmung einhergeht. Dtsch Arch Klin Med 1:484, 1866.

295. Zeek PM: Periarteritis nodosa and other forms of necrotizing angiitis. N Engl J Med 18:764, 1953.

296. Lieb ES, Restivo C, Paulus HE: Immunosuppressive and corticosteroid therapy for polyarteritis nodosa. Am J Med 67:941, 1979.

297. Kurland LT, Chuang TY, Hunder GG: The epidemiology of systemic arteritis. In Laurence RE, Shulman LE (Eds): Current Topics in Rheumatology: Epidemiology of the Rheumatic Diseases. Gower Medical Publishers, New York, 1984, pp 196–205.

298. Cupps TR, Fauci AS: The Vasculitides. W.B. Saunders, Philadelphia, 1981.

299. Cohen RD, Conn DL, Ilstrup DM: Clinical features, prognosis, and response to treatment in polyarteritis. Mayo Clin Proc 55:146, 1980.

300. Goldstein I, Wexler D: The ocular pathology of periarteritis nodosa. Arch Ophthalmol 2:288, 1929.

301. Friedenwald JS, Rones B: Ocular lesions in septicemia. Arch Ophthalmol 5:175, 1931.

302. Gaynon IE, Asbury MK: Ocular findings in a case of periarteritis nodosa. Am J Ophthalmol 23:1072, 1943.

303. Goldsmith J: Periarteritis nodosa with involvement of the choroidal and retinal arteries. Am J Ophthalmol 29:435, 1946.

304. Goar EL, Smith LS: Polyarteritis nodosa of the eye. Am J Ophthalmol 35:1619, 1952.

305. Sheehan B, Harriman DG, Bradshaw JP: Polyarteritis nodosa with ophthalmic and neurological complications. Arch Ophthalmol 60: 537, 1958.

306. King RT: Ocular involvement in a case of periarteritis nodosa. Trans Ophthalmol Soc UK 55:246, 1935.

307. Ford RG, Siekert RG: Central nervous system manifestations of periarteritis nodosa. Neurology 15:114, 1965.

308. Kimbrell OC Jr, Wheliss JA: Polyarteritis nodosa complicated by bilateral optic neuropathy. JAMA 201:61, 1967.

309. Van Wien S, Merz EH: Exophthalmos secondary to periarteritis nodosa. Am J Ophthalmol 56:204, 1963.

310. Purcell JJ Jr, Birkenkamp R, Tsai CC: Conjunctival lesions in periarteritis nodosa, a clinical and immunopathologic study. Arch Ophthalmol 102:736, 1984.

311. Harbert F, McPherson SD: Scleral necrosis in periarteritis nodosa. Am J Ophthalmol 30:727, 1947.

312. Wise GN: Ocular periarteritis nodosa. AMA Arch Ophthalmol 48:1, 1952.

313. Cogan DG: Corneoscleral lesions in periarteritis nodosa and Wegener's granulomatosis. Trans Am Acad Ophthalmol 53:321, 1955.

314. Moore JG, Sevel D: Corneoscleral ulceration in periarteritis nodosa. Br J Ophthalmol 50: 651, 1966.

315. Longstreth PL, Lorobkin M, Palubinskas AJ: Renal microaneurysms in a patient with systemic lupus erythematosus. Radiology 113:65, 1974.

316. McKusick VA: Buerger's disease: a distinct clinical and pathologic entity. JAMA 181:93, 1962.

317. Diaz-Perez JL, Winkelmann RK: Cutaneous periarteritis nodosa. Arch Dermatol 110:407, 1974.

318. Sack M, Cassidy JT, Bole GG: Prognostic factors in polyarteritis. J Rheumatol 2:411, 1975.

319. Dyck PJ, Conn DL, Okazaki H: Necrotizing angiopathic neuropathy: three-dimensional morphology of fiber degeneration related to sites of occluded vessels. Mayo Clin Proc 47:461, 1972.

320. Churg J, Strauss L: Allergic granulomatosis, allergic angiitis, and periarteritis nodosa. Am J Pathol 27:277, 1951.

321. Chumbley LC, Harrison EG Jr, Deremee RA: Allergic granulomatosis and angiitis (Churg–

Strauss syndrome). Report and analysis of 30 cases. Mayo Clin Proc 52:477, 1977.

322. Lanham JG, Elkon KB, Pusey CD, Hughes GR: Systemic vasculitis with asthma and eosinophilia: a clinical approach to the Churg–Strauss syndrome. Medicine (Baltimore) 63: 65, 1984.

323. Nissim F, Von der Valde J, Czernobilsky B: A limited form of Churg–Strauss syndrome. Arch Pathol Lab Med 106:305, 1982.

324. Cury D, Breakey AS, Payne BF: Allergic granulomatous angiitis associated with uveoscleritis and papilledema. Arch Ophthalmol 55:261, 1950.

325. Dicken CH, Winkelmann RK: The Churg–Strauss granuloma: cutaneous, necrotizing, palisading granuloma in vasculitis syndromes. Arch Pathol Lab Med 102:576, 1978.

326. Strauss L, Churg J, Zak FG: Cutaneous lesions of allergic granulomatosis. A histopathologic study. J Invest Dermatol 17:349, 1951.

327. Crotty CP, Deremee RA, Winkelmann RK: Cutaneous clinicopathologic correlation of allergic granulomatosis. J Am Acad Dermatol 5:571, 1981.

328. Wegener F: Über generalisierte, septische Gefässerkrankungen. Verh Dtsch Ges Pathol 29:202, 1936.

329. Wegener F: Über eine eigenartige rhinogene Granulomatose mit besonderer Beteilingung des Arteriensystems und der Nieren. Beitr Pathol Anat Allg Pathol 102:36, 1939.

330. Godman GC, Churg J: Wegener's granulomatosis: pathology and review of the literature. Arch Pathol 58:533, 1954.

331. Walton EW: Giant cell granuloma of the respiratory tract (Wegener's granulomatosis). Br Med J 2:265, 1958.

332. Carrington CB, Leibow AA: Limited forms of angiitis and granulomatosis of Wegener's type. Am J Med 41:497, 1966.

333. Gross WL: Wegener's granulomatosis. New aspects of the disease course, immunodiagnostic procedures, and stage-adapted treatment. Sarcoidosis 6:15, 1989.

334. Coutu RE, Klein M, Lessell S, Friedman E, Snider GL: Limited form of Wegener granulomatosis. Eye involvement as a major sign. JAMA 233:868, 1975.

335. Spalton DJ, Graham EM, Page NGR, Sanders MD: Ocular changes in limited forms of Wegener's granulomatosis. Br J Ophthalmol 65:553, 1981.

336. McDonald TJ, DeRemee RA: Wegener's granulomatosis. Laryngoscope 93:220, 1983.

337. DeRemee RA, McDonald TJ, Harrison EG Jr, Coles DT: Wegener's granulomatosis. Anatomic correlates, a proposed classification. Mayo Clin Proc 51:777, 1976.

338. Fauci AS, Haynes BF, Katz P, Wolff SM: Wegener's granulomatosis: prospective clinical and therapeutic experience with 85 patients over 21 years. Ann Intern Med 98:76, 1983.

339. Niffenegger JH, Jakobiec FA, Raizman MB, Foster CS: Pathologic diagnosis of very limited (ocular or orbital) Wegener's granulomatosis (in press).

340. Hall SL, Miller LC, Duggan E, Mauer SM, Beatty EC, Hellerstein S: Wegener's granulomatosis in pediatric patients. J Pediatr 106: 739, 1985.

341. Nölle B, Specks U, Lüdemann J, Rohrbach MS, DeRemee RA, Gross WL: Anticytoplasmic autoantibodies: their immunodiagnostic value in Wegener's granulomatosis. Ann Intern Med 111:28, 1989.

342. Pinching AJ, Lockwood CM, Pussell BA, Rees A, Swaney P, Evans D, Bowley N, Peters D: Wegener's granulomatosis: observations on 18 patients with severe renal disease. Q J Med 52:435, 1983.

343. Bullen CL, Liesegang TJ, McDonald TJ, DeRemee RA: Ocular complications of Wegener's granulomatosis. Ophthalmology 90:279, 1983.

344. Haynes BF, Fishman ML, Fauci AS, Wolff SM: The ocular manifestations of Wegener's granulomatosis. Fifteen years experience and review of the literature. Am J Med 63:131, 1977.

345. Straatsma BR: Ocular manifestations of Wegener's granulomatosis. Am J Ophthalmol 44:789, 1957.

346. Kinyoun JL, Kalina RE, Klein ML: Choroidal involvement in systemic necrotizing vasculitis. Arch Ophthalmol 105:939, 1987.

347. Schmidt R, Koderisch J, Krastel H, Zeier M, Andrassy K: Sicca syndrome in patients with Wegener's granulomatosis. Lancet 1:904, 1989.

348. Leveille AS, Morse PH: Combined detachments in Wegener's granulomatosis. Br J Ophthalmol 65:564, 1981.

349. Brubacker R, Font RL, Shepherd EM: Granulomatous sclerouveitis. Regression of ocular lesions with cyclophosphamide and prednisone. Arch Ophthalmol 86:517, 1971.

350. Sacks RD, Stock EL, Crawford SE, Greenwald MJ, O'Grady RB: Scleritis and Wegener's granulomatosis in children. Am J Ophthalmol 111:430, 1991.

351. Kalina PH, Garrity JA, Herman DC, De-Remee RA, Specks U: Role of testing for anticytoplasmic autoantibodies in the differential diagnosis of scleritis and orbital pseudotumor. Mayo Clin Proc 65:1110, 1990.

352. Charles SJ, Meyer PAR, Watson PG: Diagnosis and management of systemic Wegener's granulomatosis presenting with anterior ocular inflammatory disease. Br J Ophthalmol 75:201, 1991.

353. van der Woude FJ, Rasmussen N, Lobatto S, Wiik A, Permin H, van Es LA, van der Giessen M, van der Hem GK, The TH: Autoantibodies against neutrophils and monocytes; tool for diagnosis and marker of disease activity in Wegener's granulomatosis. Lancet 1:425, 1985.

354. Ludemann G, Gross WL: Autoantibodies against cytoplasmic structures of neutrophil granulocytes in Wegener's granulomatosis. Clin Exp Immunol 69:350, 1987.

355. Savage CS, Winearls CG, Jones S, Marshall PD, Lockwood CM: Prospective study of radioimmunoassay for antibodies against neutrophil cytoplasm in diagnosis of systemic vasculitis. Lancet 1:1389, 1987.

356. Falk RJ, Jennette JC: Antineutrophil cytoplasmic autoantibodies with specificity for myeloperoxidase in patients with systemic vasculitis and idiopathic necrotizing and crescentic glomerulonephritis. N Engl J Med 318:1651, 1988.

357. Niles JL, McCluskey RT, Ahmad MF, Arnaout MA: Wegener's granulomatosis autoantigen is a novel neutrophil serine protease. Blood 74:1888, 1989.

358. Jennette JC, Wilkman AS, Falk RJ: Antineutrophil cytoplasmic autoantibody-associated glomerulonephritis and vasculitis. Am J Pathol 135:921, 1989.

359. Cohen Tervaert JW, Goldschmeding R, Elema JD, Limburg PC, van der Giessen M, Huitema MG, Koolen MI, Hené RJ, The TH, van der Hem GK, von der Borne AEGKr, Kallenberg CGM: Association of autoantibodies to myeloperoxidase with different forms of vasculitis. Arthritis Rheum 33:1264, 1990.

360. Cohen Tervaert JW, Elema JD, Kallenberg CGM: Clinical and histopathological association of 29kD-ANCA and MPO-ANCA. APMIS 98(Suppl 19):35, 1990.

361. Pulido JS, Goeken JA, Nerad JA, Sobol WM, Folberg R: Ocular manifestations of patients with circulating antineutrophil cytoplasmic antibodies. Arch Ophthalmol 108:845, 1990.

362. Soukiasian SH, Foster CS, Niles JL, Raizman MB: Diagnostic value of anti-neutrophil cytoplasmic antibodies (ANCA) in scleritis associated with Wegener's granulomatosis. Ophthalmology 99(1):125, 1992.

363. Leavitt RY, Fauci AS, Bloch DA, Michel BA, Hunder GG, Arend WP, Calabrese LH, Fries JF, Lie JT, Lightfoot RW Jr, Masi AT, McShane DJ, Mills JA, Stevens MB, Wallace SL, Zvaifler NJ: The American College of Rheumatology 1990 criteria for the classification of WG. Arthritis Rheum 33:1101, 1990.

364. Feigenbaum A: Description of Behçet's syndrome in the hippocratic third book of endemic diseases. Br J Ophthalmol 40:355, 1956.

365. Behçet H: Ueber rezidivieerende, aphthose, durch ein Virus verursachte Geschwure am Mund, am Auge and an den Genitalien. Dermatol Wochenschr 105:1152, 1937.

366. Yamamoto S, Toyokawa H, Matsubara J, et al.: A nation-wide survey of Behçet disease in Japan. 1. Epidemiological survey. Jpn J Ophthalmol 18:282, 1974.

367. Foster CS, Baer JC, Raizman MB: Therapeutic responses to systemic immunosuppressive chemotherapy agents in patients with Behçet's syndrome affecting the eyes. Proc. Fifth International Congress on Behçet's Disease, Rochester, MN, 1989.

368. Atmaca LS: Fundus changes associated with Behçet's disease. Graefe's Arch Clin Exp Ophthalmol 227:340, 1989.

369. BenEzra D, Cohen E: Treatment and visual prognosis in Behçet's disease. Br J Ophthalmol 70:589, 1986.

370. Mishima S, Masuda K, Izawa Y, Mochizuki M, Namba K: Behçet's disease in Japan: ophthalmological aspects. Trans Am Ophthalmol Soc 77:225, 1979.

371. Colvard DM, Robertson DM, O'Duffy JD: The ocular manifestations of Behçet's disease. Arch Ophthalmol 95:1813, 1977.

372. Yazici H, Tuzun Y, Pazarli H, Yurdakul S, Ozyazgan Y, Ozdogan H, Serdaroglu S, Ersani M, Ulku BY, Muftuoglu AU: Influence of age on onset and patients' sex on the prevalence and severity of manifestations of Behçet's syndrome. Ann Rheum Dis 43:783, 1984.

373. Ohno S, Ohguchi M, Hirose S, Matsuda H, Wakisaka A, Aizawa M: Close association of HLA-Bw51 with Behçet's disease. Arch Ophthalmol 100:1455, 1982.

374. Baricordi OR, Sensi A, Pivetti-Pezzi P, Perrone S, Balboni A, Catarinelli G, Filippl F, Melchiouri R, Moncada A, Mattiuz PL: Behçet's disease associated with HLA-B51 and DRw52 antigens in Italians. Hum Immunol 17:297, 1986.

375. Yazici H, Chamberlain MA, Schreuder I, D'Amaro J, Muftuoglu M: HLA antigens in Behçet's disease: a reappraisal by a comparative study of Turkish and British patients. Ann Rheum Dis 39:344, 1980.

376. O'Duffy JD, Taswell HF, Elvebeck LR: HL-A antigens in Behçet's disease. J Rheumatol 3:1, 1976.

377. Davies PG, Fordham JN, Kirwan JR, Barnes CG, Dinning WS: The pathergy test and Behçet's syndrome in Britain. Ann Rheum Dis 43:70, 1984.

378. James DG, Spiteri MA: Behçet's disease. Ophthalmology 89:1279, 1982.

379. O'Duffy JD: Suggested criteria for the diagnosis of Behçet's disease. J Rheumatol 1(Suppl 1):18, 1974.

380. Wechsler B, Davatchi F, Mizushima Y, Hamza M, Dilsen N, Kansu E, Yazici H, Barnes CG, Chamberlain MA, James DG, Lehner T, O'Duffy JD: (International Study Group for Behçet's disease): Criteria for diagnosis of Behçet's disease. Lancet 335:1078, 1990.

381. Wilkinson IMS, Russell RWR: Arteries of the head and neck in giant cell arteritis. Arch Neurol 27:378, 1972.

382. Klein RG, Hunder GG, Stanson AW, Sheps SG: Large artery involvement in giant cell (temporal) arteritis. Ann Intern Med 83:806, 1975.

383. Hunder GG, Bloch DA, Michel BA, Steuens MB, Arend WP, Calabrese LH, Edworthy SM, Fauci AS, Leavitt, RY, Lie JT, et al.: The American College of Rheumatology 1990 criteria for the classification of giant cell arteritis. Arthritis Rheum 33:8, 1990.

384. Bengtsson BA, Malmvall BE: The epidemiology of giant cell arteritis including temporal arteritis and polymyalgia rheumatica. Arthritis Rheum 24:899, 1981.

385. Friedman G, Friedman B, Benbassat J: Epidemiology of temporal arteritis in Israel. Isr J Med Sci 18:241, 1982.

386. Machado EBV, Michet C, Ballard DJ, Hunder GG, Beard CM, Chu CP, O'Fallon WM: Trends in incidence and clinical presentation of temporal arteritis in Olmsted County, Minnesota, 1950–1985. Athritis Rheum 31:745, 1988.

387. Hazleman B, Goldstone A, Voak D: Association of polymyalgia rheumatica and giant-cell arteritis with HLA-B8. Br Med J 2:989, 1977.

388. Barrier J, Bignon JD, Soulillou JP, Grollean J: Increase prevalence of HLA-DR4 in giant-cell arteritis [Letter]. N Engl J Med 305:104, 1981.

389. Malmvall B, Bentsson B, Rydberg L: HLA antigens in patients with giant cell arteritis, compared with two control groups of different ages. Scand J Rheumatol 9:65, 1980.

390. Hunder GG, Taswell HF, Pineda AA, Elveback LR: HLA antigens in patients with giant cell arteritis and polymyalgia rheumatica. J Rheumatol 4:321, 1977.

391. Huston KA, Hunder GG, Lie JT, Kennedy RH, Elveback LR: Temporal arteritis. A 25-year epidemiologic, clinical, and pathologic study. Ann Intern Med 89:162, 1978.

392. Whitfield AGW, Bateman M, Trevor-Cooke W: Temporal arteritis. Br J Ophthalmol 47:555, 1963.

393. Hunder GG: Giant cell (temporal) arteritis. Rheum Dis Clin N Am 16:399, 1990.

394. Caselli RJ, Hunder GG, Whisnant JP: Neurologic disease in biopsy-proven giant cell (temporal) arteritis. Neurology 38:352, 1988.

395. Reich KA, Giansiracusa DF, Strongwater SL: Neurologic manifestations of giant cell arteritis. Am J Med 89:67, 1990.

396. Cohen MD, Ginsburg WW: Polymyalgia rheumatica. Rheum Dis Clin N Am 16:325, 1990.

397. Hunder GG, Allen GL: Giant cell arteritis: a review. Bull Rheum Dis 29:980, 1978–1979.

398. Chuang T, Hunder GG, Ilstrup DM, Kurland LT: Polymyalgia rheumatica. A 10-year epidemiological and clinical study. Ann Intern Med 97:672, 1982.

399. Rynes RI, Mika P, Bartholomew LE: Development of giant cell (temporal) arteritis in a patient "adequately" treated for polymyalgia rheumatica. Ann Rheum Dis 36:88, 1977.

400. Birkhead NC, Wagener HP, Shick RM: Treatment of temporal arteritis with adrenal corticosteroids: results in 55 cases in which the lesion was proved at biopsy. JAMA 163:821, 1975.

401. Hollenhorst RW, Brown JR, Wagener HP, Schick RM: Neurologic aspects of temporal arteritis. Neurology 10:490, 1960.

402. Graham E, Holland A, Avery A, Russell RW: Prognosis in giant-cell arteritis. Br Med J 282:269, 1981.

403. Hayreh HH: Anterior ischemic optic neuropathy. Differentiation of arteritis from non-arteritic type and its management. Eye 4:25, 1990.

404. Daiker B, Keller HH: Riesenallarteriitis mit endookulärer Ausbreitung und Hypotonia bulbi dolorosa. Klin Monatsbl Augenheilk 158:358, 1971.

405. Wong RL, Korn JH: Temporal arteritis without an elevated erythrocyte sedimentation rate. Am J Med 80:959, 1986.

406. Andersson R, Malmvall B, Bengtsson B: Acute phase reactants in the initial phase of giant cell arteritis. Acta Med Scand 220:365, 1986.

407. Kyle V, Cawston TE, Hazleman BL: Erythrocyte sedimentation rate and C reactive protein in the assessment of polymyalgia rheumatica/giant cell arteritis on presentation and during followup. Ann Rheum Dis 48:667, 1989.

408. Desmet GD, Knockaert DC, Bobbaers HJ: Temporal arteritis: the silent presentation and delay in diagnosis. J Intern Med 227:237, 1990.

409. Dasgupta B, Duke O, Timms AM, Pitzalis C, Panayi GS: Selective depletion and activation of $CD8^+$ lymphocytes from peripheral blood of patients with polymyalgia rheumatica and giant cell arteritis. Ann Rheum Dis 48:307, 1989.

410. Hall S, Hunder GG: Is temporal artery biopsy prudent? Mayo Clin Proc 59:793, 1984.

411. Albert DM, Ruchman MC, Keltner JL: Skip areas in temporal arteritis. Arch Ophthalmol 94:2072, 1979.

412. Allison MC, Gallagher PJ: Temporal artery biopsy and corticosteroid treatment. Ann Rheum Dis 43:416, 1984.

413. Hedges TR, Geiger GL, Albert DM: The clinical value of negative temporal artery biopsy specimens. Arch Ophthalmol 101:1251, 1983.

414. Hall S, Persellin S, Lie JT, O'Brien PC, Kurland LT, Hunder GG: The therapeutic impact of temporal artery biopsy. Lancet 2:1217, 1983.

415. Cogan DG: Syndrome of nonsyphilitic interstitial keratitis with vestibuloauditory symptoms. Arch Ophthalmol 33:144, 1945.

416. Cogan DG: Nonsyphilitic keratitis and vestibuloauditory symptoms: four additional cases. Arch Ophthalmol 42:42, 1949.

417. Cobo LM, Haynes BF: Early corneal findings in Cogan's syndrome. Ophthalmology 91:903, 1980.

418. Norton EW, Cogan DG: Syndrome of nonsyphilitic interstitial keratitis and vestibulo-auditory symptoms. Arch Ophthalmol 61:695, 1959.

419. Roberts J: Cogan's syndrome. Med J Aust 1:186, 1965.

420. Cheson BD, Bluming AZ, Alroy J: Cogan's syndrome: a systemic vasculitis. Am J Med 60:549, 1976.

421. Cogan DG, Dickerson GR: Nonsyphilitic interstitial keratitis with vestibuloauditory syndrome: a case with fatal aortitis. Arch Ophthalmol 71:172, 1964.

422. Haynes BF, Kaiser-Kupfer MI, Mason P, Fauci AS: Cogan's syndrome: studies in thirteen patients, long-term followup, and a review of the literature. Medicine 59:426, 1980.

423. Eisenstein B, Taubenhaus M: Nonsyphilitic interstitial keratitis and bilateral deafness (Cogan's syndrome) associated with cardiovascular disease. N Engl J Med 258:1074, 1958.

424. Fisher ER, Hellstrom HR: Cogan's syndrome and systemic vascular disease. Arch Pathol 72:572, 1961.

425. Gelfand ML, Kantor T, Gorstein F: Cogan's syndrome with cardiovascular involvement; aortic insufficiency. Bull NY Acad Med 48:647, 1972.

426. Haynes BF, Pikus A, Kaiser-Kupfer MI, Fauci AS: Successful treatment of sudden hearing loss in Cogan's syndrome with corticosteroids. Arthritis Rheum 24:501, 1981.

427. Bennet FM: Bilateral recurrent episcleritis associated with posterior corneal changes, vestibulo-auditory symptoms and rheumatoid arthritis. Am J Ophthalmol 55:815, 1963.

428. Watson PG: Management of scleral disease. Trans Ophthalmol Soc UK 86:151, 1966.

429. Gilbert WS, Talbot FJ: Cogan's syndrome. Signs of periarteritis nodosa and cerebral venous sinus thrombosis. Arch Ophthalmol 82:633, 1969.

430. Holt-Wilson AD, Watson PG: Nonsyphilitic deep interstitial keratitis associated with scleritis. Trans Ophthalmol Soc UK 94:52, 1974.

431. Hedges TR, Taylor GW: Uveal and vestibulo-auditory disease with sarcoid. Arch Ophthalmol 48:88, 1952.

432. McGavin DDM, McNeill J: Scleritis and perceptive deafness: case report. Ann Ophthalmol 48:1287, 1979.

433. Coca AF, Cooke RA: On the classification of the phenomena of hypersensitiveness. J Immunol 8:163, 1923.

434. Duke-Elder S, Leigh AG: Diseases of the outer eye. Cornea and sclera. In Duke-Elder S (Ed): System of Ophthalmology, Vol 8, Part 2. C.V. Mosby, St. Louis, 1965, p 1034.

435. Braude LS, Chandler JW: Atopic corneal disease. Int Ophthalmol Clin 24(2):145, 1984.

436. Buckley RJ: Atopic disease of the corneal. In Cavanagh HD (Ed): The Cornea: Transactions of the World Congress of the Cornea III. Raven, New York, 1988, pp 435–437.

437. Cassidy JT, Levinson JE, Bass JC, Baum J, Brewer EJ Jr, Fink CW, Hanson V, Jacobs JC, Masi AT, Schaller JG et al.: A study of classification criteria for a diagnosis of juvenile

rheumatoid arthritis. Arthritis Rheum 29:274, 1986.

438. Kanski JJ: Juvenile arthritis and uveitis. Surv Ophthalmol 34:253, 1990.

439. Lyne AJ, Rosen ES: Still's disease and rheumatoid nodules of the sclera. Br J Ophthalmol 52:853, 1968.

440. Watson P: Diseases of the sclera and episclera. In Duane TD, Jaeger EA (Eds): *Clinical Ophthalmology*, Vol 4. Harper & Row, Philadelphia, 1985, Chap 23.

441. Ide T, Inoue K: Case of unilateral episcleral sarcoid tubercle. Folia Ophthalmologica Japonica 19:632, 1968.

442. James DG, Anderson R, Langley D, Ainslie D: Ocular sarcoidosis. Br J Ophthalmol 48: 461, 1964.

443. Friedman AH, Henkind P: Unusual cases of episcleritis. Trans Am Acad Ophthalmol Otolaryngol 78:890, 1974.

444. Klein M, Calvert RJ, Joseph WE, Smith E: Rarities in ocular sarcoidosis. Br J Ophthalmol 39:416, 1955.

445. Donaldson DD: Sarcoid nodules of iris and of paralimbal sclera. Arch Ophthalmol 71:246, 1964.

446. Zeiter JH, Bhavsar A, McDermott ML, Siegel MJ: Ocular sarcoidosis manifesting as an anterior staphyloma. Am J Ophthalmol 112:3, 1991.

447. Tabbara KF: Scleromalacia associated with Vogt-Koyanagi–Harada syndrome. Am J Ophthalmol 105:6, 1988.

448. Sainz de la Maza M, Foster CS: Necrotizing scleritis after ocular surgery: a clinicopathologic study. Ophthalmology 98:1720, 1991.

449. Mamalis N, Johnson MD, Haines JM, Teske MP, Olson RJ: Corneal-scleral melt in association with cataract surgery and intraocular lenses: a report of four cases. J Cataract Refract Surg 16:109, 1990.

450. Yang HK, Kline OR Jr: Corneal melting with intraocular lenses. Arch Ophthalmol 100:1272, 1982.

451. Insler MS, Boutros G, Boulware DW: Corneal ulceration following cataract surgery in patients with rheumatoid arthritis. Am Intraocular Implant Soc J 11:594, 1985.

452. Bloomfield SE, Becker CG, Christian CL, Nauheim JS: Bilateral necrotising scleritis with marginal corneal ulceration after cataract surgery in a patient with vasculitis. Br J Ophthalmol 64:170, 1980.

453. Rao NA, Marak GE, Hidayat AA: Necrotizing scleritis. A clinicopathologic study of 41 cases. Ophthalmology 92:1542, 1985.

454. Collins DH: The subcutaneous nodule of rheumatoid arthritis. J Pathol Bacteriol 45:97, 1937.

455. Bennett GA, Zeller JW, Bauer W: Subcutaneous nodules of rheumatoid arthritis and rheumatic fever: a pathologic study. Arch Pathol 30:70, 1940.

456. Kaye BR, Kaye RL, Bobrove A: Rheumatoid nodules. Review of the spectrum of associated conditions and proposal of a new classification, with a report of four seronegative cases. Am Rheum Dis 23:345, 1964.

457. Soter NA, Austen KF: Cutaneous necrotizing venulitis. In Samter M, Talmage DW, Frank MM, Austen KF, Claman HN (Eds): *Immunological Diseases*. Little, Brown, Boston, 1978, pp 1267–1280.

458. McDuffee FD, Sams WM Jr, Maldonado JE: Hypocomplementemia with cutaneous vasculitis and arthritis: possible immune complex syndrome. Mayo Clin Proc 48:340, 1973.

459. Lyons CJ, Dart JKG, Aclimandos WA, Lightman S, Buckley RJ: Sclerokeratitis after keratoplasty in atopy. Ophthalmology 97:729, 1990.

460. Episcleritis and secondary glaucoma after transcleral fixation of a posterior chamber intraocular lens. Arch Ophthalmol 109:617, 1991.

461. Browning DJ, Proia AD: Ocular rosacea. Surg Ophthalmol 31:145, 1986.

462. Osgood JK, Dougherty JM, McCulley JP: The role of wax and sterol esters of meibomian secretions in chronic blepharitis. Invest Ophthalmol Vis Sci 30:1958, 1989.

463. Borrie P: Rosacea with special reference to its ocular manifestations. Br J Dermatol 65:458, 1953.

464. Richter S: Skleraperforation bei Rosaceokeratitis. Klin Monatsbl Augenheilk 146: 422, 1965.

465. Hoang-Xuan T, Rodriguez A, Zaltas MM, Rice BA, Foster CS: Ocular rosacea. A histologic and immunopathologic study. Ophthalmology 97:1468, 1990.

466. Scharf J, Nahir M, Sharf J: Scleritis associated with hyperuricaemia. Rheumatol Tindall 14: 251, 1975.

467. McWilliams JR: Ocular findings in gout. Am J Ophthalmol 35:1778, 1952.

468. Wood DJ: Inflammatory disease in the eye caused by gout. Br J Ophthalmol 20:510, 1936.

469. Heinz K: Ocular findings in cases of gout and hyperuricemia. Wien Klin Wochenschr 83:42, 1971.

470. Fishman RS, Sunderman FW: Band keratopathy in gout. Arch Ophthalmol 75:367, 1966.

7
Infectious Scleritis: The Massachusetts Eye and Ear Infirmary Experience

Although systemic immune-mediated diseases are the main possibilities in the differential diagnosis of scleritis, other unusual etiologies such as infectious diseases must also be considered. Infectious scleritis, either endogenous or exogenous, may be caused either by a direct invasion of organisms that cause the systemic and local signs, or by an immune response induced by the infectious agent.

All classes of microbial organisms can infect the sclera, including bacteria, fungi, viruses, and parasites (Table 7.1). As the scleritis caused by these conditions may be identical to that caused by immune-mediated diseases, the challenge for the ophthalmologist is to distinguish infectious scleritis from other inflammatory conditions of the sclera. The differential diagnosis between both groups of diseases is important because infectious etiologies are usually treatable by specific therapy, and because corticosteroid therapy or immunosuppressive therapy, often used in scleritis associated with immune-mediated diseases, is contraindicated in active infection; if topical or systemic corticosteroids are started because it is thought the scleritis has an immunological basis, scleral destruction and extension of the microbial process may progress.

In evaluating a patient with scleritis, it is important to take a history not only for evidence of underlying systemic diseases, but also for trauma, contact lens effects, past ocular conditions, topical therapy, and surgical procedures. There are no specific clinical signs that confirm scleral infection. When the diagnosis is suspected, laboratory studies are required to establish the causative agent. Appropriate therapy is initiated on the basis of clinical suspicion, the results of initial laboratory studies, and a knowledge of the most likely organisms responsible. The plan may be modified later, depending on the clinical response and laboratory results. With advanced infection or with a severe host inflammatory response, devastating

TABLE 7.1. Classification of organisms causing infectious scleritis.

Bacteria
  Gram-positive cocci
  Gram-negative rods
  Atypical mycobacteria
    Mycobacterium tuberculosis
    Mycobacterium leprae
  Spirochetes
    Treponema pallidum
    Borrelia burgdorferi
  Chlamydiae
  Actinomycetes
    Nocardia asteroides
Fungi
  Filamentous fungi
  Dimorphic fungi
Viruses
  Herpes zoster
  Herpes simplex type 1
  Mumps
Parasites
  Protozoa
    Acanthamoeba
    Toxoplasma gondii
  Helminths
    Toxocara canis

complications can occur, resulting in structural alterations such as thinning, perforation, or extension to adjacent structures.

In theory, any infectious agent that induces an immune response can cause vasculitis. Bacteria such as *Pseudomonas*, *Streptococcus*, *Staphylococcus*, or viruses such as herpes simplex or varicella-zoster virus, may be associated with small-sized vessel vasculitis. Syphilis and tuberculosis may cause large-sized vessel vasculitis (aortitis). Vascular damage is commonly incurred by direct invasion of the vessel by the organism, or by embolization, both of which result in an inflammatory response and immune complex formation and deposition.

This chapter focuses on the infectious diseases that may be associated with scleritis. Recommendations for an approach to the management and therapy of infectious scleritis are presented.

7.1. Bacterial Scleritis

7.1.1. Gram-Positive Coccus and Gram-Negative Rod Scleritis

7.1.1.1. Pathogenesis

Bacteria are capable of establishing a focus of infection in the sclera if normal host barriers or defense mechanisms are compromised. The presence of exogenous bacteria in scleral tissue leads to an inflammatory response. Bacterial scleritis is usually the result of scleral extension of primary corneal infections.[1-6] Risk factors in these cases include contact lens wear, recent ocular surgery or suture removal, use of topical medications (corticosteroids, beta blockers), neovascular or phacomorphic glaucomas, adnexal disease, corneal tissue devitalization (recurrent attacks of herpes simplex or herpes zoster keratitis, corneal exposure), and debilitating systemic diseases (AIDS, diabetes). However, primary bacterial scleritis with or without keratitis may occur, in which case they may follow accidental or surgical injury, or a severe endophthalmitis.[1,7-18] Surgical injuries include pterygium excision followed by β irradiation or topical thiotepa, retinal detach-

ment repair with buckling procedures and/or diathermy, or strabismus surgery.

Scleritis also may be the result of immune-mediated scleral or episcleral vascular damage caused by infectious agents. Bacteria such as *Pseudomonas*, *Streptococcus*, or *Staphylococcus* may cause an inflammatory microangiopathy in sclera by inducing immune-mediated responses in the vessel wall, such as formation and deposition of immune complexes containing bacterial products. The scleritis then becomes autoimmune, and thereafter independent of the presence of the initiating organism.

7.1.1.2. Organisms

Certain bacterial groups are most frequently encounted in scleral infections. These include the Pseudomonadaceae (*Pseudomonas*), Streptococcaceae (*Streptococcus*), Micrococcaceae (*Staphylococcus*), and Enterobacteriaceae (*Proteus*).

Pseudomonas aeruginosa is the most common cause of exogenous scleral infection. It is usually associated with primary corneal infection and subsequent scleral extension in a compromised host.[1-6] It also may appear after pterygium excision followed by either β irradiation or topical thiotepa (reported range, 6 weeks to 10 years)[1,7-11]; persistent bare sclera due to failure of conjunctival regrowth contributes to chronic scleral exposure and subsequent infection.[11]

Streptococcus pneumoniae scleritis also has been described as an extension of corneal infection[1] or after pterigium removal followed by β radiation.[7,13] *Staphylococcus aureus*,[1,19] *Staphylococcus epidermidis*,[1] and *Proteus* scleritis[14] also have been reported.

7.1.1.3. Management

Bacterial scleritis should be suspected in cases of indolent progressive scleral necrosis with suppuration, especially if there is a history of accidental trauma, debilitating ocular or systemic disease, chronic topical medication use (including corticosteroids), or surgical procedures. Scrapings for smears (Gram, Giemsa) and cultures (blood agar, chocolate agar, Sabouraud dextrose agar, thioglycollate broth)

TABLE 7.2. Selection of initial antibiotic for infectious scleritis or keratoscleritis on the basis of smear morphology.

Smear morphology	Topical[a]	Subconjunctival[b]	Systemic[c]
Gram-positive cocci	Cefazolin (133 mg/ml)	Cefazolin (100 mg)	Methicillin, iv (200 mg/kg per day)
Gram-negative rods	Tobramycin (14 mg/ml)	Tobramycin (40 mg)	Tobramycin, iv (3.0–7.0 mg/kg per day)
Acid-fast bacilli	Amikacin (10 mg/ml)	Amikacin (25–50 mg)	Amikacin, iv (5 mg/kg per day)
No microorganisms but infectious suspect	Cefazolin (133 mg/ml) and tobramycin (14 mg/ml)	Cefazolin (100 mg) and tobramycin (40 mg)	Methicillin, iv (200 mg/kg per day) and tobramycin (3.0–7.0 mg/kg per day)
Hyphal fragments[d]	Natamycin (5%)	Miconazole (10 mg)	Ketoconazole, PO (400 mg per day–1.0 gm per day)[e]
Yeast or pseudohyphae[d]	Amphotericin B (0.075–0.3%)	Miconazole (10 mg)	Ketoconazole, PO (400 mg per day–1.0 gm per day)[e]
Cysts or trophozoites	Controversial[f]		

[a] Topical solutions should be used hourly; cefazolin, tobramycin, and amikacin are tapered over 1 to 2 weeks to four times a day for 2 more weeks. Natamycin and amphotericin are tapered over several weeks, depending on clinical response.
[b] Cefazolin, tobramycin, and amikacin subconjunctival therapy should be used every 24 h and miconazole every 48 h. Although two or three doses are commonly given, length of therapy depends on process severity.
[c] Length of therapy depends on process severity.
[d] If scleral or corneal perforation threatens or occurs, intravenous amphotericin B should be added to topical and subconjunctival therapy: 1 mg in 500 ml of 5% D/W iv over 2 to 4 h test dose; work up by 5 to 10 mg total dose per day to maintenance of 0.3 to 0.5 mg/kg (4 to 6 h infusion); amphotericin B should not be used with ketoconazole because they are antagonists; amphotericin B iv and flucytosine PO (150 mg/kg per day in four divided doses) are synergistic. Therapy should be continued for 2 to 4 weeks before tapering.
[e] Single dose.
[f] 1% topical propamidine isethionate (Brolene), one drop followed 5 min later by one drop of neomycin–polymyxin B–gramicidin (Neotricin, AK-spore) every 15 min to 1 h, 18 h per day, and slowly tapered over a year; 1% miconazol nitrate or 2% clotrimazole one drop every hour and oral ketoconazole 400 mg per day to 1.0 mg per day may be added.

must be obtained and fortified antibacterial therapy, depending on smear results, must be initiated as soon as possible. Infection around implants used in retinal detachment surgery, or around stitches in any type of scleral surgery, mandate removal of the foreign body. If bacterial infection is the primary clinical suspicion, but smears and cultures (at 48 h) are negative, and the patient is not improving on the initial broad-spectrum antibacterial therapy chosen, scleral or corneoscleral biopsy is recommended. Biopsied tissue is then bisected and half is transported immediately to the microbiology laboratory for homogenization and culture in the usual medium. The remaining half is placed in formalin and transported to the pathology laboratory for histopathology with special stains (periodic acid–Schiff [PAS], Gomori methenamine silver, acid fast, calcofluor white) for identification of infectious agents.

7.1.1.4. Therapy

A classification of bacteria based on Gram stain findings from scleral or corneoscleral smears permits organization of therapy (Table 7.2). Aggressive and prolonged topical, subconjunctival, and intravenous antibiotics must be instituted, particularly if keratoscleritis occurs. As soon as the bacteria are isolated by culture, therapy may be refined with antibiotic sensitivity results. Topical corticosteroids should not be included in the initial therapy of bacterial keratoscleritis or scleritis, but may be of benefit after several days of aggressive antibiotic therapy if the infection is coming under control, or if the histopathological study reveals an inflammatory microangiopathy. An exception to this includes *Pseudomonas* infection, because steroid therapy has almost always been associated with persistence and progression of infection. Corticosteroids act as modulators of the inflammatory response associated with the infection, which also may be destructive to the sclera. Patients with prolonged corticosteroid therapy must be carefully monitored, particularly if antibiotics are discontinued, because they may have recurrences of the infection.[20]

Strong consideration should be given to surgical management if the patient is not improving within the first few days of antibacterial therapy. Surgical procedures include conjunctival resection and cryotherapy to the immediate underlying sclera.[1] Some of the possible mechanisms for efficacy of cryotherapy include mechanical destruction of microorganisms, osmotic changes, or disruption of DNA. Cryotherapy may enhance antibiotic penetration through bacterial cell walls or into the sclera as well.[5,21] Surgical intervention also may include definitive excisional biopsy for therapeutic and isolation purposes. Definitive excisional biopsy includes deep scleral dissection with subsequent scleral graft and/or lamellar or penetrating keratoplasty. If bacteria are not isolated and histopathological study reveals an inflammatory microangiopathy, immune-mediated responses associated with previous bacterial infection or with systemic autoimmune vasculitic diseases must be suspected and therapy with corticosteroids or immunosuppressive agents must be considered; continued antibiotic coverage is recommended.

7.1.1.5. Prognosis

Bacterial scleritis is generally associated with a poor prognosis. Poor penetration of antibiotics into the tightly bound collagen fibers of the scleral coat may account, at least partially, for that. Tarr and Constable[10,11] reported one eye with light perception and two eyes enucleated in their series of four patients with *Pseudomonas* scleritis complicating pterygium excision with adjunctive β irradiation. The remaining eye, which retained useful vision, was associated with little delay in the institution of aggressive anti-*Pseudomonas* therapy. Alfonso and co-workers,[2] reviewing their series of 3 patients and another series of 9 patients, noted

that in 7 of 12 patients with *Pseudomonas* keratoscleritis who had predisposing conditions, the involved eye was enucleated. Those eyes receiving early, appropriate, and prolonged anti-*Pseudomonas* therapy retained useful vision. Farrell and Smith[7] showed the devastating visual outcome (no light perception) of a case with *S. pneumoniae* keratoscleritis and endophthalmitis that appeared 2 weeks after pterygium excision with β irradiation. They also reported on a patient with *Pseudomonas* keratoscleritis that appeared 6 weeks after pterygium excision and topical thiotepa therapy; the final visual acuity was light perception only. Both patients waited several days after symptoms began before seeking medical care. Reynolds and Alfonso[1] noted that whereas 9 of their 17 cases (52%) of bacterial keratoscleritis were either enucleated or eviscerated, none of the 8 cases of bacterial scleritis required enucleation. These findings suggest that isolated bacterial scleritis has a better prognosis than bacterial keratoscleritis,[13] and that early, aggressive, and prolonged appropriate antibacterial therapy may improve final visual acuity. Early diagnosis, therefore, is essential in order to institute early treatment to halt the progression of the corneal and/or scleral bacterial infection.

7.1.1.6. Massachusetts Eye and Ear Infirmary Experience

In our series of 172 patients with scleritis, 2 patients had primary bacterial scleritis (1.16%). One of these was a 70-year-old white male with Graves' ophthalmopathy, diabetes mellitus, hypertension, anemia, and atherosclerotic heart disease, who developed a suppurative necrotizing anterior scleritis and posterior scleritis in his left eye 2 weeks after strabismus surgery.[14] Visual acuity at that time was 20/70. Biopsy of the sclera showed perivascular neutrophilic and lymphocytic infiltration; Gram's stain showed gram-negative rods, and periodic acid–Schiff stain, acid-fast stain, and Gomori methenamine silver stain were negative. *Proteus mirabilis* was identified from cultures of the scleral tissue after biopsy and homogenization. This *Proteus* scleritis responded well

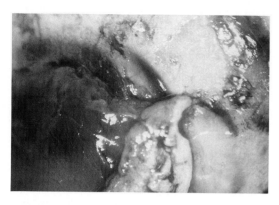

FIGURE 7.1. Intraoperative photograph of excisional biopsy of sclera. Lamellar dissection has been carried out down to healthy-appearing sclera, and the entire geographic extent of the area affected by the infection is excised.

to early and aggressive therapy with topical and intravenous vancomycin and gentamicin. Visual acuity improved to 20/30 and there were no recurrences of infection.

Our second patient was a 60-year-old woman with quiescent ulcerative colitis who developed necrotizing scleritis in her left eye after recurrent and persistent S. aureus infections following a scleral buckling procedure for retinal detachment. Prolonged treatment with aggressive topical bacitracin and oral erythromycin decreased suppuration but did not halt the progression of the scleral necrosis. Visual acuity at that time was hand motions. Excisional scleral biopsy with scleral homografting was performed (Fig. 7.1). Cultures from scleral tissue were negative but histopathological study showed a granulomatous inflammatory reaction, inflammatory microangiopathy, perivascular eosinophils, and a large mast cell population. Immunosuppressive therapy and antibiotic coverage were instituted. The scleral graft remained stable without further scleral melting, although the patient did not regain vision because of retinal problems. Whether necrotizing scleritis was the result of an immune-mediated response induced by S. aureus products, by the potentially vasculitic disease ulcerative colitis after surgical trauma, or by both, is unknown.

7.1.2. Mycobacterial Scleritis

Although ocular lesions, including scleritis and episcleritis, are now rarely caused by *Mycobacterium tuberculosis*, the number of ocular infections caused by atypical mycobacteria such as *Mycobacterium chelonai*, *Mycobacterium marinum*, *Mycobacterium fortuitum*, or *Mycobacterium gordonae* has increased over the past decade.[1,22–29] Keratitis and scleritis are the most common ocular manifestations caused by atypical mycobacteria.

7.1.2.1. Atypical Mycobacterial Disease

Atypical mycobacterial scleritis has been reported following extension of severe infectious keratitis into the sclera, resulting in keratoscleritis,[1,29] or following procedures done on an outpatient basis such as removal of an extruded scleral buckle.[28] Certain concentrations of standard disinfectants used in minor office procedures have been shown to permit *Mycobacterium* growth; some of these are 2% aqueous formaldehyde, 2% alkaline glutaraldehyde, and 0.3 to 0.7 µg of free chlorine/ml.[30] Atypical mycobacterial scleritis with or without keratitis is characterized by nodular or necrotizing slowly progressive lesions over several months, often accompanied by mild mucopurulent discharge. The most common *Mycobacterium* causing scleritis is *M. chelonai*,[1,29] a rapid-growing *Mycobacterium* (Runyon group IV), which may be associated with minor office ophthalmic procedures,[25,29] or abscesses following intramuscular injections. Scleritis also may be caused by *M. marinum*,[28] a slow-growing *Mycobacterium* (Runyon group I) that is often linked with skin diseases such as swimming pool, aquarium, or fish tank granuloma[31,32]; *M. marinum* keratoscleritis has also been associated with systemic *Mycobacterium leprae* infections.[33]

Standard smears and cultures are not helpful in the isolation of mycobacteria from corneal and scleral biopsy specimens; however, Ziehl–Neelsen stain demonstrates the presence of acid-fast bacilli, and culture on Löwenstein–Jensen culture medium at 30°C (poor growth at 37°C) yields the organisms.[34,35] Because cultures on Löwenstein–Jensen culture medium may take several weeks to become positive, the finding of characteristic acid-fast bacilli in the biopsy is sufficient for making the diagnosis of mycobacterial infection. Thus, treatment with amikacin may be undertaken weeks before definitive mycobacterial identification by culture is achieved (Table 7.2). Although intradermal skin tests may be positive for a specific atypical *Mycobacterium* and negative for others, a tuberculin protein-purified derivative (PPD) skin test often turns positive. Tissue debridement associated with topical and systemic medical therapy may be effective in curing mycobacterial scleritis and keratitis. Pharmacological possibilities after definitive mycobacterial identification include rifampin, ethambutol, isoniazid, streptomycin, kanamycin, minocycline, cefoxitin, or sulfamethoxazol singly or in combination; the choice depends on in vitro sensitivity laboratory studies.

Differential diagnosis of infectious scleritis with or without keratitis must include atypical mycobacteria, particularly if the scleritis appears following either minor office ophthalmic procedures, or ocular injuries associated with soil or contaminated water (swimming pool, aquarium, other water containers). Laboratory studies of scleral or corneal biopsy specimens from patients with infectious scleritis must include acid-fast stain and cultures at 30°C for exclusion of atypical mycobacterial disease.

7.1.2.2. Tuberculosis

Although the incidence of pulmonary and extrapulmonary tuberculosis has decreased in the United States since the last century, infection by *M. tuberculosis* still remains a major medical problem in certain inmigrant and underprivileged groups. The apices of the lungs are involved commonly in pulmonary tuberculosis, but the lower lobes or any other site may be affected. Most cases are believed to be a reactivation of *M. tuberculosis* that was acquired months to years earlier rather than reinfection or initial infection by this *Mycobacterium*. Pulmonary tuberculosis may spread to distant organs such as the eye by lymphatics or via the blood stream, causing scleritis and episcleritis. Only about 40% of patients with extrapul-

monary tuberculosis have clinical or radiographic evidence of lung disease.

The incidence of ocular involvement in a tuberculosis sanatorium ranged from 0.5 to 1.4% from 1940 to 1966 (14 cases with scleral tuberculosis)[36] and the incidence of tuberculosis in patients with scleritis was 1.92% in 1976.[37] Occasional cases have been reported more recently.[17,38] Tuberculous scleritis may be the result either of a direct *M. tuberculosis* scleral invasion or of an immune-mediated reaction to circulating tuberculoproteins. Early diagnosis may minimize ocular and systemic complications.

Direct *M. tuberculosis* scleral invasion is usually due to hematogenous miliary spread of pulmonary tuberculosis[36,39–42]; occasionally, scleritis may occur from local infection caused by direct injury[43] or by extension of lesions in adjacent tissues such as cornea, conjunctiva, or iris.[44,45] Direct *M. tuberculosis* scleral invasion may appear as nodular scleritis that, untreated, may progress to necrotizing scleritis.[42,43,46,47] Tuberculous posterior scleritis has also been described.[48] The marginal cornea may be secondarily involved with infiltrates and neovascularization, and there may be mucopurulent discharge. Occasionally, *M. tuberculosis* may involve episclera, causing simple or nodular episcleritis.[37,49] Tuberculosis may be diagnosed from sputum, urine, ocular tissue, or other body fluids by demonstrating acid-fast bacilli on Ziehl–Neelsen stain and by identification of *M. tuberculosis* on Löwenstein–Jensen culture medium at a temperature optimum of 37°C. Intradermal skin testing (PPD) and chest X rays may aid in the diagnosis. Diagnosis of tuberculous scleritis requires scleral biopsy; scleral specimens show caseating granulomas with multinucleated giant cells and characteristic acid-fast bacilli. Because cultures may become positive after several weeks, detection of acid-fast bacilli in scleral tissue and in sputum enables the presumptive diagnosis of systemic tuberculosis, allowing institution of adequate therapy with ethambutol (400 mg orally twice a day), isoniazid (300 mg orally once a day), rifampin (600 mg orally once a day), and pyridoxine (50 mg orally once a day) for 6 to 12 months.[18] Detection of acid-fast bacilli in scleral tissue but not in sputum or other body fluid is regarded as characteristic of localized mycobacterial disease, allowing institution of amikacin before definitive mycobacterial identification by culture (Table 7.2). If *M. tuberculosis* is identified, therapy should include concomitant use of two or more systemic drugs (isoniazid, rifampin, ethambutol, streptomycin, pyridoxine), depending on antibiotic sensitivities. Streptomycin may be applied topically and subconjunctivally.[42] Systemic or topical steroids may worsen the active infection.[38]

Immune-mediated tuberculous scleritis, usually with interstitial or phlyctenular keratitis or phlyctenular keratoconjunctivitis, is considered to be a host immune response to cell wall components of *M. tuberculosis* proteins. Occasionally, episcleritis may occur.[37] The pathogenesis appears to be related to a cell-mediated type IV hypersensitivity reaction to these antigens. Although there is no mycobacterial invasion of sclera, immune-mediated tuberculous scleritis often occurs in conjunction with active systemic disease. Histologically, scleral specimens show a granulomatous reaction without acid-fast bacilli. Interstitial keratitis associated with scleritis tends to be peripheral and sectorial. Unlike luetic interstitial keratitis, in which the deep stroma is involved, tuberculous interstitial keratitis affects the superficial and midstromal layers. There are often nodular infiltrates with superficial stromal vascularization. The clinical course is prolonged, with residual corneal scarring. Phlyctenular keratoconjunctivitis develops as a small vesicle in peripheral cornea, bulbar conjunctiva, or tarsal conjunctiva. The vesicle progresses to a nodule, which degenerates and heals. Resolution of corneal phlyctenules involves scarring and neovascularization; resolution of conjunctival phlyctenules does not involve scarring. Corneal phlyctenules may spread centrally, leaving a characteristic leash of vessels from the central lesions to the healed peripheral areas marking its path. The diagnosis of tuberculosis as the cause of immune-mediated scleritis with or without keratitis is in most cases difficult or impossible to confirm. It depends on the associated ocular findings and evidence of previous or present systemic tuberculosis demonstrated by a positive PPD test,

chest X ray-compatible findings, and positive sputum culture. Treatment must include topical corticosteroids with meticulous tapering and systemic tuberculostatic drugs if there is evidence of active disease.[50,51]

In our series of 172 patients with scleritis, 1 patient had scleritis associated with systemic tuberculosis (0.57%). The patient was a 55-year-old black Haitian female with a 4-year history of intermittent redness without pain and gradual decrease in vision in her right eye. Past family history disclosed a member with tuberculosis and review of systems revealed constitutional symptoms and productive cough. At the moment of her first visit with us, the visual acuity was hand motions in the right eye and 20/50 in the left eye. Slit-lamp examination showed diffuse scleritis associated with adjacent interstitial keratitis in the right eye. A PPD intradermal skin test was reactive and the chest X ray showed extensive left lower and middle lobe infiltrates. Her sputum contained acid-fast bacilli and *M. tuberculosis* grew when cultured. Systemic tuberculosis was diagnosed and systemic tuberculostatic agents were instituted. Sclerokeratitis was believed to be due to tuberculosis, probably secondary to an immune-mediated reaction, and topical steroids were begun. Ocular inflammation subsided 2 months after the initiation of systemic and topical treatment. Visual acuity was at the level of counting fingers at 4 ft, due to corneal scarring. Tapering and discontinuation of topical steroids was followed by a recurrence of the sclerokeratitis; reinstitution of topical steroids with a slow taper halted the process without further recurrences.

7.1.2.3. Leprosy

Leprosy is a chronic granulomatous infection caused by *M. leprae*, an acid-fast bacillus. The disease is characterized by lesions in skin, mucous membranes, nerves, and eyes. The ocular lesions include keratitis, uveitis, scleritis, and episcleritis. *Mycobacterium leprae* was first recognized by Hansen in 1874 but to date has never been cultured in vitro and requires a host, such as the human, or experimental animals, such as the mouse (foot pads), for propagation.[52] *Mycobacterium leprae* infections are uncommon in western societies but have significant prevalence in central Africa, the Middle East, and Southeast Asia, including India and Indonesia, and some countries of temperate climate such as North and South Korea, Argentina, and Central Mexico.[53] Susceptibility to *M. leprae* varies according to the sex, race, and geographic distribution of the involved population.[54] According to the Madrid classification, there are three clinical forms of the disease, depending on the immune response of the host: tuberculoid, borderline, and lepromatous.[55] Patients with tuberculoid leprosy exhibit only a few discrete demarcated, hypopigmented, and hypoesthetic skin lesions that histologically consist of granulomas, resembling those of tuberculosis, and a few acid-fast bacilli. The dermal nerves also are involved, usually in a symmetrical pattern. Patients with lepromatous leprosy exhibit multiple diffuse skin lesions and peripheral nerve involvement. Cell-mediated immunity is impaired in these patients.[56] Histologically, the lesions contain many macrophages and histiocytes with many intracellular, extracellular, and intravascular acid-fast bacilli. Thickening of the facial skin leads to the characteristic leonine facies. Eye involvement is more common in this type of leprosy than in the tuberculoid form.[57] Borderline leprosy shares characteristics of tuberculoid and lepromatous types of leprosy.

Scleritis, episcleritis, and anterior uveitis are the initial manifestations in up to 16% of leprosy patients[58] and are more commonly seen in lepromatous leprosy than in tuberculoid leprosy. Scleritis and episcleritis in leprosy may be initiated by a direct *M. leprae* invasion, but an immune-mediated reaction to the products from the destroyed bacilli may also produce inflammation. The episcleritis may be simple or nodular. The scleritis is usually nodular, but it may progress to necrotizing scleritis. Direct *M. leprae* scleral invasion usually arises de novo although it may result as an extension of lesions in adjacent tissues such as lids or uveal tract. Scleritis is characterized by miliary lepromas with macrophages and *M. leprae*, is usually bilateral, and often is accompanied by mucopurulent discharge. Scleritis is usually recurrent over many years, with exacerbations lasting 3 to 4 weeks. Chronic or recurrent

scleritis in leprosy may lead to scleral thinning and staphyloma formation.

Mycobacterium leprae bacilli migrate from sclera into the cornea, causing superficial avascular keratitis characterized by whitish, subepithelial corneal opacities that usually begin in the superior or supratemporal quadrant and spread from peripheral to central areas; corneal opacities eventually coalesce and cause gradual decrease of vision. Superficial neovascularization occurs later in the disease and forms the classic superior or supratemporal leprous pannus. Edematous corneal nerves resembling beads on a string are pathognomonic of leprosy.[59] Corneal invasion from scleral *M. leprae* bacilli also may cause interstitial keratitis, which usually appears in the superior quadrants as deep stromal inflammation with progressive vascularization.[59,60] In some cases, interstitial keratitis is secondary to the deeper extension of the superficial avascular keratitis. When the inflammation subsides, the vascular flow diminishes, leaving behind ghost vessels in mid- to deep stroma. Scleritis also may be associated with anterior uveitis, which is characterized by iris pearls or creamy white particles consisting of bacilli and monocytes,[61] by iris atrophy or loss of iris stroma, and by small, nonreactive pupils.[62] Iris pearls are pathognomonic of ocular leprosy. Angle-closure glaucoma may result from seclusion of the pupil by posterior synechiae.

The diagnosis of leprous scleritis is made on the basis of clinical and histopathological findings. Dermatological and ocular findings substantiate the diagnosis, which is confirmed by the finding of granulomatous inflammation with acid-fast bacilli on scleral biopsy specimen. Therapy consists of a combination of oral dapsone, clofazimine, and rifampin. This is supplemented by prolonged treatment with local steroids, which must be carefully monitored and slowly tapered.

7.1.3. Spirochetal Scleritis

The spirochetes that most frequently cause scleritis or episcleritis are *Treponema pallidum* and *Borrelia burgdorferi*, etiological agents of syphilis and Lyme disease, respectively. Because syphilis and Lyme disease have increasingly been detected for the past decade in the United States and Europe, both entities must be included in the differential diagnosis of patients with scleritis and episcleritis. Past history, review of systems, and laboratory testing are important contributors to the diagnosis of spirochetal scleritis or episcleritis.

7.1.3.1. Syphilis

Scleritis and episcleritis may be ocular manifestations of syphilis, a sexually transmitted disease caused by the spirochete *T. pallidum*.

7.1.3.1.1. Epidemiology

Syphilis was considered to be one of the most common causes of intraocular inflammation before 1925. The advent of antibiotic therapy led to a marked decrease in syphilitic infections and, in 1955, it was believed that syphilis had been eradicated.[63] However, since the late 1970s the incidence of syphilis, and therefore of its ocular manifestations, has been steadily increasing in the United States.[64] Syphilis now accounts for approximately 100,000 new sexually transmitted diseases annually. The association of ocular syphilis, particularly uveitis, retinitis, or optic neuritis, and human immunodeficiency virus (HIV) infection has been reported.[65–76]

7.1.3.1.2. Pathogenesis and Clinical Features

Syphilis is transmitted either by venereal contact or transplacentally by an infected mother to her unborn child (congenital syphilis).[77] Primary syphilis appears as an ulcerated, painless chancre at the point of *T. pallidum* inoculation, usually in the genital area, with regional lymphadenopathy. One month to 3 years later, hematogenous spread of *T. pallidum* leads to secondary syphilis characterized by skin and mucous membrane lesions, as well as generalized lymphadenopathy. The humoral and cellular immune responses can suppress the treponemes in an immunocompetent individual, resulting in a latent stage. In one-third of affected individuals, often after latent periods of 1 to 30 years, tertiary syphilis develops. Tertiary syphilis consists of an immune-mediated response to *T. pallidum* and its metabolic products, leading to formation of gummas. Although gummas may appear in any organ, they usually cause cardiovascular lesions (aortic aneurysms) and central nervous system involvement (paralysis). Treponemes may be found in the gummas.

Treponema pallidum dissemination through transplacental passage from an infected mother, followed by hypersensitivity reactions, causes congenital syphilis. Interstitial keratitis, peg top teeth, and deafness, considered the cardinal signs, are late manifestations of the disease. Other, less common manifestations are saddle nose deformity, skull abnormalities, and arched palate.

7.1.3.1.3. Scleritis and Episcleritis

The reported incidence of syphilis in patients with scleritis is 2.89%.[37] Not infrequently, scleritis is the initial manifestation of the disease.[65,78] Scleritis usually occurs during the course of secondary, tertiary, or congenital syphilis. Episcleritis also may occur during the primary stage. Therefore the pathogenesis of syphilitic scleritis or episcleritis may be related either to a direct invasion of *Treponema* (primary or secondary) or to an immune-mediated response to *Treponema* or its metabolic products (tertiary or congenital).

1. *Primary syphilis*: Episcleritis during primary syphilis is usually secondary to an overlying conjunctival chancre. Preauricular and submaxillary lymphadenopathy also may occur.[79]

2. *Secondary syphilis*: Scleritis and episcleritis during secondary syphilis appear at the same time as or after the onset of skin rash. They are often associated with conjunctival involvement. Scleritis or episcleritis and conjunctivitis are characteristically localized at the limbus. Limbal swelling may overlap the corneal margin.

3. *Tertiary syphilis*: Scleritis and episcleritis during tertiary syphilis are not clinically different from that caused by any other disease. Scleritis in this stage has an insidious onset, may be of the diffuse anterior, nodular anterior, necrotizing anterior, or posterior type, and is

often recurrent.[78–80] Immune-mediated mechanisms lead to scleral granulomatous inflammation and inflammatory microangiopathy.[81] Occasionally, scleritis is associated with interstitial keratitis. Interstitial keratitis often is unilateral, localizes in the superior sector, and appears as tiny stromal opacities, mild endothelial edema, and keratic precipitates 5 months to 10 years following primary infection. Stromal opacities may coalesce, affecting either a localized area or the entire cornea, giving a ground-glass appearance. Later, vessels arrive and invade the deep stroma. Once the inflammation subsides, vascular flow diminishes, leaving behind the empty ghost vessels. Anterior uveitis may occasionally occur. Episcleritis in this stage may be simple or nodular.[78] The presence of ocular involvement in tertiary syphilis may be associated with other systemic lesions characteristic of this stage, such as neurosyphilis[65] or cardiovascular involvement.

4. *Congenital syphilis*: Scleritis in congenital syphilis develops many years after the cardinal characteristics appear and is usually of long duration, mild severity, and resistant to treatment. Scleritis is usually of the diffuse anterior or posterior type.[80] Interstitial keratitis in congenital syphilis usually begins between the ages of 5 and 20 years and may reappear at the same time as the onset of scleritis. It is eventually bilateral and is more severe and diffuse than the interstitial keratitis seen in tertiary syphilis.[82] Anterior uveitis is often associated.

In our series of 172 patients with scleritis, 1 patient had syphilis (0.58%). The patient was a 63-year-old black female with a 1-year history of nodular scleritis in her right eye, which was unresponsive to systemic prednisone and azathioprine and to local steroid therapy. At the moment of her first examination by us, visual acuity was 20/25 in the right eye and 20/20 in the left and slit-lamp examination revealed nodular scleritis and mild anterior uveitis. Past history review did not reveal any prior disease or specific treatment, and review of systems did not disclose teeth, hearing, skull, or nose abnormalities. Serological tests were unremarkable and scleral biopsy disclosed only subacute inflammation. No silver stains or immunostains were performed on the specimen. Prednisone was slowly tapered and oxyphenbutazone was begun. The inflammation resolved but the patient returned again 3 months later with a nodular scleritis in her left eye. This new episode prompted repeat laboratory studies, including tests for syphilis. The fluorescent treponemal antibody absorption (FTA-ABS) test was positive. Retrospective indirect immunofluoresce testing in an attempt to demonstrate *T. pallidum* in the prior scleral biopsy (rabbit anti-treponemal antibody and fluorescein-labeled sheep anti-rabbit antibody) was negative. The patient was advised to begin therapy for syphilis but she did not return until 7 months later, when she had a nodular scleritis recurrence in her left eye. She refused spinal tap. The patient was hospitalized and treated with intravenous penicillin (24 million units of aqueous penicillin G daily for 10 days), topical prednisolone acetate (1%, four times daily), and scopolamine (0.25%, twice daily). Therapy was continued on an outpatient basis with penicillin (2.4 million units of penicillin G benzathine, intramuscular, once a week for 3 weeks); topical steroid was tapered and discontinued after 8 weeks. The scleritis resolved within 2 weeks after the onset of therapy. The patient did not have recurrences of her scleritis during the following 2 years. The presence of scleritis in this patient was the first manifestation whose study led to the diagnosis and treatment of syphilis.

7.1.3.1.4. Diagnosis

Because treponemes may be scant in sclera, particularly in tertiary or congenital syphilis, their identification with silver stains (Levaditi's stain or Warthin–Starry stain) or by immunological methods (direct or indirect immunofluorescence or immunoperoxidase testing) may be difficult.[83–86]

The presumed diagnosis of acquired syphilitic scleritis when scleral treponemes cannot be demonstrated is made on the basis of the histological conjunctival or scleral granulomatous inflammatory reaction with obliterative endarteritis,[80,87,88] associated with a positive FTA-

ABS test or microhemagglutination assay for *T. pallidum* (MHA-TP). Past history of venereal disease and signs of CNS or cardiovascular involvement also support the diagnosis.

Scleritis due to congenital syphilis is suggested by a history of ocular inflammation in childhood, previous therapy for syphilis, a maternal history of a positive syphilis serology, other ocular signs such as salt-and-pepper chorioretinitis or optic atrophy, or presence of late clinical manifestations of syphilis, such as deafness, teeth abnormalities, palatal perforation, or saddle nose deformity, and a positive FTA-ABS test or MHA-TP.

The FTA-ABS and MHA-TP tests are the most sensitive tests for any stage of syphilis except primary, early secondary, and early congenital forms. The FTA-ABS test is 98% sensitive and the MHA-TP test is 98 to 100% sensitive in tertiary syphilis.[63,89–91] The MHA-TP is more specific than the FTA-ABS, with only 1% or less of false-positive reactions in leprosy, relapsing fever, systemic lupus erythematosus, rheumatoid arthritis, or yaws.[91] The Venereal Disease Research Laboratory (VDRL) quantitative test is not reliable in late congenital or tertiary syphilis and has a high incidence of false-positive reactions.[89,90] Therefore the FTA-ABS and MHA-TP tests are preferred for episcleritis and scleritis suspected to be caused by syphilis. However, the FTA-ABS and MHA-TP tests do not indicate active, as opposed to previous, disease; patients with scleritis or episcleritis and positive FTA-ABS and MHA-TP tests could have had syphilis in the past, which was treated, or could have latent syphilis and coincidentally develop idiopathic scleral or episcleral inflammation. The clinical response after adequate therapy for syphilis suggests that scleritis or episcleritis in patients with positive FTA-ABS and MHA-TP tests is caused by syphilis.

The presence of ocular lesions, including scleritis and episcleritis, in tertiary syphilis requires a careful search for evidence of neurosysphilis through a cerebrospinal fluid examination for cells and protein, and a VDRL test.[63]

Because ocular syphilis may occur concomitantly with HIV infection, we believe that all patients with ocular syphilis should now be evaluated for HIV and vice versa.[63]

7.1.3.1.5. Therapy

Once the diagnosis of syphilitic scleritis or episcleritis has been established and a history of possible penicillin allergy discarded, therapy with penicillin G benzathine (2.4 million units, intramuscular once a week for 2 weeks in secondary syphilis; the same regimen for 3 weeks in tertiary or congenital syphilis) may be instituted. However, because of previous reports of therapeutic failures with intramuscular penicillin G benzathine and experimental data suggesting that complete spirochetal sterilization from the eye may be impossible unless high dosages and prolonged periods of treatment are used,[92] we prefer to treat patients, particularly those with tertiary syphilis, with the neurosyphilis regimen of intravenous penicillin (24 million units of aqueous penicillin G, intravenous, daily for 10 days) followed by intramuscular penicillin (2.4 million units of penicillin G benzathine, intramuscular, once a week for 3 weeks).[89] Tetracyclin or eythromycin (500 mg, four times a day for 4 weeks) has been used in penicillin-allergic patients; there are no properly controlled studies to test the efficacy of these treatments. We prefer instead to have penicillin-allergic patients undergo penicillin desensitization before treating with penicillin. Some patients who give a history of penicillin allergy prove negative when skin tested for immediate hypersensitivity to penicillin and could be given aqueous crystalline penicillin G under close supervision in the hospital.

Scleritis in tertiary or congenital syphilis with or without interstitial keratitis requires topical corticosteroids with careful clinical monitoring and slowly progressive dose reduction.

There is evidence that syphilis may pursue a more aggressive course in patients who are concurrently infected with HIV, rendering standard intramuscular therapy inadequate.[67] Therefore a patient with primary, secondary, tertiary, or congenital syphilis and concurrent HIV infection needs intravenous antibiotic therapy.

7.1.3.2. Lyme Disease

Scleritis and episcleritis may be ocular manifestations of Lyme disease, a tick-borne illness caused by *Borrelia burgdorferi*, a larger spirochete than *T. pallidum*.

7.1.3.2.1. Epidemiology

Lyme disease was first described in 1977 by Steere et al.[93] in three Connecticut communities. Since then it has been increasingly recognized in the United States, particularly in the northeast, upper midwest, and California, as well as in certain areas of the Pacific Northwest and midwest.[94,95] Lyme disease has also been detected in Europe.[96]

7.1.3.2.2. Pathogenesis and Clinical Features

Lyme disease is acquired by the bite of *Ixodes dammini*, a well-recognized tick vector for the spirochete *B. burgdorferi*.[97,98] However, only approximately 30% of persons recall being bitten.[99] Lyme disease has three defined clinical stages.[100–102] Stage 1 appears within 1 month of an infected tick bite, usually in the summer, and is characterized by a skin macular rash of varying severity, often with a clear center at the area of the bite, known as erythema chronicum migrans. There may be associated stiff neck, fever, headache, malaise, fatigue, myalgias, and/or arthralgias.[99]

Stage 2 begins several weeks to months after the tick bite and is characterized by neurological (meningitis, radiculoneuropathies, severe headache) and cardiac (atrioventricular block, myopericarditis) manifestations.[103–109]

Stage 3 occurs up to 2 years after the tick bite and is characterized by a migratory oligoarthritis.[103,110–112] Neurological manifestations (encephalopathy, seizure, dementia, myelitis, spastic paraparesis, psychiatric disturbances, ataxia) also may occur in this stage.[113–118] Other manifestations include fatigue, lymphadenopathy, splenomegaly, sore throat, dry cough, nephritis, hepatitis, or testicular swelling.

Ocular manifestations of Lyme disease may appear at any stage but are more common in the last two stages. They include neuroophthalmic findings such as involvement of third, sixth, and seventh cranial nerves, optic nerve (optic neuritis and perineuritis, papilledema, ischemic optic neuropathy, optic nerve atrophy), and retina (retinal hemorrhages, exudative retinal detachments, cystoid macular edema).[96,114,119–123] Other ocular findings are anterior and posterior uveitis, endophthalmitis, keratitis, conjunctivitis, blepharitis, scleritis, and episcleritis.[124–133] Keratitis may manifest as stromal opacities, punctate superficial keratitis, or peripheral ulcerative keratitis. Ocular manifestations also may indicate recrudescence of the Lyme disease after inadequate treatment of the infection.[130,132]

7.1.3.2.3. Scleritis and Episcleritis

Scleritis and episcleritis may occur in Lyme disease. Their pathogenesis may be related either with direct invasion of the *Borrelia* species or to an immune-mediated response to *Borrelia* or its metabolic products. Scleritis has not been previously reported in Lyme disease.

In our series of 172 patients with scleritis, 1 patient had Lyme disease (0.58%). The patient was a 57-year-old female who had been living in New England for the past 5 years. She had had recurrent episodes of diffuse scleritis in her left eye along with mild anterior uveitis, disk edema, and cystoid macular edema. The patient did not recall being bitten and no systemic clinical abnormalities were found. Laboratory tests revealed a Lyme titer of 1:640 by enzyme-linked immunosorbent assay (ELISA) and elevated circulating immune complexes by Raji cell assay; an FTA-ABS test was negative. No scleral biopsy for silver stains or immunostains was performed. Therapy with intravenous ceftriaxone (2 mg a day for 14 days) and topical steroids controlled the scleritis without further recurrences.

Lyme disease must always be considered in the differential diagnosis of scleritis associated with neuroophthalmological findings.

Episcleritis also may appear in Lyme disease,[132,133] usually after other ocular manifestations, such as follicular conjunctivitis or stromal keratitis. Episcleritis may indicate a recurrence of the infection after inadequate treatment for Lyme disease.[132]

7.1.3.2.4. Diagnosis

In the absence of histological detection of *B. burgdorferi* in scleral or episcleral tissue specimens, criteria for suggesting that scleritis or episcleritis is caused by Lyme disease include lack of evidence of other disease, including multiple sclerosis, clinical findings consistent with Lyme disease, the occurrence in patients living in an endemic area, positive serology, and, in most cases, response to treatment. The ELISA is usually negative in stage 1, but is positive in approximately 90% of patients in stage 2 and in almost 100% of patients in stage 3. It tests both IgM and IgG levels with IgM rising early and IgG later. The ELISA is the most sensitive and most specific of the routinely available tests.[119] The indirect fluorescent antibody (IFA) method is also a reliable test. A Lyme titer of 1:256 as determined by ELISA or IFA is diagnostic of Lyme disease. Patients with chronic Lyme disease may not have antibodies against *B. burgdorferi* if there was earlier inadequate oral antibiotic treatment or if the patient is immunosuppressed. Immunoblotting (Western blot) is helpful in differentiating false positives occurring in patients with syphilis, Rocky Mountain spotted fever, autoimmune disease, or other neurological disorders, but it is not routinely available. Culture is generally not useful because the spirochete is difficult to grow from sites of infection, culture media are expensive, and culture conditions are not standardized. The use of T lymphocyte assays, urine antigen assays, and the polymerase chain reaction may prove helpful, but the tests need further studies for corroboration. Histological staining of *B. burgdorferi* with silver stains or immunostains in tissue biopsy has been shown to be positive in skin or brain.[119] There are no data on histological stainings in scleral or episcleral tissue specimens from patients with Lyme disease.

7.1.3.2.5. Treatment

Although still controversial, therapy for definitive ocular, neuroophthalmic, neurological, or cardiac disease in adults includes penicillin G (24 million units, intravenous, daily in four divided doses for 21 days) or intravenous cef-triaxone (2 mg daily in two divided doses for 21 days).[134] Therapy for children consists of intravenous penicillin G (250,000 units/kg per day in four divided doses for 21 days) or intravenous ceftriaxone (100 mg/kg per day in two divided doses for 21 days). Scleritis and episcleritis require topical corticosteroids with careful clinical monitoring and slowly progressive dose reduction.

Nonspecific symptoms with positive Lyme titers may be treated with oral doxycycline (100 mg twice daily for 4 to 6 weeks) or oral tetracycline (500 mg four times a day for 4 to 6 weeks). Children may receive oral penicillin V potassium (50 mg/kg per day in four divided doses) oral amoxicillin (125 to 250 mg three times a day), or erythromycin (40 mg/kg per day in four divided doses) each regimen for 3 to 4 weeks.

7.1.4. Chlamydial Scleritis

It is possible that *Chlamydia trachomatis*, the etiological agent of neonatal inclusion conjunctivitis, adult inclusion conjunctivitis, and trachoma causes scleritis or episcleritis,[80] but there are no reported cases of either scleral or episcleral inflammation during chlamydial keratoconjunctivitis, or of idiopathic scleritis or episcleritis with positive Giemsa stains or immunostains from scleral or episcleral tissue specimens. Scleritis has been produced by intracorneal injection of chlamydiae.[135]

7.1.5. Actinomycetic Scleritis

Scleritis is an uncommon manifestation of actinomycetic infections. Actinomycetic organisms superficially resemble fungi but are related to the true bacteria. They most frequently cause disease in patients with malignancies and in those undergoing immunosuppressive therapy.

7.1.5.1. Nocardiosis

Nocardia asteroides is an actinomycetic organism that is gram positive, filamentous, and may stain acid fast.[136] The organism grows aerobically, slowly, on many simple media. *Nocardia* is part of the normal soil microflora and is considered an opportunistic organism usually affecting immunosuppressed patients or patients after trauma.[136–138] Systemically, it can involve lungs, brain, kidney, skin, and less commonly other organs such as heart, liver, spleen, and bone. Ocular manifestations include scleritis, conjunctivitis, keratitis, endophthalmitis, and orbital involvement.[139–145]

Nocardial scleritis has been reported as necrotizing scleritis with mucopurulent discharge in association with a silicone scleral buckle due to retinal detachment. In spite of culture isolation and institution of adequate therapy, progression of scleral necrosis could not be halted and the eye was enucleated.[143] Nocardial scleral involvement has also been shown histologically after nocardial endophthalmitis that required evisceration.[145]

Diagnosis can be established by histological identification of the characteristic hyphal forms with Gram's stain, overstained Gomori methenamine silver stain, or modified acid-fast stain. The latter, coupled with the fact that fragmented hyphae resemble bacillary forms, could lead to a erroneous diagnosis of tuberculosis. Diagnosis also can be established by culture of the bacteria in blood agar or in Sabouraud dextrose agar; the organism may appear in culture after a long period of time (as late as 14 days).[146]

Trimethoprim with sulfamethoxazole is the drug combination of choice. In case of resistance or drug reaction, amikacin or minocycline may be used as an alternative.[143]

7.2. Fungal Scleritis

Fungal scleritis is a rare entity usually caused by an exogenous infection. Occasionally, however, it may be the result of hematogenous spread of a systemic fungal disease.[147] Fungal scleritis, often associated with keratitis, poses a threat to the eye, not only because of the damage caused by the organism, but also because the available antifungal agents penetrate the sclera poorly.

7.2.1. Filamentous and Dimorphic Fungal Scleritis

7.2.1.1. Pathogenesis

As in bacterial scleritis, fungal infections of the sclera often follow an accidental injury, especially with vegetable matter or soil, surgical procedures such as pterygium excision followed by β irradiation[148] or retinal detachment repair with buckling procedures,[149,150] or panophthalmitis.[151] Debilitating ocular or systemic diseases, contact lens use, intravenous narcotic addiction,[147] and chronic topical medication use, including corticosteroids, also are risk factors.

7.2.1.2. Organisms

Fungi are eukaryotic organisms that may be classified as yeasts, molds, and dimorphic. Yeasts are oval structures that grow as single cells and reproduce by asexual budding, producing structures resembling hyphae (pseudohyphae). Molds grow as long multicellular filamentous strands (mycelia) that may reproduce either by cellular division or by elaboration of fruiting bodies called sporangia. Some pathogenic fungi are termed *dimorphic* because they exist as yeast forms in host tissues while behaving as molds in the saprophytic state. The most common fungi that may cause scleritis are the filamentous fungi such as *Aspergillus*,[147,148,152] *Acremonium*,[1] or Sphaeropsidales (*Lasiodiplodia theobromae*).[151] Another fungus implicated in scleral infection is the dimorphic fungus *Sporothrix schenckii*.[153] *Rhinosporidium seeberi*, an organism of uncertain taxonomic position although most probably a fungus, also may cause scleral ulceration.[154–156]

7.2.1.3. Management

Fungal scleritis should be suspected in cases of slow but progressive scleral necrosis with suppuration, especially if there is a history of accidental trauma (especially involving vegetable matter or soil), debilitating ocular or systemic disease, contact lens use chronic topical medication use (including corticosteroids), or surgical procedures. If there is adjacent fungal keratitis, clinical characteristics include feathery borders of a corneal stromal white blood cell infiltrate, satellite lesions, hypopyon, or endothelial plaque. Infected scleral buckles need to be removed. Material from vigorous scraping of the infected scleral or corneoscleral area with a surgical blade should be smeared onto glass slides for staining (Gram and Giemsa) and onto agar plates or broth for cultures two blood agarpreparations [one kept at room temperature for isolation of fungi, the other at 35°C for routine culture] chocolate agar, Sabouraud dextrose agar, thioglycollate broth, brain–heart infusion medium). Because Gram's stain may identify fungal forms, particularly yeasts (oval structures or pseudohyphae), and alkaline Giemsa and calcofluor white stains are more likely to show the morphology of filamentous fungi (septate hyphal fragments), antifungal therapy must be initiated if the smears detect fungi. If the smears are negative, a topical broad-spectrum antibacterial therapy must be instituted.

If fungal infection is the primary clinical suspicion, but smears and cultures (at 48 h) are negative and the patient is not improving on the initial broad-spectrum antibacterial therapy chosen, scleral or corneoscleral biopsy is recommended. Our technique for this includes dissection of conjunctiva, Tenon's capsule, and episcleral tissue and careful removal of necrotic scleral tissue under the operating microscope (Fig. 7.1). In case of corneal biopsy, we perform a partial thickness trephination with a depth and diameter depending on the corneal area affected, followed by a lamellar dissection. The scleral or corneoscleral biopsy specimen is bisected and half is sent to the microbiology laboratory, where it is placed in 1 ml of meat broth and homogenized with a tissue grinder. One-drop samples are cultured in different media, including blood agar at room temperature, Sabouraud dextrose agar, thioglycollate broth, and brain–heart infusion medium for fungus isolation. The remaining half is placed in formalin and transported to the pathology laboratory for histopathology with special stains, including PAS, Gomori methenamine silver, and calcofluor white for fungus identification.

Anterior chamber paracentesis is indicated in cases of corneoscleral involvement with hypopyon and primary clinical suspicion of fungal keratoscleritis, in which smears, cultures, and scleral or corneoscleral biopsies are negative, and in which no patient improvement on the initial broad-spectrum antibacterial therapy chosen has occurred. The hypopyon present in a patient with bacterial keratitis is a sterile hypopyon, provided the cornea has not perforated. Indeed, performing a paracentesis in a patient with bacterial keratitis carries with it the potential for inoculation of microorganisms into the anterior chamber. However, fungi may invade the anterior chamber through an intact Descemet's membrane. Anterior chamber paracentesis must be performed with an adequate-sized needle (usually at least 22 gauge) for vacuuming the hypopyon, through a beveled wound created with a sharp, thin blade. The harvested material should be immediately transported to the microbiology laboratory for culture on blood agar (room temperature), Sabouraud dextrose agar, thyoglycollate broth, and brain–heart infusion medium.

As soon as the fungi are identified by culture, therapy may be modified on the basis of results. Because sensitivities of isolated fungi to the various antifungal agents can be determined in only a few specialized centers, such as the Centers for Disease Control (Atlanta, GA), standard antifungal sensitivity studies are generally not performed. However, it is recommended that any fungus isolated be propagated rather than discarded so that additional studies by such centers can be performed in the event the case does not evolve to a cure.

7.2.1.4. Therapy

A definitive diagnosis should be made before starting therapy. In the absence of laboratory confirmation, it is best to defer fungal treatment until isolation is achieved, because unusual organisms such as *Mycobacterium*, *Acanthamoeba*, or anaerobes could be the etiological agents of scleritis or keratoscleritis.

A classification of fungi as yeasts and molds, on the basis of smear findings, permits organization of therapy (Table 7.2). Aggressive and prolonged topical, subconjunctival, and oral antifungal treatment must be instituted, particularly if keratoscleritis occurs. More selective antifungal treatment may be indicated after fungus identification by culture. Medical therapy is limited by the paucity of approved antifungal drugs and by the poor ocular penetration of available agents. Most of the recommendations for treatment are derived largely from uncontrolled clinical studies.

Therapy for confirmed fungal scleritis or keratoscleritis is initially medical, although surgery may be required if progressive melting continues in spite of antifungal drug therapy. Surgical intervention may include scleral or keratoscleral excisional biopsy for therapeutic purposes; this procedure may be effective in removing a concentrated abscess and facilitating topical antifungal penetration. Definitive excisional biopsy includes deep scleral dissection, sometimes with subsequent scleral graft and/or lamellar or penetrating keratoplasty after adequate antifungal therapy.

Corticosteroids are contraindicated in fungal scleritis or keratoscleritis because of unequivocal enhancement of fungal growth.

7.2.1.5. Massachusetts Eye and Ear Infirmary Experience

In our series of 172 patients with scleritis, 1 patient had fungal scleritis (0.58%) (see Section 5.2.2.1.8.2). The patient developed a necro-

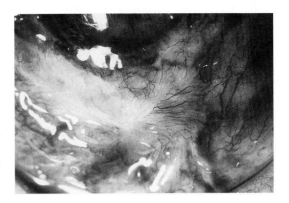

FIGURE 7.3. Inferior sclera of the same patient as in Figs. 7.2.

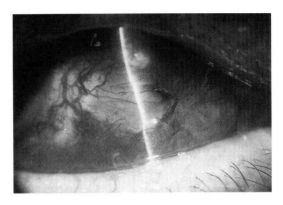

FIGURE 7.4. Same patient as in Figs. 7.2 and 7.3, showing the extensive involvement of the scleritic process, with necrotizing lesions nasally as well as inferiorally and supratemporally.

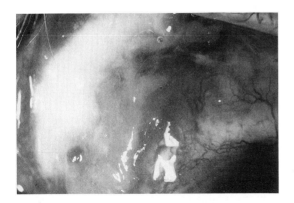

FIGURE 7.2. Extensive necrotizing scleritis in a patient following trauma from a cow's tail.

tizing scleritis in his right eye a few days after being struck by a cow's tail (Figs. 7.2 –7.4). Initial cultures were negative but specimens from scleral biopsy stained with Giemsa and Gomori methenamine silver (Fig. 5.33; see color insert) revealed the presence of fungal forms with septate hyphae forming acute angles, a morphology consistent with *Aspergillus*. *Aspergillus fumigatus* was later recovered in culture. Prolonged systemic and topical therapy cured the infection without further recurrence (Fig. 7.5; see color insert; Figs. 7.6–7.8).

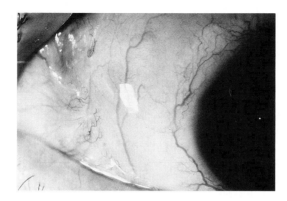

FIGURE 7.6. Same patient as in Figs. 7.2 through 7.5, 3 months into aggressive topical and systemic antifungal therapy.

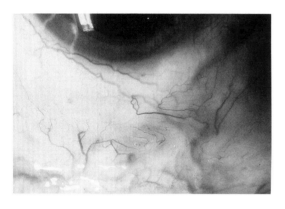

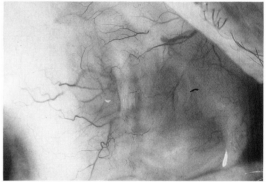

FIGURE 7.7. Same eye as in Figs. 7.2 through 7.6, showing the inferior scleral area, now without evidence of active scleritis.

FIGURE 7.8. Same eye as in Figs. 7.2 through 7.7, showing the nasal area, again demonstrating total quiescence of the scleritic process.

7.3. Viral Scleritis

Viral scleritis and episcleritis are rare entities occurring either as a direct viral invasion during the course of a viral infection, or as a result of an autoimmune response to the virus, months after the initial viral encounter. The most frequent viruses that may cause scleritis are varicella-zoster virus (VZV), herpes simplex virus type 1 (HSV-1), and mumps.

7.3.1. Herpes Zoster Scleritis

Herpes zoster is the most common systemic infection that may involve the sclera. Herpes zoster scleritis is often progressively destructive, sometimes leading to the loss of the eye from deteriorating vision, severe pain, or even (occasionally) perforation of the globe. Scleritis during the acute episode of herpes zoster ophthalmicus is easily associated with VZV infection. However, because scleritis often occurs months after the onset of the VZV infection, herpes zoster scleritis is sometimes difficult to diagnose. A careful past history review and meticulous facial and ocular examination are essential for early diagnosis of herpes zoster scleritis. Subsequent aggressive and prolonged treatment may halt the progression of the scleral destruction.

7.3.1.1. Epidemiology

Herpes zoster may occur in any age group, but is most common in individuals over age 60. That the aging process enhances the risk of developing herpes zoster infection can be judged from the fact that herpes zoster has an incidence of 3 cases per 1000 population per year for ages 20 to 49 years, and of 10 cases per 1000 population per year for ages 80 to 89 years.[157,158] Immunosuppressed patients, such as patients with acquired immune deficiency syndrome, organ transplantation, neoplasia, or blood dyscrasia, are also at great risk for developing herpes zoster infection.[159]

7.3.1.2. Pathogenesis

Varicella (chickenpox) and herpes zoster are different clinical conditions caused by the same virus. Primary infection with VZV results in chickenpox. In the United States, over 90% of adults have serological evidence of previous infection by VZV and most of them have VZV in a latent state.[160] About 20% of these adults may have a reactivation of VZV occurring as herpes zoster.[161]

Ocular herpes zoster is thought to represent a reactivation of latent VZV left in the trigeminal ganglion following a previous attack of chickenpox[162]; this involves a partial immune response after first exposure to the virus: the immune system is not capable of effectively eliminating the virus but is capable of producing immunopathology. There is no convincing evidence that herpes zoster can occur after contact with exogenous VZV from a patient suffering active chickenpox or zoster. Herpes zoster most commonly involves the thoracic nerves; however, the trigeminal nerve is involved in 9 to 16% of patients.[163–166] Of the three divisions

of the trigeminal nerve (ophthalmic, maxillary, and mandibular), the first or ophthalmic is the most frequently affected.

The ophthalmic division of the trigeminal nerve has three branches: the frontal, the lacrimal, and the nasociliary. The frontal branch, supplying the upper lid, forehead, and superior conjunctiva, is the most commonly involved. The lacrimal branch supplies the lacrimal gland, the conjunctiva, and the skin of the temporal angle of the eye. The nasociliary branch is the sensory nerve that supplies the eyeball. This branch divides into the infratrochlear and the nasal nerves. The infratrochlear nerve goes to the lacrimal sac, conjunctiva, skin of both lids, and root of the nose. The nasal nerve goes to the most critical structures: the sclera, cornea, uveal tract, and the tip of the nose. Because VZV most commonly affects all three branches of the ophthalmic division, ocular involvement in herpes zoster may lead to devastating ocular pathology.

Skin papules, pustules, or vesicles, conjunctival or episcleral vesicles, and corneal dendritic ulcers are caused by direct invasion of the virus. Scleritis, sometimes episcleritis, keratitis, trabeculitis, and anterior uveitis are most commonly caused by immune-mediated reactions triggered by the virus[167]; recurrences are independent of the presence of the virus.

7.3.1.3. Clinical Features

Herpes zoster is a disease characterized by an intensely painful, vesicular eruption involving the skin or mucous membrane in the distribution of a single sensory nerve. Although the incubation period after reactivation of endogenous virus is not known, the incubation period after contact with exogenous virus ranges from a few days to 2 weeks.[168] Headache, malaise, fever, and chills may precede the skin eruption by 4 or 5 days; neuralgia may precede the skin eruption by 2 or 3 days. The skin eruptions begin as papules, which rapidly become vesicles and pustules; vesicles subside within 2 weeks, often leaving permanent scars, variable degrees of hypoesthesia, or severe post-zoster neuralgia.[169] Eye lesions occur in about 50% of these cases.[170] Rarely, the ocular manifestations may appear without the skin eruption; a careful search for subtle papules, pustules, or vesicles in scalp or serial VZV blood titers may contribute greatly to the diagnosis.

Ocular involvement in VZV infection often includes conjunctivitis, episcleritis, scleritis, keratitis, uveitis, and glaucoma; scarred lid retraction, paralytic ptosis, retinitis, acute retinal necrosis, disk edema, pupil abnormalities, and extraocular nerve palsies also may occur.[170,171] Hypopyon, hemorrhage into the anterior chamber, and phthisis bulbi may result from herpes zoster vasculitis and ischemia (anterior segment necrosis).

Postherpetic neuralgia may be defined as pain in the involved dermatome persisting for more than 2 months following the onset of zoster dermatitis. It is more common in patients over 60 years of age (about 50% of these). It may be the result of herpes zoster vasculitis and neuritis.

7.3.1.3.1. Scleritis

The reported incidence of scleritis in herpes zoster ophthalmicus ranges from 0.68 to 8%.[37,80,172–174] Although scleritis may occur during the acute disease (about 10 to 15 days after the onset of skin lesions), it most commonly appears months or years after an episode of herpes zoster ophthalmicus,[175] sometimes triggered by ocular surgery. Zoster scleritis is of immune etiology and, although it may be diffuse or nodular, it often is necrotizing, with painful, persistent, circumscribed nodules with translucent centers, and risk of perforation or staphyloma formation.[176–179] It requires aggressive and prolonged therapy or even adjunctive procedures such as scleral homografting to maintain the integrity of the globe. Scleritis may take months to resolve and often leaves extensive scleral thinning. Recurrences, sometimes occurring not at the same site as the previous attack of scleritis, may be frequent, even after many years. Zoster scleritis may be accompanied by stromal keratitis, either immune disciform or white necrotic interstitial keratitis, which may progress to sclerosing keratitis or even to peripheral ulcerative kera-

titis. It also may be associated with anterior uveitis, which may cause a sectorial iris atrophy and/or trabeculitis, which in turn may cause glaucoma. Decreased corneal sensation in the affected area and sectorial iris atrophy are helpful indicators for the diagnosis of herpes zoster ophthalmicus.

In our series of 172 patients with scleritis, 2 patients had scleritis secondary to herpes zoster infection (1.16%). The first patient was an 85-year-old white female who developed necrotizing scleritis and sclerosing keratitis near the superior limbus in her right eye. Visual acuity at presentation was at the count fingers level in the right eye and corneal sensation was markedly decreased. Six months prior to the onset of scleritis she had had an episode of herpes zoster ophthalmicus with skin lesions and dendritic keratitis, which was treated with oral acyclovir and oral steroids. She had also had an uncomplicated extraocular cataract extraction with implantation of an intraocular lens 9 months prior to the onset of scleritis. An extensive laboratory investigation revealed only circulating immune complexes. A diagnosis of herpes zoster necrotizing scleritis with marked scleral destruction and uveal show associated with sclerosing keratitis was made (Fig. 7.9), treatment with oral prednisone was initiated, and scleral debridement and homografting were performed (Fig. 7.10). Pathological examination of the sclera showed chronic granulomatous inflammation with multinucleated giant cells and epithelioid cells, and inflammatory microangiopathy. Immunohistochemical studies with anti-VZV antibodies did not detect varicella-zoster antigen. The patient could not tolerate oral prednisone and oral acyclovir, and she developed progressive melting of the scleral graft and peripheral ulcerative keratitis (Fig. 7.11). Institution of oral methotrexate initially reduced scleral and corneal inflammation but, after 3 weeks, progressively destructive inflammatory activity again increased. Extensive scleral and corneal melting, and hemorrhage into the anterior chamber with a profound fibrin-type reaction, indicated anterior segment necrosis. Enucleation was performed by her local ophthalmologist and we did not obtain the pathology

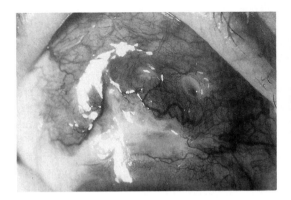

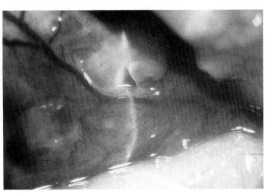

FIGURE 7.9. Necrotizing scleritis in a patient with herpes zoster ophthalmicus. Note the intense degree of inflammation and the associated scleral necrosis with uveal show. Also note the area of peripheral ulcerative keratitis at the far edge of the superior corneal periphery.

FIGURE 7.11. Same patient as in Figs. 7.9 and 7.10: Necrotizing scleritis and peripheral ulcerative keratitis have recurred following discontinuation of the oral prednisone and acyclovir, which had been used to achieve quiescence prior to grafting.

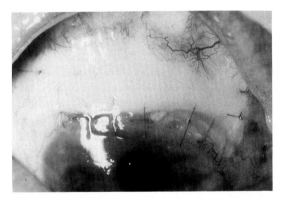

FIGURE 7.10. Same patient as in Fig. 7.9, following following quieting of the active inflammatory process through treatment with systemic prednisone and acyclovir and scleral grafting.

report. Varicella-zoster virus infection in this elderly patient triggered an immune-mediated necrotizing scleritis with peripheral ulcerative keratitis, presumably through deposition of circulating immune complexes in the area previously traumatized by ocular surgery. Cyclophosphamide might have been more effective than was methotrexate.

The second patient was a 75-year-old male who developed necrotizing scleritis with uveal prolapse and peripheral ulcerative keratitis at 12 o'clock in his left eye 6 years after a herpes zoster ophthalmicus infection and 9 months after an extracapsular cataract extraction. The patient had developed recurrent anterior uveitis, glaucoma, and cataract 3 months after the onset of acute VZV infection and had undergone extracapsular cataract extraction 5 years after the onset of anterior uveitis. Therapy for the destructive sclerocorneal process included oral cyclophosphamide, oral acyclovir, and scleral homografting. Pathological examination of the resected necrotic tissue revealed granulomas and inflammatory microangiopathy. Immunohistochemical studies did not detect VZV antigen. The scleral graft and peripheral cornea remained stable without further melting. Necrotizing scleritis and peripheral ulcerative keratitis developed as a result of an VZV-induced immune-mediated reaction in the area traumatized by ocular surgery.

7.3.1.3.2. Episcleritis

Simple or nodular episcleritis, often accompanied by vesicles in conjunctiva and episclera, or dendrites in cornea, may appear before or early in the course of the skin eruption. Episcleritis in this case is the result of direct viral invasion and usually resolves in 3 or 4 weeks without sequelae.[17] Immune-mediated episcleritis may develop between 10 and 15 days after the onset of skin lesions.

In our series of 94 patients with episcleritis, 1 patient had episcleritis associated with herpes zoster ophthalmicus infection (1.06%). The patient developed simple episcleritis and dendritic keratitis 2 days after the onset of skin vesicles. Skin and ocular lesions recovered without sequelae with oral acyclovir and there were no recurrences.

7.3.1.4. Diagnosis

Diagnosis of herpes zoster is basically clinical. However, because zosteriform herpes simplex virus infection, contact dermatitis, impetigo, and hypersensitivity reactions may resemble herpes zoster, laboratory tests sometimes may be crucial for diagnosis.[175,180,181]

Viral particles may be identified from skin or conjunctival vesicles or dendritic corneal ulcers for 3 days after their appearance (Tzanck technique); alkaline Giemsa, hematoxylin–eosin, Wright's, Papanicolaou's, Paragon, or methylene blue stains can show the presence of viral cytoplasmic or intranuclear inclusion bodies without distinguishing between VZV and herpes simplex virus. There also may be a ballooning degeneration of dendritic epithelial cells with multinucleated giant cells and infiltration of mononuclear cells.[182]

Herpes-like particles have been observed intraocularly by direct electron microscopy but they have never been found in sclera.[183,184] Again, electron microscopy cannot distinguish between VZV and herpes simplex virus.

Immunofluorescence (direct and indirect), immunoperoxidase, radioimmunoassay, countercurrent immunoelectrophoresis, agar gel immunodiffusion, and enzyme-linked immunosorbent assay testing may detect the VZV antigen in involved tissues[185–188]; these tests can detect VZV antigens when cultures are no longer positive.[185]

Culture from skin lesions on human embryonic lung diploid cells, human fetal diploid kidney cells, or human foreskin fibroblasts may show a cytopathic effect characteristic of VZV that becomes evident 3 to 5 days after inoculation[189]; viral shedding may be tested sub-sequently with immunofluorescence-specific probes. Varicella-zoster virus is labile and does not grow at room temperature or cooler. Culture from epithelial dendrites is difficult.

Initial VZV infection (chickenpox) produces cellular immune responses and IgG, IgM, and IgA anti-VZV antibodies[190]; high levels of IgG anti-VZV persist throughout childhood. Recurrent VZV infection (herpes zoster) produces a rapid increase in antibodies detectable by complement fixation, enzyme immunoassay, or fluorescent antibody to viral-associated membrane antigen. Herpes zoster diagnosis is confirmed by an increase or fall of fourfold or greater when comparing two samples: one taken during infection and another taken before or after infection. Herpes zoster diagnosis is suggested by a single high titer ($>1:640$) of IgG antibody against VZV.

Herpes zoster must be strongly considered in a patient with scleritis and a previous history of herpes zoster ophthalmicus, particularly if the patient has decreased corneal sensation and iris atrophy. Because scleritis in herpes zoster is a viral-induced immune-mediated manifestation, Giemsa staining, immunofluorescence techniques, electron microscopy studies, and cultures from involved scleral tissue will be negative for evidence of VZV.

7.3.1.5. Treatment

The treatment for active VZV infection must be vigorous to prevent severe complications. Acyclovir is a guanosine analog that inhibits viral replication by phosphorylating and activating the virus-encoded thymidine kinase and by inhibiting the viral deoxyribonucleic acid polymerase. Systemic acyclovir decreases pain, stops viral shedding, speeds acute resolution of skin lesions and ocular manifestations such as episcleritis, conjunctivitis, or epithelial keratitis, and reduces the incidence and severity of scleritis with or without stromal keratitis or anterior uveitis[191–193]; however, it may not be effective in reducing postherpetic neuralgia. The dose of acyclovir needed to inhibit VZV is 10 times higher than that needed to inhibit herpes simplex virus. Controlled clinical trials suggest oral acyclovir should be given within

72 h of the onset of skin lesions with a dosage of 800 mg five times a day (4000 mg/day) during 10 days in immunocompetent adults; intravenous acyclovir (15 mg/kg per day for 7 days or until 2 days beyond last new skin lesion) should be used in immunodeficient individuals, including patients with AIDS. Because side effects are mild and uncommon, acyclovir is considered a fairly safe drug.[194]

The role of systemic steroids in preventing postherpetic neuralgia is controversial[195–197]; however, they reduce the incidence and severity of ocular complications such as scleritis, keratitis, anterior uveitis, or glaucoma.[169,197] Systemic steroids may be reserved for immunocompetent adults over age 60 years, because they are at greatest risk for severe or permanent pain. The suggested dosage is 40 to 60 mg/day for 5 to 7 days, 30 to 40 mg/day for 5 to 7 days, and 20 mg for 5 to 7 days.

Capsaicin (a 0.025% topical skin cream applied three to six times daily in the involved dermatome after the skin has healed) relieves pain in 75% of patients (after 2 to 6 weeks of treatment) through depletion of substance P from the sensory peripheral neurons.[198,199] Tricyclic antidepressants, especially amitriptyline hydrochloride, may also relieve postherpetic neuralgia.[200–203]

Systemic nonsteroidal antiinflammatory drugs may be helpful in patients with immune-mediated ophthalmic complications such as scleritis (diffuse or nodular) with or without keratitis or anterior uveitis. If systemic nonsteroidal antiinflammatory agents are not effective in diffuse or nodular scleritis, systemic steroids may be used. Oral acyclovir should be added for prevention of acute VZV infection or if the diagnosis is not completely clear in terms of differentiating herpes zoster from herpes simplex. Topical steroid therapy has little effect on scleral inflammation. Immunosuppressive agents (alone or in combination with systemic steroids) are indicated if there is a necrotizing scleritis, if the scleritis is steroid unresponsive, or if the scleritis is steroid responsive but requires prolonged toxic doses of systemic steroids. Addition of oral acyclovir is recommended for prevention of recurrent VZV infection or if the diagnosis is not completely

clear in terms of differentiating herpes zoster from herpes simplex.

7.3.2. Herpes Simplex Scleritis

Herpes simplex virus (HSV) may occasionally cause episcleritis and scleritis. Episcleritis most often occurs as a result of direct viral invasion during the active HSV infection. Scleritis may occur during the active HSV infection as a result of direct viral invasion, or months after the initial viral encounter as a result of an immune-mediated reaction induced by the virus.

7.3.2.1. Epidemiology

Herpes simplex virus is ubiquitous and primary infection usually occurs between 6 months and 5 years of age. More than 70% of individuals have been infected with HSV by age 15 to 25 years and, therefore, have HSV antibodies; this percentage progressively increases with age to about 97% of individuals 60 years of age being infected.[204] Because only about 1 to 6% of patients with primary HSV infection experience some form of clinical disease,[205] most primary HSV infections are subclinical and, therefore, more than 95% of HSV-related clinical manifestations are the result of recurrences that develop long after a primary infection.[206]

7.3.2.2. Pathogenesis

Viral transmission in primary HSV seems to be by direct contact from infected individuals. The virus infects a peripheral end organ and travels to the ganglia, where it becomes latent. The virus may be reactivated by different stimuli such as fever, sunlight, trauma, or stress, presumably through cyclic nucleotide concentration changes[207]; it travels to the peripheral end organ via the neuronal network and produces recurrent HSV disease. Immunosuppressed individuals such as patients with leukemia, malignancies, or transplanted organs are at high risk for reactivation of latent HSV.[208,209]

Clinical disease and frequency of recurrences seem to depend on the type of virus strain (viral genome) of the primary HSV infection[210,211]: although most people are colonized by a "good" virus incapable of producing disease except under extreme conditions (leukemia, malignancies, etc.), some patients are colonized by a more virulent virus that causes clinical manifestations with varying frequencies of recurrence.[206] Viral genome and neuronal stimuli, therefore, are important factors in the development of viral reactivation and subsequent clinical recurrent disease.

7.3.2.3. Clinical Features

Primary ocular HSV usually occurs as an acute follicular conjunctivitis with preauricular adenopathy, with or without vesicular ulcerative blepharitis or periocular cutaneous involvement, and punctate or branching epithelial keratitis. The virus establishes a latent infection, which may recur under different types of neuronal stimuli.

Recurrent ocular HSV is mainly characterized by keratitis, including epithelial keratitis (dendritic ulcers, geographic ulcers, and metaherpetic ulcers), stromal keratitis (necrotizing, interstitial, or disciform keratitis, immune rings, and limbal vasculitis), and endotheliitis. Dendritic or geographic ulcers are caused by direct viral invasion; necrotizing stromal keratitis is caused by direct viral invasion and by immune complex hypersensitivity immune disease[206,212]; interstitial stromal keratitis, immune rings, limbal vasculitis, and peripheral ulcerative keratitis are caused by immune complex hypersensitivity immune disease; disciform keratitis is caused by delayed hypersensitivity immune disease; endotheliitis may be caused by active viral invasion or by immune disease; metaherpetic ulcers are caused by trophic factors.[206]

Uveitis and retinitis also may occur in recurrent HSV. Episcleritis and scleritis are uncommon.

7.3.2.3.1. Scleritis

Direct HSV invasion (often with epithelial infectious ulceration or necrotizing stromal disease) or the host immune reaction to the virus (often with necrotizing or interstitial stromal keratitis, immune rings, limbal vasculitis, disciform keratitis, or peripheral ulcerative keratitis) may cause scleritis. Active infectious

scleritis is usually of the diffuse or nodular type[37]; immune-mediated scleritis is most often of the necrotizing type.

In our series of 172 patients with scleritis, 2 patients had scleritis associated with HSV infection (1.16%). One patient was a 49-year-old white male with a maxilla osteosarcoma that required bone removal and multiple debridement and bone grafts because of secondary osteomyelitis (see Section 5.2.2.1.8.1). While receiving antibiotics via a continuous intravenous central line antibiotic pump, the patient developed blotchy white infiltrates in the corneal stroma and diffuse scleritis adjacent to the corneal infiltration. Immunofluorescence studies of the corneo–conjunctiva–scleral biopsy, using anti-HSV type 1 antibodies, revealed positive detection of HSV type 1 antigens in cornea, conjunctiva, and sclera. Treatment with acyclovir and steroids resolved the process.

The second patient was a 77-year-old white male with multiple recurrences of HSV dendritic keratitis who developed necrotizing scleritis and peripheral ulcerative keratitis in his right eye 1 month after the last active infectious episode. An extensive systemic review of systems was negative. Histopathological examination of the conjunctiva and scleral biopsies revealed granulomatous inflammation with epithelioid and multinucleated giant cells, and inflammatory microangiopathy in both tissues; immunofluorescence studies with anti-immunoglobulins and anti-complement antibodies revealed immune complex deposition in the vessel walls in both tissues; immunofluorescence studies with anti-HSV type 1 antibodies were negative in both tissues. Superficial keratectomy and conjunctival-scleral debridement followed by cornescleral grafting stopped the progression of the process. Keratoscleritis in this patient seemed to have been caused by an autoimmune mechanism induced by HSV type 1.

7.3.2.3.2. Episcleritis

Episcleritis may rarely occur in HSV infection.[17,213–215] It may be simple or nodular and is often accompanied by areas of lymphocytic infiltration manifested as yellow spots in conjunctiva and episclera, or by dendrites in cornea.[17] Episcleritis is usually the result of direct viral invasion and resolves in a few weeks without sequelae. Recurrences are not unusual.

In our series of 94 patients with episcleritis, 1 patient had episcleritis associated with HSV infection (1.06%). The patient was a 64-year-old white female who developed a follicular conjunctivitis; there were also vesicles in bulbar conjunctiva and episclera with surrounding redness and edema in the absence of keratitis. Treatment with trifluridine resolved the inflammation completely in 1 week. Visual acuity was not affected. Unfortunately, scrapings for cytology, antigen detection, or cultures were not taken.

7.3.2.4. Diagnosis

Although often clinically characteristic, diagnosis of either primary or recurrent active ocular HSV infection can be assisted with laboratory techniques. Giemsa or Papanicolaou staining may show eosinophilic intranuclear inclusions, ballooning degeneration, multinucleated giant cells, and monocytic infiltration (indistinguishable from VZV) from corneal dendrite or skin vesicle scrapings; conjunctival swabbing is not usually helpful, unless there is follicular conjunctivitis with or without episcleritis. Herpes simplex virus type 1 antigen may be detected by immunofluorescence assays performed on scrapings (corneal dendrite, upper palpebral conjunctiva, and skin vesicle) or tissue biopsies (skin, cornea, conjunctiva, episclera, and sclera). Herpes simplex virus causes a cytopathic effect in ordinary tissue cultures (HeLa cells, human amnion cells, or Vero cells). Herpes virus also may be detected by electron microscopy studies, but HSV and VZV are indistinguishable. Serology may differentiate primary HSV infection from recurrent HSV infection, because only primary infection shows an increase in HSV type 1 antibody titer: negligible titers are found during the acute phase and considerably higher titers are found 4 to 6 weeks later. Because most adults have developed an anti-HSV antibody titer indicating prior, usually asymptomatic or subclinical, primary infection, absence of antibody can help to exclude HSV as a cause of atypical keratitis.

Herpes simplex virus immune-mediated keratitis and/or scleritis diagnosis is suggested by clinical findings in a patient with a prior history of herpetic epithelial keratitis. There is no current laboratory method available to substantiate HSV as the responsible agent of the immune damage.

7.3.2.5. Therapy

Active HSV infection, including epithelial keratitis, scleritis, or episcleritis, may be treated with topical antiviral agents such as idoxuridine, vidarabine, trifluridine, or acyclovir.[206] Trifluridine (1% drops, one drop 9 times a day for 14 to 21 days) and acyclovir (3% ophthalmic ointment, one application five times a day), are the most effective agents in clinical trials,[216,217] although acyclovir ointment is available only on a compassionate plea basis in the United States. Idoxuridine and vidarabine remain effective agents and can be used in the absence of a history of drug failure or intolerance. Preliminary results from a current prospective multicenter trial concerning the effect of oral acyclovir on recurrent infectious dendritic or geographic herpes ulcerative keratitis show that long-term oral acyclovir (200 mg, five times a day) significantly reduces recurrences of HSV epithelial keratitis[218]; we may assume that long-term oral acyclovir may also decrease recurrences of episcleritis or scleritis due to active viral invasion. Results on the effect of long-term oral acyclovir on herpes stromal keratouveitis are not available yet. Long-term oral acyclovir has been shown to reduce recurrences of HSV keratitis following penetrating keratoplasty.[219]

Therapeutically, the same rules apply to treatment of immune-mediated scleritis secondary to HSV as to immune-mediated scleritis secondary to VZV (see Section 7.3.1.5). If systemic or topical steroids are used, concomitant prophylactic antiviral agents such as topical trifluridine drops (four times a day) or oral acyclovir (200 mg, five times a day) should be used.

7.3.3. Mumps Scleritis

Mumps may affect the eye, leading to catarrhal conjunctivitis, punctate epithelial keratitis, or severe stromal keratitis. Occasionally, scleritis, episcleritis, uveitis, optic neuritis, glaucoma, retinitis, and extraocular muscle palsies may occur.[220–224] Diagnosis is usually made by the presence of systemic manifestations of mumps, although isolation of virus and rising antibody titers confirm the disease. Mumps ocular manifestations usually resolve spontaneously without recurrences. No specific therapy is recommended.

7.4. Parasitic Scleritis

Parasites are generally seen by doctors as exotic organisms that infect individuals from underdeveloped countries. However, the increased interchange of people from different parts of the world through international travel, and the improved diagnostic skills of doctors, have contributed to an increased recognition of these microorganisms as the cause of parasitic infections of the ocular structures, including the sclera.

7.4.1. Protozoal Scleritis

7.4.1.1. Acanthamoeba

Acanthamoeba is a small amoeba that may be found in soil, contaminated water (distilled water, tap water, well water, hot tube water, brackish water, swimming pools, water baths, and sea water), contact lenses (hard and soft lenses), and solutions used to rinse contact lenses (tap water, saliva, well water, homemade nonsterile saline).[225] Scleritis due to *Acanthamoeba* is usually the result of scleral extension of primary corneal infections.[226,227] Scleritis may be caused by either a direct infection by the microorganism or by an immune-mediated reaction to killed microorganisms.[226] *Acanthamoeba* keratitis with or without scleritis is a potentially devastating infection that has been recognized increasingly in recent years.[228] Patients with keratoscleritis due to *Acanthamoeba* are usually young, healthy,

immunocompetent individuals, with at least one of the following risk factors: (1) history of minor corneal trauma, (2) direct exposure to soil or contaminated fluids, or (3) contact lens wear.[228–230] Scleritis is usually diffuse or nodular, although it may progress to necrotizing, and lead to scleral ectasia,[226] and is accompanied by a ring-shaped infiltrative stromal keratitis,[231] sometimes with persistent or recurrent pseudodendritic or punctate epithelial erosions; anterior uveitis rarely with hypopyon also may be present. Herpes simplex keratitis is the initial diagnosis in about 65% of the patients. Standard cultures are usually negative for bacteria, fungi, and viruses and the course is chronic and progressive in spite of treatment with antimicrobial agents. Many patients present with intense ocular pain, usually out of proportion to the stromal keratitis; the pain is probably due to predilection of the amoeba for neural tissue.[232]

The diagnosis of keratoscleritis due to *Acanthamoeba* is usually missed because the infection is uncommon; herpes simplex keratoscleritis is the most frequent misdiagnosis. However, even if the infection is considered initially, diagnosis of *Acanthamoeba* may still be difficult to confirm. Superficial scrapings of the cornea may not include the parasite if it is located only in corneal stroma. Corneal scrapings or corneal and scleral tissue from biopsy may be stained with calcofluor white stain[233,234]; Gram's, Giemsa, Masson trichrome, Gomori methenamine silver, and Wright's stains as well as fluorescent antibodies also may be used.[235] Culture from corneal scrapings or corneoscleral biopsy, or from contact lenses or contact lens solutions, can be done in confluent layers of coliform bacteria (*Escherichia coli, Enterobacter aerogenes*, or *Klebsiella pneumoniae*)[236]; the specimen may be transferred directly into the plate or may be placed in Page's saline solution for transportation, kept at room temperature, and placed in nonnutrient agar with coliform bacteria in the laboratory. Positive cultures have been seen sometimes in as little as 24 h.

Because *Acanthamoeba* keratoscleritis has a poor prognosis, a meticulous past history, slit-lamp examination, smears with calcofluor white stain, and cultures with nonnutrient agar with

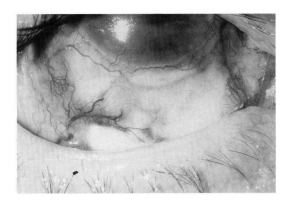

FIGURE 7.12. Necrotizing scleritis in a patient who also developed stromal keratitis, ultimately requiring corneal grafting for perforation. The keratoplasty grew *Acanthamoeba*.

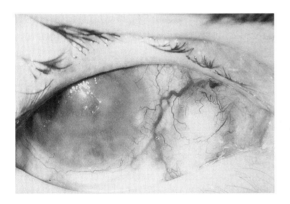

FIGURE 7.13. Additional views of the extent of the necrotizing scleritis in the patient shown in Fig. 7.12.

E. coli from scrapings or biopsy may be contributory to early diagnosis.

Acanthamoeba keratoscleritis therapy is controversial and sometimes unsatisfactory. The microorganism exists in both cyst and trophozoite states, thus requiring extremely prolonged therapy. The medical regimen for *Acanthamoeba* keratoscleritis includes 1% propamidine isethionate (Brolene), neomycin–polymyxin B–gramicidin (Neotricin), and topical 1% miconazole nitrate[225,237]; oral ketoconazole or itraconazole also may be added. Corticosteroid use is controversial. Penetrating keratoplasty with or without scleral

debridement may be needed to eradicate persistent active keratoscleritis despite medical therapy or in actual or threatened corneal perforation.

In our series of 172 patients with scleritis, one patient had scleritis due to *Acanthamoeba* (0.58%). The patient was a 51-year-old male with a presumed past history of herpes keratitis who developed a persistent corneal epithelial defect, a suppurative stromal keratitis, and a nodular scleritis in his right eye (Figs. 7.12 and 7.13). Nodular scleritis rapidly progressed to necrotizing scleritis. Review of systems was unrevealing. Corneal scrapings were taken for Gram's stain and standard cultures, which were negative. Conjunctival and episcleral biopsy showed nongranulomatous inflammation; Gram's stain was negative. Progressive corneal thinning necessitated penetrating keratoplasty (Fig. 7.14). Corneal button histopathological examination disclosed numerous basophilic cysts with darkly staining capsules, clear periphery, and darkly staining centers compatible with *Acanthamoeba* cysts (Fig. 7.15) as well as stromal necrosis. Culture on nonnutrient agar with *E. coli* identified *Acanthamoeba polyphaga*. Therapy with intensive topical 1% propamidine isethionate (Brolene), neomycin, miconazole, and oral ketoconazole was instituted. The postoperative course was complicated by glaucoma. Two weeks after surgery the patient developed progressive graft tissue necrosis with wound leak and further scleral thinning (Fig. 7.16). Penetrating keratoplasty was repeated and therapy for *Acanthamoeba* keratoscleritis was continued; 2 months later the eye became phthisical.

7.4.1.2. Toxoplasmosis

Although the most frequent ocular manifestation in toxoplasmosis is retinochoroiditis, scleritis and episcleritis occasionally may occur.[238–240] Scleritis in toxoplasmosis, usually associated with retinochoroiditis, is probably the result of scleral extension of severe toxoplasmic retinitis and choroiditis.[241] Either nongranulomatous or granulomatous inflammation of the sclera has been found.[241] Toxoplasmosis is a disease caused by the protozoan *Toxo-*

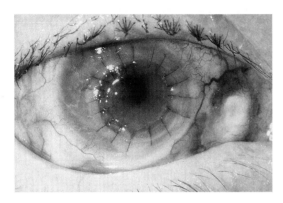

FIGURE 7.14. Same patient as in Figs. 7.12 and 7.13: Status postpenetrating keratoplasty.

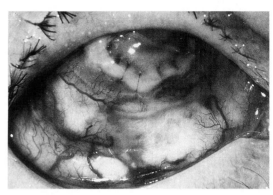

FIGURE 7.16. Same patient as in Figs. 7.12 through 7.15: Progressive necrotizing scleritis in spite of aggressive topical and systemic therapy for *Acanthamoeba*. The eye was eventually enucleated because of an unsightly phthisical eye.

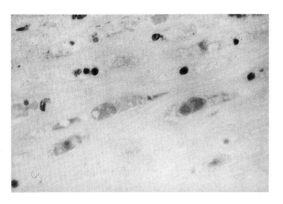

FIGURE 7.15. Same patient as in Figs. 7.12 through 7.14: Corneal button examination. Note the numerous basophilic cysts with darkly staining capsules, clear periphery, and darkly staining centers. (Magnification, ×63; hematoxylin–eosin stain.)

Although a definitive diagnosis of ocular toxoplasmosis can be made only by identifying the protozoa histologically, a supportive diagnosis is made on the basis of the clinical picture and serological tests. The serological tests most commonly used are the ELISA and the indirect fluorescent antibody test. The presence of high IgM anti-*Toxoplasma* titers indicates a recent infection.

Treatment of toxoplasmosis retinochoroiditis with or without scleritis includes oral corticosteroids and antitoxoplasmic agents such as sulfadiazine, pyrimethamine, and clindamycin; folinic acid should be added to avoid toxic depression of the bone marrow by pyrimethamine.

Any patient with scleritis and retinochoroiditis should be examined for toxoplasmosis.

7.4.2. Helminthic Scleritis

7.4.2.1. Toxocariasis

Toxocariasis is a common parasitic disease in the United States; humans are infected after ingestion of the helminth *Toxocara canis*. The natural host for this parasite is the dog; droppings from which can contaminate sand and earth, which is later inadvertently ingested, primarily by children at play. Ocular manifestations, usually affecting individuals 6 to 40 years of age, include posterior pole and retinal

plasma gondii; ocular damage may occur either from direct invasion of the protozoan or from immunological reactions against protozoan products. Toxoplasmosis is almost always congenital but may be acquired through inhalation of oocytes in cat feces or ingestion of contaminated pork or lamb meat. In both forms, an acute focal chorioretinitis lesion develops between ages 10 and 40 years. The lesions are usually single, posterior to the equator, and are often about one disk diameter in size; they commonly occur next to an area of scar.

periphery granulomas and chronic endophthalmitis.[242] Although a definitive diagnosis of ocular toxocariasis can be made only by identifying the larva histologically, supportive diagnosis is made on the basis of the clinical picture and ELISA blood tests. Treatment includes corticosteroids, either systemic or transeptal; thiabendazole also may be added.

Scleritis has not previously been described as a presenting manifestation of ocular toxocariasis.[18,242] In our series of 172 patients with scleritis, 1 patient had toxocariasis (0.58%). The patient was a 70-year-old white female who developed recurrent nodular scleritis, anterior uveitis, dense cataract, and 360° posterior synechiae in her left eye. Visual acuity in the left eye was at the level of hand motions only. Because adequate examination of the posterior segment of the eye could not be done, ultrasonography was performed; this showed a temporal mass and vitreous membranes in the left eye. Review of systems disclosed a history of cervical cancer. Given the patient's age, history of cervical cancer, and the presence of an intraocular mass, a metastatic lesion versus a primary ocular melanoma was considered. Extracapsular cataract extraction, sphincterotomy, and pars plana vitrectomy were performed to improve visualization of the posterior segment. A granuloma temporal to the disk, subretinal exudates, and a tractional detachment of the retina were found. Biopsy of the scleral nodule and fine needle biopsy of the intraocular mass were performed; nongranulomatous inflammation of the scleral specimen and granulomatous inflammation of the intraocular mass specimen were found with absence of tumor cells from either lesion. An ELISA test for *Toxocara* was positive (titer, 1:64) and ocular toxocariasis was diagnosed. The patient was subsequently treated with topical and systemic corticosteroids; ocular inflammation, including scleritis was controlled, but the visual acuity did not improve.

Results of serology, and clinical and histological granuloma in the posterior segment of the eye, supported the diagnosis of toxocariasis in spite of the organism not being isolated, and the patient was beyond the age group normally associated with ocular toxocariasis.

Any patient who develops scleritis and posterior pole or peripheral retinal granuloma should be examined for toxocariasis.

Summary

Although immune-mediated diseases are the main disorders associated with scleritis, other, less common etiologies such as infections must also be considered. Infectious agents such as bacteria, fungi, viruses, and parasites may cause scleritis through a direct invasion or through an immune response. Infectious scleritis should be suspected in cases of indolent progressive scleral necrosis with suppuration, especially if the past and present history reveals an accidental trauma, chronic topical medication use (including corticosteroids), surgical procedures, or debilitating ocular or systemic disease; they also should be suspected if the review of systems reveals multisystem findings compatible with a systemic infection.

In exogenous and endogenous infections, scrapings for smears and cultures must be obtained and fortified antimicrobial therapy, depending on smear results, must be initiated as soon as possible. If scleral infection is the primary clinical suspicion, but smears and cultures (at 48 h) are negative, and the patient is not improving on the initial broad-spectrum antimicrobial therapy chosen, scleral or corneoscleral biopsy is recommended. Biopsied tissue may be homogenized and cultured in the usual media, evaluated histopathologically with special stains, or analyzed by immunofluorescence techniques.

In endogenous infections, serological tests and radiographic studies also may be helpful in suggesting the diagnosis of a specific scleral infection.

Because infectious etiologies are usually treatable with antimicrobial therapy, early diagnosis improves the ocular and systemic prognoses.

References

1. Reynolds MG, Alfonso E: Infectious scleritis and keratoscleritis: management and outcome. Am J Ophthalmol 112:543, 1991.

2. Alfonso E, Kenyon KR, Ormerod LD, Stevens R, Wagoner MD, Albert DM: *Pseudomonas* corneoscleritis. Am J Ophthalmol 103:90, 1987.
3. Codère F, Brownstein S, Jackson WB: *Pseudomonas aeruginosa* scleritis. Am J Ophthalmol 91:706, 1981.
4. Raber IM, Laibson PR, Kurz GH, Bernardino VB: *Pseudomonas* corneoscleral ulcers. Am J Ophthalmol 92:353, 1981.
5. Eiferman RA: Cryotherapy of *Pseudomonas* keratitis and scleritis. Arch Ophthalmol 97:1637, 1979.
6. Nanda M, Pflugfelder SC, Holland S: Fulminant pseudomonal keratitis and scleritis in human immunodeficiency virus-infected patients. Arch Ophthalmol 109:503, 1991.
7. Farrell PLR, Smith RE: Bacterial corneoscleritis complicating pterygium excision. Am J Ophthalmol 107:515, 1989.
8. Cameron ME: Preventable complications of pterygium excision with beta-irradiation. Br J Ophthalmol 56:52, 1972.
9. Tarr KH, Constable IJ: Late complications of pterygium treatment. Br J Ophthalmol 64:496, 1980.
10. Tarr KH, Constable IJ: *Pseudomonas* endophthalmitis associated with scleral necrosis. Br J Ophthalmol 64:676, 1980.
11. Tarr KH, Constable IJ: Radiation damage after pterygium treatment. Aust J Ophthalmol 9:97, 1981.
12. Berler DK, Alper MG: Scleral abscesses and ectasia cased by *Pseudomonas aeruginosa*. Ann Ophthalmol 14:665, 1982.
13. Altman AJ, Cohen EJ, Berger ST, Mondino BJ: Scleritis and *Streptococcus pneumoniae*. Cornea 10(4):341, 1991.
14. Sainz de la Maza M, Foster CS: Necrotizing scleritis after ocular surgery. Ophthalmology 98:1720, 1991.
15. Duke-Elder S: *System of Ophthalmology*, Vol 3. Kimpton, London, 1964, p 825.
16. Zinn KM, Ferry AP: Massive scleral necrosis from a *Pseudomonas* infection following scleral buckling and pars plana vitrectomy surgery. Mt Sinai J Med 47:618, 1980.
17. Watson P: Diseases of the sclera and episclera. In Duane TD, Jaeger EA (Eds): *Clinical Ophthalmology*, Vol 4. Harper & Row, Philadelphia, 1985, Chap 23.
18. Jackson WB: Infections of the sclera. In Tabbara KF, Hyndiuk RA (Eds): *Infections of the Eye*. Little, Brown, Boston, 1986, Chap 28.
19. Friedman AH, Henkind P: Unusual cases of episcleritis. Trans Am Acad Ophthalmol Otolaryngol 78:890, 1974.
20. Harbin T: Recurrence of a corneal pseudomonal infection. Am J Ophthalmol 58:670, 1964.
21. Alpren TVP, Hyndiuk RA, Davis SD, Starff LD: Cryotherapy for experimental *Pseudomonas* keratitis. Arch Ophthalmol 97:711, 1979.
22. Turner L, Stinson I: *Mycobacterium fortuitum* as a cause of corneal ulcer. Am J Ophthalmol 60:329, 1965.
23. Zimmerman LE, Turner L, McTigue JW: *Mycobacterium fortuitum* infection of the cornea. Arch Ophthalmol 82:596, 1969.
24. Gangadharam PRJ, Lanier JD, Jones DE: Keratitis due to *Mycobacterium chelonei*. Tubercle 59:55, 1978.
25. Newman PE, Goodman RA, Waring GO III, Finton RJ, Wilson LA, Wrigh TJ, Cavanagh HD: A cluster of cases of *Mycobacterium chelonei* keratitis associated with outpatient office procedures. Am J Ophthalmol 97:344, 1984.
26. Moore MB, Newton C, Kaufman HE: Chronic keratitis caused by *Mycobacterium gordonae*. Am J Ophthalmol 102:516, 1986.
27. Laflamme MY, Poisson M, Chéhadé N: *Mycobacterium chelonei* keratitis following penetrating keratoplasty. Can J Ophthalmol 22:178, 1987.
28. Pope J, Sternberg P, McLane NJ, Potts DW, Stulting RD: *Mycobacterium chelonei* scleral abcess after removal of a scleral buckle. Am J Ophthalmol 107:557, 1989.
29. Schönherr U, Naumann GOH, Lang GK, Bialasiewicz AA: Sclerokeratitis by *Mycobacterium marinum*. Am J Ophthalmol 108:607, 1989.
30. Carson LA, Peterson NJ, Favero MS, Aguero SM. Growth characteristics of atypical mycobacteria in water and their comparative resistance to disinfectants. Appl Environ Microbiol 36:839, 1978.
31. Jolly HW, Seabury JH: Infections with *Mycobacterium marinum*. Arch Dermatol 106:32, 1972.
32. Zeligman I: *Mycobacterium marinum* granuloma. Arch Dermatol 106:26, 1972.
33. Spencer WH: *Ophthalmic Pathology. An Atlas and Textbook*, 3rd ed. W.B. Saunders, Philadelphia, 1985, pp 275–277.
34. Kubica GP: Differential identification of mycobacteria. VII. Key features for identification of clinically significant mycobacteria. Am Rev ιesp Dis 107:9, 1973.
35. Wolinsky E: Nontuberculous mycobacterial infections of man. Med Clin N Am 58:639, 1974.

36. Donahue HC: Ophthalmologic experience in a tuberculosis sanatorium. Am J Ophthalmol 64:742, 1967.

37. Watson PG, Hayreh SS: Scleritis and episcleritis. Br J Ophthalmol 60:163, 1976.

38. Nanda M, Pflugfelder SC, Holland S: *Mycobacterium tuberculosis* scleritis. Am J Ophthalmol 108:736, 1989.

39. Glassroth J, Robins AG, Snider DE Jr: Tuberculosis in the 1980's. N Engl J Med 302:1441, 1980.

40. Shumomura Y, Tader R, Yuam T: Ocular disorders in pulmonary tuberculosis. Folia Ophthalmol Jpn 30:1973, 1979.

41. Phillips S, Williams ML, Maiden SD: Chronic miliary tuberculosis. Am Rev Tuberculosis 62:549, 1950.

42. Bloomfield SE, Mondino B, Gray GF: Scleral tuberculosis. Arch Ophthalmol 94:954, 1976.

43. Bell GH: Report of a case of tuberculosis of the sclera of probable primary origin. Trans Am Ophthalmol Soc 13:787, 1914.

44. Swan KC: Some contemporary concepts of scleral disease. Arch Ophthalmol 45:630, 1951.

45. Finnoff WC: Tuberculosis in etiology of acute iritis. Am J Ophthalmol 14:127, 1931.

46. Brini A, Quéré M, Achard M: Sclérite nodulaire nécrosante (presence de bacille de Koch). Bull Soc Ophthalmol Fr 7:822, 1953.

47. Andreani DG: Tuberculoma of the sclera. Giornale Italiano di Oftalmologia 7:506, 1954.

48. Woods AC: Ocular tuberculosis. In Sorsby A (Ed): *Modern Ophthalmology*. Lippincott, Philadelphia, 1972, p 105.

49. Sarda RP, Mehrotra AS, Asnani K: Nodular episcleritis (a proved case of tubercular origin). Indian J Ocular Pathol 3:24, 1969.

50. Thygeson PL: The etiology and treatment of phlyctenular keratoconjunctivitis. Am J Ophthalmol 9:446, 1975.

51. Smith RE, Dippe DW, Miller SD: Phlyctenular keratoconjunctivitis. Results of penetrating keratoplasty in Alaskan natives. Ophthalmic Surg 6:62, 1975.

52. Shepard CC: The experimental disease that follows the injection of human leprosy bacilli into footpads of mice. J Exp Med 112:445, 1960.

53. Bechelli LM, Dominguez UM: The leprosy problem in the world. Bull WHO 34:811, 1966.

54. Shepard CC: Leprosy. In Harrison TR (Ed): *Principles of Internal Medicine*, McGraw-Hill, New York, 1980, pp 711–714.

55. Memoria del VI Congreso Internacional de Leprología, Madrid, October 1953.

56. Van Voorhis WC, Kaplan G, Sarno EN, Horwitz MA, Steinman RM, Levis WR, Nogueira N, Hair LS, Gattass, Arrick BA, Cohn ZA: The cutaneous infiltrates of leprosy: cellular characteristics and the predominant T-cell phenotypes. N Engl J Med 307:1593, 1982.

57. De Barros JM: Aspectos clinicos do comprolimento ocular da lepra. Companhia Melhoramentos, Sao Paulo, 1939.

58. Brand ME: Early ocular changes in leprosy. IXth International Leprosy Conference, London, 1968.

59. Schwab IR: Ocular leprosy. In Tabbara JF, Hyndiuk RA (Eds): *Infections of the Eye*. Little, Brown, Boston, 1986, pp 613–624.

60. King EF: Eye in leprosy. Br J Ophthalmol 20:561, 1936.

61. Allen JH, Byers JL: The pathology of ocular leprosy. Arch Ophthalmol 64:216, 1960.

62. Ffytche TJ: Role of iris changes as a cause of blindness in lepromatous leprosy. Br J Ophthalmol 65:231, 1981.

63. Holmes, KK, Lukehart SA: Syphilis. In Braunwald E, Isselbacher KJ, Petersdorf RG, Wilson JD, Martin JB, Fanci AS (Eds): *Harrison's Principles of Internal Medicine*, 11th ed, Vol 1. McGraw-Hill, New York, 1987, pp 639–649.

64. Centers for Disease Control: Summary-cases of specified notifiable diseases, United States. MMWR 37:802, 1989.

65. Tamesis RR, Foster CS: Ocular syphilis. Ophthalmology 97:1281, 1990.

66. Johns DR, Tierney M, Felsenstein D: Alteration in the natural history of neurosyphilis by concurrent infection with the human immunodeficiency virus. N Engl J Med 316:1569, 1987.

67. Berry CD, Hooton TM, Collier AC, Lukehart SA: Neurologic relapse after benzathine penicillin therapy for secondary syphilis in a patient with HIV infection. N Engl J Med 316:1587, 1987.

68. Richards BW, Hessburg TJ, Nussbaum JN: Recurrent syphilitic uveitis. N Engl J Med 320:62, 1989.

69. Levy JH, Liss RA, Maguire AM: Neurosyphilis and ocular syphilis in patients with concurrent human immunodeficient virus infection. Retina 9:175, 1989.

70. Zaidman GW: Neurosyphilis and retrobulbar neuritis in a patient with AIDS. Ann Ophthalmol 18:260, 1986.

71. Carter JB, Hamill RJ, Matoba AY: Bilateral syphilitic optic neuritis in a patient with a positive test for HIV. Arch Ophthalmol 105:1485, 1987.

72. Kleiner RC, Najarian L, Levenson J, Kaplan HJ: AIDS complicated by syphilis can mimick uveitis and Crohn's disease [Letter]. Arch Ophthalmol 105:1486, 1987.

73. Zambrano W, Perez GM, Smith JL: Acute syphilitic blindness in AIDS. J Clin Neurol Ophthalmol 7:1, 1987.

74. Stoumbos VD, Klein ML: Syphilitic retinitis in a patient with acquired immunodeficiency syndrome-related complex [Letter]. Am J Ophthalmol 103:103, 1987.

75. Radolf JD, Kaplan RP: Unusual manifestations of secondary syphilis and abnormal humoral immune response to *Treponema pallidum* antigens in a homosexual man with asymptomatic human immunodeficiency virus infection. J Am Acad Dermatol 18:423, 1988.

76. Passo MS, Rosembaum JT: Ocular syphilis in patients with human immunodeficiency virus infection. Am J Ophthalmol 106:1, 1988.

77. Wilhelmus KR: Syphilis. In Insler MS (Ed): *AIDS and Other Sexually Transmitted Diseases and the Eye*. Grune & Stratton, Orlando, FL, 1987, pp 73–104.

78. Wilhelmus KR, Yokoyama CM: Syphilitic episcleritis and scleritis. Am J Ophthalmol 104: 595, 1987.

79. Evans JJ: Diffuse gummatous infiltration of scleral and episcleral tissues. Trans Ophthalmol Soc UK 25:188, 1905.

80. Watson PG, Hazleman BL: *The Sclera and Systemic Disorders*. W.B. Saunders, Philadelphia, 1976, pp 206–346.

81. Deodati F, Bec P, Labro JB, Barrioulet Y: Sclérite syphilitique. Aspect clinique et angiographique. Bull Soc Ophtalmol Fr 71:63, 1971.

82. Spicer WTH: Parenchymatous keratitis; interstitial keratitis; uveitis anterior. Br J Ophthalmol (Monogr Suppl I) 1, 1924.

83. Yobs AR, Brown, L, Hunter EF: Fluorescent antibody technique in early syphilis. Arch Pathol 77:220, 1964.

84. Tourville DR, Byrd LH, Kim DU, Zajd D, Lee I, Reichman LB, Baskin S: Treponemal antigen in immunopathogenesis of syphilitic glomerulonephritis. Am J Pathol 82:479, 1976.

85. Bansal RC, Cohn H, Fani K, Lynfield YL: Nephrotic syndrome and granulomatous hepatitis. Arch Dermatol 114:1228, 1978.

86. Beckett JH, Bigbee JW: Immunoperoxidase localization of *Treponema pallidum*. Arch Pathol 103:135, 1979.

87. Trantas M: Bourrelet périkératique syphilitique. Arch Ophtalmol (Paris) 31:320, 1911.

88. Bhaduri BN, Basu SK: Scleral gumma. Br J Ophthalmol 40:504, 1956.

89. Spoor TC, Wynn P, Hartel WC, Bryan CS: Ocular syphilis: acute and chronic. J Clin Neurol Ophthalmol 3:197, 1983.

90. Harner RE, Smith JL, Israel CW: The FTA-ABS in late syphilis. A serological study in 1985 cases. JAMA 203:545, 1968.

91. Hart G: Syphilis tests in diagnostic and therapeutic decision making. Ann Intern Med 104:368, 1986.

92. Collart P, Poitevin M: Is penicillin therapy always infallible in syphilis? J Clin Neurol Ophthalmol 2:77, 1982.

93. Steere AC, Malawista SE, Snydman DR, Shope RE, Andiman WA, Ross MR, Steele FM: Lyme arthritis: an epidemic of oligoarticular arthritis in children and adults in three Connecticut communities. Arthritis Rheum 20:7, 1977.

94. Steere AC, Taylor E, Wilson ML, Levine JF, Spielman A: Longitudinal assessment of the clinical and epidemiological features of Lyme disease in a defined population. J Infect Dis 154:295, 1986.

95. Hanrahan JP, Benach JL, Coleman JL, Bosler EM, Morse DL, Cameron DJ, Edelman R, Kaslow RA: Incidence and cumulative frequency of endemic Lyme disease in a community. J Infect Dis 150:489, 1984.

96. MacDonald AB: Lyme disease: a neuro-ophthalmologic view. J Clin Neurol Ophthalmol 7:185, 1987.

97. Steere AC, Malawista SE: Cases of Lyme disease in the United States. locations correlated with the distribution of *Ixodes dammini*. Ann Intern Med 91:730, 1979.

98. Burgdorfer W, Keirans JE: Ticks and Lyme disease in the United States. Ann Intern Med 99:121, 1983.

99. Steere AC, Broderick TE, Malawista SE: Erythema chronicum migrans and Lyme arthritis: epidemiologic evidence for a tick vector. Am J Epidemiol 108:312, 1978.

100. Burgdorfer W, Barbour AG, Hayes SF, Benach JL, Grunwaldt E, Davis JP: Lyme disease—a tick-borne spirochetosis? Science 216:1317, 1982.

101. Steere AC, Grodzicki RL, Kornblatt AN, Craft JE, Barbour AG, Burgdofer W, Schmid GP, Johnson E, Malawista SE: The spirochetal etiology of Lyme disease. N Engl J Med 308: 740, 1983.

102. Benach JL, Bosler EM, Hanrahan JP, Coleman JL, Habicht GS, Bast TF, Cameron DJ,

Ziegler JL, Barbour AG, Burgdorfer W, Edelman R, Kaslow RA: Spirochetes isolated from the blood of two patients with Lyme disease. N Engl J Med 308:740, 1983.

103. Steere AC, Malawista SE, Hardin JA, Ruddy S, Askenase PW, Andiman WA: Erythema chronicum migrans and Lyme arthritis: the enlarging clinical spectrum. Ann Intern Med 86:685, 1977.

104. Steere AC, Bartenhagen NH, Craft JE, Hutchinson GJ, Newman JH, Rahn DW, Sigal LH, Spieler PN, Stenn KS, Malawista SE: The early clinical manifestations of Lyme disease. Ann Intern Med 99:76, 1983.

105. Reik L, Steere AC, Bartenhagen NH, Shope RE, Malawista SE: Neurologic abnormalities of Lyme disease. Medicine 58:281, 1979.

106. Steere AC, Batsford WP, Weinberg M, Alexander J, Berger HJ, Wolfson S, Malawista SE: Lyme carditis: cardiac abnormalities of Lyme disease. Ann Intern Med 93:8, 1980.

107. Halperin JJ, Pass HL, Anand AK, Luft BJ, Valkman DJ, Dattwyler RJ: Nervous system abnormalities in Lyme disease. Ann NY Acad Sci 539:24, 1988.

108. Schmutzhard E, Pohl P, Stockhammer G, et al.: Unusual neurological manifestations of second-stage Lyme borreliosis. Ann NY Acad Sci 539:495, 1988.

109. Schmutzhard E, Pohl P, Stanek G: Involvement of Borrelia burgdorferi in cranial nerve affection. Zentralbl Bakteriol Mikrobiol Hyg 263:328, 1986.

110. Wallis RC, Brown SE, Kloter KO, Main AJ Jr: Erythema chronicum migrans and Lyme arthritis: field study of ticks. Am J Epidemiol 108:322, 1978.

111. Steere AC, Gibofsky A, Patarroyo ME, Winchester RJ, Hardin JA, Malawista SE: Chronic Lyme arthritis: clinical and immunogenetic differentiation from rheumatoid arthritis. Ann Intern Med 90:896, 1979.

112. Steere AC, Brinckerhoff CE, Miller DJ, Drinker H, Harris ED Jr, Malawista SE: Elevated levels of collagenase and prostaglandin E_2 from synovium associated with erosion of cartilage and bone in a patient with chronic Lyme arthritis. Arthritis Rheum 23:591, 1980.

113. Pachner AR, Steere AC: CNS manifestations of third stage Lyme disease. Zentralbl Bakteriol Mikrobiol Hyg 263:301, 1986.

114. Stiernstedt G, Gustafsson R, Karlsson M, Svenungsson B, Skoldenberg B: Clinical manifestations and diagnosis of neuroborreliosis. Ann NY Acad Sci 539:46, 1988.

115. Kristoferitsch W, Sluga E, Graf M, Partsch H, Neumann R, Stanek G, Budka H: Neuropathy associated with acrodermatitis chronica atrophicans. Ann NY Acad Sci 539:35, 1988.

116. Ackermann R, Rehse-Küpper B, Gollmer E, Schmidt R: Chronic neurologic manifestations of erythema migrans borreliosis. Ann NY Acad Sci 539:16, 1988.

117. Pachner AR, Duray P, Steere AC: Central nervous system manifestations of Lyme disease. Arch Neurol 46:790, 1989.

118. Mandell H, Steere AC, Reinhardt BN, Yoshinari N, Munsat TL, Brod SA, Clapshaw PA: Lack of antibodies to Borrelia burgdorferi in patients with amyotrophic lateral sclerosis [Letter]. N Engl J Med 320:255, 1989.

119. Lesser RL, Kornmehl EW, Pachner AR, Kattah J, Hedges TR, Newman NM, Ecker PA, Glassman MI: Neuroophthalmologic manifestations of Lyme disease. Ophthalmology 97:699, 1990.

120. Farris BK, Webb RM: Lyme disease and optic neuritis. J Clin Neurol Ophthalmol 8:73, 1988.

121. Finkel MF: Lyme disease and its neurologic complications. Arch Neurol 45:99, 1988.

122. Wu G, Lincoff H, Ellsworth RM, Haik BG: Optic disc edema and Lyme disease. Ann Ophthalmol 18:252, 1986.

123. Schechter SL: Lyme disease associated with optic neuropathy. Am J Med 81:143, 1986.

124. Bialasiewicz AA, Ruprecht KW, Naumann GOH, Blenk H: Bilateral diffuse choroiditis and exudative retinal detachments with evidence of Lyme disease. Am J Ophthalmol 105:419, 1988.

125. Damrow T, Freedman H, Lane R, Preston KL: Is Ixodes (Ixodiopsis) angustus a vector of Lyme disease in Washington State? West J Med 150:580, 1989.

126. Bruhn FW: Lyme disease. Am J Dis Child 138:467, 1984.

127. Baum J, Barza M, Weinstein P, Groden J, Aswad M: Bilateral keratitis as a manifestation of Lyme disease. Am J Ophthalmol 105:75, 1988.

128. Steere AC, Malawista SE, Bartenhagen NH, Spieler PN, Newman JH, Rahn AW, Hutchinson GJ, Green J, Snydman DR, Taylor E: The clinical spectrum and treatment of Lyme disease. Yale J Biol Med 57:453, 1984.

129. Bertuch AW, Rocco E, Schwartz EG: Lyme disease: ocular manifestations. Ann Ophthalmol 20:376, 1988.

130. Orlin SE, Lauffer JL: Lyme disease keratitis. Am J Ophthalmol 107:678, 1989.

131. Kornmehl EW, Lesser RL, Jaros P, Rocco E, Steere AC: Bilateral keratitis in Lyme disease. Ophthalmology 96:1194, 1989.

132. Flach AJ, Lavoie PE: Episcleritis, conjunctivitis, and keratitis as ocular manifestations of Lyme disease. Ophthalmology 97:973, 1990.

133. Zaidman GW: Episcleritis and symblepharon associated with Lyme disease. Am J Ophthalmol 109:487, 1990.

134. Pavan-Langston D: *Manual of Ocular Diagnosis and Therapy*, 2rd ed. Little, Brown, Boston, 1991.

135. Jones BR, Al-Hussaini KM, Dunlop EC: Infection by tric agent and other menbers of the Bedsonia group, with a note on Reiter's disease. Trans Ophthalmol Soc UK 86:291, 1966.

136. Gordon MA: Aerobic pathogenic Actinomycetaceae. In Lennette EH, Balows A, Hausler WJ, Shadomy HJ (Eds): *Manual of Clinical Microbiology*, 4th ed. American Society for Microbiology, Washington DC, 1985, pp 249–262.

137. Rifkind D, Marchioro TL, Schneck SA, Hill RB Jr: Systemic fungal infections complicating renal transplantation and immunosuppressive therapy. Am J Med 43:28, 1967.

138. Young LS, Armstrong D, Blevins A, Lieberman P: *Nocardia asteroides* infection complicating neoplastic disease. Am J Med 50:356, 1971.

139. Francois J, Pysselaere M: *Oculomycosis*. Charles C Thomas, Springfield, IL, 1972.

140. Burpee JC, Strarke WR: Bilateral metastatic intraocular nocardiosis. Arch Ophthalmol 86:666, 1971.

141. Jampol LM, Strauch BS, Albert DM: Intraocular nocardiosis. Am J Ophthalmol 76:568, 1973.

142. Panijayanond P, Olsson CA, Spivack ML, Schmitt GW, Idelson BA, Sachs BJ, Mabseth DC: Intraocular nocardiosis in a renal transplant patient. Arch Surg 104:845, 1972.

143. Kattan HM, Pflugfelder SC: *Nocardia* scleritis. Am J Ophthalmol 110:446, 1990.

144. Davidson S, Foerster HC: Intraocular nocardial abscess, endogenous. Trans Am Acad Ophthalmol Otolaryngol 71:847, 1967.

145. Meyer SL, Font RL, Shaver RP: Intraocular nocardiosis: report of three cases. Arch Ophthalmol 83:536, 1970.

146. Hoeprich PD, Brandt D, Parker RH: Nocardial brain abscess cured with cycloserine and sulfonamides. Am J Med Sci 255:208, 1968.

147. Stenson S, Brookner A, Rosenthal S: Bilateral endogenous necrotizing scleritis due to *Aspergillus oryzae*. Ann Ophthalmol 14:67, 1982.

148. Margo CE, Polack FM, Mood CI: *Aspergillus* panophthalmitis complicating treatment of pterygium. Cornea 7:285, 1988.

149. Lincoff HA, McLean JM, Nano H: Scleral abscess. I. A complication of retinal detachment buckling procedures. Arch Ophthalmol 74:641, 1965.

150. Milauskas AT, Duke JR: Mycotic scleral abscess: report of a case following a scleral buckling operation for retinal detachment. Am J Ophthalmol 63:951, 1967.

151. Slomovic AR, Forster RK, Gelender H: *Hasiodiplodia theobromae* panophthalmitis. Can J Ophthalmol 20:225, 1985.

152. Köllner H: Schimmelpilzerkrankung der Sklera. Z Augenheilk 16:441, 1906.

153. Sporotrichose gommeuse disseminée, gomme intra-oculaire, perforation de la sclérotique. Ann d'Oculistique, 148:321, 1912.

154. Kuriakose ET: Oculosporidiosis. Rhinosporidi osis of the eye. Br J Ophthalmol 47:346, 1963.

155. Lamba PA, Shucka KN, Ganapathy M: Rhinosporidium granuloma of the conjunctiva with scleral ectasia. Br J Ophthalmol 54:565, 1970.

156. De Doncker RML, de Keizer RJW, Oosterhuis JA: Scleral melting in a patient with conjunctival rhinosporidiosis. Br J Ophthalmol 74:635, 1990.

157. Hope-Simpson R: The nature of herpes zoster: a long-term study and a new hypothesis. Proc Soc Exp Biol Med 58:9, 1965.

158. Weller T: Varicella and herpes zoster: changing concepts of the natural history, control, and importance of not so benign virus (part 1). N Engl J Med 309:1362, 1983.

159. Dolin R, Reichman RC, Mazur MH, Whitley RJ: NIH conference. Herpes zoster-varicella infections in immunosuppressed patients. Ann Intern Med 89:375, 1978.

160. Gershon AA, Steinberg SP: Antibody responses to varicella-zoster virus and the role of antibody in host defense. Am J Med Sci 282:12, 1981.

161. Straus SE, Ostrove JM, Inchauspe G, Felser JM, Freifeld A, Croen KD, Sawyer MH: NIH conference. Varicella-zoster virus infections. Biology, natural history, treatment, and prevention. Ann Intern Med 108:221, 1988.

162. Weller T: Varicella and herpes zoster (part 2). N Engl J Med 309:1434, 1983.

163. Kurland L: Descriptive epidemiology of selected neurological and myopathic disorders with particular reference to a survey in Rochester, Minnesota. J Chronic Dis 8:378, 1958.

164. Ragozzino M: Population based study of herpes zoster and its sequelae. Medicine 61:310, 1982.

165. Mahalingam R, Wellish M, Wolf W, Dueland AN, Cohrs R, Vafai A, Gilden D: Latent varicella-zoster viral DNA in human trigeminal and thoracic ganglia. N Engl J Med 323:627, 1990.

166. Hyman RW, Ecker JR, Tenser RB: Varicella-zoster virus RNA in human trigeminal ganglia. Lancet 2:814, 1983.

167. Liesegang TJ: Corneal complications from herpes zoster ophthalmicus. Ophthalmology 92:316, 1985.

168. Harding SP, Lipton JR, Wells JCD: Natural history of herpes zoster ophthalmicus: predictors of postherpetic neuralgia and ocular involvement. Br J Ophthalmol 71:353, 1987.

169. Scheie HG: Herpes zoster ophthalmicus. Trans Ophthalmol Soc UK 90:899, 1970.

170. Pavan-Langston D: Varicella-zoster ophthalmicus. Int Ophthalmol Clin 15(4):171, 1975.

171. Liesegang T: The varicella zoster virus: systemic and ocular features. J Am Acad Dermatol 11:165, 1984.

172. Womack LW, Liesegang TJ: Complications of herpes zoster ophthalmicus. Arch Ophthalmol 101:42, 1983.

173. Tuft SJ, Watson PG: Progression of scleral disease. Ophthalmology 98:467, 1991.

174. Lyne AJ, Pitkeathley DA: Episcleritis and scleritis. Arch Ophthalmol 80:171, 1968.

175. Liesegang TJ: Diagnosis and therapy of herpes zoster ophthalmicus. Ophthalmology 98:1216, 1991.

176. Penman GG: Scleritis as a sequel of herpes ophthalmicus. Br J Ophthalmol 15:585, 1931.

177. Levy R, Lobstein A: Une complication rare du zona ophthalmique; l'atrophie sclérale avec perforation. Bull Soc Ophthalmol Fr 3:256, 1952.

178. Adelung JC: Skleralstaphylom nach Herpes zoster ophthalmicus. Klin Monatsbl Augenheilk 118:620, 1951.

179. Arducci F, Capelli I: Scleral staphyloma after scleritis caused by herpes zoster. Annal Ottalmologia 94:187, 1968.

180. Solomon AR: New diagnostic tests for herpes simplex and varicella-zoster infections. J Am Acad Dermatol 18:218, 1988.

181. Koneman EW, Allen SD, Dowell VR Jr, et al.: Color Atlas and Textbook of Diagnostic Microbiology. Lippincott, Philadelphia, 1988, pp 691–764.

182. Solomon AR, Rasmussen RE, Weiss JS: A comparison of the Tzanck smear and viral isolation in varicella and herpes zoster. Arch Dermatol 122:282, 1986.

183. Schwartz JN, Cashwell F, Hawkins HK, Klintworth GK: Necrotizing retinopathy with herpes zoster ophthalmicus: a light and electron microscopical study. Arch Pathol Lab Med 100:386, 1976.

184. Witmer R, Iwamoto T: Electron microscope observation of herpes-like particles in the iris. Arch Ophthalmol 79:331, 1968; and Witmer R: Personal communication, 1980.

185. Drew WL, Mintz L: Rapid diagnosis of varicella-zoster virus infection by direct immunofluorescence. Am J Clin Pathol 73:699, 1980.

186. Folkers E, Vreeswijk J, Oranje AP, Duivenvoorden JN: Rapid diagnosis in varicella and herpes zoster: re-evaluation of direct smears (Tzanck test) and electron microscopy including colloidal gold immuno-electron microscopy in comparison with virus isolation. Br J Dermatol 121:287, 1989.

187. Frey HM, Steinberg SP, Gershon AA: Rapid diagnosis of varicella-zoster virus infections by countercurrent immunoelectrophoresis. J Infect Dis 143:274, 1981.

188. Richman DD, Cleveland PH, Redfield DC, Oxman MN, Wahl GM: Rapid viral diagnosis. J Infect Dis 149:298, 1984.

189. Schmidt NJ: Varicella-zoster virus. In Lennette EH, Balows A, Hausler WJ Jr, Shadomy HJ (Eds): Manual of Clinical Microbiology, 4th ed. American Society for Microbiology, Washington DC, 1985, pp 720–727.

190. Harper DR, Grose C: IgM and IgG responses to varicella-zoster virus p32/p36 complex after chickenpox and zoster, congenital and subclinical infectios, and vaccination. J Infect Dis 159:444, 1989.

191. Cobo LM, Foulks GN, Lyesegang T, Lass J, Sutphin JE, Wilhelmus K, Jones DB, Chapman S, Segreti AC, King DH: Oral acyclovir in the treatment of acute herpes zoster ophthalmicus. Ophthalmology 93:763, 1986.

192. Cobo LM: Reduction of the ocular complications of herpes zoster ophthalmicus by oral acyclovir. Am J Med 85(Suppl 2A):90, 1988.

193. Zaal MJW, Maudga PC, Rietveld E, Suir EPE: Chronic ocular zoster. Current Eye Res 10(suppl):125, 1991.

194. Tilson HH: Monitoring the safety of antivirals. The example of the acyclovir experience. Am J Med 85(Suppl 2A):116, 1988.

195. Keczkes K, Basheer A: Do corticosteroids prevent postherpetic neuralgia? Br J Dermatol 102:551, 1980.

196. Post BT, Philbrick JT: Do corticosteroids prevent postherpetic neuralgia? A review of the evidence. J Am Acad Derm 18:605, 1988.

197. Esman V, Kroon S, Peterslund NA, Ronne-Rasmussen JO, Geil JP, Fogh H, Petersen CS, Danielsen L: Prednisolone does not prevent post-herpetic neuralgia. Lancet 2:126, 1987.

198. Bernstein JE, Bickers DR, Dahl NV: Treatment of chronic postherpetic neuralgia with topical capsaicin. A preliminary report. J Am Acad Dermatol 17:93, 1987.

199. Bucci FA Jr, Gabriels CF, Krohel GB: Successful treatment of postherpetic neuralgia with capsaicin. Am J Ophthalmol 106:758, 1988.

200. Watson PN, Evans RJ: Postherpetic neuralgia. A review. Arch Neurol 43:836, 1986.

201. Walsh TD: Antidepressants in chronic pain. Clin Neuropharmacol 6:271, 1983.

202. Max MB, Schafer SC, Culnane M, Smoller B, Dubner R, Gracely RH: Amitriptyline, but not lorazepam, relieves postherpetic neuralgia. Neurology 38:1427, 1988.

203. Watson CP, Evans RJ, Reed K, Merskey H, Goldsmith L, Warsh J: Amitriptyline versus placebo in postherpetic neuralgia. Neurology 32:671, 1982.

204. Scott T: Epidemiology of herpetic infection. Am J Ophthalmol 43:134, 1957.

205. Lehner T, Wilton J, Shillitoe E: Immunological basis for latency, recurrences, and putative oncogenicity of herpes simplex virus. Lancet 2:60, 1975.

206. Kaufman HE, Rayfield MA: Viral conjunctivitis and keratitis. In Kaufman HE, Barron BA, McDonald MB, Waltman SR (Eds): The Cornea. Churchill Livingstone, New York, 1988, pp 299–331.

207. Sainz de la Maza M, Wells PA, Foster CS: Cyclic nucleotide modulation of herpes simplex virus latency and reactivation. Invest Ophthalmol Vis Sci 30:2154, 1989.

208. Lam MT, Pazin GJ, Armstrong JA, Ho M: Herpes simplex infection in acute myelogenous leukemia and other hematologic malignancies. Cancer 48:2168, 1981.

209. Leming PD, Martin SE, Zwelling LA: Atypical herpes simplex infection in a patient with Hodgkin's disease. Cancer 54:3043, 1984.

210. Centifanto-Fitzgerald YM, Yamaguchi T, Kaufman HE, Toghon M, Roizman B: Ocular disease pattern induced by herpes simplex virus is genetically determined by a specific region of viral DNA. J Exp Med 155:475, 1982.

211. Gerdes JC, Smith DS: Recurrence phenotypes and establishment of latency following rabbit keratitis produced by multiple herpes simplex virus strains. J Gen Virol 64:2441, 1983.

212. Sanitato JJ, Asbell PA, Varnell ED, Kissling GE, Kaufman HE: Acyclovir in the treatment of herpetic stromal disease. Am J Ophthalmol 98:537, 1984.

213. Panzardi D: Contributo alla conoscenza delle lesioni erpetishe oculari: su di un particolare caso di compromissiono della conjunctiva, cornea ed episclera da virus erpetico. Bolletino d'Oculistica 26:465, 1947.

214. Saba V: Sullo episcleriti erpetishe: contributo clinico. Annal Ottalmol Clin Oculistica 73:168, 1947.

215. Sanna M: Episclerite erpetica. Bolletino d'Oculistica 29:173, 1950.

216. La Lau C, Oosterhuis JA, Versteeg J, van Rij G, Renardel de Lavalette JG, Craandijk A, Lamers WR, Mierlobensteyn T: Acyclovir and trifluorothymidine in herpetic keratitis. Preliminary report of a multicentered trial. Doc Ophthalmol 50:287, 1981.

217. La Lau C, Oosterhuis JA, Versteeg J, van Rij G, Renardel de Lavalette JG, Craandijk A, Lamers WR, Mierlobensteyn T: Multicenter trial of acyclovir and trifluorothymidine in herpetic keratitis. Am J Med 73(1A):305, 1982.

218. Pavan Langston D: Systemic acyclovir in herpes simplex keratitis. Personal communication. New England Ophthalmological Society Meeting, September 13, 1991.

219. Foster CS, Barney NP: Systemic acyclovir and penetrating keratoplasty for herpes simplex keratitis. Doc Ophthalmol 80(4):363, 1992.

220. Meyer RF, Sullivan JH, Oh JO: Mumps conjunctivitis. Am J Ophthalmol 78:1022, 1974.

221. Berg F: Scleritis pericornealis nach Parotitis epidemica. Berichte uber die Versammlungen der deutschen ophthalmologischen. Gesellschaft 46:368, 1927.

222. Rieger M: Uber subconjunctivitis epibulbaris metastatica bei Parotitis epidemica. Archiv Ophthalmologie, 133:505, 1935.

223. North DP: Ocular complications of mumps. Br J Ophthalmol 37:99, 1953.

224. Swan KC, Penn RF: Scleritis following mumps. Report of a case. Am J Ophthalmol 53:366, 1962.

225. Berger ST, Mondino BJ, Hoft RH, Donzis PB, Holland GN, Farley MK, Levenson JE: Successful medical management of Acanthamoeba keratitis. Am J Ophthalmol 110:395, 1990.

226. Lindquist TD, Fritsche TR, Grutzmacher RD: Scleral ectasia secondary to Acanthamoeba keratitis. Cornea 9:74, 1990.

227. Mannis MJ, Tamaru R, Roth AM: *Acanthamoeba* sclerokeratitis. Determining diagnostic criteria. Arch Ophthalmol 104:1313, 1986.

228. Sterh-Green JK, Bailey TM, Visversvara GS: The epidemiology of *Acanthamoeba* keratitis in the United States. Am J Ophthalmol 107:331, 1989.

229. Chang PCT, Soong HK: *Acanthamoeba* keratitis in non-contact lens wearers. Arch Ophthalmol 109:463, 1991.

230. Sharma S, Srinivasan M, George C: *Acanthamoeba* keratitis in non-contact lens wearers. Arch Ophthalmol 108:676, 1990.

231. Theodore FH, Jakobiec FA, Juechter KB, Pearl M, Troutman RC, Pang PM, Iwamoto T: The diagnostic value of a ring infiltrate in *Acanthamoeba* keratitis. Ophthalmology 92:1471, 1985.

232. Moore MB, McCulley JP, Kaufman HE, Robin JB: Radial keratoneuritis as a presenting sign in *Acanthamoeba* keratitis. Ophthalmology 93:1310, 1986.

233. Wilhelmus KR, Osato MS, Font RL, Robinson NM, Jones DB: Rapid diagnosis of *Acanthamoeba* keratitis using calcofluor white. Arch Ophthalmol 104:1309, 1986.

234. Marines HM, Osato MS, Font RL: The value of calcofluor white in the diagnosis of mycotic and *Acanthamoeba* infections of the eye and ocular adnexa. Ophthalmology 94:23, 1987.

235. Epstein RJ, Wilson LA, Visvesvara GS: Rapid diagnosis of *Acanthamoeba* keratitis from corneal scrapings using indirect fluorescent antibody staining. Arch Ophthalmol 104:1318, 1986.

236. Hoft RH, Mondino BJ: The diagnosis and clinical management of *Acanthamoeba* keratitis. Semin Ophthalmol 6:106, 1991.

237. Ishibashi Y, Matsumoto Y, Kabata T: Oral itraconazol and topical miconazol with debridement for *Acanthamoeba* keratitis. Am J Ophthalmol 109:121, 1990.

238. Wilder HC: Toxocara chorioretinitis in adults. Arch Ophthalmol 48:127, 1952.

239. Zimmerman LE: Ocular pathology of toxoplasmosis. Surv Ophthalmol 6:832, 1961.

240. Tokuda H, Okamura R, Kamano H: A case of brawny scleritis caused by *Toxoplasma gondii*. Rinsho Ganka 24:565, 1970.

241. Schuman JS, Weinberg RS, Ferry AP, Guerry RK: Toxoplasmic scleritis. Ophthalmology 95:1399, 1988.

242. Raistrick ER, Hart JCD: Ocular toxocariasis in adults. Br J Ophthalmol 60:365, 1976.

8
Noninflammatory Diseases of the Sclera

Noninflammatory diseases of the sclera are encountered infrequently in ophthalmic practice. Their detection is easily overlooked by the ophthalmologist because of this and because of the absence of inflammation. Furthermore, major textbooks of ophthalmology usually do not include discussions of the differential diagnosis of noninflammatory diseases of the sclera, and so ophthalmologists are generally unaware that distinguishing features such as deposits, thinning, thickening, and masses of the sclera can be diagnostically valuable (Table 8.1).

Like scleritis and episcleritis, noninflammatory diseases of the sclera cannot be properly understood as isolated entities but must be seen in relation to the larger picture of a patient's general health. Noninflammatory diseases of the sclera may be signs of systemic diseases such as metabolic disorders, connective tissue abnormalities, or hematological disturbances. Noninflammatory diseases of the sclera also may be signs of ocular diseases such as inherited or congenital connective tissue abnormalities, degenerations, or tumors. In many instances, the attributes of the scleral abnormalities are sufficiently distinctive that the diagnosis of the associated illness is first suspected by the ocular presentation.

This chapter reviews the clinical features and pathophysiology of the diseases associated with noninflammatory diseases of the sclera. The aim is to stimulate the readers to search for them and to pursue the appropriate course of action should such abnormalities be discovered.

8.1. Scleral Deposits

Scleral deposition of abnormal substances is caused either by systemic inherited or acquired metabolic abnormalities, or by ocular degenerative processes. For organizational purposes, these disorders will be discussed in groups based on the biochemical substance accumulated (Table 8.1). Scleral changes characteristic of the different metabolic diseases are shown in Table 8.2.

8.1.1. Scleral Protein Deposition
8.1.1.1. Porphyria

The porphyrias are characterized by the excessive excretion of one or more fluorescent pigments known as porphyrins. The porphyrias are inherited disorders that can be divided into two major types: erythropoietic, in which porphyrins accumulate in red blood cells, and hepatic porphyria, in which porphyrins accumulate in the liver. The former may be subdivided into erythropoietic uroporphyria (congenital porphyria) and erythropoietic protoporphyria; the latter may be subdivided into acute intermittent porphyria, porphyria cutanea tarda, porphyria variegata, and hereditary coproporphyria. Exposure to sunlight, certain drugs, hormones, or nutritional alterations are essential in determining the clinical expression of the porphyrias.

Scleral involvement may be a complication (although rare) of congenital porphyria,

TABLE 8.1. Classification of noninflammatory diseases of the sclera.

Scleral deposits
  Protein
    Porphyrias
    Cystinosis
    Alkaptonuria
    Amyloidosis
  Lipid
    Familial hypercholesterolemia
    Histiocytosis X
    Age-related degeneration
  Carbohydrate
    Mucopolysaccharidosis
  Mineral (calcium)
    Hyperparathyroidism
    Hypervitaminosis D
    Idiopathic hypercalcemia of infancy
    Sarcoidosis
    Hypophosphatasia
    Age-related degeneration
      Senile hyaline plaques
  Pigment (bilirubin)
    Jaundice
Scleral thinning (blue scleras)
  Inherited or congenital diseases
    Systemic
      Marfan syndrome
      Osteogenesis imperfecta
      Pseudoxanthoma elasticum
      Ehlers–Danols syndrome
    Ocular
      Keratoconus
      Buphthalmos
      Colobomas
      Myopia
  Acquired diseases
    Systemic
      Iron deficiency anemia
      Myasthenia gravis
    Ocular
      Paralimbic scleromalacia
Scleral thickening
  Nanophthalmos
  Scleropachynsis
  Phthisis bulbi
Scleral masses
  Dermoid choristomas
  Epithelial tumors
    Papillomas
    Intraepithelial epitheliomas
    Squamous cell carcinoma
  Dense connective tissue tumors
    Nodular fasciitis
    Fibromas
    Fibrous histiocytoma
    Sarcoma

TABLE 8.1. *Continued*

  Vascular tumors
    Hemangioma
    Lymphangioma
  Blood cell tumors
    Leukemia
    Lymphoma
    Lymphosarcoma
  Nervous tumors
    Neurofibroma
    Neurilemoma (Schwannoma)
  Pigmented tumors
    Nevus
    Melanocytoma
  Secondary tumors

TABLE 8.2. Scleral deposits and metabolic disease.

Scleral change	Metabolic disease
Scleromalacia	Porphyria
Crystal deposits	Gout (urate)
	Cystinosis (cystine)
Pigmented deposits (gray-bluish black)	Alkaptonuria
Lipid deposits (yellow-white)	Familial hypercholesterolemia
	Hand–Schüller–Christian disease
	Letterer–Siwe disease
Calcium deposits (white translucent)	Hyperparathyroidism
	Hypervitaminosis D

porphyria cutanea tarda, and porphyria variegata.[1–7] Acute intermittent porphyria, erythropoietic protoporphyria, and hereditary coproporphyria do not produce scleral lesions at all.

Congenital porphyria becomes manifest within a few days of birth as blisters on skin surfaces exposed to light, eventually leading to scarring and mutilation. The disease is caused by excessive deposition of porphyrins in the tissues, leading to severe photosensitization. Uroporphyrin I, derived from bone marrow normoblasts, is excreted in the urine. Progression of the disease leads to early death, usually as a result of infection or hemolytic anemia.

Porphyria cutanea tarda, the most common form of porphyria seen in Europe and in the United States, is characterized by cutaneous photosensitivity, formation of bullae, ulcers, and scars on areas exposed to light, hyperpigmentation of the skin, liver disease, and hypertrichosis.[8] The disease is caused by a partial deficiency of the enzyme uroporphyrinogen decarboxylase. Uroporphyrin I, derived from excessive synthesis in the liver, is excreted in the urine. Although the disease may be inherited in an autosomal dominant manner, a positive family history is usually not obtained. Porphyria cutanea tarda may be latent for many years but may be precipitated by excessive alcohol consumption.

Porphyria variegata is characterized by cutaneous photosensitivity, jaundice, colic, and psychosis during acute attacks. It may be asymptomatic between attacks. Coproporphyrins and protophorphyrins are excreted in the feces.

Scleral involvement in congenital porphyria, porphyria cutanea tarda, and porphyria variegata is often described as painless, bilateral, symmetric areas of scleral thinning without surrounding inflammation, with a bluish color in the base and calcareous degeneration in the adjacent areas.[1,2,9–11] These areas of scleromalacia perforans are usually localized to the sun-exposed interpalpebral fissures. The adjacent cornea may become secondarily involved with corneal opacification, thinning, or perforation.[10] Areas of active scleral inflammation, either acute diffuse anterior scleritis or posterior scleritis, also may occur.[4,10] The pathogenesis of the scleral involvement is unknown but presumably it is the result of oxidative or fluorochemical reactions. Uroporphyrin and 7-carboxylporphyrin have been found by thin-layer chromatographic analysis in conjunctiva and sclera.[2] Treatment of patients with porphyria should include general treatment of porphyria and specific treatment of acute scleritis.

The diagnosis of scleral involvement due to porphyria is made on the basis of the presence of bilateral scleral thinning, sometimes with acute scleritis, associated with characteristic cutaneous lesions and with excessive urine or feces excretion of pigments.

8.1.1.2. Cystinosis

Cystinosis is a presumably genetically determined defect of amino acid metabolism that gives rise to intracellular deposition of crystalline cystine in the reticuloendothelial cells of

the bone marrow, lymphatics, liver, spleen, and kidney. The eye also can be affected. There are three clinical forms: the infantile form, the benign adult form, and the intermediate adolescent form.[12] The infantile form (also known as Fanconi's disease or Toni–Fanconi–Lignac disease) begins in infancy and is characterized by growth retardation, rickets, secondary hyperparathyroidism, polyruria, glucosuria, urinary loss of potassium and amino acids, and progressive renal failure leading to death, usually by the age of 10 years.[13] The benign adult form is asymptomatic, with normal renal function and normal life expectancy.[14] The adolescent form appears in the second decade of life with rickets or renal failure; life expectancy depends on the degree of renal dysfunction.[15]

All three forms of cystinosis may present with ocular findings, including the deposition of glistening, polychromatic, and needlelike or fusiform cystine crystals in cornea, conjunctiva, iris, episclera, and superficial scleral tissues; crystals have also been observed in ciliary body, choroid, and retinal pigment epithelium.[16,17] The deposition of crystals progresses with the disease, but never seems to cause any inflammatory reaction within the episclera or sclera. Peripheral retinal abnormalities may be present in the infantile form, consisting of generalized depigmentation; they occasionally may precede the corneal, conjunctival, iris, episcleral, and scleral findings.[18] Corneal deposits are diagnostic; they appear as a layer of homogeneously distributed iridescent crystals that are dispersed through the entire stroma peripherally while centrally only the anterior half to two-thirds is involved.[19] In the infantile form, corneal crystals appear as early as 6 months of age, can cause intense photophobia, and do not impair vision. In the adult form or adolescent form, corneal crystals may be the only manifestation of cystinosis.

The presence of episcleral or scleral polychromatic crystals associated with the characteristic corneal involvement is suggestive of cystinosis. The diagnosis of cystinosis can be confirmed by conjunctival biopsy and analysis of cystine by column chromatography.[20] Long-term oral administration of cystamine is effective in improving renal function and growth in young patients,[21] but it does not prevent corneal crystal deposition. Frequent instillation of topical cystamine (0.1%) may reverse the deposition of crystals in the central cornea.[22]

8.1.1.3. Alkaptonuria

Alkaptonuria (ochronosis) is a rare autosomal recessive disorder characterized by the absence of the enzyme homogentisate 1,2-dioxygenase normally present in liver and kidney.[23] As a result of this error of metabolism, homogentisate, a normal intermediary in the metabolism of phenylalanine and tyrosine, accumulates in tissues, including the episclera and sclera, and is excreted in the urine.

Alkaptonuria is usually diagnosed on the basis of the urine-containing homogentisate that darkens (slowly if left to stand, or rapidly with the addition of strong alkali [alkapton]), the pigmentation of cartilage of the ear, trachea, nose, tendons, heart valves, and prostate (ochronosis), and, in later years, arthritis. In the infant, a first sign of alkaptonuria may be the presence of dark urine in a wet diaper. Ocular findings are helpful in suspecting the diagnosis of alkaptonuria. They include scleral pigmentation, seen as triangular patches in the interpalpebral area at the insertion of the horizontal rectus muscles (areas exposed to light), and episcleral pigmentation, seen as pinguecular-like masses between the limbus and the insertion of horizontal rectus muscles.[24–27] Occasionally, pigmentation may involve the whole sclera. The pigment is gray or bluish black (although microscopically it appears ochre), and it increases with age. More diffuse pigmentation, seen as oil drop-like globules when examined by retroillumination, may be found in the subepithelium and in Bowman's membrane of the peripheral cornea.[26,27] Conjunctiva and lid pigmentation also may be seen.

Any patient who develops scleral or episcleral pigmentation should be questioned and examined for urine and cartilage abnormalities.

8.1.1.4. Amyloidosis

Amyloid is an eosinophilic hyaline extracellular material made up of sheets of fibrous protein that may be deposited in various tissues of the body, including the sclera. Although foreign-body cell reactions occasionally may be seen, amyloid does not produce any inflammatory response by its presence in tissues. Several classifications of the amyloidoses by various criteria have been only partially successful because of the overlapping of the different categories. One of the classifications differentiates amyloidosis into primary and secondary amyloidosis, depending on the absence or presence of a preexisting disease, respectively. Both categories are further classified into familial and nonfamilial types. Primary amyloidosis, particularly the familial type, is the form most commonly associated with deposition of amyloid in the lid, cornea (lattice corneal dystrophy), conjunctiva, iris, choroid, retina, vitreous, ciliary nerves, extraocular muscles, orbit, and sclera.[28–30] Scleral amyloidosis is asymptomatic and does not show any specific lesion. Amyloidosis is suspected clinically, and confirmed by biopsy of appropriate tissues.

Although there are no detectable clinical changes, histological studies show that amyloid deposition in sclera occurs more often as age increases.[31] Amyloid deposition in sclera also may occur following severe scleral inflammation at any age.[32,33]

Amyloid stains brown with Congo red and exhibits dichroism and birefringence with polarized light. It also shows metachromasia with crystal violet, fluorescence with thioflavine T, and positive staining with hematoxylin–eosin, periodic acid–Schiff (PAS), iodine, and Sirius red.

8.1.2. Scleral Lipid Deposition

8.1.2.1. Familial Hypercholesterolemia and Histiocytosis X

Disorders of lipid and lipoprotein metabolism may lead to xanthomas: depositions of lipid-containing histiocytic foam cells in tissues. Xanthomas can be seen in conjunctiva or episclera of normal individuals without abnormalities in their serum lipids. Xanthomas can be seen in sclera of individuals with xanthoma disseminatum without abnormalities in their serum lipids; they appear as dark mahogany-brown papules over sclera as well as over flexion creases, mucous membranes, and cornea.[32,34]

Scleral xanthomas also may appear in association with diseases such as type II hyperlipoproteinemia (hyperbetalipoproteinemia) or familial hypercholesterolemia, and with histiocytosis X (a combination of eosinophilic granuloma, Hand–Schüller–Christian disease, and Letterer–Siwe disease).[32] Any patient with scleral xanthomas should be examined for serum lipid abnormalities.

8.1.2.2. Age-Related Degeneration

With advancing age, the sclera becomes slightly yellow from the deposition of lipids, including cholesterol esters, cholesterol, free fatty acids, triglycerides, and sphingomyelin.[35,36] Collagen acts as a trap for these lipid fractions. The lipid fractions that show the greatest increase in concentration with age are cholesterol esters and sphingomyelin.[35] The lipid deposition may be particularly obvious in old scars.

Lipid deposition in sclera also may occur following severe scleral inflammation at any age.[32,33]

8.1.3. Scleral Carbohydrate Deposition

8.1.3.1. Mucopolysaccharidosis

Histopathological scleral involvement may occasionally occur as a result of mucopolysaccharide deposition.

Mucopolysaccharide deposition between the collagen fibers of the posterior sclera may occur in mucopolysaccharidosis type VI or Maroteaux–Lamy syndrome.[37] Mucopolysaccharidosis type VI is a recessively inherited syndrome characterized by accumulation of the glycosaminoglycan dermatan sulfate (mucopolysaccharide) in several tissues of the body; this accumulation results from deficiency of the enzyme N-acetylgalactosamine-4-sulfate sulfatase (arylsulfatase B). Other systemic and ocular manifestations in mucopolysaccharidosis type VI are gargoyle-like facial dysmorphism, skeletal dysplasia, aortic stenosis, umbilical hernia, corneal clouding, and optic atrophy. Patients with the severe form die in their teens from hydrocephalus due to meningeal involvement.

Mucopolysaccharide deposition between the collagen fibers of the posterior sclera adjacent to the macula was detected in a 50-year-old man with bilateral mottling of the retinal pigment epithelium in the macular region[38]; mucopolysaccharide accumulation was thought to be the cause of choroidal compression and maculopathy.

Corneal and scleral deposits of an unusual glycosaminoglycan (mucopolysaccharide) were detected histopathologically in a 68-year-old patient with clinical corneal stromal opacities since infancy[39]; there were no deposits in other ocular or extraocular tissues. The authors suggested the possibility of a diffusion-like process from cornea to sclera.

8.1.4. Scleral Mineral Deposition: Calcium

8.1.4.1. Hyperparathyroidism

Calcium deposition in cornea, conjunctiva, and sclera may occur as a result of the calcium and phosphorus imbalance seen either in primary causes of hyperparathyroidism, such as benign adenoma or hyperplasia of the parathyroid glands,[40-44] or in secondary causes of hyperparathyroidism, such as chronic renal disease.[42,44,45] The calcium is deposited in the form of hydroxyapatite crystals in the nucleus and cytoplasm of the stromal cells of the sclera.[43]

The most frequent ocular manifestation in hyperparathyroidism is band keratopathy, a bilateral and symmetrical peripheral corneal calcification with tiny Swiss cheese-like holes and a clear interval between the band and the limbus.[43,44] Extension of the band keratopathy may involve the conjunctiva and the sclera. Conjunctival calcification is described as white flecks or glasslike crystals near the limbus. Scleral calcification appears as white translucent plaques.[32]

8.1.4.2. Other Causes of Hypercalcemia

Other diseases that may cause calcium deposition in the sclera are hypervitaminosis D,[41,46,47] idiopathic hypercalcemia of infancy,[44] Boeck's sarcoidosis, and hypophosphatasia.[40,41]

Hypophosphatasia is a rare inborn metabolic bone disease characterized by hypercalcemia, low serum and tissue alkaline phosphatase concentrations, and increased blood and urine levels of phosphoethanolamine and inorganic pyrophosphate. In hypophosphatasia bone maturation is prevented because osteoblasts cannot incorporate calcium into otherwise normal bone matrix. Abnormalities in bone maturation lead to rickets in children and osteomalacia in adults. The disease may be classified as infantile, childhood, or adult. Ocular manifestations are uncommon and are present only in the infantile and childhood forms. They include band keratopathy, conjunctival calcification, cataracts, harlequin orbits, papilledema, optic atrophy, retinitis pigmentosa, and blue sclerae.[48–52]

8.1.4.3. Age-Related Degeneration

Certain scleral areas may become translucent with increasing age, due to calcium deposition between the scleral fibers[53]; scleral calcium deposition would occur in all individuals if they lived long enough and generally occurs posterior to the equator.[54] The calcium deposition may be particularly obvious in areas that have previously been inflamed. If the calcium concentration is high, these scleral areas become completely translucent and form senile hyaline plaques.

8.1.4.3.1. Senile Scleral Hyaline Plaques

Senile scleral plaques, occurring in individuals over 60 years of age (either sex), appear as a dark oval nonprogressive patch about 2 mm in diameter surrounded by a dense calcareous yellowish ring; the center of the patch appears translucent, allowing the underlying uvea to be seen.[32,55–62] The lesion, usually bilateral and symmetrical, is localized to the interpalpebral region, anterior to the insertion of the horizontal recti muscles. The central translucent area can be transilluminated by directing the light through the pupil, but although the sclera is thinned (from 0.6 to 0.3 mm)[61] the wall is resistant, with no tendency to perforation. Histologically, plaques show decreased cellularity, replacement of the superficial layers of

the sclera by large masses of hyaline degeneration, loss of birefringence, deposition of calcium, and fragmentation of scleral fibers; the latter may account for the scleral weakness. The location of the plaque therefore may be determined by the maximal stresses of the muscles. Differential diagnosis of senile scleral hyaline plaques should include scleromalacia perforans, because both lesions have loss of scleral substance, lack of inflammatory reaction, and painless development.[63–65] Unlike in scleromalacia perforans, in senile scleral plaques there is no evidence of rheumatoid arthritis, there is no progression, males are affected as often as females, there is no histopathological necrosis, and prognosis is good without treatment (Table 4.13).

Calcium deposition in sclera may also occur following severe scleral inflammation at any age.[32,33]

8.1.5. Scleral Pigment Deposition: Bilirubin

8.1.5.1. Jaundice

Yellow discoloration of the conjunctiva and sclera is a clinical manifestation of jaundice, a condition associated with an increased blood bilirubin concentration due either to excessive breakdown of hemoglobin (hemolytic) or to biliary obstruction (hepatic). Yellow discoloration of the sclera occurs when the concentration of free bilirubin in blood rises above 1.5 mg/100 ml; bilirubin binds strongly to the elastin fibers of the sclera.

Unilateral yellow discoloration of the sclera may appear after choroidal hemorrhage following surgery for retinal detachment[66]; the yellow staining is caused by accumulation of unconjugated bilirubin derived from the breakdown of hemoglobin from the hemorrhage; bilirubin binds weakly to the elastin and to the collagen fibers of the sclera.

8.2. Scleral Thinning (Blue Sclerae)

Bluish sclera, although considered normal in premature infants and in white newborns, is pathological if it persists beyond the first months of infancy. Several inherited or congenital disorders may be associated with blue sclerae. The blue color is caused by translucency of the sclera as a result of scleral thinning, allowing the uveal pigment to show through.

Other causes of blue sclerae are acquired disorders, the most common being iron-deficiency anemia.[67-72] Iron is an important cofactor in the hydroxylation of proline and lysine residues in collagen synthesis. Fibroblasts in culture do not synthesize collagen in the presence of iron-chelating agents.[70] Iron deficiency in vivo may lead to impaired collagen synthesis and a thin sclera through which the choroid can be seen, making the sclerae appear blue. Blue sclerae also may be seen in association with myasthenia gravis.[73]

8.2.1. Scleral Thinning in Inherited or Congenital Diseases

8.2.1.1. Marfan Syndrome

Marfan syndrome is a congenital mesodermal dystrophy classically characterized by the triad of subluxated lenses, skeletal abnormalities, and cardiovascular disease. Marfan syndrome may also involve lungs, muscles, genitourinary system, skin, and nearly every structure of the eye, including the sclera.[74,75] This autosomal dominant condition affects both sexes equally and is seen in all races. Although the exact biochemical defect is not known, the disorder is thought to be caused by a basic anomaly of connective tissue.

The most conspicuous physical features of a patient with Marfan syndrome are the musculoskeletal defects. There is a generalized overgrowth of long bones; patients are tall and have long slender fingers and toes (arachnodactyly). Prognathism, high arched palate, kyphoscoliosis, pectus excavatum, muscular hypoplasia, and hypotony also are characteristic. Cardiovascular anomalies include degeneration of the tunica media of the aortic valve and ascending aorta, which may cause dissecting aneurysms.

Other ocular manifestations aside from subluxated lenses include myopia, ptosis, mega-

locornea, strabismus, hypoplasia of the iris dilator muscle, spherophakia, glaucoma, peripheral retinal degeneration, and blue sclerae. Because the anomalous scleral connective tissue is unable to resist elevated intraocular pressure, it allows the intraocular contents of the globe to bulge, producing a staphyloma. Cataract formation, lens dislocation, and glaucoma may necessitate ocular surgery, but surgical complications such as vitreous loss and incarceration in the wound, iris prolapse, hyphema, persistent anterior uveitis, and corneal edema are seen more often in these patients than in the general population.

The diagnosis is clinical; approximately 50% of patients with Marfan syndrome are diagnosed by the ophthalmologist, usually because of myopia not adequately corrected by eyeglasses. The differential diagnosis is principally from homocystinuria, an inborn error of amino acid metabolism that is also characterized by subluxated lenses, myopia, strabismus, spherophakia, glaucoma, peripheral retinal degeneration, long slender extremities, kyphoscoliosis, and pectus excavatum; however, scleral connective tissue in homocystinuria is thicker and more resistant to high intraocular pressure than in Marfan syndrome. The diagnosis in homocystinuria is established by amino acid electrophoresis and chromatography of urine and plasma.[76]

Any patient with congenital blue sclerae should be questioned and examined for skeletal anomalies and cardiovascular disease. The immediate family also should be evaluated.

8.2.1.2. Osteogenesis Imperfecta

Osteogenesis imperfecta (van der Hoeve's syndrome) is a genetically determined defect in the synthesis of extracellular matrix leading to abnormalities in connective tissue, primarily collagen and proteoglycans. Partially described in 1896 by Spurway[77] and in 1900 by Eddowes,[78] and completely described in 1918 by van der Hoeve and de Kleyn,[79] osteogenesis imperfecta is characterized by the triad of blue sclerae, brittle bones, and deafness (otosclerosis). It may be inherited as either an autosomal dominant or autosomal recessive condition; the autosomal recessive form is associated with more severe skeletal abnormalities. Osteogenesis imperfecta has an incidence of 1 in 20,000 births, affects both sexes equally, and is seen in all races.[80] The disorder is caused by anomalies at the level of the type I collagen genes, which result in the failure of type I collagen fibers to mature to their normal diameters. Individual variants result from a structural or regulatory abnormality of the α_1 or α_2 chains of type I collagen.

Two classifications have been proposed for osteogenesis imperfecta. The oldest one classifies the disease into the congenital form, which is manifest at birth, leading to early death, and the tarda form, which is manifest early in childhood and has a relatively benign course.[81,82] In the congenital form, musculoskeletal defects, including extremity deformities, rib fractures, and muscular hypotony, may be detectable at birth. In the tarda form, fractures may occur at 2 to 4 years of age, and skeletal deformities such as scoliosis may become manifest early in life. Some patients with osteogenesis imperfecta tarda do not have gross bony abnormalities and go through life without a fracture; the disease is limited to minimal radiological defects associated with ear manifestations and blue sclerae. Deafness occurs in 30% of these patients. Other ear abnormalities may include tinnitus and vertigo.

Osteogenesis imperfecta also may be classified into types I, II, III, and IV, on the basis of inheritance, clinical features, and severity.[80]

Blue sclerae, the most characteristic ocular manifestation in all types of osteogenesis imperfecta,[80,82] are the result of increased thinness of the scleral wall, allowing the visualization of the underlying uveal layer. Ocular histopathological examination reveals a 50 to 75% thinning of the sclera. Osteogenesis imperfecta patients with blue sclerae have significantly lower ocular rigidity measurements than do patients without the disease.[83] The Saturn ring, a white ring in the paralimbal sclera, is a common finding; the lack of uvea behind the sclera in the paralimbal area gives a comparative whitening aspect. The corneas also are thin and vulnerable to perforation from minor trauma. Sclera and cornea can usually with-

stand the normal intraocular pressure, but elevated pressures will produce a staphyloma.

Ultrastructurally, the scleral and corneal fibers in eyes of patients with osteogenesis imperfecta appear immature. There have been some reports showing either a decreased number,[84,85] or a reduced diameter,[86–91] of collagen fibers in both the sclera and the cornea. An ultrastructural study revealed vacuoles in the endoplasmic reticulum of scleral fibrocytes and in keratocytes, as well as deposits (possibly chondroitin sulfate) between the scleral lamellae, suggesting a disturbance of the fibroblasts.[92] In addition to abnormalities of collagen, biochemical quantitative and qualitative defects of glycosaminoglycans also have been reported.[93] Keratoconus, megalocornea, hyperopia, posterior embryotoxon, zonular cataracts, retrobulbar neuritis, optic atrophy, and glaucoma may develop.

The diagnosis of osteogenesis imperfecta is clinical. Any patient with congenital blue sclerae should be examined for skeletal and ear abnormalities. The immediate family also should be evaluated.

8.2.1.3. Pseudoxanthoma Elasticum

Pseudoxanthoma elasticum is an autosomal recessive disorder characterized by skin elasticity; small yellow papules and plaques eventually form redundant folds typically located on the neck, antecubital and popliteal fossae, abdomen, perineum, thighs, axillas, and groin areas.[93] Angioid streaks of the retina, gastrointestinal bleeding, and cardiovascular abnormalities also develop.[94,95] Thin blue sclerae may appear in pseudoxanthoma elasticum patients and in their relatives.[71] Pseudoxanthoma elasticum usually begins by age 30 years, although it may appear at a younger or older age, and is more common in women than in men (2:1). Although the exact biochemical defect is not known, the disorder is thought to be caused by abnormal formation of the elastic fibers of connective tissue.[96] Angioid streaks of the retina, occurring in 85% of the patients, consist of cracks in an abnormal Bruch's membrane that may interfere with visual acuity if they involve the macular area.[93,94,97,98] Angioid streaks may not be visible on fundus examination but they can be clearly seen on fluorescein angiography.

The diagnosis of pseudoxanthoma elasticum is made on the basis of clinical findings. Any patient with congenital blue sclerae should be examined for skin and retinal abnormalities. The immediate family also should be evaluated.

8.2.1.4. Ehlers–Danlos Syndrome

Ehlers–Danlos syndrome is a multisystem genetic disorder characterized by hyperelasticity and fragility of the skin; bleeding, atrophic scars, and even hemangiomatous pseudotumors often occur after minor trauma around joints or pressure points.[99] Other findings include hyperextensibility of the joints, particularly those of the fingers, toes, and knees, blood vessel fragility, with varicose veins or aneurysms and arterial ruptures, and ocular abnormalities such as marked epicanthal folds, angioid streaks, strabismus, keratoconus, keratoglobus, microcorneas, subluxated lenses, retinal detachment, severe myopia, or blue sclerae.[100–108] Ehlers–Danlos syndrome is usually an autosomal dominant condition, although it may be recessive in some families.

At least nine types of Ehlers–Danlos syndrome have been described, depending on inheritance, clinical features, severity, ultrastructural abnormalities, and biochemical defects. In the type VI or ocular–sclerotic form of Ehlers–Danlos syndrome, ocular features are prominent; it is also characterized by severe scoliosis and joint and skin disturbances. Within the ocular features, thin blue sclerae may lead to spontaneous perforation of the sclera.[109] Surgery should be avoided, if possible, because of the high incidence of complications secondary to fragility of tissues.[110] The ocular–sclerotic form of Ehlers–Danlos syndrome has been associated with a primary deficiency of the enzyme lysyl hydroxylase.[81,111,112] Lysyl hydroxylase converts lysine to hydroxylysine; aldehydes that cross-link spontaneously are formed. A deficiency in lysyl hydroxylase results in a lack of collagen cross-linking and, subsequently, in weakened connective tissue; however, normal enzyme levels have been de-

scribed, suggesting that the ocular form of Ehlers–Danlos syndrome has some degree of genetic heterogeneity.[113]

The diagnosis of Ehlers–Danlos syndrome is made on the basis of clinical findings. Any patient with congenital blue sclerae should be examined for skin and joint abnormalities, marked epicanthal folds, and retinal findings. The immediate family should also be evaluated.

8.2.1.5. Keratoconus

Blue sclerae or scleral thinning may occur in association with keratoconus.[108] Keratoconus or ectatic corneal dystrophy is a disorder characterized by thinning of the central cornea; conical ectasia or protrusion may occur, leading to a painless, progressive loss of vision due to a progressive irregular myopic astigmatism. Heredity plays a significant role in at least some keratoconus patients,[114–118] although the majority of cases show no definitive inheritance pattern. In the early form, distortion of keratometric mires or retinoscopic reflex occurs. In the advanced form, Vogt's striae or a Fleischer ring may be seen. Vogt's striae are fine vertical folds in the deep stroma and Descemet's membrane that parallel the steep axis of the cone. A Fleischer ring is a yellow brownish corneal epithelial pigment ring localized around the base of the cone; the color is caused by deposition of ferritin in the subepithelium. Breaks in Bowman's layer, enlarged corneal nerves, increased intensity of the corneal endothelial reflex, and fine subepithelial fibrillary lines also may occur.

Aside from blue sclerae, other ocular anomalies that may occur associated with keratoconus are subluxated lenses, cataract, aniridia, retinitis pigmentosa, and optic atrophy. Keratoconus has been described in association with various systemic connective tissue disorders such as Marfan syndrome,[119,120] osteogenesis imperfecta,[81,115] and Ehlers–Danlos syndrome.[108,113,121,122]

8.2.1.6. Buphthalmos

The high intraocular pressure of congenital glaucoma produces enlargement and stretching of scleral and corneal collagen fibers before maturation. This leads to a large eye or buph-thalmos with a corneal diameter greater than 10.5 mm at birth or greater than 12 mm at age 1 year.[123,124] The sclera, usually thin in premature infants and in white newborns, is even thinner at birth and persists like this beyond the first months of infancy; light transmitted through the thinned sclera strikes the uvea and is reflected outward, producing a bluish tinge. After surgical relief of congenital glaucoma there is no further stretching of scleral fibers; however, the scleral fibers that have become stretched never return to normal.

8.2.1.7. Coloboma

Cystic outpouching of the posteroinferior sclera or scleral ectasia may occur in association with a peripapillary coloboma of the choroid.[45,125] The normal vessels of the disk pass over bare ectatic sclera or atrophic choroid and then into normal retina.

Occasionally, intrauterine fetal infection such as toxoplasmosis may secondarily cause focal areas of scleral thinning and ectasia at the sites of intense retinal and choroidal inflammation.[45]

8.2.1.8. Myopia

Simple or stationary myopia develops during youth and stops after completion of body growth; this form of myopia is usually of low to moderate severity and is not associated with significant chorioretinal complications. Degenerative or pathological myopia develops during youth but progresses steadily throughout life; this form of myopia is usually severe and is associated with significant chorioretinal complications. Degenerative myopia is associated with an increase in the axial length of the posterior segment of the globe. The heredity and certain developmental abnormalities play an important role in myopia. Some investigators[126] have observed that chickens raised with translucent occluders over their eyes developed eyes with long axial lengths. Monkeys raised with unilateral lid suture or after unilateral opacification of the cornea with polystyrene beads also developed eyes with abnormal axial lengths[127,128]; this effect could be demonstrated only when the monkeys were

raised in light as opposed to dark. The investigators suggested that visual stimulation is necessary for the development of the alterations. However, small periods of normal vision (2 h) can prevent the development of axial elongation.[129] There appears to be an age window of susceptibility, during which abnormal axial length can be induced, because adult monkeys cannot be made myopic by lid occlusion[127] and monkeys at age 12 months can only be made less myopic.[130]

In degenerative myopia, the sclera is thin, particularly in the posterior segment of the globe[131,132]; posterior scleral thinning may cause posterior pole and equatorial staphylomas as a result of stretching of the fibers. However, rather than a purely mechanical stretch, the increase in axial length in myopic eyes seems also to be caused by increased scleral growth during which both the fibrocytes and the extracellular matrix overgrow; there is more DNA, collagen, protein, and proteoglycan synthesis in the myopic sclera.[133–135]

8.2.2. Scleral Thinning in Acquired Diseases

8.2.2.1. Iron Deficiency Anemia

Iron deficiency anemia is the most frequent cause of acquired blue sclerae. There are no data on the body depletion of iron stores needed before blue sclerae develop, but the presence of blue sclerae is a useful guide to iron deficiency anemia in patients with low dietary iron or chronic blood loss associated with duodenal ulcers, ulcerative colitis, and gluten enteropathy.[68]

Blue sclerae have occasionally been reported as associated with myasthenia gravis.[73]

8.2.2.2. Paralimbic Scleromalacia

Paralimbic scleromalacia or spontaneous intercalary scleral perforation is a degenerative process that appears in either one or both eyes of young individuals of either sex; it is characterized by a noninflammatory, painless thinning of the corneoscleral limbus (between the ciliary body and the limbus), which leads to a small, nonprogressive, well-defined hole with iris prolapse.[32,55,56,64,65,136–138] Sometimes the pupil may be drawn up into the hole. A small perforating scleral vessel may run through the defect to anastomose with the posterior ciliary circulation.[32] Differential diagnosis of paralimbic scleromalacia should include scleromalacia perforans, because both conditions have loss of scleral substance, lack of inflammatory reaction, and painless development. Unlike scleromalacia perforans, paralimbic scleromalacia affects individuals between 25 and 50 years of age without evidence of rheumatoid arthritis, and it has a good prognosis without treatment (Table 4.13).

8.3. Scleral Thickening

8.3.1. Nanophthalmos

The characteristics of the nanophthalmic eye include a thickened sclera (up to 2 mm), small cornea, high hyperopia (up to 20 diopters), shallow anterior chamber, and a tendency to develop uveal effusion. Nanophthalmos is usually bilateral and may be inherited, following either a dominant or a recessive pattern.[139,140] The thickening of the sclera may cause vortex vein compression, which results in impaired venous drainage; this may lead to uveal effusion and serous retinal detachment.[141–143] The ultrastructure of nanophthalmic sclera has been described, with conflicting results.[144,145] Yue and co-workers[144] found that the levels of glycosaminoglycans were markedly reduced in cell cultures of nanophthalmic scleral cells; the decreased level of glycosaminoglycans may result from either reduced synthesis, increased degradation, or a combination of both. These in vitro findings conflict with the in vivo findings of Trelstad and co-workers,[145] who reported increased quantities of Alcian blue staining material that they thought to be glycosaminoglycan in the sclera of two nanophthalmic patients. Whichever the case is, the abnormalities in glycosaminoglycan metabolism may lead to abnormal collagen fiber formation and packing of collagen bundles,[146] which may in turn contribute to the thickening of sclera and the formation of nanophthalmos. In a later study,

Yue and co-workers[147] found that the levels of fibronectin were increased.

The diagnosis of nanophthalmos is made on the basis of clinical findings. Resolution of effusions may be achieved by surgical decompression of the vortex veins.[142]

8.3.2. Scleropachynsis

Bilateral localized thickening of the inner two-thirds of the posterior temporal sclera has been reported in one case as the cause of choroidal compression and maculopathy.[38] Ultrastructurally, the collagen fibers in the inner two-thirds of the sclera in the submacular region were enlarged in diameter; mucopolysaccharide deposition was detected between the bundles of collagen.

8.3.3. Phthisis Bulbi

The term phthisis bulbi is applied to those eyes that show not only diffuse degeneration or atrophy but also shrinkage and disorganization of the ocular contents after severe injury or inflammation. The sclera becomes markedly thickened and irregular, due to scarring. The intraocular structures also are replaced by scarred tissue. It is not known whether internal fibrosis leads to the loss of intraocular pressure or the lack of ocular tension results in intraocular scarring.

8.4. Scleral Tumors

Tumors of the sclera are exceptionally rare, but when they occur they are usually the result of scleral extension of episcleral or conjunctival tumors; they also may appear secondary to intraocular or systemic neoplasms extending along vascular or neural intrascleral channels. Tumors of episclera are more common than tumors of the sclera; they may arise from episclera or from conjunctiva. Although some tumors have a characteristic clinical appearance, diagnostic confirmation can be obtained only by biopsy.

The episclera and conjunctival tissues are composed of various elements, any one of which can form tumors. Examples of these elements and tumors are (1) epithelium (intraepithelial epitheliomas, carcinomas), (2) dense connective tissue (nodular fasciitis, fibromas, fibrous histiocytoma, sarcoma), blood and lymphatic vessels (angiomas, lymphangiomas), blood cells (leukemia, lymphoma, lymphosarcoma), nerves (neurofibroma, neurilemoma), and melanocytes (nevus, melanocytoma). Dermoid choristomas are composed of elements not normally present at the episclera or conjunctiva.

Episcleral and scleral tumors pose a challenge to the ophthalmologist, because they can be easily mistaken for inflammatory abnormalities of the episclera and sclera.

8.4.1. Dermoid Choristomas

Epibulbar choristomas are easy to diagnose if they appear at the limbus in young infants; however, choristomas occurring in the conjunctiva, episclera, or sclera are difficult to distinguish from other tumors. Epibulbar episcleral choristomas, usually occurring in the lower temporal quadrant, are characterized by isolated solid or cystic nodules of variable size, which are adherent to the bulbar conjunctiva or to the sclera. They result from inclusions of epidermal and connective tissue at sites of closure of the fetal clefts that grow from birth and have a burst of activity at puberty; the connective tissue is covered by stratified epithelium with keratin, hair follicles, and sebaceous glands.[87]

Episcleral osseous choristomas usually occur in the upper temporal quadrant 5 to 10 mm behind the limbus[148] and are characterized by isolated nodules of variable size that are either freely moveable or adherent to the conjunctiva or to the sclera. They can grow very large. Although most of them are composed of mature bone, occasionally cartilage may be found[149,150]; bone or cartilage is surrounded by connective tissue with other choristomatous elements, such as meningothelial cells or hematopoietic marrow.[148,151]

Episcleral lipodermoids (dermolipomas) are solid tumors that contain fatty tissue. The are true choristomas, because fatty tissue is not normally present anterior to the orbital septum.

They are usually located laterally and may extend into the orbit. Because the excision is only for cosmetic reasons, only the superficial layer of the tumor must be removed.

8.4.2. Epithelial Tumors

8.4.2.1. Papillomas or Intraepithelial Epitheliomas

Epithelial tumors of the conjunctiva, including papillomas or intraepithelial epithelioma (Bowen's disease), tend to occur at the limbus, are confined to the superficial conjunctival layers without episcleral invasion, and ulcerate into the surface.[32] Occasionally, however, papillomas or epitheliomas can grow away from the limbus and deeply invade the episclera and sclera.

8.4.2.2. Squamous Cell Carcinoma

Intraocular invasion by squamous cell carcinoma of the conjunctiva may manifest as necrotizing scleritis, sometimes with scleral perforation and uveal prolapse.[152–154] Necrotizing scleritis appears adjacent to an enlarging, vascularized, elevated, conjunctival mass, close to the limbus. Diagnosis of the tumor is achieved after excisional biopsy of the mass. Squamous cell carcinomas have been associated with acquired immunodeficiency syndrome (AIDS), AIDS-related complex, and human immunodeficiency virus seropositivity.[152,155] Necrotizing scleritis may occasionally be the initial manifestation of the invasive tumor.[154]

8.4.3. Dense Connective Tissue Tumors

8.4.3.1. Nodular Fasciitis

Nodular fasciitis is a benign nodular reactive proliferation of fibroblasts and vascular tissue within the fascias of the trunk, upper extremities, scalp, neck, and face, including those in the eye.[156] The lesion appears as a tender, isolated, vascularized, round or oval nodule with a size ranging from 0.5 to 1.5 cm in diameter; sometimes the rapid growth suggests a malignant tumor, particularly a lymphoma or sarcoma, but excisional biopsy reveals proliferating fibroblasts varying in configuration from spindle to stellate. In the eye, the nodule may involve Tenon's capsule, eyelid, periorbital tissue, and the ligaments of the extraocular muscles.[157–159] Episcleral nodules usually occur at the limbus or under the bulbar conjunctiva anterior to the insertion of the recti muscles. Episcleral tissue heals well after excision of the nodule and there are no recurrences.

8.4.3.2. Fibroma

Fibromas of the episclera may occur anywhere but usually arise adjacent to the limbus. They are vascularized, firm, of variable size, and not adherent to the sclera. Histologically, fibroma is a tumor composed of packed fibroblasts intermingled with inflammatory cells. If extracellular matrix components outnumber the fibroblasts, the tumor may be termed a myxoma. If extracellular matrix components and fibroblasts are present in similar amounts, the tumor may be termed a myxofibroma.[87]

8.4.3.3. Fibrous Histiocytoma

Fibrous histiocytoma is a tumor composed of fibroblasts and histiocytes; it arises from primitive mesenchymal cells with the capacity to differentiate into either or both cell lines. The orbit is one of the most common locations of the tumor. Rarely, fibrous histiocytoma may originate in the episclera and, although it usually remains localized, metastasis may occur. Excisional biopsy is essential for diagnosis and therapy. Histologically, there may be interweaving fascicles of fibroblasts (storiform pattern) and stellate deposits of dense collagen with fibroblasts intermingling with lipid-laden histiocytes.[45] Recurrences may occur after excision.

8.4.3.4. Sarcomas

Although primary sarcomas of the episclera and sclera are exceptionally rare,[32,160] secondary invasion from adjacent ocular structures occasionally may occur.[161] Rhabdomyosarcoma in a child has been reported to manifest as nodular episcleritis.[32]

8.4.4. Vascular Tumors

8.4.4.1. Hemangiomas

Episcleral capillary hemangioma occurs early in life, may grow rapidly, and often regresses before the child is 5 years old. Sometimes, however, the small and circumscribed tumor may be present for many years without any further growth, in which case it can be mistaken for nodular episcleritis; in the episcleral capillary hemangioma the new vessels appear to radiate from the mass rather than skirt it, as in inflammatory conditions.[32] Episcleral capillary hemangioma may be the only external manifestation of Sturge–Weber syndrome, which usually presents with facial (port-wine stain, nevus flammeus) and leptomeningeal angiomas. Because of its small size it usually does not require removal.

Episcleral cavernous hemangiomas are often a peripheral manifestation of an orbital cavernous hemangioma. They present as a mass of vessels associated with an overlying conjunctival overgrowth that may bleed spontaneously and severely. Both episclera and conjunctiva are readily moveable over the underlying sclera. Episcleral cavernous hemangiomas are present at birth, grow rapidly, and often regress before the child is 5 years old. Conservative therapy is advised unless it is cosmetically intolerable, in which case surgical removal is the proper treatment.

8.4.4.2. Lymphangiomas

Lymphangiomas are benign but slowly progressive tumors that are present from birth and may involve the orbits, the lids, and the conjunctiva. They can appear either as a red or white mass at the limbus or on the bulbar conjunctiva and extend back into the orbit; the tumor rarely may involve the episclera. Coexisting lymphangiomas of facial structures such as nasal cavity, paranasal sinuses, or palate may be present. Because hemorrhages into the lymphatic channels are common, lymphangioma may be mistaken for hemangioma. Treatment is not necessary unless the lesions are large. Repeated partial excisions to obtain satisfactory cosmetic and functional results may be needed.

8.4.5. Blood Cell Tumors

8.4.5.1. Leukemia

Most clinical and pathological studies suggest that 50 to 70% of the eyes of leukemic patients are affected. Acute leukemia involves the eye four times as often as chronic leukemia, but there is no way to distinguish between the various forms of leukemia on the basis of clinical involvement. Although the choroid is the ocular tissue most commonly involved in leukemia, episcleral and intrascleral infiltration occur frequently, particularly around the aqueous and emissary veins. Episcleral and intrascleral involvement may be either clinically undetectable or may manifest as hemorrhages, focal nodules, or diffuse infiltrates. Other ocular tissues that may be involved are conjunctiva, iris, retina, optic nerve, and extraocular muscles. Various combined immunosuppressive regimens are employed in the management of the different types of leukemia.[162–165]

8.4.5.2. Lymphoma and Lymphosarcoma

Lymphomas are malignant tumors that can be classified as lymphoblastic, lymphocytic, and histiocytic, according to cell type. They can affect episclera primarily or as a result of an extension from an orbital mass. Episcleral lymphoma may easily be mistaken for episcleritis because both may appear as small red nodules. However, the color of the tumor is dull red as opposed to the bright red of episcleritis; the posterior edge of the tumor is ill defined as opposed to the sharp margins of the episcleritis; the tumor grows slowly as opposed to disappearing after an acute attack of episcleritis; the tumor shows a yellow infiltrated area with red-free light; episcleritis gives the appearance of a solid mass.[32] Although these clinical characteristics are helpful, diagnostic confirmation of lymphoma can be made only by biopsy. Any patient with episcleral lymphoma should be examined for systemic involvement of the tumor. Lymphosarcomas resemble lymphomas but they are larger and exhibit greater systemic extension.[87]

Radiotherapy and combined immunosuppressive regimens are used to treat the different types of lymphoma.

8.4.6. Nervous Tissue Tumors

8.4.6.1. Neurofibroma

Neurofibromas may occur as hard tumors arising from the episclera and superficial sclera adherent to the underlying structures.[166,167] Histologically, Schwann cells and fibroblasts may be seen. The differential diagnosis must include tuberous sclerosis, intrascleral nerve loops of Axenfeld, and neurilemomas. Occasionally, episcleral or scleral neurofibromas are part of neurofibromatosis or Recklinghausen's disease.

8.4.6.2. Neurilemoma (Schwannoma)

Neurilemomas are benign tumors composed of proliferating Schwann cells arising from ciliary nerves. They are usually not associated with neurofibromatosis. Although the orbit is the most common location of neurilemomas, the uveal tract, and less often, the sclera, also may be involved.[168–171]

Differentiating neurilemomas from neurofibromas may be difficult, because both are formed by Schwann cells; the diagnosis requires detailed histological examination, including specialized staining techniques and electron microscopy. The S-100 stain, characteristic of Schwann cells, is positive for both neurilemomas and neurofibromas; however, neurilemomas show a more generalized and stronger staining pattern than do neurofibromas, because S-100 stain does not stain fibroblasts. Under electron microscopy examination, the Lüse bodies are seen in neurilemomas and not in neurofibromas; Lüse bodies are aggregates of long-spaced or broad-banded collagen with an axial periodicity of 130 nm.[171] They were considered in the past as pathognomonic of neurilemomas, but it is now known that they occur in other tumors such as basal and squamous carcinomas and nevoid tumors.

Because surgical removal of neurilemoma may lead to rupture, the possibility of donor sclera homografting must always be kept in mind.[171]

8.4.7. Pigmented Tumors

Pigmented tumors of the episclera are common. The differential diagnosis must include congenital episcleral melanosis, acquired episcleral melanosis, and nerve loops of Axenfeld. Melanocytes are normally present in the episclera and in scleral lamellae adjacent to and along the course of vascular and neuronal transcleral channels. An increased number of melanocytes may exist in these locations in association with these congenital and acquired benign pigmentations.

Ocular melanocytosis (melanosis oculi) is a congenital unilateral pigmentation of episclera, sclera, and uveal tract. There is an increased incidence of uveal melanomas in the involved eye. Oculodermal melanocytosis (nevus of Ota) is ocular melanocytosis associated with ipsilateral pigmentation of the periocular tissues. It occurs more often in the nonwhite races. Malignant transformation is not common.

Acquired melanosis is a flat, diffuse, and slowly growing melanotic lesion that may appear either in the skin or in the conjunctiva–episclera. Biopsy should be performed before therapy is planned. Management is conservative unless there is malignant transformation. In the conjunctiva–episclera, 17% of the melanosis may progress to melanoma; mortality in patients with these melanomas is up to 40%.[172]

A branch of the long posterior ciliary nerve (intrascleral nerve loop of Axenfeld) may loop out through the sclera in the region between the limbus and the insertions of the recti muscles, forming a nodule that is often darkened with melanocytes. The nerve loop, may be mistaken clinically for a melanotic tumor or for a foreign body,[173] and histologically for a neurofibroma, especially when the nerve is associated with neurilemmal or connective tissue proliferation.

8.4.7.1. Nevus

Nevi are present at birth but may not be noticed until middle childhood. Approximately 33% of conjunctival–episcleral nevi are not pigmented. Both pigmented and nonpigmented nevi are diffuse and flat lesions localized close to the limbus; they may look like nodular episcleritis. More than 50% of conjunctival–episcleral nevi

have epithelial cysts, which can be clinically evident.[174] Increased melanogenesis in nevi can result from pituitary stimulation (puberty, pregnancy, adrenal insufficiency), physical irritation (sun exposure, trauma, inflammation), and coexisting malignant melanoma. Malignant transformation of nevi to melanomas is rare; a great increase in vascularity without obvious growing and increase in pigmentation may be the first signs before extension in the conjunctiva–episclera and to the sclera occurs. The episcleral vessels radiate from the mass rather than skirt it, as in inflammatory conditions such as necrotizing scleritis.[32] Biopsy should be performed before therapy is planned. Management of nevi requires photography at regular intervals to look for the possibility of malignant transformation. Therapy is conservative unless it is cosmetically intolerable, in which case surgical removal is the proper treatment. Surgical removal also eliminates the remote chance of malignant change.

8.4.7.2. Melanocytoma

Melanocytomas of the conjunctiva–episclera may arise from nevi, from acquired melanosis, or without any preexisting lesion. They may also result from extension of melanoma arising in ciliary body, or the skin or mucous membranes anywhere in the body. Occasionally, it may be localized to the episclera and sclera and may be mistaken for scleromalacia perforans.[175] Biopsy of melanocytoma does not seem to increase its lethality, and may prevent unnecessary mutilation.[176] Treatment consists of either exenteration or wide local excision, depending on location; radiotherapy may be effective in those melanocytomas arising from acquired melanosis.

8.4.8. Secondary Tumors

Although episcleral and scleral secondary tumors from conjunctiva are not uncommon, episcleral and scleral secondary tumors from anywhere in the body are rare.[32] Occasional cases have been reported arising from seminoma, breast carcinoma, skin melanoma, or generalized systemic lymphomatous disease.[87,177,178]

Summary

Noninflammatory diseases of the sclera may be manifestations of ocular diseases such as connective tissue abnormalities, degenerations, or tumors. They may also be signs of systemic diseases such as metabolic disorders, connective tissue abnormalities, or hematological disorders. In many cases, the characteristics of the scleral abnormality (deposit, thinning, thickening, or mass) are sufficiently distinctive that the ocular or systemic diagnosis is first suspected by the ocular presentation. Ophthalmologists must be able to recognize these interconnections, and therefore to diagnose promptly and, if possible, treat the underlying ocular or systemic disease.

References

1. Barnes HD, Boshoff PH: Ocular lesions in patients with porphyria. Arch Ophthalmol 48: 567, 1952.
2. Sevel D, Burger D: Ocular involvement in cutaneous porphyria. A clinical and histological report. Arch Ophthalmol 85:581, 1971.
3. Douglas WHG: Congenital porphyria. General and ocular manifestations. Trans Ophthalmol Soc UK 92:541, 1972.
4. Salmon JF, Strauss PC, Todd G, Murray ADN: Acute scleritis in porphyria cutanea tarda. Am J Ophthalmol 109:400, 1990.
5. Miani P: Ocular manifestations in congenital porphyria. Giornale Italiano di Oftalmologica 11:381, 1958.
6. Girod P: Les signes ophthalmologiques de la porphyrie congénitale. Ann Oculist (Paris) 202:937, 1969.
7. Hamard H, Guillem AD, Onfray B, Guillaumat L: Complications oculaires des porphyries. A propos d'un cas de maladie de Günther. J Fr Ophthalmol 5:771, 1982.
8. Waldenström J: Studien über Porphyrie. Acta Med Scand 82(suppl):1, 1937.
9. Urrets-Zavalia A, Allende IM, Oliva RO: Escleromalacia observada en el curso de una porfirinuria cronica. Arch Oftalmol Buenos Aires 12:115, 1937.
10. Chumbley LC: Scleral involvement in symptomatic porphyria. Am J Ophthalmol 84:729, 1977.
11. Calmettes L, Deodati F, Bec P, Delpech J: Ocular manifestations of chronic porphyria. Bull Mem Soc Fr Ophthalmol 79:569, 1966.
12. Goldman H, Scriver CR, Aaron K, Delvin E, Canlas Z: Adolescent cystinosis: comparisons with infantile and adult forms. Pediatrics 47: 979, 1971.
13. Seegmiller JE, Friedmann T, Harrison HE, Wong VG, Schneider JA: Cystinosis: combined clinical staff conference at the National Institutes of Health. Ann Intern Med 68:883, 1968.
14. Lietman PS, Frazier PD, Wong VG, Shotton D, Seegmiller JE: Adult cystinosis: a benign disorder. Am J Med 40:511, 1966.
15. Zimmerman TJ, Hood I, Gasset AR: "Adolescent" cystinosis: a case presentation and review of the recent literature. Arch Ophthalmol 92: 265, 1974.
16. Kenyon KR, Sensenbrenner JA: Electron microscopy of cornea and conjunctiva in childhood cystinosis. Am J Ophthalmol 78:68, 1974.
17. Sanderson PO, Kuwabara T, Stark WJ, Wong VG, Collins E: Cystinosis: a clinical, histopathologic, and ultrastructural study. Arch Ophthalmol 91:270, 1974.
18. Wong VG, Lietman PE, Seegmiller JE: Alterations of pigment epithelium in cystinosis. Arch Ophthalmol 77:361, 1967.
19. Wong VG: Ocular manifestations in cystinosis. Birth Defects 12(3):181, 1976.
20. Wong VG, Schulman JD, Seegmiller JE: Conjunctival biopsy for the biochemical diagnosis of cystinosis. Am J Ophthalmol 70:278, 1970.
21. Gahl WA, Reed GF, Thoene JG, Schulman JD, Rizzo WB, Jonas AJ, Denman DW, Schlesselman JJ, Corden BJ, Schneider JA: Cysteamine therapy for children with nephropathic cystinosis. N Engl J Med 316:971, 1987.
22. Kaiser-Kupfer MI, Fujikawa L, Kuwabara T, Jain S, Gahl WA: Removal of corneal crystals by topical cysteamine in nephropathic cystinosis. N Engl J Med 316:775, 1987.
23. Garrod AE: The incidence of alkaptonuria: a study in chemical individuality. Lancet 2:1616, 1902.
24. Smith JW: Ochronosis of the sclera and cornea complicating alkaptonuria: review of the literature and report of four cases. JAMA 120:1282, 1942.
25. Ashton N, Kirker JG, Lavery FS: Ocular findings in a case of hereditary ochronosis. Br J Ophthalmol 48:405, 1964.
26. Wirtschafter JD: The eye in alkaptonuria. Birth Defects 12(3):279, 1976.

27. Allen RA, O'Malley C, Straatsma BR: Ocular findings in hereditary ochronosis. Arch Ophthalmol 65:657, 1961.
28. Paton D, Duke JR: Primary familial amyloidosis. Ocular manifestations with histopathological observations. Am J Ophthalmol 61:736, 1966.
29. Brownstein MH, Elliot R, Helwig EB: Ophthalmologic aspects of amyloidosis. Am J Ophthalmol 69:423, 1970.
30. Schwartz MF, Green WR, Michels RG, Kincaid MC, Fogle J: An unusual case of ocular involvement in primary systemic nonfamilial amyloidosis. Ophthalmology 89:394, 1982.
31. Wright JR, Calkins E, Breen WJ, Stolte G, Schultz RT: Relationship of amyloid to ageing. Medicine 48:39, 1969.
32. Watson P: Diseases of the sclera and episclera. In Duane TD, Jaeger EA (Eds): Clinical Ophthalmology, Vol 4. Harper & Row, Philadelphia, 1985, Chap 23.
33. Coats G: Hyperplasia, with colloid and amyloid degeneration, of the episcleral and circumdural fibrous tissue. Trans Ophthalmol Soc UK 35:257, 1915.
34. Parker F: Xanthomas and hyperlipidemias. J Am Acad Dermatol 13:1, 1985.
35. Broekhuyse RM, Kuhlmann ED: Lipids in tissues of the eye. VI. Sphingomyelins and cholesterol esters in human sclera. Exp Eye Res 14:111, 1972.
36. Broekhuyse RM: The lipid composition of aging sclera and cornea. Ophthalmologica 171:82, 1975.
37. Kenyon KR, Topping TM, Green WR, Maumenee AE: Ocular pathology of the Maroteaux–Lamy syndrome (systemic mucopolysaccharidosis type VI); histologic and ultrastructural report of two cases. Am J Ophthalmol 73:718, 1972.
38. Conn H, Green WR, de la Cruz ZC, Hillis A: Scleropachynsis maculopathy: a clinicopathologic case report. Arch Ophthalmol 95:497, 1977.
39. Winterbotham CTC, Torczynski E, Horwitz AL, Yue BYJT, Font RL: Unusual mucopolysaccharide disorder with corneal and scleral involvement. Am J Ophthalmol 109:544, 1990.
40. Walsh FB, Murray RG: Ocular manifestations of disturbances in calcium metabolism. The Ninth Sanford R. Gifford Lecture. Am J Ophthalmol 36:1657, 1953.
41. Cogan DG, Albright F, Bartter FC: Hypercalcemia and band keratopathy. Report of nineteen cases. Arch Ophthalmol 40:624, 1940.
42. Porter R, Crombie AL: Corneal calcification as a presenting and diagnostic sign in hyperparathyroidism. Br J Ophthalmol 57:665, 1973.
43. Berkow JW, Fine BS, Zimmerman LE: Unusual ocular calcification in hyperparathyroidism. Am J Ophthalmol 66:812, 1968.
44. Jensen OA: Ocular calcifications in primary hyperparathyroidism. Acta Ophthalmol (Copenhagen) 53:173, 1975.
45. Spencer WH: Sclera. In Spencer WH (Ed): Ophthalmic Pathology, 3rd ed. W.B. Saunders, Philadelphia, 1985, pp 389–422.
46. Gartner S, Rubner K: Calcified scleral nodules in hypervitaminosis D. Am J Ophthalmol 39:658, 1955.
47. Heat P: Calcinosis oculi. Trans Am Ophthalmol Soc 59:141, 1961.
48. Brenner RL, Smith JL, Cleveland WW, Bejar RL, Lockhart WS Jr: Eye signs of hypophosphatasia. Arch Ophthalmol 81:614, 1969.
49. Fraser D: Hypophosphatasia. Am J Med 22:730, 1957.
50. Bethune JE, Dent CE: Hypophosphatasia in the adult. Am J Med 28:615, 1960.
51. Lessel S, Norton EWD: Band keratopathy and conjunctival calcification in hypophosphatasia. Arch Ophthalmol 71:497, 1964.
52. Roxburgh STD: Atypical retinitis pigmentosa with hypophosphatasia. Trans Ophthalmol Soc UK 103:513, 1983.
53. Pagenstecher A: Beitrage zur pathologischen Anatomie des Auges. Graefes Arch Ophthalmol 7:92, 1860.
54. Watson PG, Hazleman BL: The Sclera and Systemic Disorders, W.B. Saunders, Philadelphia, 1976, pp 347–381.
55. Duke-Elder S, Leigh AG: Diseases of the outer eye. Cornea and sclera. In Duke-Elder S (Ed): System of Ophthalmology, Vol 8, Part 2. C.V. Mosby, St. Louis, 1965, p 1042.
56. Franceschetti A, Bischler V: La sclérite nodulaire nécrosante et ses rapports avec la scléromalacie. Ann d'Oculist 183:737, 1950.
57. Kiss J: Fall von seniler Sklerverdünnung. Klin Monatsbl Augenheilk 92:121, 1934.
58. Roper KL: Senile hyaline scleral plaques. Arch Ophthalmol 34:283, 1945.
59. Graves B: Bilateral mesial superficial deficiency of the sclera: scleral plaques. Br J Ophthalmol 25:35, 1941.
60. Katz D: A localized area of calcareous degeneration in the sclera. Arch Ophthalmol 2:30, 1929.
61. Culler AM: The pathology of scleral plaques; report of 5 cases of degenerative plaques in the

sclera mesially, one studied histologically. Br J Ophthalmol 23:44, 1939.

62. Drescher EP, Henderson JW: Senile hyaline scleral plaques; report of 3 cases. Proc Staff Meet Mayo Clin 24:334, 1949.

63. van der Hoeve J: Scleromalacia perforans. Arch Ophthalmol 11:111, 1934.

64. François J: Scleromalacia perforans, arthritis deformans and pemphigus. Trans Ophthalmol Soc UK 71:61, 1951.

65. Sorensen TB: Paralimbal scleromalacia. Acta Ophthalmol 53:901, 1975.

66. Tolentino FI, Brockhurst RJ: Unilateral scleral icterus due to choroidal hemorrhage. Arch Ophthalmol 70:358, 1963.

67. Hall GH: Blue sclerotics in iron deficiency. Lancet ii:1377, 1971.

68. Kalra L, Hamlyn AN, Jones BJM: Blue sclerae: a common sign of iron deficiency? Lancet ii:1267, 1986.

69. Agnoleto A: Blue sclerotics in iron deficiency. Lancet ii:1160, 1971.

70. Walter FB, Israel MS: *General Pathology*, 5th ed. Churchill Livingstone, Edinburgh, 1979, pp 63–65.

71. Bennet RM: Blue sclerotics in iron deficiency. Lancet ii:1100, 1971.

72. Pope FM: Blue sclerotics in iron deficiency. Lancet ii:1160, 1971.

73. Wiernik PH: Blue sclerae. Lancet ii:1199, 1972.

74. Allen RA, Straatsma BR, Apt L, Hall MD: Ocular manifestations of the Marfan syndrome. Trans Am Acad Ophthalmol Otolaryngol 71:18, 1967.

75. Cross HE, Jensen AD: Ocular manifestations in the Marfan syndrome and homocystinuria. Am J Ophthalmol 75:405, 1973.

76. Gerritsen T, Waisman H: Homocystinuria. In Stanbury J, Wyngaarden J, Fredrickson D (Eds): *The Metabolic Basis of Inherited Disease*, 3rd ed. McGraw-Hill, New York, 1972, p 404.

77. Spurway J: Hereditary tendency to fracture. Br Med J 2:844, 1896.

78. Eddowes A: Dark sclerotics and fragilitas ossium. Br Med J 2:222, 1900.

79. van der Hoeve J, de Kleyn A: Blaue Sclera, Knochenbruchigkeit und Schwerhorigkeit. Graefes Arch Klin Exp Ophthalmol 95:81, 1918.

80. Rowe DW: Osteogenesis imperfecta. In Wyngaarden JB, Smith LH Jr (Eds): *Cecil Textbook of Medicine*, 17th ed. W.B. Saunders, Philadelphia, 1985, pp 1151–1152.

81. McKusick VA: *Heritable Disorders of Connective Tissue*, 4th ed. C.V. Mosby, St. Louis, 1972.

82. Shoenfeld T, Fried A, Ehrenfeld NE: Osteogenesis imperfecta: review of the literature and presentation of 29 cases. Am J Dis Child 129:679, 1975.

83. Kaiser-Kupfer MI, McCain L, Shapiro JR, Podgor MJ, Kupfer C, Rowe D: Low ocular rigidity in patients with osteogenesis imperfecta. Invest Ophthalmol Vis Sci 20:807, 1981.

84. Ruedemann AD: Osteogenesis imperfecta congenita and blue sclerotics. Arch Ophthalmol 49:6, 1953.

85. Leonibus F, Gemolotto G: Rilievi istologici su di un caso di sclera blu. Boll Oculistica 33:789, 1954.

86. Buchanan L: Case of congenital maldevelopment of the cornea and sclerotic. Trans Ophthalmol Soc UK 23:267, 1903.

87. Casanovas J: Blue scleras and fragilitas osseum. Am J Dis Child 50:1298, 1935.

88. Follis RJ Jr: Osteogenesis imperfecta congenita: a connective tissue diathesis. J Pediatr 44:713, 1953.

89. Haebara H, Yamasaki Y, Kyogoku M: An autopsy case of osteogenesis imperfecta. Acta Pathol Jpn 19:377, 1969.

90. Blumcke S, Niedorf HR, Theil HJ, Langness U: Histochemical and fine structural studies on the cornea in osteogenesis imperfecta congenita. Virchows Arch Abt B Zellpath 11:124, 1972.

91. Chan CC, Green WR, Zenaida C, Dela C, Hillis A: Ocular findings in osteogenesis imperfecta congenita. Arch Ophthalmol 100:1459, 1982.

92. Eichholtz W, Mueller D: Electron microscopy findings on the cornea and sclera in osteogenesis imperfecta. Klin Monatsbl Augenheilk 161:646, 1972.

93. Connor J, Juergens J, Perry H, Hollenhorst R, Edwards J: Pseudoxanthoma elasticum and angioid streaks: a review of 106 cases. Am J Med 30:537, 1961.

94. Clarkson JG, Altman RD: Angioid streaks. Surv Ophthalmol 26(5):235, 1982.

95. Lebwohl MG, Distefano D, Prioleau PG, Uram M, Yannuzzi LA, Fleischmajer R: Pseudoxanthoma elasticum and mitral valve prolapse. N Engl J Med 307:228, 1982.

96. Huang S, Steele H, Kumar G, Parker J: Ultrastructural changes of elastic fibers in pseudoxanthoma elasticum: a study of histogenesis. Arch Pathol 83:108, 1967.

97. Goodman R, Smith E, Paton D, Bergman R, Siegel C, Ottesen E, Shelley W, Pusch A, McKusick V: Pseudoxanthoma elasticum: a clinical and histopathological study. Medicine 42:297, 1963.

98. Paton D: *The Relation of Angioid Streaks to Systemic Disease*. Charles C Thomas, Springfield, IL, 1972, pp 13–31.

99. Lorincz A: Ehlers–Danlos syndrome. In Demis D (Ed): *Clinical Dermatology*. Harper & Row, Hagerstown, MD, 1979.

100. Beighton P: Serious ophthalmological complications in the Ehlers–Danlos syndrome. Br J Ophthalmol 54:263, 1970.

101. Green W, Friedman-Kien A, Banfield W: Angioid streaks in Ehlers–Danlos syndrome. Arch Ophthalmol 76:197, 1966.

102. Pemberton J, Freeman HM, Schepens C: Familial retinal detachment and the Ehlers–Danlos syndrome. Arch Ophthalmol 76:817, 1966.

103. Biglan AW, Brown SI, Johnson BC: Keratoglobus and blue sclera. Am J Ophthalmol 83:225, 1977.

104. Babel J, Houber J: Keratocone et sclerotiques bleues dans one anomalie congenitale de tissue conjuncti. J Genet Hum 17:241, 1969.

105. Gregoratos N, Bartoscocas C, Papas K: Blue sclera with keratoglobus and brittle cornea. Br J Ophthalmol 55:424, 1971.

106. Hymas SW, Dar H, Newman E: Blue sclera keratoglobus. Br J Ophthalmol 53:53, 1969.

107. Stein R, Lazar M, Adam A: Brittle cornea. A familial trait associated with blue sclera. Am J Ophthalmol 66:67, 1968.

108. Greenfield G, Stein R, Romano A, Goodman RM: Blue sclera and keratoconus. Key features of a distinct heritable disorder of connective tissue. Clin Genet 4:8, 1973.

109. McKusick VA: Multiple forms of the Ehlers–Danlos syndrome. Arch Surg 109:475, 1974.

110. Watson PG, Hazleman BL: *The Sclera and Systemic Disorders*, W.B. Saunders, Philadelphia, 1976, pp 306–346.

111. Pinnell SR, Krane SM, Kenzora JE, Glimcher MJ: Heritable disorder with hydroxylysine-deficient collagen. Hydroxylysine-deficient collagen disease. N Engl J Med 286:1013, 1972.

112. Maumenee IH: Hereditary connective tissue diseases involving the eye. Trans Ophthalmol Soc UK 94:753, 1974.

113. Judisch G, Waziri M, Krachmer J: Ocular Ehlers–Danlos syndrome with normal lysyl hydroxylase activity. Arch Ophthalmol 94: 1489, 1976.

114. Falls HF, Allen AW: Dominantly inherited keratoconus. Report of a family. J Genet Hum 17:317, 1969.

115. Hammerstein W: Zur Genetik des Keratoconus. Graefes Arch Klin Exp Ophthalmol 190:293, 1974.

116. Hallermann W, Wilson EJ: Genetishe Betrachtungen uber den Keratokonus. Klin Monatsbl Augenheilk 170:906, 1977.

117. Redmond KB: The role of heredity in keratoconus. Trans Ophthalmol Soc NZ 27:52, 1968.

118. Woillez M, Razemon PH, Constantinides G: A propos d'un nouveau cas de keratocone chez des juneaux univitellins. Bull Soc Ophthalmol France 76:279, 1976.

119. Austin MG, Shaefer RF: Marfan syndrome with unusual blood vessel manifestations; primary medionecrosis, dissection of the right inominate. Arch Pathol Lab Med 64:205, 1957.

120. Storch H: Ein Fall von Arachnodaktylie (Dystrophia mesodermalis congenita), Typus Marfan. Dermatologica 104:322, 1952.

121. Blandau RJ: Morphogenesis and malformations of the skin. Birth Defects 17:155, 1981.

122. Robertson I: Keratoconus and the Ehlers–Danlos syndrome. Med J Aust 1:571, 1975.

123. Shaffer RN, Weiss DI: *Congenital and Pediatric Glaucomas*. C.V. Mosby, St. Louis, 1970.

124. Sampaolesi R: Corneal diameter and axial length in congenital glaucoma. Can J Ophthalmol 23:42, 1988.

125. Donaldson DD, Bennett N, Anderson DR, Eckelhoff R: Peripapillary staphyloma. Arch Ophthalmol 82:704, 1969.

126. Wallman J, Turkel J: Extreme myopia produced by modest change in early visual experience. Science 201:1249, 1978.

127. Raviola E, Weisel TN: An animal model of myopia. N Engl J Med 312:1609, 1985.

128. Wiesel TN, Raviola E: Increase in axial length of the macaque monkey eye after corneal opacification. Invest Ophthalmol Vis Sci 18: 1232, 1979.

129. Judge SJ: Does the eye grow into focus. Nature (London) 345:477, 1990.

130. Wallman J, Adams JI: Developmental aspects of experimental myopia in chicks: susceptibility, recovery, and relation to emmetropization. Vision Res 27:1139, 1987.

131. Curtin BJ, Teng CC: Scleral changes in pathological myopia. Trans Am Acad Ophthalmol 62:777, 1958.

132. Heine L: Beitrage zur Anatomie des myopischen Auges. Arch Augenheilk 38:277, 1899.

133. Christensen AM, Wallman J: Increased DNA and protein synthesis in scleras of eyes with visual-deprivation myopia. Invest Ophthalmol Vis Sci Suppl 30:402, 1989.

134. Rada JA, Thoft RA, Hassell JR: Extracellular matrix changes in the sclera of chickens with experimental myopia. Invest Ophthalmol Vis Sci Suppl 31:253, 1990.

135. Wu YR: DNA, collagen, and uronic acid in form deprivation myopia. Invest Ophthalmol Vis Sci 31:254, 1990.

136. Anderson B, Margolis C: Scleromalacia: clinical and pathologic study of a case with consideration of differential diagnosis, relationship of collagen disease, and effect of ACTH and cortisone therapy. Am J Ophthalmol 35:917, 1952.

137. Arkle JS, Ingram HV: Scleromalacia perforans. Trans Ophthalmol Soc UK 55:552, 1935.

138. Mader TH, Stulting RD, Crosswell HH: Bilateral paralimbal scleromalacia perforans. Am J Ophthalmol 109:233, 1990.

139. Black M: Twins with high hyperopia. Am J Ophthalmol 7:375, 1924.

140. Wolff E: A family with microphthalmos. Proc R Soc Med 23:45, 1930.

141. Schaffer RN: The management of glaucoma in nanophthalmos. Trans Am Ophthalmol Soc 73:119, 1975.

142. Brockhurst RJ: Vortex vein decompression for nanophthalmic uveal effusion. Arch Ophthalmol 98:1987, 1980.

143. Gass JDM: Uveal effusion syndrome; a new hypothesis concerning pathogenesis and technique of surgical treatment. Retina 3:159, 1983.

144. Yue BYJT, Duvall J, Goldberg MF: Nanophthalmic sclera. Morphologic and tissue culture studies. Ophthalmology 93:534, 1986.

145. Trelstad RL, Silbermann NN, Brockhurst RJ: Nanophthalmic sclera; ultrastructural, histochemical, and biochemical observations. Arch Ophthalmol 100:1935, 1982.

146. Stewart DH, Streeten BW, Brockhurst RJ: Abnormal scleral collagen in nanophthalmos. An ultrastructural study. Arch Ophthalmol 109:1017, 1991.

147. Yue BYJT, Kurosawa A, Duvall J, Goldberg MF, Tso MOM, Sugar J: Nanophthalmic sclera: fibronectin studies. Ophthalmology 95:56, 1988.

148. Boniuk M, Zimmerman LE: Episcleral osseous choristoma. Am J Ophthalmol 53:290, 1961.

149. Pittke EC, Marquardt R, Mohr W: Cartilage choristoma of the eye. Arch Ophthalmol 101: 1569, 1983.

150. Bengisu U, Tahsinoglu M, Toker G: Neurofibromatosis associated with cartilaginous choristoma of the episclera. Ann d'Oculist 206:401, 1973.

151. Ferry AP, Hein HF: Epibulbar osseous choristoma within an epibulbar dermoid. Am J Ophthalmol 70:764, 1970.

152. Kim RY, Seiff SR, Howes EL, O'Donnell JJ: Necrotizing scleritis secondary to conjunctival squamous cell carcinoma in acquired immunodeficiency syndrome. Am J Ophthalmol 109: 231, 1990.

153. Stokes JJ: Intraocular extension of epibulbar squamous cell carcinoma of the limbus. Trans Am Acad Ophthalmol Otolaryngol 59:143, 1955.

154. Lindenmuth KA, Sugar A, Kincaid KC, Nelson CC, Comstock CP: Invasive squamous cell carcinoma of the conjunctiva presenting as necrotizing scleritis with scleral perforation and uveal prolapse. Surv Ophthalmol 33:50, 1988.

155. Overly WL, Jakubek DJ: Multiple squamous cell carcinomas and human immunodeficiency virus infection. Ann Intern Med 106:334, 1987.

156. Konwaler BE, Keasby L, Kaplan L: Subcutaneous pseudosarcomatous fibromatosis (fasciitis). Am J Clin Pathol 25:241, 1955.

157. Font RL, Zimmerman LE: Nodular fasciitis of the eye and adnexa. A report of ten cases. Arch Ophthalmol 75:475, 1966.

158. Tolls RE, Mohr S, Spencer WH: Benign nodular fasciitis originating in Tenon's capsule. Arch Ophthalmol 75:482, 1966.

159. Ferry AP, Sherman SE: Nodular fasciitis of the conjunctiva apparently originating in the fascia bulbi (Tenon's capsule). Am J Ophthalmol 78:514, 1974.

160. Hirschberg J: Casuistiche Mittheilungen uber Geschwulste der orbita und des bulbus. Klin Monatsbl Augenheilk 6:153, 1868.

161. Betteto G, Amidei B: Fibrous sarcoma of the sclera. Ann Ottalmol 80:495, 1954.

162. Ninane J: The eye as a sanctuary in acute lymphoblastic leukemia. Lancet 1:452, 1980.

163. Allen R, Straatsma B: Ocular involvement in leukemia and allied disorders. Arch Ophthalmol 66:490, 1961.

164. Kincaid M, Green W, Kelley J: Acute ocular leukemia. Am J Ophthalmol 87:698, 1979.

165. Murray K, Paolino F, Goldman J, Galton DA, Grlindle CF: Ocular involvement in leukaemia. Report of three cases. Lancet 1:829, 1977.

166. Nitsch M: Neurofibromatose des Auges. Z Augenheilk 69:117, 1929.

167. Dabezies OH, Penner R: Neurofibroma and neurilemmoma of the bulbar conjunctiva. Arch Ophthalmol 66:73, 1961.

168. Quintana M, Lee WR: Intrascleral schwannoma. Ophthalmologica 173:64, 1976.

169. Kyrieleis W: Ein Neurinom am Limbus corneae. Graefes Arch Clin Exp Ophthalmol 119:119, 1927.

170. Szabo G, Cseh E: Sklera-Neurinom in der Nähe des Limbus. Ophthalmologica 106:14, 1943.

171. Graham CM, McCartney ACE, Buckley RJ: Intrascleral neurilemmoma. Br J Ophthalmol 73:378, 1989.

172. Reese AB: Precancerous and cancerous melanosis. Am J Ophthalmol 61:1272, 1966.

173. Crandall AS, Yanoff M, Schaffer DB: Intrascleral nerve loop mistakenly identified as a foreign body. Arch Ophthalmol 95:497, 1977.

174. Jay B: Naevi and melanomata of the conjunctiva. Br J Ophthalmol 49:169, 1965.

175. Lee JS, Smith RE, Minckler DS: Scleral melanocytoma. Ophthalmology 89:178, 1982.

176. Epstein E, Bragg K, Linden G: Biopsy and prognosis of malignant melanoma. JAMA 208:1369, 1969.

177. Garret M: Ocular metastasis from seminoma. Br J Ophthalmol 43:759, 1959.

178. Sacks I: Kaposi's disease manifesting in the eye. Br J Ophthalmol 40:574, 1956.

9

Treatment: The Massachusetts Eye and Ear Infirmary Experience

9.1. Treatment of Episcleritis

Episcleritis may or may not require treatment; scleritis always does. Although simple, diffuse episcleritis may produce low-grade aggravation and temporary cosmetic consequences for the patient, it does not absolutely require therapy, because untreated it will eventually resolve leaving no sequelae. Regrettably, topical steroid therapy appears to be the reflex treatment prescribed by many physicians in developed countries. This is regrettable not simply because of the potential side effects of such treatment, but because experience suggests that such treatment actually prolongs the overall duration of the patient's problem: the number of recurrences following discontinuation of each episode of steroid therapy appears to be greater, and a so-called "rebound effect," in which the episcleritis intensifies with each recurrent episode after discontinuation of steroid therapy, has been observed. Our philosophy, and that of Watson,[1] is to leave simple episcleritis untreated except for comfort and supportive therapy, such as cold compresses and iced artificial tears. It appears that, on the basis of the results of a randomized double-masked placebo-controlled clinical trial, nonsteroidal antiinflammatory therapy is not effective.[2]

If the patient demands treatment, or if the patient's occupation is such that withholding treatment would produce a vocational disability (actor, television personality, etc.), we suggest treating the patient with episcleritis in the same way in which the patient with scleritis is initially treated, that is, with systemic nonsteroidal antiinflammatory drug (NSAID) therapy. A substantial proportion of those individuals with nodular episcleritis will require treatment, and the systemic NSAIDs are typically effective. Table 9.1 lists the currently available NSAIDs, along with suggested initial dosage. As usual, package insert directions should be followed from the standpoint of frequency of hematological monitoring, and so on. We advise uninterrupted therapy for a minimum of 6 months, followed by subsequent attempts to taper and discontinue the medicine while observing for recurrence.

Episcleritis associated with some specific disease may, of course, require systemic NSAID therapy, but also typically requires addressing the specific etiology of the episcleritis. Atopic individuals require appropriate environmental controls and systemic antihistamine therapy. Patients with gout require allopurinol. Patients with rosacea require one of the systemic tetracyclines. Patients with a specific connective tissue disease who have episcleritis may or may not require systemic therapy with medications other than NSAIDs. Plaquenil (hydroxychloroquine; 200 mg twice daily by mouth), is often effective in treating the dermatological and superficial ocular (e.g., episcleritis) consequences of systemic lupus erythematosus. Patients with nodular episcleritis associated with rheumatoid arthritis usually respond to one systemic NSAID or another; however, one may have to experiment sequentially with two or more NSAIDs before finding the one to which

TABLE 9.1. Nonsteroidal antiinflammatory drugs available for treatment of episcleritis and scleritis.

Trade name	Generic name	Dosage
Dolobid	Diflunisal	500 mg bid
Naprosyn	Naproxen	250–500 mg bid
Indocin	Indomethacin	75 mg SR bid[a]
Motrin	Ibuprophen	800 mg tid
Feldene	Piroxicam	20 mg qid
Butazolidin	Phenylbutazone	100 mg tid
Nalfon	Fenoprofen	600 mg tid
Voltaren	Diclofenac	75 mg bid
Tolectin	Tolmetin	400 mg tid
Meclomen	Meclofenamate	100 mg qid
Ansaid	Flurbiprofen	100 mg tid
Orudis	Ketoprofen	100 mg tid

[a] SR, sustained-release preparation.

the patient responds. We have also cared for three patients with rheumatoid arthritis associated with nodular episcleritis over the past 10 years whose nodular episcleritis did not respond to NSAIDs; low-dose methotrexate once a week was required. The efficacy of topical cyclosporine A is unclear, and appropriate studies to test this agent as applied topically will be required to answer the question of efficacy.

Five of our 94 patients with episcleritis had rheumatoid arthritis, 1 had systemic lupus erythematosis, 7 had rosacea, 1 had gout, and 64 had idiopathic episcleritis. The patient with systemic lupus erythematosus responded completely to hydroxychloroquine therapy (400 mg /day). The patients with rosacea responded to oral doxycycline (100 to 200 mg/day), and two of the patients with rheumatoid arthritis responded to NSAID therapy; the other three, with nodular episcleritis, required 5 to 7.5 mg of methotrexate once weekly for 6 months. Ten patients with idiopathic episcleritis required therapy. Each had suffered from recurrent episcleritis for prolonged periods (6 to 24 months) and each had been treated with topical steroids, with the predictable result: recurrence of episcleritis more severe than prior to steroid therapy after steroids were discontinued. Each of these patients responded well to oral NSAID therapy, with no recurrence of episcleritis after drug withdrawal.

9.2. Treatment of Scleritis

9.2.1. Medical Treatment

Patients with simple, diffuse, or even nodular scleritis rarely require cytotoxic drug therapy for successful control of their inflammation. Systemic NSAID therapy is almost invariably effective, although as mentioned above, sequential trials of several NSAIDs may be required before one that is completely effective is found. We habitually treat our scleritis patients who have responded to an NSAID for a minimum of 1 year before attempting to taper and discontinue the medicine. Patients with an associated disease, such as rosacea, gout, or atopy, will require specific treatment for those diseases as described above. Fourteen of our 25 patients with idiopathic nodular scleritis responded to oral NSAID therapy. Five patients required the addition of systemic prednisone, and four required the addition of an immunosuppressive medication.

The treatment of patients with scleritis associated with connective tissue or collagen vascular diseases requires slightly more consideration in that control of their scleral inflammation often needs more potent therapy, and vigilance for extraocular, "silent" inflammatory foci requires extra effort. For example, we were once consulted about a patient with limited Wegener's granulomatosis (scleritis, sinus involvement, and a positive anti-neutrophil cytoplasmic antibody [ANCA] test) whose scleritis responded to systemic NSAID therapy, prompting the patient's ophthalmologist and rheumatologist to settle for this treatment and to become less vigilant for a transformation of the patient's limited form of Wegener's granulomatosis into the lethal generalized form, despite our advice to treat the patient with cyclophosphamide. The patient died of renal complications of Wegener's granulomatosis 2 years later.

We believe, quite strongly, that NSAID therapy alone is unacceptable in the care of an individual with scleritis in whom the diagnosis of Wegener's granulomatosis or polyarteritis nodosa has been made. It is our frank view that such therapy represents negligence. The published evidence on this point of appropriate therapy for these two lethal diseases is too abundant and the conclusions are unarguable. Regardless of other therapy these patients might be receiving, the 5-year death rate of patients with polyarteritis nodosa who are not receiving cytotoxic immunosuppressive therapy is 87%,[3] and the 5-year mortality rate of patients with Wegener's granulomatosis who are not receiving cytotoxic chemotherapy is 95%.[4] Furthermore, we would extend this therapeutic attitude to patients with necrotizing scleritis associated with rheumatoid arthritis or with relapsing polychondritis. Multiple studies have now shown that, in the rheumatoid arthritis patient who develops necrotizing scleritis and who is not treated with an immunosuppressive agent, the 5-year mortality rate from extraocular vasculitic lesions is approximately 50%.[5-7] Patients with relapsing polychondritis who develop

necrotizing scleritis may also die, either from the tracheal complications of this disease or from the eventual emergence of renal pathology.

Therefore our recommendations for the treatment of patients with the various collagen vascular diseases who develop scleritis are as follow (see Table 9.2 for summary).

9.2.1.1. Rheumatoid Arthritis

We suggest treating rheumatoid arthritis patients who develop simple, diffuse scleritis with an oral nonsteroidal antiinflammatory drug, with or without the concomitant use of topical corticosteroids. If the scleritis does not respond, or if it recurs with attempted discontinuation of the topical corticosteroid, we generally switch to a different NSAID, treat once again with topical corticosteroids, taper the steroids, and

TABLE 9.2. Treatment summary for patients with collagen vascular disease and scleritis.

Disease	Scleritis		
	Diffuse	Nodular	Necrotizing
Rheumatoid arthritis	Oral NSAID Topical steroids Topical cyclosporine A (?) Systemic corticosteroids	Oral NSAID Topical cyclosporine A (?) Systemic corticosteroids Low-dose (once a week) methotrexate	Methotrexate Azathioprine Cyclophosphamide Systemic cyclosporine A Systemic corticosteroids
Systemic lupus erythematosus	Oral NSAID Plaquenil Systemic corticosteroids	Oral NSAID Plaquenil Systemic corticosteroids Low-dose (once a week) methotrexate	Oral corticosteroids Intravenous pulse corticosteroids Azathioprine Cyclophosphamide, oral or intravenous pulse
Polyarteritis nodosa	Cyclophosphamide and prednisone	Cyclophosphamide and prednisone	Cyclophosphamide and prednisone Azathioprine, methotrexate, cyclosporine alternatives
Wegener's granulomatosis	Cyclophosphamide and prednisone	Cyclophosphamide and prednisone	Cyclophosphamide and prednisone Azathioprine, methotrexate, cyclosporine alternatives
Relapsing polychondritis	Oral NSAID Dapsone Systemic corticosteroids Low-dose (once a week) methotrexate Azathioprine	Oral NSAID Dapsone Systemic corticosteroids Low-dose (once a week) methotrexate Azathioprine	Cyclophosphamide and prednisone Azathioprine and prednisone
Behçet's disease	Oral NSAID Colchicine	Oral NSAID Colchicine Systemic corticosteroids	Prednisone and chlorambucil Prednisone and cyclophosphamide Prednisone and cyclosporine A

observe for recurrence. We go through these steps at least three times, that is, with three different NSAIDs, before concluding that additional systemic medication is required. Our next step, if additional systemic medication is deemed necessary, is to treat the patient with a short course of systemic prednisone. We typically start with 1 mg/kg per day, rapidly taper when the scleritis has resolved totally (usually within 7 to 14 days), and then switch to alternate-day therapy once the dose of the prednisone is down to 20 mg/day. If the patient has had no recurrence of the scleritis with topical steroid discontinuation and tapering of the systemic steroid to 20 mg/day, our next therapeutic step is to switch the systemic prednisone to 40 mg every other day. This dose is continued for 2 weeks, after which it is further tapered to 30 mg every other day for the following 2 weeks. If there is still is no relapse of the scleritis, the drug is tapered to 20 mg every other day for an additional 2 weeks, with further tapering on an every-other-week basis to 15 mg every other day, 10 mg every other day, 7.5 mg every other day, and 5 mg every other day, after which the drug is discontinued. This is the usual withdrawal program we use for systemic prednisone. It is the rare rheumatoid arthritis patient with diffuse scleritis who does not respond to this program and who requires low-dose methotrexate once a week.

Although the vast majority of rheumatoid arthritis patients with nodular scleritis respond well to the systemic prednisone program described above for diffuse scleritis, some require low-dose, once-a-week methothrexate therapy. We always go through these steps first with our nodular scleritis patients, but in a small number of cases we have discovered that the scleritis does not respond completely or that it continues to recur with steroid tapering. We treat these patients with methotrexate, generally beginning with 7.5 mg given once a week (5 mg once a week for an individual weighing less than 50 kg); the drug dosage is generally advanced, every 3 to 4 weeks, if the scleritis does not resolve completely, with a maximum dose in our practice of 25 mg/week.

Patients with necrotizing scleritis, we believe, must be treated with a systemic immunosup-

pressant. Systemic prednisone is generally appropriate as well, concommitant with the nonsteroidal immunosuppressive medication. If the necrotizing scleritis is unilateral, is not severe, and is not rapidly progressive, our first-choice therapy once again is once-a-week methotrexate, with the usual caveats vis-à-vis liver, bone marrow, and appropriate monitoring.[8,9] The dose used is the same as stated above for nodular scleritis. If the disease is bilateral, not severe, or rapidly progressive, or if the patient has not responded to the methotrexate, we generally use azathioprine at a starting dose of 2 mg/kg per day, with dosage adjusted on the basis of clinical response and systemic tolerance. Systemic cyclosporine A is an alternative medication under this circumstance. If the patient fails to respond to these medications, cyclophosphamide is used. This is also the drug immediately used in patients with severe or rapidly progressive necrotizing scleritis, unilateral or bilateral. The dosage is 2 mg/kg per day, restricted to morning and noontime, with high fluid intake in afternoons and evenings. Hematological, urological, and systemic monitoring is as previously described, with the usual caveats (see Section 9.2.3).[8,9]

9.2.1.2. Systemic Lupus Erythematosus

Patients with systemic lupus erythematosus (SLE) who have diffuse scleritis are treated by us with an oral NSAID as described above for diffuse scleritis associated with rheumatoid arthritis. We typically add hydroxychloroquine (Plaquenil; 200 to 400 mg once daily) if the response to the oral NSAID is not complete. Systemic prednisone is added if these first two steps are inadequate to bring about a complete resolution of the scleritis. The strategy for the use of the systemic steroid is the same as that described above for the care of patients with diffuse or nodular scleritis associated with rheumatoid arthritis. Our strategy for treating patients with SLE who have nodular scleritis is the same as for treating those with diffuse scleritis, with the additional recommendation that low-dose methotrexate be given once a week for those rare patients that do not adequately respond to oral NSAID, Plaquenil, and/or systemic corticosteroids. In the extremely rare event that a patient with SLE develops necrotizing scleritis, our first-choice therapy would be high-dose oral corticosteroids and/or intravenous pulse corticosteroid therapy. We would, unlike in every other instance of systemic steroid use in our practice, use a split-dosing regime for the SLE patients, as is generally used in the care of paients with serious systemic manifestations of SLE. We might give, for example, 20 mg of prednisone four times daily to a 60- to 80-kg woman, with one to three intravenous pulse doses of 500 mg of hydrocortisone to bring about a rapid resolution of the destructive inflammation. Azathioprine (2 mg/kg per day) could be added for those patients who do not completely respond, although oral or intravenous pulse cyclophosphamide would probably be a better choice, at least if one extrapolates from the experience in treating lupus nephritis.[10]

9.2.1.3. Polyarteritis Nodosa

Patients with scleritis associated with polyarteritis nodosa must be treated with systemic cyclophosphamide and prednisone. This is true regardless of the form of scleritis the patient has. Not to treat the patient in this way, in our view, represents frank negligence, given the mortality data associated with alternative therapies.[3] If the patient is intolerant to cyclophosphamide, other immunosuppressants should be used in an effort to save not only the patient's eye but the patient's life as well. Such alternatives include azathioprine, methotrexate, and cyclosporine A.

9.2.1.4. Wegener's Granulomatosis

The comments just made about polyarteritis nodosa can be repeated verbatim regarding scleritis associated with Wegener's granulomatosis.

9.2.1.5. Relapsing Polychondritis

Some of the manifestations of relapsing polychondritis are responsive to dapsone. For this reason, we recommend that the relapsing polychondritis patient who is not sulfa sensitive or glucose-6-phosphate dehydrogenase deficient be given dapsone, along with an oral NSAID for diffuse or nodular scleritis. Because most patients receiving dapsone will experience low-grade hemolysis, which is typically compensated by reticulocytosis, we generally start with low-dose dapsone therapy, that is, 25 mg twice daily. Monitoring of liver enzymes and peripheral hemograms then allow us to judge whether a slow escalation in the dose is acceptable. We advance, as clinically needed and systemically tolerated, to as high as 150 mg/day with dapsone. For the patient with relapsing polychondritis who is not responding to a combination of oral NSAID and dapsone, we add systemic corticosteroid therapy, using the same kind of dosing technique as described above for rheumatoid arthritis. If the scleritis does not respond to the combination oral NSAID plus dapsone plus systemic corticosteroid we add low-dose methotrexate (7.5 to 15 mg/week) or daily azathioprine (2 mg/kg per day). This approach is used for both diffuse and nodular scleritis in the relapsing polychondritis patient.

The relapsing polychondritis patient who develops necrotizing scleritis, however, represents one of the most difficult therapeutic challenges that the ophthalmologist and chemotherapist ever encounter. Indeed, the authors and Mr. Watson have independently concluded that, of all the potential etiologies for necrotizing scleritis, necrotizing scleritis associated with relapsing polychondritis is the most intransigent and most difficult to place into full, permanent remission (unpublished observations and personal communication). Combination high-dose systemic corticosteroid and cyclophosphamide therapy is the strategy we most commonly use, as described for polyarteritis nodosa. In some patients we have resorted to once-a-week pulse cyclophosphamide therapy. We use 1 g/cm^2 body surface area, intravenous in 250 cc of normal saline, piggybacked onto 1 liter of 0.5% dextrose in water, infused over a period of 2 h, for intravenous pulse therapy. These infusions are repeated every 3 to 6 weeks, depending on the nadir of the leukocyte count and the rate of recovery.

9.2.1.6. Behçet's Disease

Diffuse scleritis associated with Behçet's disease usually responds to an oral NSAID plus colchicine, 0.6 mg twice daily. The nodular scleritis associated with Behçet's disease, however, almost always requires the addition of a short course of systemic corticosteroids as described above for rheumatoid arthritis. Necrotizing scleritis associated with Behçet's disease is extraordinarily rare, but like the retinal vasculitis associated with this disease, it too requires the addition of a major immunosuppressive agent such as chlorambucil (0.01 mg/kg body weight per day), cyclophosphamide (oral or intravenous pulse), or cyclosporine A (5 mg/kg body weight per day).

9.2.1.7. Posterior Scleritis

Posterior scleritis is usually idiopathic and almost never requires the use of a chemotherapeutic drug. Our approach to this disorder has been combination oral NSAID and corticosteroid therapy. Such a combination approach, described in Section 9.2.1.1, requires special attention to the gastrointestinal tract (see Section 9.2.2). In those instances of posterior scleritis that have not responded to this combination NSAID and systemic corticosteroid therapy, we have used, judicially and with reluctance, retrobulbar orbital floor steroid injections. We have used triamcinolone (40 mg) in an effort to judge the effect of such regional steroid therapy, and have continued such injections to a maximum of eight. We have not been willing to inject sustained-release (depo) preparations of corticosteroids.

9.2.1.8. Infectious Scleritis

Our experience in treating infectious scleritis with antimicrobial agents specific for the microbe causing the scleritis is described in Chapter 7.

Ancillary antiinflammatory therapy may be required. For example, the patient with scleritis associated with syphilis may require not only the intravenous penicillin therapy appropriate for the syphilis but also systemic nonsteroidal antiinflammatory drug therapy and/or corti-costeroids for control of the debilitating inflammation. A major caveat in this regard is that any patient with fungal scleritis must not, under any circumstances, be treated with corticosteroids, and a patient with bacterial scleritis may be treated judicially with steroids only after the physician is certain that the infectious agent has been properly identified, specific antibiotic therapy to which the agent is susceptible has been instituted, and the infectious process has begun to respond.

9.2.2. Ancillary Therapy

It is not uncommon for patients who require prolonged therapy with oral NSAIDs to require ancillary treatment for the gastrointestinal side effects caused by this class of drugs. Patients who take systemic steroid and NSAIDs are at high risk for gastrointestinal mucosal ulceration, and fatal gastrointestinal bleeding or peritonitis from ulcer perforation can occur. We use a "step-ladder" approach to ancillary therapy so as to prevent these side effects, beginning with the use of oral antacids and gastric mucosal coating materials such as Carafate (sucralfate). We add an H_2 receptor blocker, such as Zantac (ranitidine hydrochloride), when treating a patient with gastrointestinal mucosal irritation symptoms or a patient with a past history of such symptoms, and we add Cytotec (misoprostol) to the regimen of any patient with a past history of a documented peptic ulcer or any patient who is taking NSAIDs while also taking systemic steroids.

9.2.3. Drug Management Responsibility

We have emphasized repeatedly over the past 17 years that the responsibility for the details of management of the medications of patients requiring the use of multiple medications or in patients who are taking immunosuppressive drugs must lie with an individual who is, by virtue of training and experience, truly expert in the use of these multiple drugs, and in the anticipation of, recognition of, and treatment of side effects produced by the drugs. Few ophthalmologists are trained to do this and, happily, few are inclined to take on the responsibility. A "hand-in-glove" collaboration between the ophthalmologist and a chemotherapist works well in the management of patients requiring these medications. Timely communication is essential, with the ophthalmologist apprising the chemotherapist of the ocular condition, for example, whether or not the ocular inflammatory lesions are under total control or not, and the chemotherapist deciding whether or not the current dose of medications employed can be safely continued or, if the ocular inflammatory lesions are not completely controlled, whether it is safe and prudent to increase the dose of medication. Rheumatologists and dermatologists, as well as oncology and hematology chemotherapists, *must* collaborate with the ophthalmologist vis-à-vis the ocular needs of the patient for more or less therapy.

9.2.4. Surgical Treatment

Surgical therapy is rarely necessary in the care of patients with scleritis. It is virtually never necessary except in instances of necrotizing scleritis that have advanced to the point of perforation of the globe or to such a point of threatened perforation that prudent physicians would deem to require scleral reinforcement. The central, critical element in the successful surgical plan in these cases of necrotizing scleritis requiring scleral grafting is, in fact, not surgical: The ophthalmologist must understand that the immunological processes that resulted in destruction of the patient's sclera will invariably result in destruction of any graft material, scleral or otherwise (periosteum, fascia lata, etc.), used to reestablish the integrity of the globe unless such immunological proesses are suppressed. Therefore the most essential element of the successful surgical plan for treating a patient with necrotizing scleritis is the institution of the appropriate systemic medical therapy to interrupt the destructive immune phenomenon.

We have successfully treated patients with peripheral ulcerative keratitis and/or necrotizing scleritis by using allograft ocular material, without additional nonocular materials.[11] For patients with necrotizing scleritis associated with peripheral ulcerative keratitis we prefer a preserved (frozen) whole globe. Evidence suggests that the immunoreactivity of such tissue without living cells is extremely low, and we know of no instance in which rejection of such material has complicated the course of the patient with peripheral ulcerative keratitis and necrotizing scleritis who required grafting and surgical reinforcement of the globe. The recipient surgical bed is prepared, first by a generous conjunctival resection surrounding the area of peripheral ulcerative keratitis, then by removal of the ulcerating corneal lamellae, then by removal of the thin border of necrotic conjuncitva surrounding the focus of scleral necrosis, and finally by removal of necrotic sclera itself (Figs. 9.1 through 9.3). This latter step can be extremely tedious, and carries with it the potential risk of perforation of the choroid with subsequent ocular hemorrhage. We have not personally encountered this, but in instances in which the choroid is exposed or in which the only tissue overlying the choroid is the necrotic sclera to be removed (lest it remain a stimulant for nonspecific inflammation) the scleral dissection requires great care, patience, and often a great deal of time.

Once the limits of the surgical bed to be reinforced with donor material have been defined, we create a template, using a piece of plastic surgical drape, of the surgical bed; this template is then used to outline the size of the graft to be excised from the donor eye. The outlined graft material is excised, trimmed of nonscleral material, trimmed to fit the surgical recipient bed (Fig. 9.4), and secured with interrupted 10-0 and/or 9-0 nylon sutures (Fig. 9.5). The knots are rotated into the tissue (buried) and, if possible, conjunctiva surrounding the surgical site is undermined and advanced over the graft and secured with 7-0 Vicryl sutures (Fig. 9.6). In instances in which uveal ectasia is pronounced, securing the graft into the graft bed can be facilitated by first performing an anterior chamber paracentesis to partially decompress the globe.

In instances in which peripheral ulcerative keratitis is not part of the destructive lesion either frozen sclera, a frozen globe, or glycerin-preserved sclera can serve as a source for the

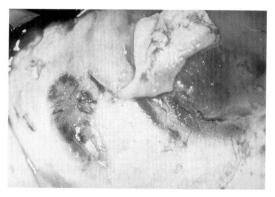

FIGURE 9.1. Keratectomy and sclerectomy in a patient with necrotizing scleritis and associated peripheral ulcerative keratitis.

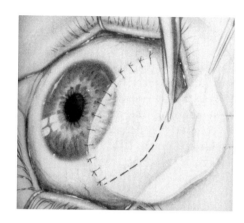

FIGURE 9.4. Diagrammatic illustration of the fitting of a corneoscleral graft to the surgical bed previously prepared (see Fig. 9.3).

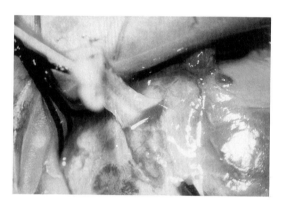

FIGURE 9.2. A lamella of corneoscleral tissue being elevated by forceps, disclosing occult areas of tissue digestion not observable prior to surgery.

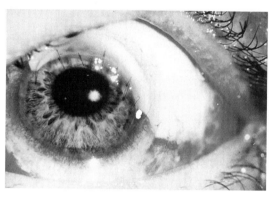

FIGURE 9.5. Same eye as in Figs. 9.1 through 9.3, after securing of the corneoscleral graft.

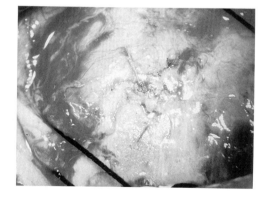

FIGURE 9.3. Same eye as in Figs. 9.1 and 9.2: The necrotic tissue has been resected and the surgical bed prepared for receiving graft tissue.

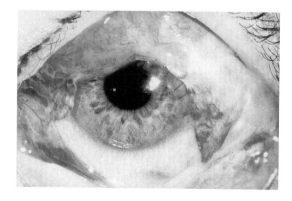

FIGURE 9.6. Same patient as in Fig. 9.5, after mobilizing a conjunctival flap over the corneoscleral graft.

graft material. Glycerin-preserved sclera must be thoroughly washed and allowed to rehydrate in balanced salt solution for approximately 10 min prior to grafting.

Vascularization of the graft and repopulation of it by recipient fibroblasts may take many months. We tend not to use topical steroids postoperatively, in order not to inhibit this process.

drug. The cure rate in such instances following 1 year of freedom from any evidence of recurrent inflammation is high. Surgical treatment through tectonic scleral and peripheral corneal grafting is rarely, although sometimes, indicated. It is to be emphasized, however, that such treatment alone will virtually never solve the patient's problem; the essential ingredient for success is control or cure of the underlying immunoregulatory dysfunction that has created the destruction in the first place.

Summary

The treatment of episcleritis can usually be strictly supportive, although in some instances systemic nonsteroidal antiinflammatory drug therapy is indicated. Such treatment can usually be tapered and discontinued after 6 months of freedom from an attack of episcleritis. Diffuse and nodular scleritis can usually be effectively treated in the same way, that is, with nonsteroidal antiinflammatory drugs, although auxiliary therapy, dictated by the specific underlying disease causing the scleritis, is also always indicated (e.g., tetracycline in patients with rosacea, allopurinol in patients with gout, etc.). If NSAID therapy fails to control the inflammation, a limited course of systemic corticosteroid therapy is indicated, provided there are no contraindications to this approach. Subsequent taper and switch to alternate-day administration can usually begin as soon as 7 to 14 days after initiation of systemic steroid treatment, but discontinuation of the medication may not be possible (without recurrence of the scleritis) for several months. If the scleritis continues to recur with each attempt to discontinue steroid therapy after 6 months of treatment, we believe immunosuppressive therapy should be considered. The same applies for patients who develop serious steroid-induced side effects. Patients with an established, potentially lethal systemic vasculitis as the cause of the scleritis (e.g., polyarteritis nodosa or Wegener's granulomatosis), and patients with necrotizing scleritis, always require treatment with an immunosuppressive chemotherapeutic

References

1. Watson PG, Hazleman DL: *The Sclera and Systemic Disorders*. W.B. Saunders, Philadelphia, 1976, Chap 10, p 398.
2. Lyons CJ, Hakin KN, Watson PG: Topical flurbiprophen: An effective treatment for episcleritis? Eye 4:521–525, 1990.
3. Fronert PP, Scheps FG: Long term follow up study of patients with periarteritis nodosa. Am J Med 43:8, 1967.
4. Fauci AS: Vasculitis. In Parker CW (Ed): *Clinical Immunology*. W.B. Saunders, Philadelphia, 1980, pp 473–519.
5. McGavin DDM, Williamson J, Forrester JV, Foulds WS, Buchanan WW, Dick WC, Lee P, MacSween RNM, Whaley K: Episcleritis and scleritis. Br J Ophthalmol 60:192, 1976.
6. Watson PG, Hayreh SS: Scleritis and episcleritis. Br J Ophthalmol 60:163, 1976.
7. Jones P, Jayson MIV: Rheumatoid arthritis of the eye. Proc Royal Soc Med 66:1161, 1973.
8. Foster CS: Nonsteroidal antiinflammatory and immunosuppressive agents. In Lambert DW, Potter DE (Eds): *Clinical Ophthalmic Pharmacology*. Little, Brown, Boston, 1987, pp 173–192.
9. Hemady R, Tauber J, Foster CS: Immunosuppressive drugs in immune and inflammatory ocular disease. Surv Ophthalmol 35:369–385, 1991.
10. McCune WJ, Golbus J, Zeldes W, Bohlke P, Dunne R, Fox DA: Clinical and immunologic effects of monthly administration of intravenous cyclophosphamide in severe lupus erythematous. N Engl J Med 318:1423–1431, 1988.
11. Raizman MB, Sainz de la Maza M, Foster CS: Tectonic keratoplasty for peripheral ulcerative keratitis. Cornea 10:312–316, 1991.

Index